Facial Plastic and Reconstructive Surgery

Concepts, Questions, Answers

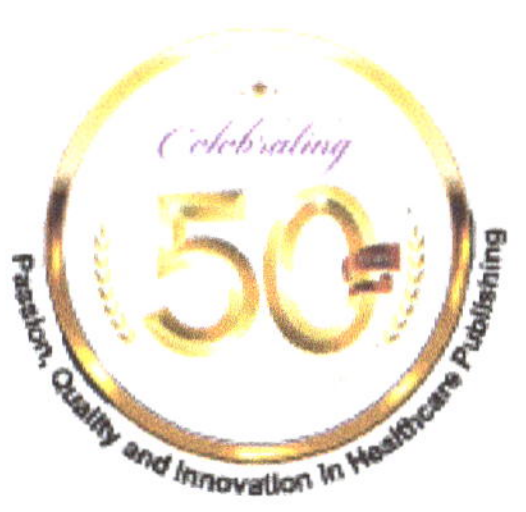

Facial Plastic and Reconstructive Surgery
Concepts, Questions, Answers

Sami P Moubayed MD
Montreal, QC, Canada

Moustafa W Mourad MD
New York, NY, USA

Antoni Riera-March MD
Puerto Rico, PR, USA

Foreword

Sam P Most MD

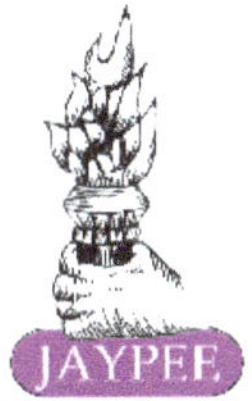

JAYPEE BROTHERS MEDICAL PUBLISHERS
The Health Sciences Publisher
New Delhi | London

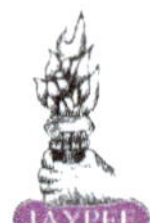 **Jaypee Brothers Medical Publishers (P) Ltd**

Headquarters

Jaypee Brothers Medical Publishers (P) Ltd
4838/24, Ansari Road, Daryaganj
New Delhi 110 002, India
Phone: +91-11-43574357
Fax: +91-11-43574314
Email: jaypee@jaypeebrothers.com

Overseas Office

J.P. Medical Ltd
83 Victoria Street, London
SW1H 0HW (UK)
Phone: +44 20 3170 8910
Fax: +44 (0)20 3008 6180
Email: info@jpmedpub.com

Website: www.jaypeebrothers.com
Website: www.jaypeedigital.com

Facial Plastic and Reconstructive Surgery: Concepts, Questions, Answers

First Edition: **2020**

ISBN 978-93-5270-292-3

Dedicated to

My mother, father, and sister who have always provided me unconditional love and support.

— Sami P Moubayed

My beautiful wife Sarah, and my son Ilyas
My incredible parents Walid and Hala
My wonderful siblings Youssef, Adam, Mariam, and Ismail
and
To my dearest friend, Dr Sami P Moubayed.

— Moustafa W Mourad

I wish to dedicate this book to the readers. My hope is that our efforts in some way, large or small, contribute to their formation in the field of Facial Plastic and Reconstructive Surgery. It is a beautiful and interesting field, as well as a challenging one, and will provide practitioners great joy and satisfaction throughout their professional lives.

— Antoni Riera-March

Contributors

Amani Ben Moussa
Medical Student
University of Montreal
Montreal, QC, Canada

Anastasios Maniakas MD
Resident in Otolaryngology—Head
and Neck Surgery
University of Montreal
Montreal, QC, Canada

Angelique M Berens MD
Fellow in Facial Plastic and
Reconstructive Surgery
University of California
Los Angeles, CA, USA

Anisha R Noble MD
Resident in Otolaryngology—Head
and Neck Surgery
University of Washington
Seattle, WA, USA

Antoni Riera-March MD
Otolaryngologist—Head and Neck
Surgeon
University of Puerto Rico
Puerto Rico, PR, USA

Arvind K Badhey MD
Resident in Otolaryngology—Head
and Neck Surgery
New York Eye and Ear Infirmary of
Mount Sinai
New York, NY, USA

Badr Ibrahim MD
Resident in Otolaryngology—Head
and Neck Surgery
University of Montreal
Montreal, QC, Canada

Beatrice Voizard MD
Resident in Otolaryngology—Head
and Neck Surgery
University of Montreal
Montreal, QC, Canada

Brittany Barber MD
Fellow in Head and Neck Surgery
Mount Sinai Hospital
New York, NY, USA

Catherine Dufour-Fournier MD
Resident in Otolaryngology—Head
and Neck Surgery
University of Montreal
Montreal, QC, Canada

Cinzia L Marchica, MD
Resident in Otolaryngology—Head
and Neck Surgery
McGill University
Montreal, QC, Canada

Daniel O'Connell MD
Head and Neck Surgeon
University of Alberta
Edmonton, AB, Canada

Dina Moubayed MD
Medical Student
University of Montreal
Montreal, QC, Canada

Elizabeth Jasso-Ramirez MD
Facial Plastic and Reconstructive
Surgeon
Private Practice
Mexico City, Mexico

Erika Mercier MD
Resident in Otolaryngology—Head
and Neck Surgery
University of Montreal
Montreal, QC, Canada

Grace Wandell
Medical Student
University of Washington
Seattle, WA, USA

Gregory S Dibelius MD
Facial Plastic and Reconstructive
Surgeon
Private Practice
Boca Raton, FL, USA

Hadi Seikaly MD
Head and Neck Surgeon
University of Alberta
Edmonton, AB, Canada

Jamil Manji
Medical Student
University of Melbourne
Melbourne, Australia

Jay J Agarwal MD
Resident in Otolaryngology—Head
and Neck Surgery
New York Eye and Ear Infirmary of
Mount Sinai
New York, NY, USA

Jeffrey Cranford MD
Resident in Otolaryngology—Head
and Neck Surgery
New York Eye and Ear Infirmary of
Mount Sinai
New York, NY, USA

José Juan Montes-Bracchini MD
Facial Plastic and Reconstructive
Surgeon
Private Practice
Mexico City, Mexico

Kaete A Archer MD
Facial Plastic and Reconstructive
Surgeon
Private Practice
Melbourne, FL, USA

Kaitlin Wiseman MD
Medical Student
University of Montreal
Montreal, QC, Canada

Kaitlyn B Zenner MD
Resident in Otolaryngology—Head
and Neck Surgery
University of Washington
Seattle, WA, USA

Ketan Mehta
Resident Physician
Division of Plastic Surgery
Montefiore Medical Center
Bronx, NY, USA

Khalid Ansari MD
Facial Plastic and Reconstructive
Surgeon
University of Alberta
Edmonton, AB, Canada

Kirkland N Lozada MD
Resident in Otolaryngology—Head
and Neck Surgery
New York Eye and Ear Infirmary of
Mount Sinai
New York, NY, USA

Lina Zahra Benamira MD
Resident in Otolaryngology—Head
and Neck Surgery
McGill University
Montreal, QC, Canada

Marie-Renée Atallah MD
Resident in Otolaryngology—Head
and Neck Surgery
University of Montreal
Montreal, QC, Canada

Matthew Brace MD
Facial Plastic and Reconstructive
Surgeon
Private Practice
Guelph, ON, Canada

Michael Duyzend PhD
Medical Student
University of Washington
Seattle, WA, USA

Michael G Roskies MD
Resident in Otolaryngology—Head
and Neck Surgery
McGill University
Montreal, QC, Canada

Moustafa W Mourad MD
Facial Plastic and Reconstructive
Surgeon
Private Practice
New York, NY, USA

Nathalie Gabra MD
Resident in Otolaryngology—Head
and Neck Surgery
McGill University
Montreal, QC, Canada

Neha A Patel MD
Pediatric Otolaryngologist
Cohen Children's Medical Center
New Hyde Park, NY, USA

Noor G Shah
Medical Student
Robert Wood Johnson Medical
School—Rutgers University
New Brunswick, NJ, USA

Paul Covello DDS MD
Fellow in Head and Neck Oncologic
Surgery and Microvascular
Reconstruction
LSU Health Sciences Center
Shreveport, LA, USA

Paul Tabet MD
Resident in Otolaryngology—Head
and Neck Surgery
University of Montreal
Montreal, QC, Canada

Sameep Kadakia MD
Fellow in Facial Plastic and
Reconstructive Surgery
Private Practice
Fort Worth, TX, USA

Sami P Moubayed MD
Facial Plastic and Reconstructive
Surgeon
University of Montreal
Montreal, QC, Canada

Samuel N Helman MD
Resident in Otolaryngology—Head
and Neck Surgery
New York Eye and Ear Infirmary of
Mount Sinai
New York, NY, USA

Sapna A Patel MD
Facial Plastic and Reconstructive
Surgeon
Private Practice
Seattle, WA, USA

Sarah M Kidwai MD
Resident in Otolaryngology—Head
and Neck Surgery
Mount Sinai Hospital
New York, NY, USA

Scott W Smith MD
Resident in Otolaryngology—Head
and Neck Surgery
Ohio State University
Columbus, OH, USA

Yadranko Ducic MD FRCSC FACS
Director
Baylor Scott and White Neuroscience
Skull Base Program
Methodist Dallas Face Trauma Program
Dallas, TX, USA

Foreword

Facial plastic surgery is a multidisciplinary field, encompassing subject matter that exists at the intersection of Otolaryngology—Head and Neck Surgery, Plastic Surgery, Oculoplastic Surgery and Oral/Maxillofacial Surgery. To date, no comprehensive review book for Facial Plastic and Reconstructive Surgery has existed. Preparation for board examinations covering this material was thus quite an adventure! As an academic Facial Plastic Surgeon and Fellowship Director in Facial Plastic and Reconstructive Surgery, I have seen countless residents and fellows struggle to prepare for both in-service and board examinations that cover facial plastic surgery. Thankfully, we now have a comprehensive review manual, with review questions, to aid in mastery of this topic.

In the following text, Moubayed, Mourad, and Riera-March have organized this diverse subject matter in a concise manner for rapid review. The text is first divided into five sections: (1) Basic principles, (2) Rhinoplasty (both esthetic and functional), (3) Esthetic facial surgery, (4) Nonsurgical cosmetic procedures, (5) Reconstructive surgery (including pediatric and craniofacial surgery). Each section contains multiple pertinent chapters with choice tables and figures for reviewers to use for reference and rapid recall. Furthermore, an essential component review and recall is testing. Recognizing this, the authors have organized a question bank of over 1,250 questions that the student will find invaluable in his/her review.

As I read this text, I found that it covers facial plastic surgery quite comprehensively. Insofar as is possible, the authors have covered virtually all topics that are likely to be tested. From basic science to evidence-based medicine, from the anatomy of the face to the physics of lasers, from pediatric to adult reconstructive surgery, facial plastic surgery is well-represented in the pages of this book. The reader should find an excellent resource for rapid review in preparation for board examinations in Facial Plastic and Reconstructive Surgery, Otolaryngology—Head and Neck Surgery, and Plastic Surgery.

Today, the American Board of Facial Plastic and Reconstructive Surgery boasts over 1,000 diplomates. I know this because one of my former fellow became the 1,000th diplomate a few years ago. While preparation for this examination has traditionally been the domain of graduating fellows and residents, every diplomate since 2002 has been required to retake the examination for maintenance of certification (MOC). As such, the examination *is now the domain of recent trainees and long-time practitioners alike*. Having taken both the primary examination and the recertification examination, I can attest to the depth of information tested in both circumstances. Preparation for these examinations with materials such as this is a key component of success.

The authors are to be lauded for creating the first comprehensive review and self-test book for Facial Plastic and Reconstructive Surgery. As mentioned above, facial plastic surgery is a multidisciplinary field with material that exists at the intersection of Otolaryngology—Head and Neck Surgery, Plastic Surgery, Oculoplastic Surgery and Oral/Maxillofacial Surgery. I believe all students of the specialty, recently graduated or preparing for MOC examinations, will find this text eminently useful in preparation and review for their respective examinations.

Sam P Most MD
Professor and Chief
Division of Facial Plastic and Reconstructive Surgery
Stanford University School of Medicine
California, USA

Preface

The reason that we love Facial Plastic and Reconstructive Surgery (FPRS) so much is that it is such a diverse field. It is also for this reason that its study can be at times confusing. The best way to master a subject is simplification, classification, and self-assessment questions. There are a ton of resources available for high-yield review materials for medical school and for Otolaryngology—Head and Neck Surgery, but I found it at times frustrating that there was no definitive source for a summarized, simplified, and classified overview of FPRS that includes a large quantity of review questions.

It is with that in mind that we initially embarked on this journey with Dr Moustafa W Mourad. Our goal was to create a comprehensive, organized, yet focused textbook to serve as an introduction as well as a study guide for the FPRS Board Examination. At the same time, I was a great fan of Dr Antoni Riera-March's FPRS question bank, and I cannot overemphasize the joy and excitement that I felt when he accepted to participate in this project as a coeditor. It was a tremendous opportunity to work with Dr Riera, whose hard work, passion, and dedication to medical education is a true inspiration. He single-handedly contributed over 1,250 original questions to this book, and without his efforts this project would definitely not have been the same.

As editors, we *a priori* organized each chapter into sections and chapters that would enable the contributors to stay focused and target the essential points in each chapter. The mind of a trainee is perfectly suited to present information in a way that is aimed at maximizing retention and stressing the high-yield points. For this reason, most of the contributors are exceptional trainees who are passionate about medical education. We are eternally thankful for their hard work and collaboration. It was also a pleasure to work with M/s Jaypee Brothers Medical Publishers (P) Ltd, who facilitated this project from beginning to end.

We hope you will enjoy this textbook. As this is the first edition, we will be collecting feedback from readers to keep improving this book for future editions to come.

Sami P Moubayed
Moustafa W Mourad
Antoni Riera-March

Contents

Section 4   Nonsurgical Cosmetic Procedures

Section 5   Reconstructive Surgery

Basic Principles

Section Outlines

Chapter 1

Basic Techniques

Paul Tabet, Sami P Moubayed

NORMAL ANATOMY OF THE SKIN

Normal Skin Histology

The layers of the skin are as follows:[1-3]
- *Epidermis*
  - Outer layer
  - Five strata: (1) Corneum, (2) lucidum, (3) granulosum, (4) spinosum, and (5) basale (mnemonic: Californians Love G-String Bikinis)
  - Predominant cells: Keratinocyte, melanocytes, Langerhans cells, and Merkel cells.
- *Epidermal-dermal junction*
  - Rete pegs: Epidermal projection into dermal layer
  - Papillae: Dermal projection into epidermal layer (vascularized).
- *Dermis*
  - Predominant cells: Fibroblast, histiocytes, monocytes, lymphocytes, and Langerhans cells
  - Papillary layer: Loose connective tissue, and small vessels/nerve endings
  - Reticular layer: Dense connective tissue, blood vessels, hair follicles, sweat glands, lymphatics, nerves, sebaceous glands, and apocrine/eccrine glands.
- *Hypodermis (subcutaneous layer)*
  - Contains fat and fibrous tissue

Variations in Skin Thickness in the Head and Neck

The measure of skin thickness can help guide reconstructive choices by matching similar skin thickness between donor and recipient sites (Table 1).[4]

Skin Biomechanical Properties

The four fundamental biomechanical properties of the skin are the following:[5]
1. *Stress*: Force applied per cross-sectional area of the skin.
2. *Strain*: Change in length divided by the original length of the given tissue to which a force is applied.
3. *Creep*: Increase in strain applied to skin when it is under constant stress. Creep can occur over a brief amount of time (minutes) and is due to the extrusion of fluid from the dermis and breakdown of the dermal framework.
4. *Stress relaxation*: Decrease in stress on skin when it is held in tension at a constant strain for a given period of time.

Table 1: Variation in skin thickness in the head and neck (in ascending order).[4]	
Site	*Average skin thickness in mm*
Upper eyelid	0.4
Neck	0.5
Nasal dorsum	0.7
Lips, lower eyelids, and philtrum	0.8
Submental	0.9
Forehead	1.0
Cheek	1.0
Chin	1.1
Nasal tip	1.2

SKIN INCISION PLACEMENT

Relaxed Skin Tension Lines

Incisions parallel to relaxed skin tension lines (RSTL) result in the most favorable scars. The RSTLs are fine lines on the facial skin that are formed by the action of the underlying muscles and as a result, are perpendicular to them (Fig. 1).[6]

Facial Subunit Principle

The units and subunits are based on skin thickness, color, texture, and underlying structural contour. Precise planning of surgical incisions and reconstructions require analysis of the entire unit or subunit. Incisions within unit or subunit borders result in the most favorable scars.

The original 14 esthetic units include:[7]
1. *Forehead unit:* Central subunit, lateral subunit, and eyebrow subunit

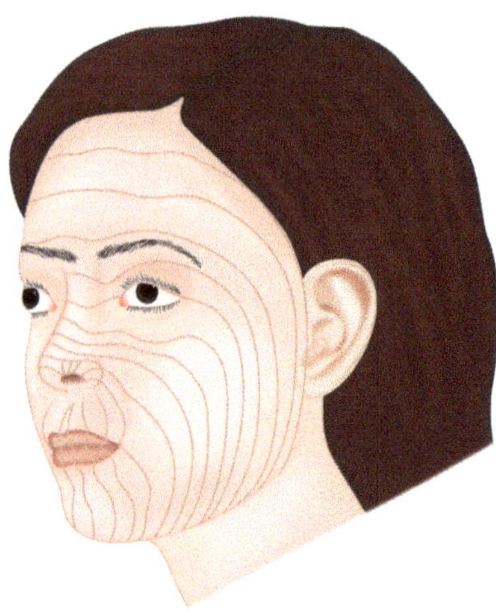

Fig. 1: Relaxed skin tension lines.

2. *Nasal unit:* Tip subunit, columellar subunit, right and left alar base subunits, right and left alar side wall subunits, dorsal subunit, and right and left dorsal side wall subunits
3. *Eye lid units:* Lower lid unit, upper lid unit, lateral canthal subunit, and medial canthal subunit
4. *Cheek unit:* Medial subunit, zygomatic subunit, lateral subunit, and buccal subunit
5. *Upper lip unit:* Philtrum subunit, lateral subunit, and mucosal subunit
6. *Lower lip unit:* Central subunit, and mucosal subunit
7. *Mental unit*
8. *Auricular unit:* Helical subunit, antihelical subunit, and triangular fossa subunit, conchal subunit, and lobe subunit.
9. *Neck unit.*

WOUND CLOSURE

Different Suture Techniques and their Characteristics

Good suturing technique should eliminate dead space in subcutaneous tissues, and minimize tension that causes wound separation. Below are the steps required in obtaining a fine line scar:[8]
- Minimizing damage to the skin edges with a traumatic technique
- Tension free closure with
- Wound edge eversion
- Prompt removal of suture material
- Clean non-infected wound
- Use of non-absorbable synthetic sutures

Table 2 outlines the most commonly employed suture techniques and their most common indications.[9-13]

SKIN APPROXIMATION MATERIAL REFERENCES

Suture Materials, Advantages, and Disadvantages

Suture materials, advantages, and disadvantages described in Tables 3 to 5.[14]

Evidence Base for Suture Removal

On the face and ears, sutures can be removed within 5–7 days, with eyelid sutures being removed in 3–5 days.[11] Neck sutures are removed within 7 days and scalp sutures in 7–10 days.[11]

WOUND HEALING

Description of Normal Wound Healing Stages[15,16]

The normal wound healing stages have been described in Table 6.

Most Common Causes of Impaired Wound Healing

Wound healing is the result of interactions among cytokines, growth factors, blood, and the extracellular matrix. The cytokines promote healing by various pathways such as stimulating the production of components of the basement membrane, preventing dehydration, increasing inflammation and the formation of granulation tissue. These pathways are affected by various local and systemic factors. Table 7 summarizes the most common causes of impaired healing.[17, 18]

DRESSINGS AND PROBLEM WOUNDS

Dressing Selection and Wound Management Principles

Based on the wound type, suitable dressing material must be used. In general, modifiable characteristics of the optimal wound environment is moist, sterile, and warm.[19] To obtain a moist environment, dry wounds should be moistened and excessively exudative wounds should be dried up.

Common Dressings

The common dressings and their characteristics are described in Table 8.[8-19]

Negative Pressure Therapy[20]

Negative pressure wound therapy (NPWT) has been shown to accelerate healing. It has become increasingly valuable in the management of chronic and acute wounds,

Table 2: Suture techniques.[9-13]

Technique	Characteristics
Simple interrupted suture	Gold standard and most commonly employed suture
Vertical mattress suture	Eversion of skin edges when not possible with simple sutures Most obvious/unsightly cross-hatching (if not removed early) For wounds under tension For wounds with edges that tend to invert
Horizontal mattress suture	Maximal eversion Hemostatic
Subcuticular suture	No need for external skin sutures No suture marks
Running suture	Not as precise as interrupted sutures Fast

Table 3: Wound closure materials.[14]

Material	Advantages	Disadvantages
Staples	Speed	Less precise tissue eversion
Adhesives	Speed Ease of use (especially in children) Immediate wound sealing Fast return to routine activities No risk of needle-stick injury No need for postoperative suture removal	Less precise tissue eversion Limited to external use
Absorbable sutures	No need for suture removal	Increased inflammatory response (except if synthetic)
Nonresorbable sutures	Decreased inflammatory response	Requires removal
Synthetic	Usually nonresorbable [except for polydioxanone (PDS)] When resorbable, hydrolytic degradation process with less inflammation	Requires removal
Natural	Usually resorbable (except for silk)	When resorbable, and proteolytic degradation process with more inflammation
Monofilament sutures	Decreased risk of harboring microorganisms	Less knot security Weaker than multifilament Sensitive to crimping and crushing
Multifilament (braided)	Better knot security Stronger than monofilament More pliable than monofilament Less sensitive to crimping and crushing	Increased risk of harboring microorganisms

Table 4: Absorbable sutures with their preferred anatomic site and tensile strength.

Suture type	Common uses	Duration of maximum strength
Plain catgut (fast absorbing)	Skin	3–4 days
Chromic gut	Mucosa	10–14 days
Polyglactin 910 (vicryl)	Mucosa, and deep dermal	14–21 days
Vicryl rapide	Skin	5–14 days
Poliglecaprone 25 (monocryl)	Skin	7–14 days
Polydioxanone (PDS)	Deep dermal, and cartilage	14–42 days

Source: Ethicon, Inc.

Table 5: Nonabsorbable sutures.

Suture type	Common uses
Silk	Drain and tube suturing
Nylon	Skin, and cartilage
Polypropylene (Surgilene, and Prolene)	Skin, and cartilage
Mersilene	Skin

Table 6: Stages of wound healing.

1. Inflammatory stage					
Hemostasis		*Cellular migration*			
		Neutrophils		*Macrophages*	*Fibroblasts*
Vasoconstriction Vasodilation Endothelial cell contraction Platelet plug formation Coagulation/complement cascade		Within 6 h Max cell influx at 24–48 h Phagocytosis		Predominant cell by 48–72 h PDGF + fibroblasts TNF-α, TNF-β, IGF-1, IL-1	Appear by 48 h Maximum at 15 days Collagen, elastin, and fibronectin Differentiation into myofibroblasts
2. Proliferative phase					
Reepithelialization	*Neovascularization*			*Collagen deposition*	*Wound contraction*
Begins in hours postinjury Epithelial cell differentiation Separation from basement membrane Dissolution of eschar matrix Fibroblast migration into wound	Granulation tissue (day 4) Fibrin, fibronectin, and hyaluronic acid in matrix	Angiogenesis Epithelial cell to perivascular space ↑ Delivery of neutrophils, macrophages, fibroblasts VEGF modulated		Type III initially, and type I later Maximum deposition 2–3 weeks ↑ tensile begins at 4–5 days	Myofibroblasts mediated Maximal at 12–15 days 0.6–0.75 mm/days
3. Remodeling (maturation) phase: ↑ in type 1 collagen					
3 weeks	*6 weeks*			*6 months*	
15% of original tensile strength	60% of original tensile strength			70–80% of original tensile strength	

Abbreviations: PDGF, platelet-derived growth factor; TNF-α, tumor necrosis factor-alpha; IGF-1, insulin-like growth factor-1; IL-1, interleukin-1, VEGF, vascular endothelial cell growth factor.

Table 7: Common causes of impaired wound healing.[17,18]

Local factors	*Medications*	*Medical conditions*	*Technical factors*
• Infection • Radiation • Hematoma • Wound desiccation • Ischemia	• Steroids • Immunosuppressants	• Diabetes • Malnutrition • Smoking • Hypothyroidism • Connective tissue disorders • Immunodeficiency	• Traumatic handling of tissues • Tension

Table 8: Common dressings and their characteristics.[8,19]

Dressing	*Advantages/disadvantages*	*Commercial name*
Wet to dry Gauze	Low material expense Frequent changes and adherent to wound	
Nonadherent	Maintains a moist environment, nonadherent to wound	Xeroform, Bactigras, and Jelonet
Occlusive and semi-occlusives	Elastic, flexible, conforms to any shape, no additional tapping, and inspection without removal Maintains the moisture content of clean wounds	Tegaderm, Opsite, and Biocclusive
Hydrogel	Suitable for all four stages of wound healing except infected/heavy drainage wounds Absorbs moderate amounts of fluid from the wound	NU-GEL
Hydrocolloids	Permeable to water vapor and impermeable to bacteria Used on light to moderate exudative wounds	DuoDERM
Foam	Used for moderate to highly exudative wounds	Allevyn, Lyofoam, and Tielle
Alginates	Used for moderate to heavy drainage wounds, not for dry wounds	Algisite, Kaltostat, Sorbsan
Skin substitutes	Useful for sites prone to contracture (neck and axilla) Enable coverage of tendons, bone, and surgical hardware	Laserskin, Biobrane

Table 9: Hyperbaric oxygen complications and contraindications.

Complications[24]	Absolute contraindications[21]	Relative contraindications[21]

• Pneumothorax
• ARDS
• Seizures
• Middle ear barotrauma
	• Untreated pneumothorax
	• Select medications
	  – Cisplatin
	  – Doxorubicin
	  – Disulfiram
	  – Mefenamic acid
	  – Steroids
		• Emphysematous blebs
		• Eustachian tube dysfunction
		• Sinusitis
		• Seizure disorder
		• History of thoracic surgery
		• Pregnancy
		• Cardiac disease

Abbreviations: ARDS, acute respiratory distress syndrome.

Box 1: Pressure and O_2

- Poisoning (carbon monoxide)
- Radiation injury
- Embolism (air or gas)
- Severe anemia
- Sudden sensorineural hearing loss (SNHL)
- Unsuccessful grafts/flaps
- Refractory osteomyelitis
- Abscess (intracranial)
- Necrotizing soft tissue infections
- Decompression sickness
- Occluded arteries
- Traumatic ischemic injury
- Warning, hot! (acute thermal injury)
- Organism (clostridial myositis-gas gangrene)

contaminated wounds, traumatic tissue loss, surgical dehiscence, ulcers from vascular insufficiency, fistulas, and other indications.

Its effect on the wound bed are the following: Extraction of exudate from the wound bed, decrease of interstitial edema, increase in vascularity, promotion of granulation formation, decrease in bacterial burden, stimulation of fibroblast and endothelial cell proliferation, and mechanical contracture of the wound bed.

Head and neck evidence: Negative pressure wound therapy in head and neck surgery is safe and has potential to be a useful tool for complex wounds in patients with a compromised ability to heal.

Hyperbaric Oxygen Therapy

Hyperbaric oxygen therapy (HBOT) is defined by the Undersea and Hyperbaric Medical Society (UHMS) as a treatment in which a patient intermittently breathes 100% oxygen while the treatment chamber is pressurized to a pressure greater than sea level (1 atmosphere absolute, or 1 ATA).

The mechanisms of HBOT when relative to wound healing are:[21]

- Hyperoxygenation
- Vasoconstriction (to reduce edema)
- Angiogenesis
- Fibroblast proliferation and collagen synthesis
- Leukocyte oxidative killing
- Toxin inhibition and antibiotic synergy

Indications of Hyperbaric Oxygen Therapy[22,23]

Indications of hyperbaric oxygen therapy illustrated in Box 1 and and complications/contraindications illustrated in Table 9.[24]

■ REFERENCES

1. Moore KL, Persaud TVN, Torchia MG. Before we are born: essentials of embryology and birth defects, 9th edition. Philadelphia, PA: Elsevier/Saunders; 2016. p. 361.
2. Carlson BM. Human embryology and developmental biology, 5th edition. 2014, Philadelphia, PA: Saunders/Elsevier; 2014. p. 506.
3. Burns T, Breathnach S, Cox N, et al. Rook's Textbook of Dermatology, 8th edition. Chichester, West Sussex, UK; Hoboken, NJ: Wiley-Blackwell; 2010.
4. Ha RY, Nojima K, Adams WP Jr, et al. Analysis of facial skin thickness: defining the relative thickness index. Plast Reconstr Surg. 2005;115:1769-73.
5. Gaboriau HP, Murakami CS. Skin anatomy and flap physiology. Otolaryngol Clin North Am. 2001;34:555-69.
6. Johnson JT, Rosen CA, Bailey BJ. Bailey's Head and Neck Surgery—Otolaryngology, 5th edition. Philadelphia: Wolters Kluwer Health /Lippincott Williams & Wilkins; 2014.
7. Fattahi TT. An overview of facial aesthetic units. J Oral Maxillofac Surg. 2003;61:1207-11.
8. Thorne C, Gurtner GC, Chung K, et al. Grabb and Smith's Plastic Surgery, 7th edition. Philadelphia: Wolters Kluwer Health/Lippincott Williams & Wilkins; 2014. p. 1030.
9. Kudur MH, Pai SB, Sripathi H,et al. Sutures and suturing techniques in skin closure. Indian J Dermatol Venereol Leprol. 2009;75:425-34.
10. Moy RL, Waldman B, Hein DW. A review of sutures and suturing techniques. J Dermatol Surg Oncol. 1992;18:785-95.
11. Zachary CB. Basic cutaneous surgery: a primer in technique. Practical Manuals in Dermatologic Surgery. New York: Churchill Livingstone, 1991. p. 134.
12. Swanson NA. Atlas of cutaneous surgery, 1st edition. Boston: Little, Brown; 1987. p. 177.
13. Borges AF. Elective incisions and scar revision, 1st edition. Boston,: Little; 1973. p. 316.

14. Janis JE. Essentials of plastic surgery, Second edition. St. Louis, Missouri Boca Raton: Quality Medical Publishing, CRC Press/ Taylor & Francis Group; 2014. xxv, p. 1336.
15. Singer AJ, Clark RA. Cutaneous wound healing. N Engl J Med. 1999;341:738-46.
16. Gurtner GC, Werner S, Barrandon Y, et al. Wound repair and regeneration. Nature. 2008;453:314-21.
17. Guo S, Dipietro LA. Factors affecting wound healing. J Dent Res. 2010;89:219-29.
18. Thomas Hess C. Checklist for factors affecting wound healing. Adv Skin Wound Care. 2011;24:192.
19. Dhivya S, Padma VV, Santhini E. Wound dressings—a review. Biomedicine (Taipei). 2015;5:22.
20. Asher SA, White HN, Golden JB, et al. Negative pressure wound therapy in head and neck surgery. JAMA Facial Plast Surg. 2014;16:120-6.
21. Kindwall EP. Hyperbaric medicine practice, 2nd edition. Flagstaff, Ariz: Best Publishing. Company;1995. p. 692.
22. Young T. Hyperbaric oxygen therapy in wound management. Br J Nurs. 1995;4:796, 798-803.
23. Broussard CL. Hyperbaric oxygenation and wound healing. J Vasc Nurs. 2004;22:42-8.
24. Plafki C, Peters P, Almeling M, et al. Complications and side effects of hyperbaric oxygen therapy. Aviat Space Environ Med. 2000;71:119-24.

Self-Assessment Exercise

Q 1. Define stress relaxation.

Ans: A decrease in stress on skin when it is held in tension at a constant strain for a given period of time.

Q 2. Name 5 local factors of impaired wound healing.

Ans:
- Infection
- Radiation
- Hematoma
- Wound desiccation
- Ischemia.

Q 3. Name all nasal subunits.

Ans:
- Tip subunit
- Columellar subunit
- Right and left alar base subunits
- Right and left alar side wall subunits
- Dorsal subunit
- Right and left dorsal side wall subunits.

Q 4. Where are the thickest and thinnest skin sites of the face?

Ans: Thinnest: upper eyelid; Thickest: nasal tip.

Q 5. Name three possible complications of HBOT.

Ans: Pneumothorax, ARDS, middle ear barotrauma.

Multiple Choice Questions

Q 1. Which of the following statements is TRUE regarding the different Skin Line Types?

A. Relaxed Skin Tension Lines (RSTL) usually run perpendicular to the wrinkles

B. Relaxed Skin Tension Lines (RSTL) usually run parallel to the contraction of muscles

C. Langer's lines are relaxation creases found in the skin of cadavers

D. Facial Langer's lines coincide with the facial wrinkle lines.

Ans: C. Langer's lines are relaxation creases found in the skin of cadavers

Q 2. Which of the following nasal subunits has a thick, immobile and sebaceous skin?

A. The lobule

B. The dorsum

C. The sidewall

D. The ala

Ans: A. The lobule

Q 3. Which of the following statements is TRUE about external nasal subunits?

A. Any subunit defect greater than 30% should be enlarged to occupy the entire subunit

B. The ala refers to the skin and soft tissue overlying the lateral crura of the lower lateral cartilages

C. The tip-defining point indicates the base of the soft triangle of the nose

D. The sill comprises the most posterior aspect of the nostril rim

Ans: D. The sill comprises the most posterior aspect of the nostril rim

Q 4. Which of the following nasal areas has the THINNEST skin?

A. Nasion

B. Rhinion

C. Supratip

D. Columella

Ans: D. Columella

Q 5. In tissue expanders, the INCREASE in skin surface when the skin is under constant stress is related to:

A. Viscoelasticity

B. Creep

C. Extensibility

D. Stress relaxation

Ans: B. Creep

Q 6. Which of the following statement regarding BIOLOGIC CREEP is FALSE?

A. It involves an overall increase in mitotic activity

B. It involves a displacement of fluids and the collagen fibers are realigned

C. It involves an increase in surface area

D. It involves permanent changes in the microanatomy of tissue

Ans: B. It involves a displacement of fluids and the collagen fibers are realign

Q 7. Which of the following terminology is related to " a DECREASE in the force necessary on the skin when is held in a contant stretch over a given period of time".

A. Viscoelasticity
B. Creep
C. Extensibility
D. Stress relaxation

Ans: D. Stress relaxation

Q 8. Which of the following cell types is MOST predominantly seen in the epidermis?:

A. Langerhan's cells
B. Keratinocytes
C. Melanocytes
D. Merkel's cells

Ans: B. Keratinocytes

Q 9. Which of the following cells have THE MOST important ROLE in the inflammatory phase of wound healing?

A. Macrophages
B. Lymphocytes
C. Monocytes
D. Neutrophils

Ans: A. Macrophages

Q 10. Which of the following cells are FIRST TO APPEAR in the wound healing process?

A. Polymorphonuclear leukocytes
B. Macrophages
C. Lymphocytes
D. Endothelial cells

Ans: A. Polymorphonuclear leukocytes

Q 11. Which of the following tissue adhesives is the LEAST histotoxic?

A. Butyl-2-cyanoacrylate
B. Methyl-α-cyanoacrylate
C. Octyl-8-cyanoacrylate
D. Fibrin glues

Ans: D. Fibrin glues

Q 12. Which of the following cells synthesizes COLLAGEN?

A. Keratinocytes
B. Melanocytes
C. Langerhans' cells
D. Fibrocytes

Ans: D. Fibrocytes

Q 13. Which of the following cells are implicated in the production of TROPOCOLLAGEN UNITS?

A. Macrophages
B. Fibroblasts
C. Lymphocytes
D. Endothelial cells

Ans: B. Fibroblasts

Q 14. Which of the following cell types have been RELATED to the mediation of immunologic responses within the skin?

A. Keratinocytes
B. Langerhans' Cells
C. Merkel's Cells
D. Melanocytes

Ans: B. Langerhans' Cells

Q 15. Which one of the following will promote FASTER reepithelialization during wound healing?

A. Desiccation
B. Occlusive wound dressing
C. Triamcinolone acetonide ointment (0.1%)
D. Anticoagulants

Ans: B. Occlusive wound dressing

Q 16. Which of the following mineral DEFICIENCIES is clinically important in wound healing?

A. Zinc
B. Iron
C. Calcium
D. Copper

Ans: A. Zinc

Q 17. Which of the following suture materials will produce LESS tissue reaction when used on the face?

A. Chromic catgut
B. Vicryl
C. Silk
D. Nylon

Ans: D. Nylon

Q 18. The main DISADVANTAGE in applying cyanoacrylate tissue adhesive to the skin is its:

A. Erythema effect
B. Foreign body effect
C. Local histotoxicity effect
D. Blister effect

Ans: C. Local histotoxicity effect

Q 19. Which of the following suture materials will induce the MOST inflammatory tissue reaction?

A. Nylon
B. Vicryl
C. Chromic catgut
D. Prolene

Ans: C. Chromic catgut

Q 20. In which layer of the skin are the "melanocytes" found?

A. The basal cell layer
B. The prickle cell layer
C. The granular cell layer
D. The stratum lucidum layer

Ans: A. The basal cell layer

Q 21. The corpuscles of "Vater-Pacini" mediate the sensation of:

A. Pressure
B. Pain
C. Temperature
D. Touch

Ans: A. Pressure

Q 22. Which of the following is TRUE regarding the phases and order of wound healing?

A. Inflammation, proliferation and differentiation
B. Inflammation, proliferation and maturation
C. Proliferation, remodeling and differentiation
D. Proliferation, remodeling and contraction

Ans: B. Inflammation, proliferation and maturation

Q 23. At the end of the remodeling phase of wound healing the scar HAS approximately:

A. 20% of the tensile strength of nonwounded normal skin
B. 40% of the tensile strength of nonwounded normal skin
C. 60% of the tensile strength of nonwounded normal skin
D. 80% of the tensile strength of nonwounded normal skin

Ans: D. 80% of the tensile strength of non-wounded normal skin

Q 24. Which of the following is the CORRECT TIMING for the appearance of the fibroblasts in the process of wound healing?

A. 24 hours
B. 3 days
C. 7 days
D. 10 days

Ans: B. 3 days

Q 25. In the wound healing process granulation tissue forms at which of the following points?

A. 24 hours
B. 48 hours
C. 4 days
D. 7 days

Ans: C. 4 days

Q 26. HOW LONG does the tensile strength chromic gut last?

A. 1 week
B. 2 weeks
C. 4 weeks
D. 6 weeks

Ans: B. 2 weeks

Q 27. When is the REMODELING PHASE in wound healing COMPLETE?

A. 3 months
B. 6 months
C. 10 months
D. 12 months

Ans: D. 12 months

Q 28. At the end of the inflammatory phase of wound healing (one week after closure) the wound HAS what percentage of unwounded normal skin?

A. 10%
B. 30%
C. 50%
D. 70%

Ans: A. 10%

Q 29. Which of the following vitamins, supplements or medications WILL NOT INTERFERE with blood clotting?

A. St. John's wort
B. Vitamin B
C. Ginkgo biloba
D. Naproxen

Ans: B. Vitamin B

Q 30. Which of the following statements about WOUND HEALING is TRUE?

A. Polymorphonuclear leukocytes appear after 72 hours
B. Macrophages are predominant in the first 36 hours
C. Granulation tissue appears on day # 4
D. Wound contraction initiates 3 weeks after injury

Ans: C. Granulation tissue appears on day # 4

Q 31. When will FAST ABSORBING SURGICAL GUT LOOSE virtually ALL TENSILE STRENGTH?

A. After 48 hours
B. After 72 hours
C. After 5 days
D. After 7 days

Ans: C. After 5 days

Q 32. In which of the following facial areas are SILK SUTURES INDICATED?

A. Eyelid margin
B. Cheek
C. Forehead
D. Ear

Ans: A. Eyelid margin

Q 33. Which of the following cells plays a KEY ROLE in the coagulation phase of wound healing?

A. Platelets
B. Neutrophils
C. Lymphocytes
D. Macrophages

Ans: A. Platelets

Q 34. When does PEAK wound contraction occur?

A. 5 days
B. 7 days
C. 14 days
D. 21 days

Ans: C. 14 days

Q 35. Which of the following cellular components in wound healing is responsible for the CONTRACTION PHASE?

A. Macrophages
B. Fibroblasts
C. Myofibroblasts
D. Lymphocytes

Ans: C. Myofibroblasts

Q 36. When in the healing process does a wound achieve the Tensile Strength of preinjured tissue?

A. 6 months
B. 1 year
C. 2 years
D. Never

Ans: D. Never

Q 37. Which of the following properties enables this condition, related to the skin: " the ability to retain the shape obtained by stretching when the deforming force is gone"?

A. Tensile strength
B. Elasticity
C. Plasticity
D. Memory

Ans: C. Plasticity

Q 38. Which of the following nonabsorbable sutures has the MOST tissue reaction?

A. Silk
B. Polypropylene (prolene)
C. Polyester (mersilene)
D. Stainless steel

Ans: A. Silk

Q 39. Which of the following statements about the suture material PLAIN CATGUT is FALSE?

A. It is derived from the submucosal layer of sheep intestine
B. It elicits a low inflammatory response
C. It loses its tensile strength by 7 days
D. It increases its tensile strength up to 21 days by treating the catgut with chromium salts (chromic gut)

Ans: B. It elicits a low inflammatory response

Q 40. Which of the following substances is produced by THE LYMPHOCYTES in the immune response to wound repair?

A. FGF (Fibroblast growth factor)
B. IGF-1(Insulin-like growth factor)
C. PDGF (Platelet derived growth factor)
D. TGF-beta (Transforming growth factor-beta)

Ans: D. TGF-beta (Transforming growth factor-beta)

Q 41. The Epidermal Growth Factor (EGF) is derived from:

A. Platelets
B. Lymphocytes
C. Macrophages
D. Neutrophils

Ans: A. Platelets

Q 42. Which of the following is the source of Interferon?
A. Fibroplasts and lymphocytes
B. Macrophages and neutrophils
C. Masts cells and lymphocytes
D. Neutrophils and lymphocytes

Ans: A. Fibroplasts and lymphocytes

Q 43. Which of following herbal and supplemental medicines used by cosmetic patients WILL INHIBIT AND PROLONG wound healing?
A. Glucosamine
B. Ginseng
C. Garlic
D. Vitamin E

Ans: D. Vitamin E

Q 44. Which of the following herbal and supplemental medicines used by cosmetic patients will most likely cause hypoglycemia?
A. Glucosamine
B. Ginseng
C. Garlic
D. Vitamin E

Ans: A. Glucosamine

Q 45. Which of the following is the INITIAL EVENT in wound healing?
A. Local vasoconstriction
B. Local vasodilatation
C. Increase microvascular permeability
D. Cellular response proliferation

Ans: A. Local vasoconstriction

Q 46. Which of the following factors WILL NOT impede wound healing?
A. Diabetes mellitus
B. Venous stasis
C. Wound moisture
D. Hyperthyroidism

Ans: C. Wound moisture

Q 47. Which of the following primary cell types are predominantly found in the DAY 6 of the wound healing process?
A. Fibroblasts
B. Red blood gell
C. Platelets
D. Neutrophils

Ans: A. Fibroblasts

Q 48. Which of the following cells synthesize COLLA-GEN?
A. Macrophages
B. Fibroblasts
C. Mast cells
D. Muscle cells

Ans: B. Fibroblasts

Q 49. Which type of collagen is the MOST common in scar tissue?
A. Type I
B. Type II
C. Type III
D. Type IV

Ans: A. Type I

Q 50. Which of the following primary cell type in the post wound healing is the ONE indicated by the rectangle? The vertical axis represents the cell type, the horizontal axis represents the time (days).

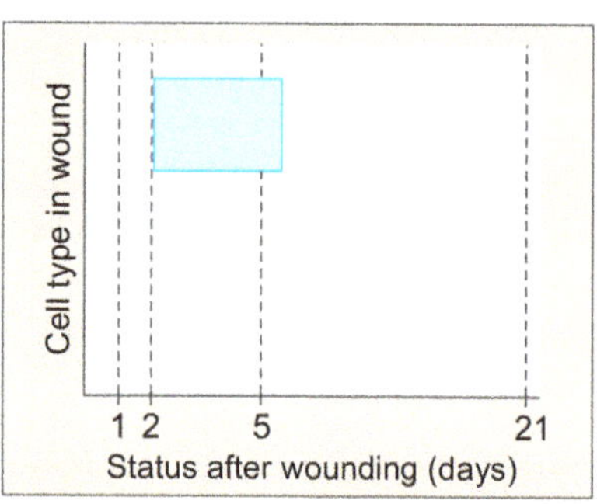

A. Red blood cells
B. Macrophages
C. Neutrophils
D. Platelets

Ans: B. Macrophages

Q 51. In wound healing the MAXIMAL CONTRACTION occurs at:
A. 1 week
B. 2 weeks
C. 3 weeks
D. 1 month

Ans: B. 2 weeks

Q 52. Which of the following components is CRITICAL in the hemostatic phase of wound healing?
A. Neutrophils
B. Macrophages
C. Platelets
D. Red blood cells

Ans: C. Platelets

Q 53. Which of the following components is CRITICAL in the synthesis of collagen?
A. Vitamin A
B. Vitamin C
C. Zinc
D. Vitamin E

Ans: B. Vitamin C

Q 54. Which of the following vitamins or trace elements in high doses has been associated with delayed wound healing ?
A. Vitamin A
B. Vitamin C
C. Vitamin E
D. Zinc

Ans: C. Vitamin E

Q 55. Which of the following percentage of the hair cycle is in the ANAGEN phase?
A. 10%
B. 50%
C. 70%
D. 90%

Ans: D. 90%

Q 56. In which of the following medical conditions in the use of synthetic tissue adhesives for wound closure INDICATED?
A. Patients with insulin-dependent diabetes
B. Patients with collagen vascular disease
C. Patients with tendency to form hypertrophic scars or keloids
D. Wound depth beyond the depth of the dermis with tendency toward skin-edge inversion

Ans: D. Wound depth beyond the depth of the dermis with tendency toward skin-edge inversion

Q 57. Which of the following statements regarding skin staples in FALSE?

A. They are made of stainless steel
B. They are used in hair-bearing of the scalp
C. They do not evert the skin edges
D. They are minimally reactive

Ans: C. They do not evert the skin edges

Q 58. Which of the following suture materials has the MOST tensile strength?

A. Polypropylene (Prolene)
B. Silk
C. Polyglactin (Vicryl)
D. Polyester (Mersilene)

Ans: D. Polyester (Mersilene)

Q 59. The IDEAL place for using staples for skin closure IS:

A. The scalp
B. The postauricular area
C. The temple area
D. The neck

Ans: A. The scalp

Q 60. You are excising a scar by the fusiform ellipse technique. The excision line is 1 cm wide. What is the value of "X" representing the LENGTH of the fusiform incision?

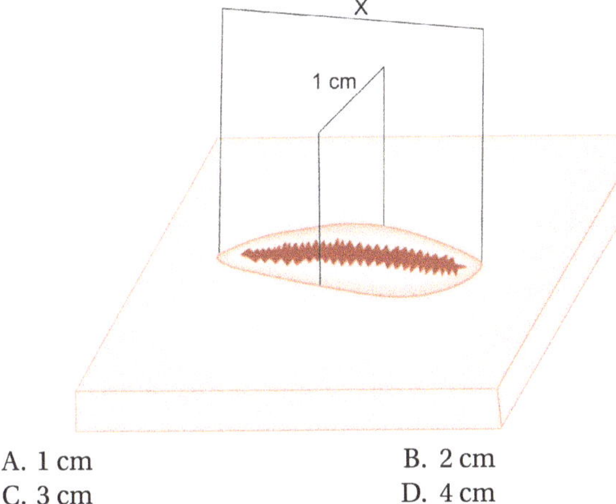

A. 1 cm
B. 2 cm
C. 3 cm
D. 4 cm

Ans: C. 3 cm

Q 61. Which of the following statements regarding tissue adhesives is TRUE?

A. BioGlue is a tissue adhesive primarily use for vascular anastamosis
B. Cyanoacrylate tissue adhesives are designed for superficial and deep tissue use
C. Butyl-cyanoacrylate is a long-chained derivatives with a slow breakdown rate of degradation
D. Fibrin tissue adhesives are contraindicated in facelift surgery

Ans: A. BioGlue is a tissue adhesive primarily use for vascular anastamosis

Q 62. Which of the following tissue adhesives is composed of purified bovine serum albumin and glutaraldehyde?

A. BioGlue
B. Tisseel
C. Butyl-cyanoacrylate
D. 2-Octyl cyanoacrylate

Ans: A. BioGlue

Q 63. Which of the following statements regarding CYANOACRYLATE tissue adhesives is FALSE?

A. Cyanoacrylate tissue adhesives are solely recommended for superficial skin closure
B. Cyanoacrylate tissue adhesives are contraindicated in children
C. Cyanoacrylate tissue adhesives can be used in wound/incision closure for blepharoplasty and facelift
D. Cyanoacrylate tissue adhesives breakdown products can produce a histotoxic reaction

Ans: B. Cyanoacrylate tissue adhesives are contraindicated in children

Q 64. Which of the following tissue adhesives is the ONE used for superficial tissue closure?

A. Tisseel
B. BioGlue
C. 2-Octyl cyanoacrylate
D. Butyl-cyanoacrylate

Ans: C. 2-Octyl cyanoacrylate

Chapter 2

Analgesia and Conscious Sedation

Noor G Shah

■ INTRODUCTION

Continuum of Sedation

Sedation and analgesia describe a continuum of states ranging from minimal sedation to general anesthesia. Each of these stages carries its own scope of practice and effects on the body. As a nonanesthesiologist an understanding of these stages is necessary in order to correctly apply them to the appropriate population. Table 1 summarizes the major effects and differences of the four major stages of sedation.

■ PREOPERATIVE ASSESSMENT

Preprocedural Evaluation

It is imperative to adequately assess each patient in the preoperative period in order to identify any factors that may lead to difficulty with administering sedation or with any complications that may arise during or after recovery from sedation. When taking a patient history, it is important to identify any abnormalities of the major organ systems, problems with prior anesthesia or sedation, sleep apnea, or history of airway obstruction. Similarly, the presence of any genetic/congenital abnormality that affects airway structure should prompt a more detailed examination of the airway. A patient's current medications and drug allergies should be scrutinized in order to identify possible reactions and potential drug-drug interactions that may occur during anesthesia induction. A history of tobacco, alcohol or substance use/abuse can also help identify potential comorbidities that may negatively affect anesthesia.

On physical examination, it is important to note a patient's body habitus as significant obesity, specifically involving the neck and facial structures, can lead to upper airway obstruction, making protecting the airway and intubation much more difficult. A though head and neck exam should also be completed in order to identify factors that are associated with a more precarious airway such as:
- Short neck
- Limited neck extension
- Decreased hyoid-mental distance (<3 cm in an adult)
- Increased neck mass
- Cervical spine disease or trauma
- Tracheal deviation and dysmorphic facial features.

The mouth should be examined to identify features that lead to a more difficult assessment of the airway and a more difficult intubation:
- Small opening (<3 cm in an adult)
- Edentulous
- Protruding incisors
- Loose or capped teeth
- Dental appliances
- High arched palate

Table 1: Continuum of sedation.

	Minimal sedation (anxiolysis)	Moderate sedation (analgesia)	Deep sedation (analgesia)	General anesthesia
Responsiveness	Intact response to verbal stimuli	Purposeful response to verbal or tactile stimulation	Purposeful response following repeated or painful stimulation	Unarousable
Airway	Unaffected	Airway patent without intervention	Intervention may be required	Intervention often required
Spontaneous ventilation	Unaffected	Adequate	May be inadequate	Frequently inadequate
Cardiovascular function	Unaffected	Maintained under normal circumstances	Maintained under normal circumstances	May be impaired

- Macroglossia
- Tonsillar hypertrophy
- High Mallampati score.

The jaw should be similarly examined to identify features that may lead to a challenging intubation:

- Micrognathia
- Retrognathia
- Trismus
- Significant malocclusion.

Laboratory Testing and Evaluation

In general, preoperative tests should not be ordered routinely, rather they may be ordered on a selective basis. Routine hemoglobin or hematocrit studies are not indicated unless there is a history or suspicion for bleeding disorder, history of liver disease or anticoagulation medication that may pose a risk due to the invasiveness of the procedure. Coagulation studies are indicated in patients with bleeding disorders, renal dysfunction, liver dysfunction and according to the type and invasiveness of the procedure. Serum chemistries are indicated in patients with endocrine disorders, patients at risk for renal and liver dysfunction, or if there is use of certain perioperative therapies.

An EKG is indicated in patients with known cardiovascular risk factors.

Similarly, chest radiographs are indicated in patients who have a significant history of smoking, recent URI, COPD and/or cardiac disease.

Preprocedural Fasting Guidelines

Sedatives and analgesics tend to impair airway reflexes in proportion to the degree of sedation-analgesia achieved. Preprocedure fasting decreases risk of aspiration during moderate sedation, while it greatly reduces risk and is strongly recommended during deep sedation. Table 2 displays the recommended preoperative fasting time for common liquids and meals.

Preoperative Specialist Consultation

A specialist may need to be consulted for evaluation of a patient's risk for a specific procedure in certain circumstances. Cardiac evaluation with a specialist may

Table 2: Recommended fasting period.

Ingested material	Minimum fasting period
Clear liquids	2 hours
Breast milk	4 hours
Infant formula	6 hours
Nonhuman milk	6 hours
Light meal	6 hours

be warranted if significant cardiac risk factors are present and the type of surgery indicates that either noninvasive screening tests, such as stress tests, or invasive screening tests, such as echocardiogram or cardiac catheterization. Pulmonary evaluation with a specialist may be indicated in patients with a history of significant pulmonary disease who are undergoing an invasive procedure. This evaluation may include pulmonary function tests, spirometry or arterial blood gases.

■ CONSCIOUS SEDATION

Patient Monitoring

Conscientious patient monitoring is essential to ensure the best outcomes for each patient during conscious sedation. Conscious sedation is a synonym for moderate sedation; also know as a state of analgesia. During this state a drug-induced depression of consciousness is induced, during which patients can respond purposefully to verbal commands, either alone or accompanied by light tactile stimulation. No interventions are required to maintain a patent airway, and spontaneous ventilation is adequate. Cardiovascular function is usually maintained.

It is important to monitor a patient's response to commands as this serves as a guide to the patient's level of consciousness. Spoken responses also provide an indication that patient is breathing and allows timely detection of complications and is thus recommended in all patients.

Monitoring of respiratory function is essential in all procedures as the airway can become unstable very quickly. Monitoring of ventilator function by observation or auscultation reduces the risk of adverse outcomes associated with sedation/analgesia. Oximetry monitoring effectively detects oxygen desaturation and hypoxemia and can decrease the likelihood of adverse outcomes, such as cardiac arrest and death. Supplemental oxygen use is recommended for use in moderate sedation to reduce risk of hypoxemia and is strongly recommended in deep sedation.

Monitoring of hemodynamics is also essential to identify any cardiorespiratory compromise. Regular monitoring of vital signs at 5-minute intervals once a stable level of sedation is established reduces the likelihood of adverse outcomes.

It is recommended that a designated individual, other than the practitioner performing the procedure, should be present to monitor the patient throughout the procedure. This individual should be educated and trained in the pharmacology of agents commonly used during sedation and should be trained in recognition of complications associated with sedation/analgesia. This individual should also be trained in basic life support skills should the need to rescue patients in distress arises. However, an individual with advanced life support skills should be immediately available (1–5 minutes), if the need arises.

Complications

Careful assessment and monitoring of the patient helps to prevent and expeditiously recognize any complications that may arise. It is imperative to possess emergency equipment in the facility should the need arise for its utilization. Pharmacologic antagonists and appropriately sized equipment for establishing a patent airway and providing positive pressure with supplemental oxygen should be present. A defibrillator should also be immediately available for unstable patients. An individual with advanced life support skills should be immediately available (1–5 minutes) to perform any life-saving maneuvers, if the need arises.

Reversal agents for common anesthetic agents should be readily available if cardiorespiratory compromise or adverse drug reactions should arise. These include:

- *Naloxone* is an antagonist of all types of opioid receptors, however, it shows high affinity for μ receptors. It acts in 1–2 minutes when it is given intravenously. Intravenous naloxone (0.4–0.8 mg) promptly antagonizes all actions of morphine. In patients with respiratory depression, an increase in respiratory rate is seen within 1 or 2 minutes.
- *Flumazenil* is used as a reversal agent for benzodiazepines. On intravenous administration, flumazenil has a half-life of about 1 hour and the duration of clinical effects usually is only 30–60 minutes. It is eliminated via liver to inactive products and excreted renally. Therefore, resedation is a possibility with longer acting BZDs and may occur within 1–2 hours after administration, which requires subsequent doses.

A dreaded complication during any procedure that uses anesthetic agents is malignant hyperthermia, which is a life-threatening clinical syndrome triggered in susceptible individuals primarily by the volatile inhalational anesthetic agents and the muscle relaxant succinylcholine, though other drugs have also been implicated. Signs and symptoms include a very high end-tidal carbon dioxide (>100 mm Hg), a low pH with a metabolic component, tachycardia and dysrhythmias, rigidity (in some cases), rapidly increasing temperature, a mottled skin color, hyperkalemia, myoglobinuria, muscle edema, sympathetic hyperactivity with eventual metabolic exhaustion, increased cellular permeability, whole body edema, disseminated intravascular coagulopathy, and cardiac and renal failure. Early diagnosis and treatment with dantrolene can improve the outcome.

Recovery Process

It is essential to continue observation and monitoring during the recovery period as delayed drug absorption and slow drug elimination may contribute to residual sedation and cardiorespiratory depression. Predetermined discharge criteria decrease the likelihood of adverse outcomes in the recovery period. Below are some general guidelines for discharge:

- Patients should be alert and oriented
- Vitals signs should be stable and in acceptable limits
- Sufficient time (up to 2 hours) should have elapse after the last administration of reversal agents to ensure that patients do not become resedated after reversal effects have worn off
- Outpatients should be discharged in the presence of a responsible adult who will accompany them home and can be given appropriate discharge and postoperative care instructions.

Pediatric Conscious Sedation

Generally, the same recommendations apply to pediatric patients, who are defined as being less than 21 years of age. Because the level of intended sedation may be exceeded in the pediatric population, the practitioner must be sufficiently skilled to provide rescue should the child progress to a level of deep sedation. The practitioner must be trained in, and capable of providing, at the minimum, bag- valve-mask ventilation, so as to be able to oxygenate a child who develops airway obstruction or apnea.

Younger patients may require immobilization devices during anesthesia administration. Immobilization devices, such as papoose boards, must be applied in such a way as to avoid airway obstruction or chest restriction. The child's head position and respiratory excursions should be checked frequently to ensure airway patency. If an immobilization device is used, a hand or foot should be kept exposed, and the child should never be left unattended.

Commonly used Agents

Table 3 displays commonly used anesthesia agents that each practitioner should be knowledgeable of before beginning any procedure requiring any level of sedation.

Table 3: Commonly used anesthetic agents.

Medication	Indication	Administration	Advantages	Disadvantages
Benzodiazepines: Diazepam, midazolam, and lorazepam	Pre-anesthesia for anxiolysis and amnesia, sedation; induction and maintenance of anesthesia	Intravenous	• Alone has limited depressant effects on cardiovascular/respiratory system • Promotes sedation and reducing anxiety • Amnestic (anterograde) in most patients	• Drowsiness occurs several minutes after administration • Can cause significant cardiovascular and respiratory depression in combination with opioids
Barbiturates: Thiopental, methohexal sodium, and thiamylal sodium	Induction and maintenance of anesthesia	Intravenous	• Unconscious in 10–20 seconds following administration • Rapid recovery • Limited cardiovascular effects	• Poor analgesic • Dose related respiratory depression, especially at higher doses
Opioids: Morphine, meperidine, and fentanyl	Analgesia, supplement to inhalation or intravenous anesthetics	Intravenous	• Respiratory depression is reversible with naloxone	• Respiratory depression • Hypotension • Postoperative nausea or vomiting
Ketamine	Anesthesia	Intravenous	• Significant amnesia and analgesia rapidly follow administration	• Arterial blood pressure, heart rate and cardiac output increase • Recovery is slow • Awakening may be associated with bad dreams and hallucinations
Propofol	Induction and maintenance of anesthesia	Intravenous	• Does not adversely affect hepatic or renal function • Emergence is rapid with minimal postoperative confusion	• Causes peripheral vasodilation which leads to a decrease in blood pressure

■ BIBLIOGRAPHY

1. Coté CJ, et al. American Academy of Pediatrics; American Academy of Pediatric Dentistry, Guidelines for monitoring and management of pediatric patients during and after sedation for diagnostic and therapeutic procedures: an update. Paediatr Anaesth. 2008;18:9-10.
2. Anderson JA. Reversal agents in sedation and anesthesia: a review. Anesth Prog. 1988;35:43-7.
3. Apfelbaum JL, Connis RT, et al. Committee on Standards and Practice Parameters. Practice Advisory for Preanesthesia Evaluation: an updated report by the American Society of Anesthesiologists Task Force on Preanesthesia Evaluation. Anesthesiology. 2012;116:522-38.
4. Hopkins PM. Malignant hyperthermia: pharmacology of triggering. Br J Anaesth. 2011;107:48-56.
5. Kennedy SK, Longnecker DE. History and Principles of Anesthesiology. In; Hardman JG, Limbird LE, Molinoff PB, Ruddon RW, Gilman AG, (Eds). Goodman and Gillman's The Pharmacological Basis of Therapeutics. New York: The McGraw-Hill Companies Inc.;1996. p. 325-6.
6. Practice guidelines for sedation and analgesia by non-anesthesiologists. A report by the American Society of Anesthesiologists Task Force on Sedation and Analgesia by Nonanesthesiologists. Anesthesiology. 1996;84:459-71.

Multiple Choice Questions

Q 1. **Which of the following anesthetic agents has an ESTER chemical structure?**

A. Lidocaine
B. Bupivacaine
C. Tetracaine
D. Mepivacaine

Ans: C. Tetracaine

Q 2. **Which of the following is the EARLIEST symptom of local anesthetic systemic toxicity?**

A. Circumoral numbness and tingling
B. Lightheadedness
C. Tinnitus and hypotension
D. Visual disturbances

Ans: A. Circumoral numbness and tingling

Q 3. **Which of the following anesthetic agents has the LONGEST duration of action?**

A. Lidocaine (plain)   B. Bupivacaine
C. Cocaine   D. Tetracaine

Ans: B. Bupivacaine

Q 4. A patient is under local anesthesia and IV sedation and suddenly develops PVC's, premature ventricular contractions with pulse above 50. Which of the following options IS INDICATED in this particular patient?

A. Atropine

B. Carotid sinus massage

C. Lidocaine

D. Verapamil

Ans: C. Lidocaine

Q 5. Which of the following anesthetic agents is MOST likely to be involved in an allergic reaction?

A. Bupivacaine

B. Mepivacaine

C. Ropivacaine

D. Tetracaine

Ans: D. Tetracaine

Q 6. Which of the following anesthetic agents is metabolized in the plasma by the cholinesterase?

A. Bupivacaine

B. Mepivacaine

C. Tetracaine

D. Ropivacaine

Ans: C. Tetracaine

Q 7. Which of the following anesthetics is MOST likely related to cardiovascular toxicity?

A. Prilocaine

B. Mepivacaine

C. Etidocaine

D. Bupivacaine

Ans: D. Bupivacaine

Q 8. Which of the following measures is BEST for the treatment of a tachycardia over 130 due to epinephrine effect?

A Midazolam

B Verapamil

C Propanolol

D Hydralazine

Ans: C. Propanolol

Q 9. The MAXIMUM total dose of lidocaine with epinephrine for a 70-kg adult man is approximately:

A. 300 mg

B. 400 mg

C. 500 mg

D. 600 mg

Ans: C. 500 mg

Q 10. Which of the following local anesthetic agents has the LONGEST duration of action?

A. Chloroprocaine

B. Lidocaine

C. Ropivacaine

D. Mepivacaine

Ans: C. Ropivacaine

Q 11. Which of the following substances is USED in conjunction with 2% lidocaine and 1: 100.000 epinephrine in order to decrease pain of local injection?

A. 0.9 saline solution

B. 0.45 saline solution

C. Ringer lactate

D. Sodium bicarbonate

Ans: D. Sodium bicarbonate

Q 12. Which of the following is the PROPER intramuscular Ketamine SEDATIVE DOSAGE used in pediatric anesthetic?

A. 0.1 mg/kg

B. 0.5 mg/kg

C. 5 mg /kg

D. 7.5 mg/kg

Ans: C. 5 mg/kg

Q 13. What is the maximum recommended dose (mg/kg) of lidocaine (with 1:100.000 epinephrine) in the adult?

A. 3

B. 6

C. 9

D. 12

Ans: B. 6

Q 14. Which of the following statements is TRUE about local anesthetics?

A. Local anesthetic agents contain a water-soluble benzene aromatic ring connected to a hydrophylic amine by an intermediate chain

B. Amides are degraded by hepatic carboxylesterase

C. Local anesthetic physiologic activity is a function of the their water solubility

D. Amides are the most common group involved in allergic reactions

Ans: B. Amides are degraded by hepatic carboxylesterase

Q 15. Which of the following statements is TRUE about the local anesthetic, lidocaine?

A. It has a vasoconstrictor action

B. It has a duration of action of approximately 120 minutes

C. The maximum single dose without epinephrine is approximately 600 mg for adults

D. It is an ester anesthetic agent

Ans: B. It has a duration of action of approximately 120 minutes

Q 16. Which of the following IONS IS BLOCKED by local anesthetic agents?

A. Potassium

B. Sodium

C. Sodium and potassium

D. Calcium

Ans: B. Sodium

Q 17. Which of the following local anesthetics is an ESTER agent?

A. Procaine

B. Lidocaine

C. Bupivacaine

D. Mepivacaine

Ans: A. Procaine

Q 18. The toxicity of local anesthetics is MOST COMMONLY RELATED to which of the following systems?

A. Cardiovascular system

B. Central nervous system

C. Respiratory system

D. Renal system

Ans: B. Central Nervous System

Q 19. Which of the following statements regarding COMPLICATIONS of local anesthesia is TRUE?

A. True allergic reactions are common

B. The amide class of local anesthetics is the most commonly implicated

C. Most fatalities are due to drug overdose rather than allergic reaction

D. The initial symptoms of local anesthetic toxicity are nystagmus and seizures

Ans: C. Most fatalities are due to drug overdose rather than allergic reaction

Q 20. Which of the following statements about local anesthetics is TRUE?

A. Lidocaine is an ester anesthetic agent
B. Ester anesthetic agents are most likely to cause allergic
C. EMLA is a mixture of lidocaine and bupivacaine and is used for topical dermal anesthesia
D. Local anesthetic agents block potassium channels

Ans: B. Ester anesthetic agents are most likely to cause allergic reactions

Q 21. Which of the following represents the EARLIEST SYMPTOM of LOCAL ANESTHETIC TOXICITY?

A. Convulsions
B. Muscular twitching
C. Respiratory system depression
D. Numbness of tongue

Ans: D. Numbness of tongue

Q 22. Which of the following statements regarding Propofol is TRUE

A. It is a benzodiazepine sedative
B. Pain at the injection site is negligible
C. The duration of action is approximately 60 minutes
D. It is related to a much faster recovery and reduced incidence of nausea and vomiting

Ans: D. It is related to a much faster recovery and reduced incidence of nausea and vomiting

Q 23. After completion of a forehead lift, blepharoplasty and rhytidectomy, with general anesthesia, a 45-year- old female patient is agitated, uncooperative and not understanding or responding to verbal commands. Which of the following is the PROBABLE CAUSE?

A. Anxiety disorder
B. Allergic reaction
C. Hypoxia
D. Severe pain

Ans: C. Hypoxia

Q 24. Which of the following statements about lidocaine (Xylocaine) as used in local anesthesia is TRUE?

A. It is an amine local anesthetic
B. It produces local anesthesia by selectively blocking the sodium ions of the axon
C. It is totally metabolized by the liver
D. Its plasma half-life is 1.5 hours

Ans: B. It produces local anesthesia by selectively blocking the sodium ions of the axon

Q 25. Which of the following mechanisms is involved in the CONDUCTION BLOCKADE of local anesthetics?

A. Sodium ion influx is directed to flow through specific channels into the cell
B. Potassium ion influx is directed to flow through specific channels into the cell
C. Sodium and potassium ions are directed to flow through specific channels into the cell
D. Potassium and calcium ions are directed to flow through specific channels into the cell

Ans: A. Sodium ion influx is directed to flow through specific channels into the cell

Q 26. Which of the following statements relating to the infraorbital foramen nerve is TRUE?

A. The infraorbital foramen is located on a vertical line dropped from the medial limbus of the iris
B. The infraorbital foramen is located approximately 20 mm below the orbital rim
C. The transcutaneous nasolabial approach is the best for blocking the infraorbital nerve
D. The areas numbed by blocking the infraorbital nerve are the nose and the upper lip

Ans: D. The areas numbed by blocking the infraorbital nerve are the nose and the upper lip

Q 27. Which of the following dosages is the MAXIMUM DOSAGE LIMIT (μg/kg) of bupivacaine without epinephrine?

A. 1.5 mg/kg
B. 2.5 mg/kg
C. 3.5 mg/kg
D. 4.0 mg/kg

Ans: B. 2.5 mg/kg

Q 28. Which of the following statement is FALSE regarding local anesthetics for facial plastic procedures?

A. Procaine is an esther anesthetic
B. Lidocaine is an amide anesthetic
C. All local anesthetics have 3 components: an aromatic portion, an intermediate chain, and an amine group
D. Ester anesthetics are rarely associated with allergic reactions

Ans: D. Ester anesthetics are rarely associated with allergic reactions

Q 29. Which of the following local anesthetic agents is NOT metabolized by the liver?

A. Procaine
B. Lidocaine
C. Bupivacaine
D. Mepivacaine

Ans: A. Procaine

Q 30. Which of the following anesthetic has been associated with METHEMOGLOBINEMIA?

A Prilocaine
B Ropivacaine
C Bupivacaine
D Cocaine

Ans: A. Prilocaine

Q 31. In which of the following sites is metabolized the Mepivacaine local anesthetic agent?

A. Plasma
B. Liver
C. Kidney
D. Spleen

Ans: B. Liver

Q 32. Which of the following local anesthetic agents has the LONGEST duration of action?

A. Lidocaine   B. Mepivacaine
C. Bupivacaine   D. Tetracaine

Ans: C. Bupivacaine

Q 33. Which of the following inhalational anesthetic agents has been MOST commonly associated with malignant hyperthermia?

A. Nitrous oxide   B. Halothane
C. Enflurane   D. Isoflurane

Ans: B. Halothane

Q 34. Which of the following statements regarding the Propofol is FALSE?

A. Rapid onset and short duration of action
B. Hypotension for peripheral vasodilation
C. Intense nausea in the awakening period
D. Venoirritation and phlebitis

Ans: C. Intense nausea in the awakening period

Q 35. Which of the following drugs are related to hallucinations during the recovery period?

A. Ketamine   B. Barbiturates
C. Etomidate   D. Propofol

Ans: A. Ketamine

Q 36. Which of the following inhalational anesthetic agents has a high risk for renal toxicity?

A. Halothane   B. Enflurane
C. Isoflurane   D. Desflurane

Ans: B. Enflurane

Q 37. During the process of general anesthesia of a pediatric patient a masseter muscle spasm occurs, followed by sustained muscle rigidity, and increase core of body temperature. The inhalation agent is stopped immediately. Which of the following pharmacology agents is usually necessary to treat this condition?

A. Diazepam   B. Dantrolene
C. Succinylcholine   D. Atropine

Ans: B. Dantrolene

Q 38. The potency of a local anesthesia is directly related to

A. Lipid solubility
B. Class/Group of local anesthetic
C. Concentration
D. Vasoconstriction effect

Ans: A. Lipid solubility

Q 39. Which of the following local anesthetic is RARELY related to allergic reaction?

A. Cocaine   B. Procaine
C. Bupivacaine   D. Chloroprocaine

Ans: C. Bupivacaine

Q 40. Which of the following intravenous pharmacologic agents has the MOST complete and longest acting amnesia effect?

A. Diazepam   B. Midazolam
C. Lorazepam   D. Oxazepam

Ans: C. Lorazepam

Q 41. Which of the following intravenous pharmacological drugs is a specific benzodiazepine antagonist?

A. Flumazenil   B. Midazolam
C. Lorazepam   D. Oxazepam

Ans: A. Flumazenil

Q 42. Which of the following accurately describes airway status during conscious sedation?

A. Patent airway
B. Inadequate airway with intervention needed
C. Unaffected airway
D. Conspicuous airway

Ans: A. Patent airway—conscious sedation minimally affects the airway and intubation is not normally needed.

Q 43. How often should vital signs be assessed in a patient under conscious sedation?

A. Every minute   B. Every 15 minutes
C. Every 5 minutes   D. Every 30 minutes

Ans: C. Every 5 minutes—Hemodynamics should be assessed every 5 minutes in patients undergoing conscious sedation.

Q 44. How long after a reversal of anesthesia during conscious sedation should a patient be monitored?

A. 1 hour   B. 30 minutes
C. 4 hours   D. 2 hours

Ans: D. 2 hours—Patient should be monitored for at least 2 hours after reversal of anesthesia before being sent home.

Q 45. Which of the following is the single MOST important vital sign to monitor in the ambulatory surgical setting?

A. Blood oxygen   B. Heart rate
C. EKG (electrocardiogram) D. Arterial blood pressure

Ans: A. Blood oxygen

Chapter 3

Evidence-based Medicine

Dina Moubayed, Sami P Moubayed

■ INTRODUCTION

Before the beginning of evidence-base medicine (EBM), clinical decisions were based on personal experience and anecdotes. Evidence-based medicine is a concept that can be traced back as early as the 1850s, in the era of Florence Nightingale, where she applied statistical analysis and gathered evidence to help guide health care reform. Archie Cochrane, a British epidemiologist, set a precedent for EBM in the 1970s by highlighting the important of randomization in clinical trials.[1] However, it is in the 1990s that the term "evidence-based medicine" appeared in literature, and its origin can be traced back to McMaster University in Canada. It was introduced to the wide medical community in a 1992 JAMA article. Now, EBM is widespread and utilized throughout the medical community in multiple ways by legislators, policy makers, clinicians, and for teaching purposes.[2] Modern EBM is defined as "the conscientious, explicit and judicious use of current best evidence, combined with individual clinical expertise and patient preference values, in making decisions about the care of individual patients". It is composed of five steps (Table 1).[2] Evidence-based medicine integrates three critical elements: best research evidence, clinical expertise, and patient values.[8]

The levels of evidence vary according to the clinical question we are trying to answer. Therefore, there has been a classification created to modify the levels according to treatment, prognosis, diagnosis, and economic/decision analysis.[3,8]

The Oxford Centre for Evidence-Based Medicine (OCEBM) levels of evidence were redesigned in 2011. The levels of evidence for treatment are adapted and summarized in Table 2. This was adapted by the editorial board of JAMA facial plastic surgery for use in facial plastic and reconstructive surgery research. Another useful tool is the level of evidence pyramid. It helps visualize the quality of evidence and the amount of evidence available (Fig. 1).[10]

There is a distinction to make between a systematic review and a meta-analysis. Although systematic reviews and meta-analysis both combine data from multiples studies, a meta-analysis is a statistical technique that combines the results of independent studies, as if the data was collected from one large study, and analyzes it in a quantitative synthesis.[1,4] Therefore, it does not take into account the quality of the data or the distinctive characteristics of the study. A systematic review may or may not include a meta-analysis, whereas a meta-analysis is always based on a systematic review of quantitative data.[4] A systematic review is thus a powerful tool for evidence-based medical practice since it takes into account the quality of the data and the distinctive characteristic of a study, and can also include a meta-analysis of quantitative data, if necessary.[4]

Table 1: Steps in evidence-based medicine (EBM) reasoning.[1,2]

Step 1	*What is the question?* Identify the clinical problem or need for information in an answerable question
Step 2	*Search for answers* Tracking down the best evidence with which to answer the question
Step 3	*Appraise the evidence* According to its validity, impact, and applicability
Step 4	*Apply the results* Integrating the results of step 3 with our clinical experience and the patient's uniqueness
Step 5	*Assess the outcome* Evaluating our effectiveness and efficiency in executing steps 1 to 4 and seeking ways to improve next time

Table 2: Level of evidence [Oxford Centre for Evidence-Based Medicine (OCEBM)].[9]

Level 1	Properly powered and conducted randomized controlled trial (RCT), and systematic review or meta-analysis of RCTs
Level 2	Well-designed controlled trial without randomization; prospective comparative cohort trial
Level 3	Case-control studies; retrospective cohort study
Level 4	Case series with or without intervention; cross-sectional study
Level 5	Opinion of respected authorities; case reports

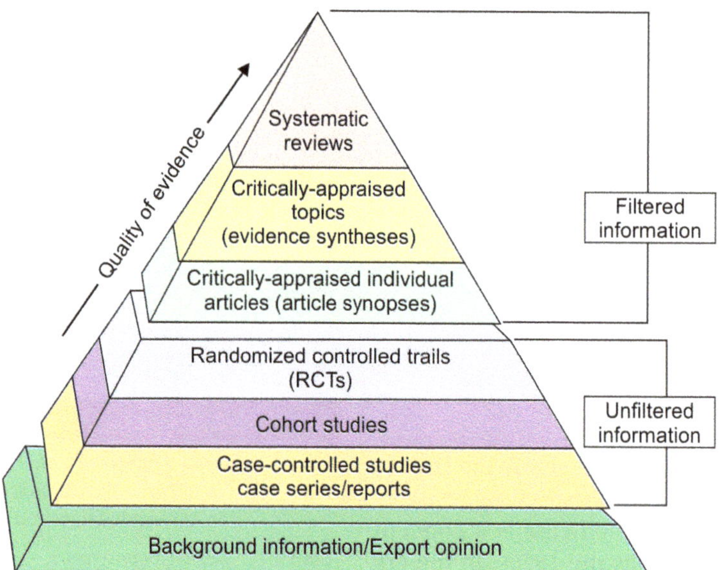

Fig. 1: Level of evidence pyramid.[10]

Table 3: Determining strength of action for key guideline statements.[9]

Statement	Definition
Strong recommendation	A strong recommendation means the benefits of the recommended approach clearly exceed the harms and that the quality of the supporting evidence is excellent
Recommendation	A recommendation means the benefits exceed the harms, but the quality of evidence is not as strong
Option	An option means that either the quality of evidence is suspect or that well-done studies show little clear advantage to one approach versus another.

Distinct from levels of evidence are recommendation grades, which are of particular interest in guideline development. The commonly used recommendation scheme in the guidelines put out by the American Academy of Otolaryngology—Head and Neck Surgery is explained in Table 3 and is based on aggregate evidence levels.[9]

Because EBM is based on the clinical use of well-constructed studies, it is important to address how to formulate a research study using the PICO method and the gold-standard research methodology, which is the randomized controlled trial (RCT). First, PICO is a tool to express the clinical problem in a focused, answerable question.[1] It contains four essential parts: patient/problem of interest, intervention, control or alternative treatment and outcome of interest. The more parts are answered, the more focused the clinical question will be.[5] Moreover, an RCT, which involves assigning patients to either an experimental group or a control group using a non-human

distribution tool, is the gold-standard research methodology because it provides the most rigorous way of determining whether cause-effect relationship exists between treatment and outcome.[6] It does so by ruling out the confounding variables or associations caused by a third factor by using randomization.[1,7]

■ REFERENCES

1. Cheung MC, Allan BJ, Yang R, et al. Evidence-based medicine and its role in plastic surgery. J Craniofac Surg. 2011;22:385-7.
2. Swanson JA, Schmitz D, Chung KC. How to practice evidence-based medicine. Plast Reconstr Surg. 2010;126:286-94.
3. Burns PB, Rohrich RJ, Chung KC. The levels of evidence and their role in evidence-based medicine. Plast Reconstr Surg. 2011;128:305-10.
4. Margaliot Z, Chung KC. Systematic reviews: a primer for plastic surgery research. Plast Reconstr Surg. 2007;120: 1834-41.
5. Burns PB, Chung KC. Developing good clinical questions and finding the best evidence to answer those questions. Plast Reconstr Surg. 2010;126:613-8.
6. Shah HM, Chung KC. Archie Cochrane and his vision for evidence-based medicine. Plast Reconstr Surg. 2009;124: 982-8.
7. McCarthy CM, Collins ED, Pusic AL. Where do we find the best evidence? Plast Reconstr Surg. 2008;122:1942-7.
8. Sackett DL, Rosenberg WM, Gray JA, et al. Evidence-based medicine: what it is and what it isn't. BMJ. 1996;312:71-2.
9. Rosenfeld RM, Shiffman RN. Clinical practice guideline development manual: a quality-driven approach for translating evidence into action. Otolaryngol Head Neck Surg. 2009;140:S1-43.
10. Glover J, Izzo D, Odato K, Wang L. "EBM Pyramid". Walden University. http://academicguides.waldenu.edu/healthevidence/evidencepyramid

Self-Assessment Exercise

Q 1. What is the modern definition of evidence-based medicine?

Ans:

The conscientious, explicit and judicious use of current best evidence, combined with individual clinical expertise and patient preference values, in making decisions about the care of individual patients.

Q 2. Name the 5 levels of evidence according to OCEBM 2011.

Ans:

Level 1 Systematic review of randomized trials or n-of-1 trials

Level 2 Randomized trial or observational study with dramatic effect

Level 3 Nonrandomized controlled cohort/follow-up study*

Level 4 Case-series, case-control studies, or historically controlled studies*

Level 5 Mechanism-based reasoning.

Q 3. What does PICO stand for?

Ans:

Patient/Problem of interest, Intervention, Control or alternative treatment and Outcome of interest.

Q 4. What two components does the level of evidence pyramid help visualize?

Ans: It helps visualize the quality of evidence and the amount of evidence available

Q 5. What are the three levels of recommendation in guidelines?

Ans:

Strong recommendation

Recommendation

Option.

Chapter 4

Legal, Ethical and Socioeconomic Issues in Facial Plastic Surgery

Kaitlin Wiseman, Anastasios Maniakas

PATIENT PHYSICIAN RELATIONSHIP AND ITS CONCEPTS

- *Concept of duty*: Physicians are required to act in such a way that social, professional, legal and ethical expectations are met, compelling a standard of performance; they have an obligation to take reasonable care of their patients, avoiding any harm that can otherwise be caused.
  - This duty is not relieved until the treatment plan, as it pertains to the appropriate standard of care, is complete, or a formal termination of the physician-patient relationship is obtained.
- The standard of care is defined as what a minimally competent physician that practices in the same field would do in a similar situation, with similar resources.
- Abandonment is defined as "the termination of a professional relationship between physician and patient at an unreasonable time and without giving the patient the chance to find an equally qualified replacement."[1,2]
- Does a physician have a duty to finish care, regardless of a patient's ability to pay? Once a formal physician-patient relationship is established and where care has been provided:
  - Treatment for that patient is the responsibility of the physician, regardless of whether the financial obligations can be met.
  - Treatment must continue until no further care is needed.[3]

INFORMED CONSENT

Informed consent is an integral part of the preoperative process. Surgeons must honestly, and in understandable terms, discuss:
- *Diagnosis*: The diagnosis or suspected diagnosis.
- *Treatment*: The nature and purpose of the proposed treatment or procedure and its benefits.
- *Risks*: The risk, complications and side effects.
- *Benefits*: The likelihood of success based on the patients preexisting condition(s).
- *Alternatives*: Reasonable and available alternatives.
- *Consequences*: Consequences, if treatment/procedural advice is not followed.[4,5]

Patient must understand that perfection may not be achieved. Expectations might not be fully satisfied, and the possibility of a secondary procedure should also be discussed.[4]

Consent is valid if:
- There is an understanding of the disease and the nature of intervention (risks and benefits).
- The patient has the ability to provide authorization to the physician.
- There is no external influence/control from others.[4]

Informed consent comprises what is called affirmative duty:
- Physician must volunteer information, such as the risks of a procedure, and must not wait for the patient to ask.
- The patient should be made aware of the most probable of known dangers as well as how frequently they occur.[2,5,6]

Details on the discussions with patients should be well-documented in patient records.

With the exception of urgent situations, treating a minor without the consent from a parent, a legal guardian, an appropriate government agency or court, leaves the physician at high risk for legal/criminal charges.[7]

COSMETIC SURGERY AND PATIENT SELECTION

Treatment: "a session of medical care or the administration of a dose of medicine". The goal of cosmetic surgery is to facilitate improvement in the patient's psychological functioning, primarily by modifying their body image; although cosmetic surgery focuses on enhancing one's appearance, it is still considered a treatment.[8,9]

Important elements in the consideration and evaluation when selecting a surgical candidate:
- Psychomorphologic analysis.
- Use of psychomorpholinguistic method.[10]

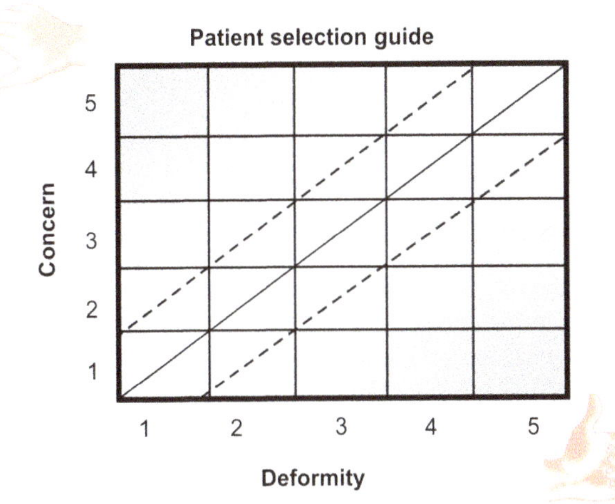

Fig. 1: Patient selection guide.

Two categories can make a patient an unlikely candidate for elective cosmetic surgery:

1. Anatomic unsuitability
2. Psychological inadequacy.

Healthy and unhealthy reasons for seeking cosmetic surgery must be well-differentiated by the surgeon.

In Figure 1 patients with a major deformity but who have minimal concern are patients who will most likely be satisfied with any degree of improvement. Patients who have a minor deformity but have a high concern are usually dissatisfied regardless of the outcome.[5]

RECORD KEEPING

Documentation of the surgical report may provide the physician with the best defense, in the case of litigation. It is imperative the surgeon record:

- A complete, adequate record of the patient's history.
- Decisions made between the physician and patient that contribute to informed consent.
- The surgical procedure described in detail, providing information about all anatomic areas treated.[4]
  - The operative report should be dictated immediately after the procedure and should contain:
    » Indication for surgery
    » Surgical procedure
    » Anesthesia used
    » Sequence of surgical steps
    » Complications/problems encountered
    » A postoperative appointment scheduled and recorded as well.
  - Preoperative and postoperative photographs should be taken as an objective form of documentation:
    » Standard pose is ideal

  » Helps avoid any suspicions of falsifying postoperative photos
  » Allows for documentation of preexisting asymmetries, irregularities or scarring.[4]

Reports dictated too long after complication lack credibility, whether or not the complication in question resulted from physician negligence.[11]

Correcting a medical record: Correction of medical records should only be made to your own entries.

- Changes must be dated and signed/initialed, or authenticated in the case of electronic records.
- The original entry must not be destroyed.
- An addendum can be added in the progress notes
  - Must be clearly labeled, include a current date, additional information and a signature.
- Electronic records
  - Most establishments require that health records management systems have an "audit trail", able to track the changes made, who they were made by and when.
  - Changes should be made without deleting the original note from view.[12]

TERMINATING THE PATIENT-PHYSICIAN RELATIONSHIP

Situations where it is acceptable to terminate a physician patient relationship:

- Nonadherence to treatment
- Nonadherence to follow-up
- Nonadherence to office policy
- *Verbal abuse*: patient or family member exhibits rude behavior, inappropriate language, violent behavior, makes threats of physical harm or uses anger to jeopardize the safety and well-being of the office personnel.
- *Nonpayment*: A patient owes many bills and has refused to work with the office to create a payment plan.[13]
- A conflict of interest that compromises the physician's duty to put the interests of his/her patient first.

It is important to terminate the relationship in an appropriate manner, reducing legislations of physician abandonment or negligence:[14]

- Give the patient written notice
- Provide the patient with a brief explanation for terminating the relationship
- Agree to continue to provide treatment and access to services for a reasonable time-frame (~30 days), giving the patient sufficient time to secure care from another physician
- Provide resources/recommendations, facilitating the search for a replacing physician
- Offer a transfer of records to the new treating physician upon patient authorization.[2]

▪ MEDICAL NEGLIGENCE

There are four principles and the scope that provide a simple and culturally neutral approach when considering ethical issues in health care:
1. Respect of autonomy
2. Beneficence
3. Nonmaleficence
4. Justice

Scope of Application[15]

When alleging medical negligence, four legal requirements need to be proven in order for a successful claim to exist:
1. Existence of a legal duty on the part of the physician to provide care or treatment to the patient
2. Breach of this duty by a failure on the part of the physician to meet the standards of care
3. Causal relationship between the breach of duty and injury to the patient
4. Existence of damages that arose from the injury, such that the legal system can provide redress.[16]

Negligence and the Borrowed Servant Theory

The borrowed servant theory, also coined the *captain of the ship doctrine*, deems the surgeon responsible/liable for the actions of those working in his operating room, whether they are part of his medical field or not.

Three key elements of negligence according to the borrowed servant theory:
1. The employee was negligent
2. The physician possessed appropriate training, supervision and control over employee
3. The negligent actions were within the scope of the employee's job description.

Further Concepts

- These elements only apply to the medical professional who is actively participating within the surgical arena during the procedure
- Any negligence outside the operating room or prior to the procedure, does not apply to the doctrine
- Surgeons are not liable for failure of hospital employees to execute reasonable instructions with respect to postoperative care.[17]

Vicarious Liability

The imposition of liability on a person or organization for the negligence of another, based entirely on the nature of their relationship.

In a medical context, historically, vicarious liability went hand in hand with the *captain of the ship doctrine*.

Currently, determining vicarious liability considers:
- Nature and extent of the attending physicians control over the environment
- Whom the resident physicians are working with (i.e. in a private setting or within a sponsoring institution).[18]

Res Ipsa Loquitur

"The thing speaks for itself."
- Negligence is inferred, there is no direct evidence of negligence or wrongdoing.

Claimant needs proof that
- The incident that occurred resulted from negligence
- It was the responsibility of the defendant

Expert testimony on the applicable standard of care and a breach in that standard of care is not needed, but the claimant needs to establish causation.[19]

▪ GUARANTEES

Reasonable expectations regarding outcome need to be discussed, considering
- Surgical candidacy
- The potential need for multiple surgical stages
- The balance of aesthetic and functional goals.

Showing photographs of similar, successful surgical procedures is not advised; each case is unique and the outcome for one patient does not translate into the outcome of another.
- Rough drawings or photographs with computerized facial analysis are helpful
  - N.B: The physician must be clear that there is no implied guarantee of success or reproducibility.[20]

Should promises be made regarding outcome, physicians could find themselves with litigations for breach of contract.[21]

▪ CONFLICT OF INTEREST

When professional judgment concerning direct patient care is inappropriately influenced by a secondary interest.[22]

The American College of Physicians suggests:
- Any gift offered to a physician from the health care industry, reducing or appearing to reduce the objectivity of professional judgment is strongly discouraged
  - Studies have documented that accepting even small gifts can affect clinical judgment and increase the perception/reality of a conflict of interest
- It is up to the physician to regularly question whether any gift relationship is ethically appropriate and how/if it will affect clinical judgment.

It is the responsibility of each physician to ensure that potential relationships with industry serve to enhance patient care as well as medical knowledge.[23]

■ REFERENCES

1. American Society of Plastic Surgeons. [online] Available from https://www.plasticsurgery.org/Documents/medical-professionals/yps/What-You-May-Not-Have-Learned-in-Residency.pdf [Accessed March, 2017].
2. Maltzman JD, Esquire BD. Can your doctor dismiss you from his/her practice—legally? Cancer Resources. The Abramson Cancer Center of the University of Pennsylvania; 2005.
3. Kroeker A. Legal, Ethical, and Socioeconomic Issues in Facial Plastic Surgery. Facial Plastic and Reconstructive Surgery. 2016;69-74.
4. Kalter PO, van der Baan B, Vuyk H. Medicolegal aspects of otolaryngologic, facial plastic, and reconstructive surgery. Facial Plast Surg. 1995;11:105-10.
5. Gorney M. Claims prevention for the aesthetic surgeon: preparing for the less-than-perfect outcome. Facial Plast Surg. 2002;18:135-42.
6. Moffett P, Moore G. The standard of care: legal history and definitions: the bad and good news. West J Emerg Med. 2011;12:109-12.
7. Coleman DL, Rosoff PM. The legal authority of mature minors to consent to general medical treatment. Pediatrics. 2013;131:786-93.
8. American Board Cosmetic Surgery. (2009). Cosmetic surgery vs plastic surgery. [online] Available from http://www.americanboardcosmeticsurgery.org/patient-resources/cosmetic-surgery-vs-plastic-surgery/ [Accessed March, 2017].
9. Pruzinsky T. Psychological factors in cosmetic plastic surgery: recent developments in patient care. Plast Surg Nurs. 1993;13:64-9.
10. Morselli PG. Plastic surgery and psychomorphology: a new tool for improving communication between physician and dysmorphopathic patient and for perfecting appropriate patient selection. Aesthetic Plast Surg. 27:485-92.
11. Medical Legal Aspects of Medical Records. [online] Available from (http://www.cpso.on.ca/policies-publications/policy/medical-records + https://www.cmpa-acpm.ca/-/the-medical-record-a-legal-document-can-it-be-corrected) [Accessed March, 2017].
12. CMPA. (2009). The medical record: a legal document—can it be corrected? [online]. Available from https://www.cmpa-acpm.ca/-/the-medical-record-a-legal-document-can-it-be-corrected-[Accessed March, 2017].
13. Thedoctors.com. [online] Available from http://www.thedoctors.com/KnowledgeCenter/PatientSafety/articles/Terminating-Patient-Relationships. [Accessed March, 2017].
14. Holder AR. Physician's abandonment of patient. American Jurisprudence Proof of Facts. 2008;3:117.
15. Gillon R. Medical ethics: four principles plus attention to scope. BMJ. 1994;309:184-8.
16. Bal BS. An introduction to medical malpractice in the United States. Clin Orthop Relat Res. 2008;467:339-47.
17. Shandell RE, Smith P, Schulman FA. The Preparation and Trial of Medical Malpractice Cases. New York, NY: Law Journal Seminars-Press; 1981.
18. Kachalia A, Studdert DM. Professional liability issues in graduate medical education. JAMA. 2004;292:1051-6.
19. Thornton RG. The limited use of inferred negligence in medical cases. Proc (Bayl Univ Med Cent). 2002;15:228-30.
20. Holt RG, Stallworth CL. Grafts and Implants in Facial, Head and Neck Surgery. In: Bailey BJ, Johnson JT, Newlands SD (Eds). Head & Neck Surgery—otolaryngology. Philadelphia: Lippincott Williams & Wilkins; 2001. pp. 2345-56.
21. Cornell Law Review. (1996). Categories and Culture: On the Rectification of Names in Comparative Law. [online] Available from http://scholarship.law.cornell.edu/cgi/viewcontent.cgi?article=1752&context=clr [Accessed March, 2017].
22. WMA. [online] Available from http://www.wma.net/en/30publications/10policies/i3/index.html.pdf?print-media-type&footer-right=[page]/[toPage] [Accessed March, 2017].
23. Lo B, Field MJ. Institute of Medicine (US) Committee on Conflict of Interest in Medical Research, Education, and Practice. Conflicts of Interest in Medical Research, Education, and Practice. National Academies Press (US). 2009;176-77.

Self-Assessment Exercise

Q 1. What are the elements of informed consent?

Ans:
- The diagnosis or suspected diagnosis
- The nature and purpose of the proposed treatment or procedure and its benefits
- The risk, complications and side effects
- The likelihood of success based on the patients pre-existing condition(s)
- Reasonable and available alternatives
- Consequences, if treatment/procedural advice is not followed.

Q 2. What is the procedure for correcting inaccuracies in the medical record?

Ans:
- Changes must be dated and signed
- Original entry must not be destroyed-notation to allow the incorrect information to be traced or information left in the record should be clearly noted as incorrect, with the additional corrected information signed and dated
- An addendum can be added in the progress notes as well-labeled, signed and dated
- *Electronic records:* Health record management systems with "audit trail", able to track the changes made, who they were made by and when. Changes should be made without deleting the original note from view.

Q 3. What are the criteria to terminate a patient-physician relationship?

Ans:
- Give the patient written notice
- Provide the patient with a brief explanation
- Agree to continue to provide treatment and access to services for a reasonable time-frame (~30 days), giving the patient sufficient time to secure care from another physician

- Provide resources/recommendations, facilitating the search for a replacing physician
- Offer a transfer of records to the new treating physician upon patient authorization.

Q 4. What are the four criteria of ethical medical practice?

Ans:
- Respect of autonomy
- Beneficence
- Nonmaleficence
- Justice
- (+ scope of application).

Q 5. What are the criteria for a physician to be considered medically negligent?

Ans:
- Existence of a legal duty on the part of the physician to provide care or treatment to the patient
- Breach of this duty by a failure on the part of the physician to meet the standards of care
- Causal relationship between the breach of duty and injury to the patient
- Existence of damages that arose from the injury, such that the legal system can provide redress.

Multiple Choice Questions

Q 1. Which of the following statements pertaining to psychological and legal considerations in revision rhinoplasty is FALSE?

A. The patient should accept improvement rather than perfection

B. Most surgeons do not charge for revisions of their own rhinoplasties

C. Most surgeons, if the patient is unhappy with the revision will refund the original surgical fee in order to avoid litigation

D. Open-ended questions are the most useful in order to understand the dissatisfaction with the initial surgery

Ans: C. Most surgeons, if the patient is unhappy with the revision will refund the original surgical fee in order to avoid litigation

Q 2. Which of the following is NOT an APPROPIATE question for the surgeon to ask when evaluating a patient for surgery?

A. What is it that prompts you to seek this surgery?

B. For what time period have you been considering this surgery?

C. What are the changes in particular that you are considering?

D. Your nose really needs work. Is that your concern?

Ans: D. Your nose really needs work. Is that your concern?

Q 3. Which of the following statements in the evaluation and management of patients for facial plastic surgery is FALSE?

A. If a patient expects perfection should not have surgery

B. Every patient is not a good candidate for surgery

C. Most faces are symmetrical

D. The goals of a patient who seeks surgical aid should be realistic

Ans: C. Most faces are symmetrical

Q 4. The cause of pediatric fractures involving ONLY the mandible is most likely related to:

A. Altercations   B. Biking accidents

C. Child abuse   D. Falls accidents

Ans: C. Child abuse

Q 5. Body dysmorphic disorder patients are most commonly concerned with the appearance of their:

A. Skin   B. Nose

C. Hair   D. Jowls

E. Eyelids

Ans: A. Skin

Q 6. The most common cosmetic surgical procedure sought out by men is:

A. Facelift   B. Blepharoplasty

C. Rhinoplasty   D. Otoplasty

E. Browlift

Ans: C. Rhinoplasty

Q 7. Considerations in the reconstruction of a total rhinectomy defect should include:

A. Nasal form

B. Nasal function

C. Nasal form and function

D. Nasal form, function, patient's social support

E. Nasal form, function patient's social support and coping skills

Ans: E. Nasal form, function patient's social support and coping skills

Q 8. Compared to the general population, body dysmorphic disorder patients have an increased risk of:

A. Noncompliance to postoperative care instructions

B. Suicide

C. Satisfaction with surgical results

D. Alcohol abuse

E. Sexually transmitted infections

Ans: B. Suicide

Q 9. Compared to females, male rhinoplasty patients have an increased risk of:

A. Depression

B. Anxiety

C. Obsessive-compulsive disorder

D. Psychosis

E. Body dysmorphic disorder

Ans: E. Body dysmorphic disorder

Chapter 5

Psychological Aspects in Plastic Surgery

Scott W Smith, Matthew Brace

INTRODUCTION

Facial plastic and reconstructive surgery is a rapidly evolving and changing field of study and practice. Fulfilling the role of surgeon is but one component of the job. Surgeons must also navigate the varying cultural and social ideals surrounding beauty and body image, while understanding the underlying psychological motivations and consequences of facial surgery.[1] A large body of research has been generated over the last 25 years supporting improved outcomes and better patient care when surgeons incorporate all of these roles into their practice. Strong communication and realistic expectations from both parties of the patient-surgeon relationship is apparent in any successful outcome.

Aesthetic and reconstructive facial plastic surgery practices have diverse patient populations catering to all age groups, genders, socioeconomic backgrounds, and ethnicities. A cancer patient with a total rhinectomy defect and a cosmetic rhinoplasty patient will have different and individualized goals. Pediatric patients and adolescents have the added complexity of physical growth and development as well as involvement of parents or guardians in decision-making. Baby boomers make up approximately half of the more than 15 million cosmetic surgical procedures performed annually in America and minorities make up an expanding number of patients with ethnically oriented surgery and acceptance of media driven westernization.[2] Although females make up approximately 87% of the cosmetic market, body dissatisfaction among men increased from 15% in 1972 to 43% in 1996 accounting for a growing proportion of male patients.[2] The practice of facial plastic and reconstructive surgery is truly diverse and surgeons must approach each patient individually, understanding their goals and motivations, in order to achieve consistently happy patients and successful results.

BODY IMAGE

Greeks were the first to quantify beauty, describing esthetic perfection with idealized symmetric mathematical proportions.[2] Darwin's *The Descent of Man and Selection in Relation to Sex* suggests that the most attractive individuals are most likely to be selected, enhancing the likelihood of passing on one's genetic material.[2] A behavioral study by Langlois et al. supports the notion of innate preprogrammed behavior; a cohort of 3–6 months old infants preferentially stared at photographs of more attractive faces longer than less attractive faces.[3] Established evidence supports that perceived attractiveness often leads to preferential treatment throughout all stages of life in a variety of social situations including better grades, jobs, and higher salaries.[4] The concept of body image is integral to the psychology behind decisions to alter appearance through means of minimally invasive procedures and surgery. Body image is defined as a person's perception of the aesthetics or attractiveness of his or her own body. The concept evolves through life responding to personal experiences, personality, various social and cultural forces, but most importantly, age. A study of patients undergoing blepharoplasty and facelift demonstrated motivation for cosmetic surgery is age dependent.[2] Subjects in their 30s endorsed motivating forces related to struggles with childhood and difficulty assuming parental roles; those in their 40s desired occupational advancement through youthful appearance; and, those greater than fifty suffering grief from loss of a close relative looking to erase physical stigmata of aging. Body dissatisfaction is so prevalent that it is considered "normative discontent" rather than psychopathologic diagnosis.[3]

GENDER DIFFERENCES

Youth, health, lustrous hair, smooth unblemished skin, and muscular physique defined attractiveness in the large International Mate Selection Project Study of over 10,000 people that included Western and non-western cultures.[5] Understanding differences in gender imagery can assist in narrowing motivating psychological factors. Women are subjected to increasingly greater societal pressures, from media, men, and themselves. In a 1989 study, American men ranked the importance of female attractiveness as 2.1 on a 0–3 scale, in contrast to 50 years earlier where it was ranked 1.5.[2] Female self-body dissatisfaction increased from 23% to 56% from 1972 to 1996.[2] More and more correlational research continues to suggest increased use of social media may be associated with higher prevalence of psychopathologies among young women, namely eating disorders. Anecdotally, an increasing number of young women are presenting with cosmetic facial concerns that they notice while using social networking phone apps.[6] The full effect of social networking apps on self-image and self-confidence remains to be seen.

Historically, male patients have a reputation of being more challenging cosmetic patients. Emotional immaturity is a common barrier to their ability to outline specific rationale for wanting to change their appearance. The acronym SIMON, coined by plastic surgeons, stands for "Single, Immature, Male, Obsessed, Narcissistic", a combination of characteristics that experienced surgeons recommend avoiding.[7] Surgeons are cautioned that bad outcomes in male cosmetic patients may provoke greater tension and more aggressive retaliation. Rhinoplasty, followed by blepharoplasty, are the two procedures most commonly requested by men. However, 2014 data from the American Society of Plastic Surgeons revealed a 64% and 49% decrease respectively in men seeking these surgeries, compared to data from 2000.[8] At the same time, procedures, such as cosmetic Botox and laser resurfacing have increased by 337% and 227% respectively.[8] This likely reflects changing societal norms and increased demand for "no downtime" procedures.

FACIAL RECONSTRUCTION

The psychological consequences of facial disfigurement caused by congenital anomalies, trauma, or cancer adds a layer of complexity to the preoperative considerations of the reconstructive surgeon. Rankin et al. demonstrated photographs of individuals with facial abnormalities like scar, burn, or cleft lip were viewed as less honest, less employable, less trustworthy, less intelligent, and less attractive than their own digitally altered photographs.[9] Research by psychologist David Sarwer, on patients with craniofacial disfigurement revealed 38% of surveyed patients with congenital disfigurement experienced discrimination in employment or social situations and 50% reported undergoing psychotherapy for issues related to their physical appearance.[10] Patients with reconstructed noses after rhinectomy were studied by Moolenburgh et al. 2009, revealing that active coping strategies and self-esteem building were associated with better psychosocial functioning.[11] These studies illustrate the critical psychological importance of form when restoring form and function in facial reconstruction. They highlight the surgeon's key role in managing patient expectations with regards to achievable outcomes as well as the importance of understanding individual patients' social support and coping skills.

COSMETIC SURGERY

Screening patients for cosmetic surgery is an art. While the overwhelming majority of patients presenting for cosmetic consultation are suitable candidates, detecting the minority with psychopathologies prior to engaging in a surgical relationship can prevent unwanted outcomes for both the patient and surgeon. Red flags during history taking include unrealistic expectations, demanding requests, inability to articulate goals, and perseverance on a minor or imagined concern. In addition, patients seeking revision surgery who make disparaging remarks regarding their previous surgeon and those patients who are difficult to develop a rapport with should be approached with caution. Utilizing a set of standard questions may ensure detection of red flags.

- What about your appearance do you dislike?
- Does your dissatisfaction prevent you from doing certain activities?
- Do you ever hide or camouflage your dislike?
- What is your motivation? Is this for you or someone else?
- What changes do you expect from surgery?
- Have you consulted with other cosmetic surgeons?
- Have you undergone prior cosmetic procedures? Are you satisfied?
- Do you currently or have you ever been treated for mental health issues?

Inability to answer the above questions may prompt the need for further questioning and perhaps consultation of a psychologist or psychiatrist, ideally experienced with body image disorders.[1] Unfortunately there is no single tool capable of revealing exact motivations and expectations of every patient who walks in the door.

BODY DYSMORPHIC DISORDER AND OTHER PSYCHOPATHOLOGY

Body dysmorphic disorder (BDD) is defined as preoccupation with slight or imagined defect in appearance that leads to significant or excessive concern, impairment in daily functioning, and not better described by another DSM-V diagnosis. Phillips et al. suggest it must consume at least an hour daily, but more commonly ranges from 3 to 8 hours per day.[12] BDD is thought to affect 1–2% of the population, and as high as 7–15% of new patients presenting for cosmetic consultation.[6] Data show that between 50% and 80% of patients with BDD have undergone some image altering procedure.[13] Skin, hair, and nose are most often the subject of preoccupation. As a group, male rhinoplasty patients have a high prevalence of BDD among other psychiatric diagnoses. Several studies support that cosmetic surgery performed on BDD patients does not confer psychological benefit, and may exacerbate symptoms. Only about 10% of BDD patients report improvement after undergoing surgery.[12]

While there are no true absolute contraindications, only patients with adequately treated conditions confirmed by mental health providers should be considered.[12] Operating on BDD patients may require investing an extraordinary amount of time and emotional effort. One study revealed that 86% of facial plastic surgeons report having operated on a BDD patient, quoting complications, such as requests for revision surgery, depression, and suicidal thoughts. Among patients with BDD, the rate of suicide has been reported as 45 times greater than the general population. Identification and treatment for this population is critical for both the patient and in rare cases the surgeon's safety. A 2011 systematic review of screening questionnaires for BDD by Picavet et al. identified two validated screening tools that best served the cosmetic surgeon: (1) the BDD Questionnaire-Dermatology Version and (2) Dysmorphic Concern Questionnaire.[14]

The next two most common presenting personality disorders to consider are (1) narcissistic and (2) histrionic, which emphasize inflation of self-importance and attention seeking behaviors, respectively. Untreated eating disorders, anorexia and bulimia, are essential to identify to mitigate against increased medical preoperative risk. Other associated psychopathologic disorders important to recognize include borderline personality, major depressive, obsessive compulsive, post-traumatic stress, acute stress, and social anxiety disorder (Table 1).

Being able to manage these challenging patients is just as important as identifying them. Having options for management can prepare the surgeon to handle varying degrees of severity. A surgeon may recommend a minimally invasive reversible office procedure, such as Botox or facial filler. Scheduling a second consultation follow-up allows a patient time to digest information discussed during the first visit. Ultimately, a surgeon must not be afraid to refer a patient to another surgeon, if there is apprehension about proceeding. Saying no and refusing to offer surgery will never be regretted.

■ OUTCOMES ASSESSMENT

The majority of cosmetic patients endorse psychological improvement after surgery.[15-17] Given the nature of research in this discipline, well-designed qualified, randomized double-blinded prospective controlled studies are impossible to create. The body of research in this field relies heavily on subjective questionnaires and surveys. The FACE-Q validated outcomes survey designed specifically for psychometric evaluation of cosmetic facial plastic surgery patients has established itself as one of the most accepted outcomes measurement tools.[18] The questionnaire is a comprehensive battery of more than 40 scales including facial appearance, adverse effects, process care, and quality of life outcomes. Others, such as the Rosenberg Self-Esteem Scale (RSES), a 10-point focused on assessment of self-esteem, have also been evaluated and accepted as validated tools in the assessment of facial plastic surgery patient outcomes. Jacono et al. used the RSES to show individuals with low preoperative self-esteem were more likely to have demonstrated postoperative improvement following rhytidectomy. Other validated scales do exist, and when utilized before and after surgery can provide great insight into an individual's coping abilities and perceived surgical outcomes.[19-24]

■ SUMMARY

- Today's facial plastic surgeon must embrace multiple roles as technical surgeon to psychosocial therapist
- Management of expectations is equally as important as surgical ability
- Understand the motivating forces for all patients regardless of age, gender, race or congenital, traumatic, oncologic, or cosmetic consultation
- Being cognizant of societal and cultural pressures allows greater insight into patient motivations and can help surgeons guide patients toward the right treatment or procedure
- Body image is an individual's perception of their own aesthetics or attractiveness, a concept that evolves with aging
- Strong communication and management techniques with challenging patients may minimize unwanted outcomes
- Awareness and early identification of psychological disorders can protect a facial plastic surgery practice saving time, resources, legal and safety consequences
- The treatment for BDD is psychiatric, rarely surgical. A relationship with a collaborating psychologist or psychiatrist can assist in getting help for those patients in need.

■ REFERENCES

1. Gossbart TA, Sarwer DB. Cosmetic surgery: surgical tools—psychosocial goals. Sem Cutan Med Surg. 1999;18:101-11.
2. Alam M, Dover JS. On beauty: evolution, psychosocial functioning, and personality: how different are adolescents and young adults applying for plastic surgery? Arch Dermatol. 2001;137:795-807.
3. Langlois JH, Roggman LA, Casey RJ, et al. Infant preferences for attractive faces: rudiments of a stereotype. Dev Psychol. 1987;23:363-9.

Table 1: Other commonly presenting psychopathologies.

Narcissistic personality disorder	Histrionic personality disorder
Anorexia nervosa	Bulimia nervosa
Borderline personality disorder	Major depressive disorder
Obsessive compulsive disorder	Posttraumatic stress disorder
Acute stress disorder	Social anxiety disorder

4. Sykes JM. Managing the psychological aspects of plastic surgery. Curr Opin Otolaryngol Head Neck Surg. 2009;17:321-5.

5. Buss DM, Abbott M, Angleitner A, et al. International preferences in selecting mates: A study of 37 cultures. J Cross-cultural Psychology. 1990;21:5-47.

6. Honrado CP, Pastorek NJ. Preventing complications in facial plastic surgery. Curr Opin Otolaryngol Head Neck Surg. 2006;14:265-9.

7. Gorney M, Martello J. Patient selection criteria. Clin Plast Surg. 1999;26:37-40.

8. American Society of Plastic Surgeons. (2014). 2014 Plastic Surgery Statistics Report. [online] Available from https://www.plasticsurgery.org/news/plastic-surgery-statistics?utm_source=vanity&%3Butm_medium=other&%3Butm_campaign=stats-2013&&&sub=2014+Plastic+Surgery+Statistics [Accessed March, 2017].

9. Rankin M, Borah GL. Perceived functional impact of abnormal facial appearance. Plast Reconstr Surg. 2003;111:2140-6.

10. Sarwer DB, Bartlett SP, Whitaker LA, et al. Adult psychological functioning of individuals born with craniofacial anomalies. Plast Reconstr Surg. 1999;103:412-8.

11. Moolenburgh SE, Mureau MA, Versnel SL, et al. The impact of nasal reconstruction following tumour resection on psychosocial functioning, a clinical empirical exploration. Psychooncology. 2009;18:747-52.

12. Ende KH, Lewis DL, Kabaker SS. Body dysmorphic disorder. Facial Plast Surg Clin North Am. 2008;16:217-23.

13. Phillips KA, Dufresne RG. Body dysmorphic disorder: a guide for dermatologists and cosmetic surgeons. Am J Clin Dermatol. 2000;1:235-43.

14. Picavet V, Gabriëls L, Jorissen M, et al. Screening tools for body dysmorphic disorder in a cosmetic surgery setting. Laryngoscope. 2011;121:2535-41.

15. Goin MK, Rees TD. A prospective study of patients' psychological reactions to rhinoplasty. Ann Plast Surg. 1991;27:210-5.

16. Rankin M, Borah GL, Perry AW, et al. Quality-of-life outcomes after cosmetic surgery. Plast Reconstr Surg. 1998;102:2139-45.

17. Honigman RJ, Phillips KA, Castle DJ. A review of psychosocial outcomes for patients seeking cosmetic surgery. Plast Reconstr Surg. 2004;113:1229-37.

18. Schwitzer JA, Sehr SR, Fan KL, et al. Assessing patient-reported satisfaction with appearance and quality of life following rhinoplasty using the FACE-Q appraisal scales. Last Reconstr Surg. 2015;135:830e-7e.

19. Jacono A, Chastant RP, Dibelius G. Association of patient self-esteem with perceived outcome after face-lift surgery. JAMA Facial Plast Surg. 2016;18:42-6.

20. Rankin M, Borah GL. Anxiety disorders in plastic surgery. Plast Reconstr Surg. 1997;100:535-42.

21. Moss TP, Harris DL. Psychological change after aesthetic plastic surgery: a prospective controlled outcome study. Psychol Health Med. 2009;14:567-72.

22. Simis KJ, Hovius SE, de Beaufort ID, et al. After plastic surgery: adolescent-reported appearance ratings and appearance-related burdens in patient and general population groups. Plast Reconstr Surg. 2002;109:9-17.

23. Sobanko JF, Sarwer DB, Zvargulis Z, et al. Importance of physical appearance in patients with skin cancer. Dermatol Surg. 2015;41:183-8.

24. Hessler JL, Moyer CA, Kim JC, et al. Predictors of satisfaction with facial plastic surgery: results of a prospective study. Arch Facial Plast Surg. 2010;12:192-6.

Multiple Choice Questions

Q 1. **Which of the following indicates MOST accurately the patient's psychological state during the period immediately following a car accident which caused him an unfavorable outcome?**

A. Depression

B. Fear

C. Anger

D. Transitory personality disorder

Ans: C. Anger

Q 2. **Which of the following patients demonstrates realistic expectations?**

A. The patient who says his nose is too large and would like you to decrease its size

B. The patient who says he wants you to tell him what he needs to have done

C. The patient who says a family member wants him to have the surgery

D. The patient who says he needs the surgery for a certain occasion

Ans: A. The patient who says his nose is too large and would like you to decrease its size

Q 3. **A patient who attempts to murder his physician MOST LIKELY has which of the following disorders?**

A. Obsessive compulsive disorder

B. Narcissistic personality disorder

C. Paranoid personality disorder

D. Maniac-depressive disorder

Ans: C. Paranoid personality disorder

Q 4. **Which of the following will trigger the MOST "concern" from a surgeon's point of view?**

A. The patient has internal motivation or personal reasons for surgery

B. The patient has external motivation or spouse related reasons for surgery

C. "Doctor, I wish that you could remove the wrinkles around my eyes and mouth"

D. The patient has seen two previous surgeons in order to collect information and make a final decision about who he will choose to do his surgery

Ans: B. The patient has external motivation or spouse related reasons for surgery

Q 5. Which of the following statements regarding identifying a potential unstable and disruptive patient prior to any facial plastic surgery is FALSE?

A. Younger patients are more prone to behave aggressively

B. Male cosmetic rhinoplasty patients are likely at increased risk of unstable behavior

C. Abuse of alcohol potentiates the risk of instability

D. Internal motivation for surgery carries a higher risk for disruptive behavior than external motivation

Ans: D. Internal motivation for surgery carries a higher risk for disruptive behavior than external motivation

Q 6. Which of the following is NOT a "red flag" when evaluating patients for cosmetic plastic surgery?

A. Overconcern with a minor deformity

B. Inability to describe problem

C. Female rhinoplasty patient

D. Surgiholic patients

Ans: C. Female rhinoplasty patient

Q 7. Which of the following statements about unstable, potentially violent patients is TRUE?

A. Men are less prone to instability than women

B. Older patients have greater frequency than younger patients in abnormal behavior

C. Rhinoplasty patients are at greater risk than facial scar patients for unstable or violent acts

D. Use and abuse of alcohol is necessary related to unstable of violent behavior

Ans: C. Rhinoplasty patients are at greater risk than facial scar patients for unstable or violent acts

Q 8. Which of the following features is NOT characteristic of a problematic rhinoplastic patient?

A. Married

B. Immature

C. Male

D. Overly expectant

Ans: A. Married

Q 9. Which of the following patients is LESS of a potential risk for dissatisfaction after a cosmetic procedure?

A. A young female who is in an active litigious process with another surgeon

B. A middle age man with a well internet cosmetic knowledge who is insisting on a rejuvenating facial procedure

C. A young male patient with an ulterior motive of solving job related problems

D. A middle age female with a great power of manipulation, flattering the office, staff and surgeon

Ans: B. Middle age man with a well internet cosmetic knowledge who is insisting on a facial rejuvenation procedure

Q 10. Which of the following issues is the LEAST important to be included in the initial consultation for rhinoplasty?

A. Dissatisfaction for nasal appearance

B. Nasal obstruction

C. Family members perception of nasal deformity

D. Medical history

Ans: C. Family members perception of nasal deformity

Q 11. Which of the following in the adult male patient represents INCORRECT motivation for cosmetic plastic surgery?

A. Internal motivation

B. Corrective surgery planned for a short time

C. A clear disfigurement noted by patient and surgeon

D. Occupational appearance important to the patient

Ans: B. Corrective surgery planned for a short time

Rhinoplasty

Section Outlines

Chapter 6

Nasal and Facial Analysis

Sami P Moubayed, Jamil Manji

INTRODUCTION

Nasal analysis must fall in the context of facial analysis, especially with regards to the forehead and the chin. As a result, a structured examination is mandatory for successful surgical planning. This chapter will focus on global examination and analysis of the nose in the general context of the face. Examination of specific components of the face (eyes and eyebrows, chin, etc.) is covered in the other sections of this book.

The face is divided into esthetic units: forehead, eyes, nose, lips, chin, ears, and neck.[1] The nose is also divided into subunits: dorsum, sidewalls, ala, tip, columella, and soft tissue triangle.[1] The subunit principle is especially important during facial reconstruction, where if 50% of a subunit is involved by a defect, the subunit must be resected entirely before reconstruction.[1] Incision planning must be performed around these subunits.[2]

Cephalometric and soft tissue landmarks are shown in the figures below (Figs. 1 to 3).[2]

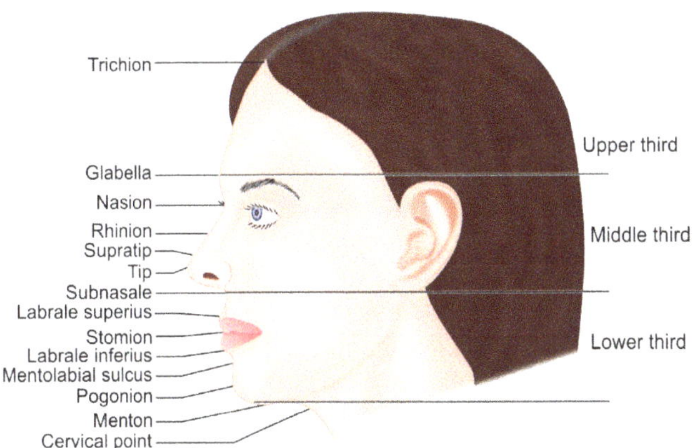

Fig. 2: Subunits of nose.

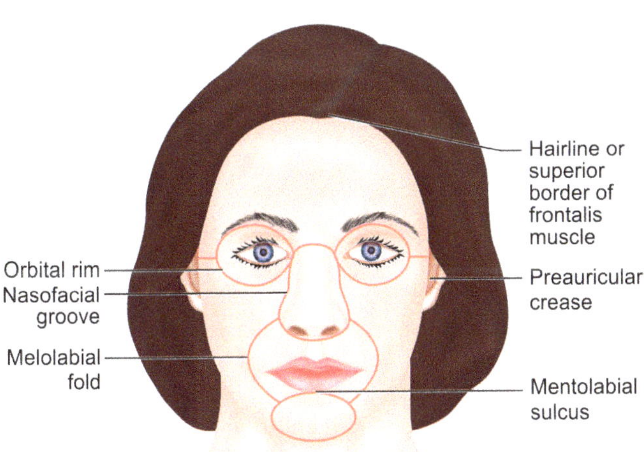

Fig. 1: Esthetic units of the face.

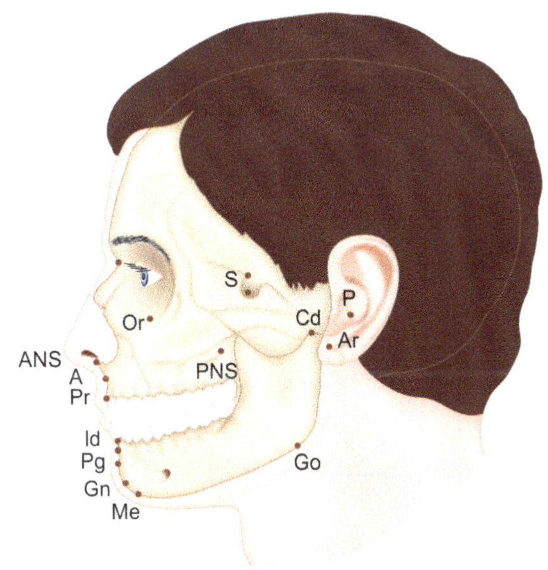

Fig. 3: Sella (S), orbitale (Or), porion (P), condylion (Cd), articulate (Ar), anterior nasal spine (ANS), posterior nasal spine (PNS), subspinale (A), prosthion (Pr), infradentale (Id), supramentale (B), pogonion (Pg), gnathion (Gn), menton (Me), and gonion (Go).

Horizontally, the face is divided into thirds: trichion to glabella, glabella to subnasale, subnasale to menton.[2] In the case of a receding hairline, an alternate subdivision is used: nasion to subnasale represent 43% and subnasale to menton represent 57% of total nasion-menton distance.[2] Vertically, the face is divided into fifths, all measuring the width of an eye.[2]

■ NASAL EXAMINATION AND ANALYSIS

Examination of the nose should be performed in the context of a complete head and neck examination. The septum, turbinates, and nasal valves must be thoroughly examined to detect functional problems, as described in "Functional Rhinoplasty" chapter. Then, palpation of the nasal bones must be performed. Short nasal bones are a contraindication to osteotomies and are defined as bones that finish less than 1 cm from the medial canthus.[3] The tip must be palpated using the recoil test to evaluate for deficient tip support which will require reconstruction in order to avoid long-term collapse.[2] The skin must be palpated to assess thickness: thin skin reveals irregularities and thick skin produces suboptimal results as it camouflages the underlying cartilaginous construct. The skin is usually thicker over the nasion, thinner over the rhinion, and thicker again over the supratip.[2]

Frontal View[4]

Ideal nasal length should measure one-third of the distance from the hairline to the inferior border of the chin and is measured from nasion to tip. The dorsum is evaluated using the "unbroken lines" method illustrated in Figure 4.

The nasal dorsum should measure approximately 75–80% of the nasal base.[1] Nasal tip contour should be evaluated. Two imaginary equilateral triangles placed base

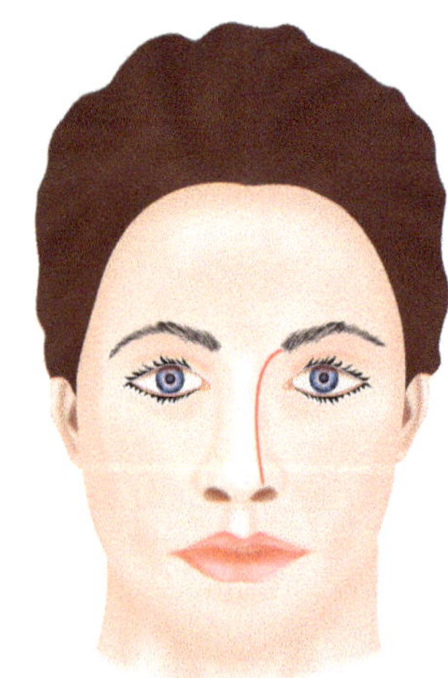

Fig. 4: The dorsum is evaluated using the "unbroken lines" method.

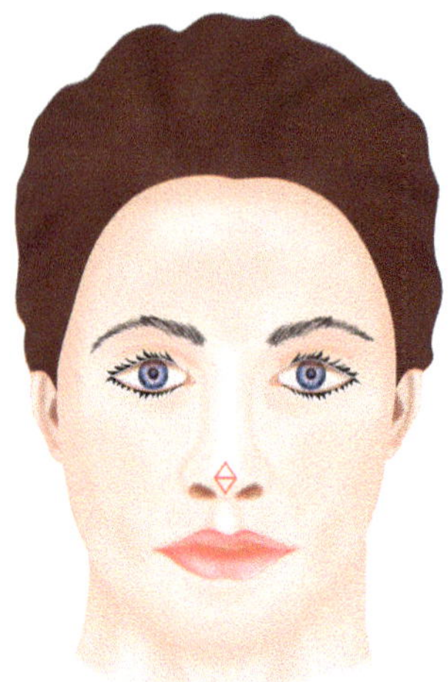

Fig. 5: Two imaginary equilateral triangles placed base to base represent the relationship between supratip break, tip defining points, and infratip break.

to base represent the relationship between supratip break, tip defining points, and infratip break (Fig. 5).

The upper rim of the nares is described as a "seagull in flight" shape with the columella is slightly lower with the nares just visible. Nasal base width should be approximately the intercanthal distance.

Lateral View[4]

The lateral view should be evaluated in the Frankfurt plane, where the superior border of the external auditory canal paralleling the infraorbital rim in a horizontal plane (Fig. 7). The nasion or nasofrontal angle is approximately at the level of the upper lid folds. The dorsum should then be evaluated for a hump or a slope. A gentle supratip break should be seen. The tip is then evaluated mainly in terms of projection and rotation. The methods to evaluate tip projection are defined in Table 1.

Tip rotation is measured using the nasofrontal and the nasolabial angles. The nasofrontal angle is formed by intersecting a line from nasion to the tip-defining-point, and a line from the nasion to glabella, and should measure 115°–135° (Fig. 8).

The nasolabial angle is formed by an intersect between a line from subnasale to the columellar break point, and another line from subnasale to upper vermilion border, and should measure 90°–95° in men, and 95°–110° in women (Figs. 9A and B).

The ala and the columella should be analyzed both separately and as a complex. The columella should have a gentle double. Ideally 2 mm or 3 mm of columellar show should be visible. The columella and the alar margins should maintain an angle to the Frankfort

Table 1: Methods to assess tip projection in the lateral view.

Method	Definition
Powell and Humphreys	Height measured from nasion (N) to subnasale (SN), perpendicular drawn through tip defining point (TDP), and ratio of N-X/X-TDP ideally 2.8:1
Nasofacial angle	Angle between a line joining N and alar-facial groove and another line joining N and TDP coursing along the dorsum, normally 36° (30°–40°)
Goode	Line drawn from the alar-facial groove to TDP measures 0.55–0.60 of the distance from N to TDP (represents the sinus of the nasofacial angle)
Crumley and Lanser	Right triangle whose sides follow a 3:4:5 ratio (Fig. 6)
Simons (Fig. 7)	Tip projection measured from TDP to SN and length of upper lip (measured from SN to upper vermilion border) should be equal (1:1)
Crumley (I)	A line is drawn from N to upper vermilion border, and a perpendicular line through the TDP is traced, and should have a 0.283:1 proportion with the longer line
Crumley (II)	A line from N through the alar-facial groove is drawn until it transects the mandibular profile, and a perpendicular line from TDP to this line should have a 0.236:1 proportion.

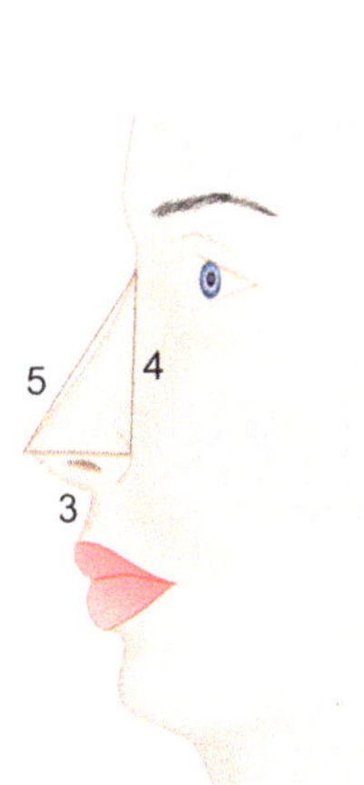

Fig. 6: The Crumley and Lanser 3-4-5 triangle method to assess tip projection.

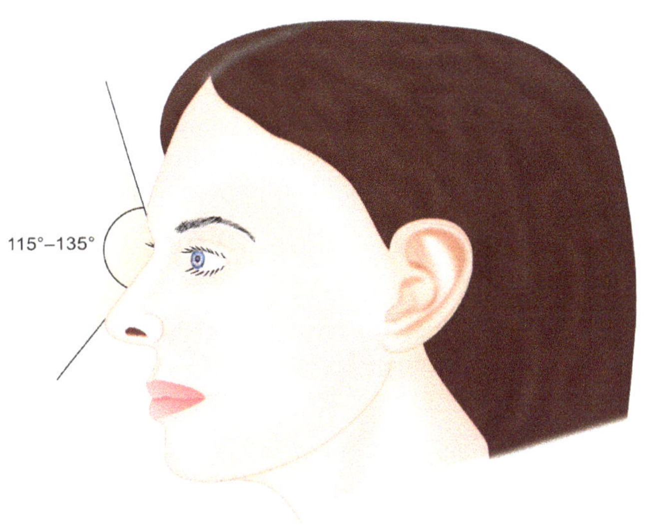

Fig. 8: The nasofrontal angle is formed by intersecting a line from the nasion to glabella and should measure 115°–135°

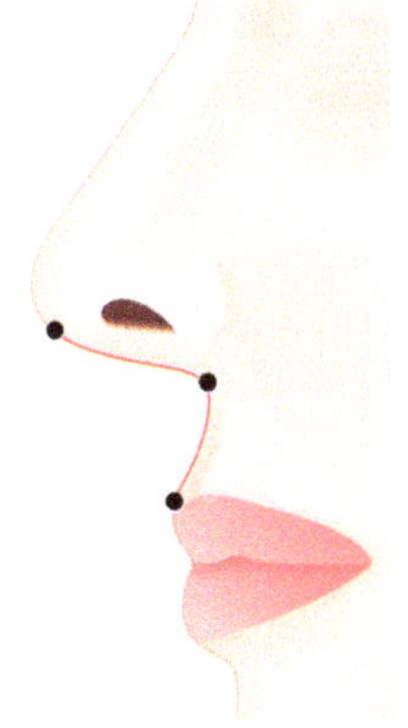

Fig. 7: Simons method.

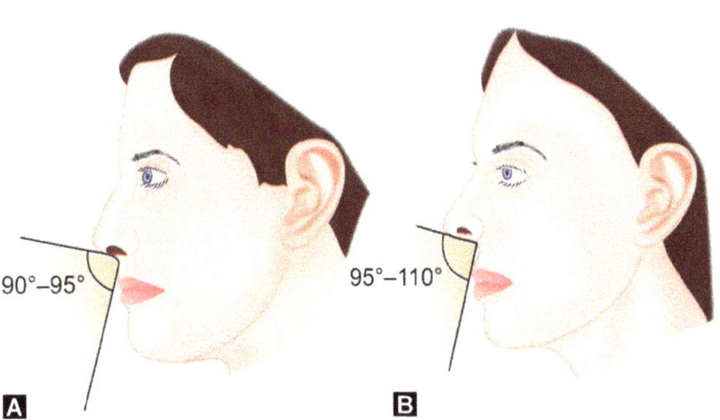

Figs. 9A and B: (A) The nasolabial angle should measure 90°–95° in men; (B) 95°–110° in women.

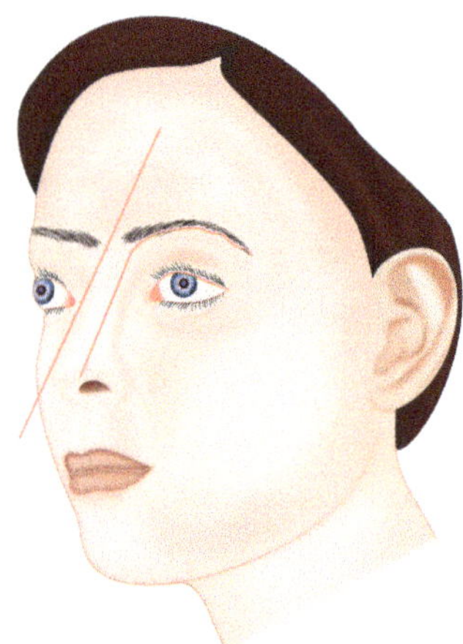

Fig. 10: The gentle curve seen from the supraorbital rim down to the dorsum.

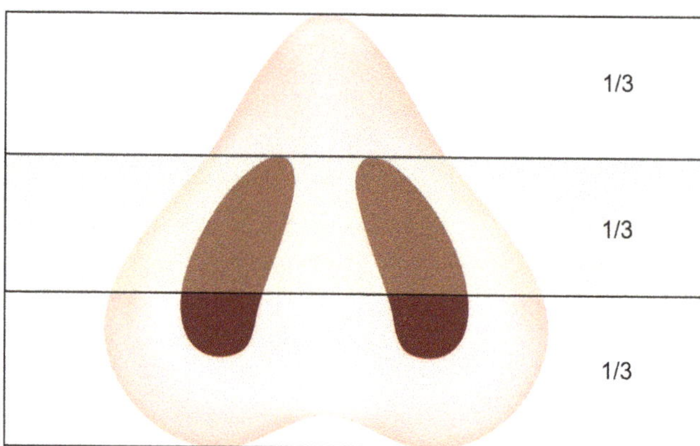

Fig. 11: The nasal base is divided into thirds.

horizontal of approximately 20° or to the facial plane of approximately 70°.

Finally, lateral nasal analysis is incomplete without analysis of chin position, where a weak chin can accentuate nasal size, and vice versa. Chin position analysis is described in "Genioplasty" chapter.

Oblique View[4]

The gentle curve seen from the supraorbital rim down to the dorsum is accentuated, and one can better appreciate the lateral contours of the dorsum (Fig. 10).

Base View[4]

The base view allows evaluation of the nostril shape and the relationship between the columella and the lobule. The nasal base is divided into thirds as follows (Fig. 11):

The general shape of the columella from the base view should resemble an equilateral triangle. The nostril should be somewhat pear shaped. The basal view also shows any caudal septal deflections and variations in the medial crural footplates.

■ REFERENCES

1. Papel ID. Facial Plastic and Reconstructive Surgery. New York: Thieme; 2016.
2. Flint PW. Cummings Otolaryngology—Head & Neck Surgery. Philadelphia, PA: Elsevier/Saunders; 2015.
3. Rohrich RJ, Adams WP, Ahmad J, et al. Dallas Rhinoplasty: Nasal Surgery by the Masters. St. Louis, MO; Boca Raton, FL: Quality Medical Publishing & CRC Press; 2014.
4. Larrabee WF Jr, Makielski KH, Henderson JL. Surgical Anatomy of the Face. Illustrated by Kathleen H. Makielski. Philadelphia: Lippincott Williams & Wilkins; 2004.

Multiple Choice Questions

Q 1. The nasolabial angle in the male IS CHARACTERIZED by which of the following?

A. It is 80 degrees
B. It is 105 degrees
C. It is more acute than the female
D. It is more obtuse than the female

Ans: C. It is more acute than the female

Q 2. Which of the following statements is TRUE about the nose?

A. The nasofrontal angle should be 120 degrees
B. The nasolabial angle should be 80 degrees
C. The thickest area of the skin is located at the rhinion
D. The basal view represents a triangle in which the lobule is one half of the height of the triangle and the columella the remaining half

Ans: A. The nasofrontal angle should be 120 degrees

Q 3. Which of the following statements about an aesthetic evaluation of the nose is TRUE?

A. The nasolabial angle is more acute in women than in men.
B. The nose with a broad, wide and flat appearance is called a leptorrhine nose
C. The nasofrontal angle is approximately 120 degrees
D. The Frankfort line extends from the superior aspect of the tragus to the margin of the lower eyelid

Ans: C. The nasofrontal angle is approximately 120 degrees

Q 4. An angle of 30 degrees PERTAINS to the:

A. Nasofacial angle
B. Nasomental angle
C. Mentocervical angle
D. Nasolabial angle

Ans: A. Nasofacial angle.

Q 5. Which of the esthetic facial proportions in the drawing below is NOT IDEAL?

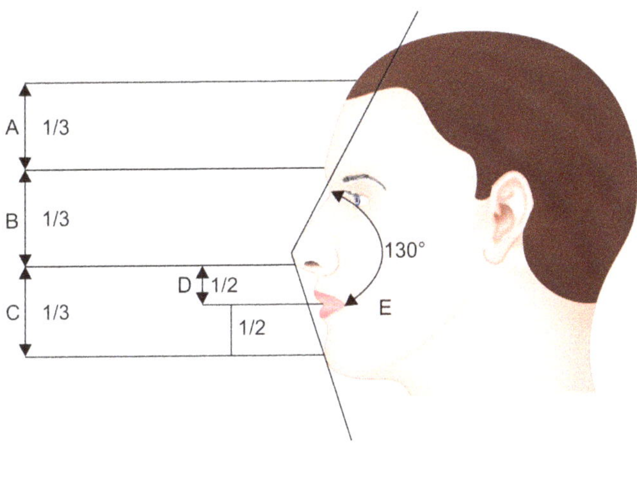

A. A
B. B
C. C
D. D

Ans: D. D

Q 6. Which following degrees represents the LEGAN facial convexity angle?

A. 15°
B. 20°
C. 25°
D. 35°

Ans: A. 15°

Q 7. Which of the following is NOT a facial characteristic typical of a 70-year-old man?

A. Drooping, elongated nasal tip complex
B. Dorsal nasal hump
C. Facial proportions (three equal third) unchanged
D. Skin and subcutaneous tissues thickened

Ans: C. Facial proportions (three equal third) unchanged

Q 8. If the entire face, from auricle to auricle, is divided by vertical lines, the nasal base width is approximately?

A. 1/3 of the face
B. 1/4 of the face
C. 1/5 of the face
D. 1/6 of the face

Ans: C. 1/5 of the face

Q 9. Which of the following anatomical terms is defined by: "the anterior hairline in the midline"?

A. The trichion
B. The glabella
C. The nasion
D. The radix

Ans: A. The trichion

Q 10. Which of the following is considered an adequate NASOFRONTAL angle?

A. 60 degrees
B. 80 degrees
C. 100 degrees
D. 130 degrees

Ans: D. 130 degrees

Q 11. Which of the following is NOT considered a esthetic subunit of the nose?

A. The tip
B. The side
C. The rhinion
D. The soft triangle

Ans: C. The rhinion

Q 12. In the lower face taking into account only the middle and lower portions: nasion to subnasale, subnasale to menton. Which of the following proportion is CORRECT?

A. Midfacial height should be 57% of the total
B. Lower facial height should be 43% of the total
C. Midfacial height should be 43% of the total
D. Lower facial height should be 65% of the total

Ans: C. Midfacial height should be 43% of the total

Q 13. Which of the following is considered an adequate NASOFACIAL angle?

A. 30 degrees
B. 45 degrees
C. 55 degrees
D. 65 degrees

Ans: A. 30 degrees

Q 14. The point of the deepest depression at the root of the nose:

A. Glabella
B. Pogonion
C. Nasion
D. Trichion

Ans: C. Nasion

Q 15. Which of the facial statements related to a female proper FACIAL PROPORTIONS is FALSE?

A. Horizontal lines are drawn through the forehead hairline, the brows, tip of the nose and the lower margin of the chin
B. The face should be five times the width of one eye
C. The chin projection should be in line with the lower lip
D. The nasolabial angle ought to measure about 105 degrees

Ans: A. Horizontal lines are drawn through the forehead hairline, the brows, tip of the nose and the lower margin of the chin

Q 16. The Frankfort Line is DEFINED by:

A. A line drawn from the inferior aspect of the bony external auditory canal to the inferior most aspect of the infraorbital rim on a lateral radiograph
B. A line drawn from the superior aspect of the bony external auditory canal to the inferior most aspect of the infraorbital rim on a lateral radiograph
C. A line drawn from the superior aspect of the bony external auditory canal to the eyelash lines on the lower eyelid
D. A line drawn from the superior aspect of the helix to the inferior most aspect of the infraorbital rim on a lateral radiograph

Ans: B. A line drawn from the superior aspect of the bony external auditory canal to the inferior most aspect of the infraorbital rim on a lateral radiograph

Q 17. Which of the following descriptions of background represents the IDEAL for photographic documentation in facial plastic surgery?

A. Light blue, single solid color, not shiny
B. White, single solid color, not shiny
C. Light blue, single solid color, shiny
D. Dark gray, single solid color, not shiny

Ans: A. Light blue, single solid color, not shiny

Q 18. Which is the BEST SLR camera lens for facial documentation photography?

A. 35 mm focal length
B. 50 mm focal length
C. 105 mm focal length
D. 135 mm focal length

Ans: C. 105 mm focal length

Chapter 7

Functional Rhinoplasty

Sami P Moubayed

BACKGROUND: NASAL VALVES AND LATERAL WALL INSUFFICIENCY

The *internal nasal valve (INV)* is located approximately 1.3 cm from the nares (nostril opening) and corresponds to the region under the upper lateral cartilages (ULCs), and its angle should measure at least 10–15° for optimal airflow. It is bound medially by the dorsal septum, inferiorly by the head of the inferior turbinate, and laterally by the ULC. The *external nasal valve* is defined as the area in the vestibule, under the nasal ala, formed by the caudal septum, medial crura of the alar cartilages, alar rim, and nasal sill.

Valve collapse may be static or dynamic. Static INV obstruction may be due to INV narrowing and midvault collapse, which is diagnosed on external inspection as either a *narrow midvault* or an *inverted V deformity*, and is associated with a positive Cottle test. The inverted V deformity appears as an overly narrow middle nasal vault with a sharp transition between the cephalic edges of the ULCs and the caudal edges of the nasal bones in patients having undergone rhinoplasty.[1] Midvault narrowing or pinching may be congenital. Midvault narrowing and the inverted V deformity may also result from either excessive ULC resection, or from inferomedial ULC displacement following rhinoplasty with inadequate midvault reconstruction.[2]

Lateral wall insufficiency (LWI) was described in 2008 by most to replace dynamic internal and external nasal valve collapse.[3] LWI is classified by the zone in which it occurs[3] (Fig. 1).

Zone 1 LWI occurs more cephalad and corresponds to dynamic movement of the nasal sidewall at the level of the ULC and scroll region. *Zone 2 LWI* occurs at the level of the ala and is what was previously termed as external valve collapse.[4] Zone 1 LWI is more often idiopathic, and sometimes due to senescence, mild to moderate trauma, or heredity, whereas zone 2 LWI is more often iatrogenic.[3]

HISTORY AND PHYSICAL EXAMINATION

Relevant patient history should include the presence of nasal obstruction, laterality, exacerbating and alleviating factors, especially the use of steroids and nasal dilator strips. Allergy symptoms, rhinosinusitis symptoms, history of previous nasal surgery, nasal trauma, and intranasal drug use should be elicited.

A functional patient-reported outcome measure, such as the NOSE (Nasal Obstruction Symptom Evaluation) scale should be administered.

Thereafter, nasal examination can proceed in the form of intranasal examination (septum and turbinates), nasal valve examination using the Cottle maneuver as well as evaluation for LWI in zones 1 and 2,[5] and palpation of the caudal septum and tip recoil. A modified Cottle maneuver can be performed using an ear curette or a cotton tipped applicator placed inside the nostril at the site of obstruction. Septal examination using inspection and palpation is performed to determine whether the deviation involves the L-strut or not. The presence of sinus disease and polyps can be identified using nasal endoscopy when the history is suggestive.

External inspection of the midvault should be performed to evaluate for pinching.

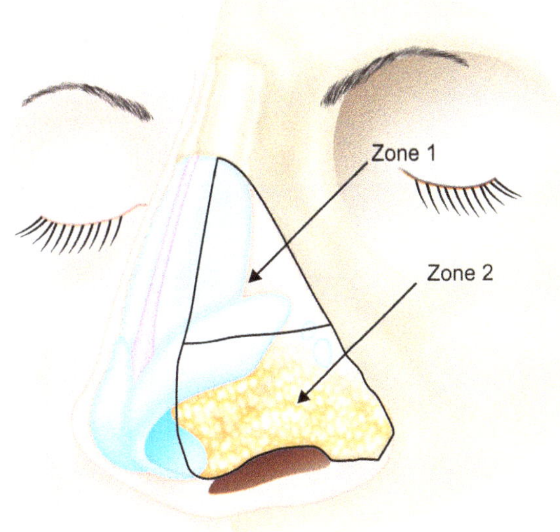

Fig. 1: Zones of lateral wall insufficiency.

■ TURBINATE HYPERTROPHY

Conservative medical management of turbinate hypertrophy includes control of allergies with intranasal corticosteroids.

Surgery is offered when medical therapy fails, and includes mucosal sparing and mucosal destructive techniques. Mucosal sparing techniques include cold-steel submucosal resection, powered submucosal resection, submucosal bone crushing, and turbinate outfracture.

Mucosal destructive techniques involve resection of the anterior third of the inferior turbinate using either through-biter forceps or a scissors, with subsequent electrocautery of the residual stump.

■ SEPTAL DEVIATION

Noninvolving the L-strut

Surgery for the deviated septum that does not involve the L-strut consists of the classic submucous resection (SMR) technique which resects the deviated septal cartilage and preserves at least 1 cm of dorsal and caudal L-strut.

Involving the L-strut

When the deviation involves the L-strut, traditional septoplasty techniques are inadequate and may result in nasal collapse.[6] Extracorporeal septoplasty involves removing the cartilaginous septum and replacing it with autologous septal cartilage, rib cartilage, or cadaveric irradiated rib cartilage.[7] A major drawback of this technique is destabilization of the junction of the quadrangular cartilage and bones (keystone area), with a potential for notching or saddling.[7]

Anterior septal reconstruction (ASR) (Fig. 2) has been developed to replace the extracorporeal septoplasty technique to minimize destabilization of the keystone (and thus preserve dorsal contour).[6] Thus, ASR is more conservative than extracorporeal septoplasty and preserves dorsal support, and concomitantly addresses nasal obstruction and the external contour deformities.[6]

■ INVERTED V DEFORMITY AND MIDVAULT PINCHING

The traditional gold standard for midvault reconstruction at the time of hump takedown is the spreader graft (Fig. 3), although the spreader flap has gained much popularity in recent years.[8] The spreader flap or autospreader graft (Fig. 4) is a technique where the medial ends ULC is turned-in and sutured to the dorsal septum in order to

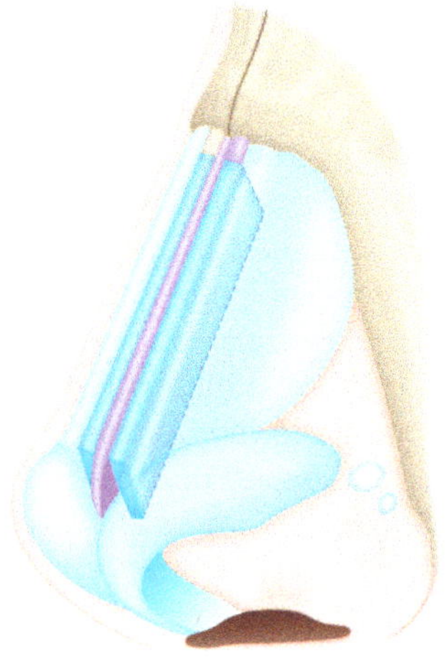

Fig. 3: Spreader graft placement (blue) on each side of the dorsal septum (purple).

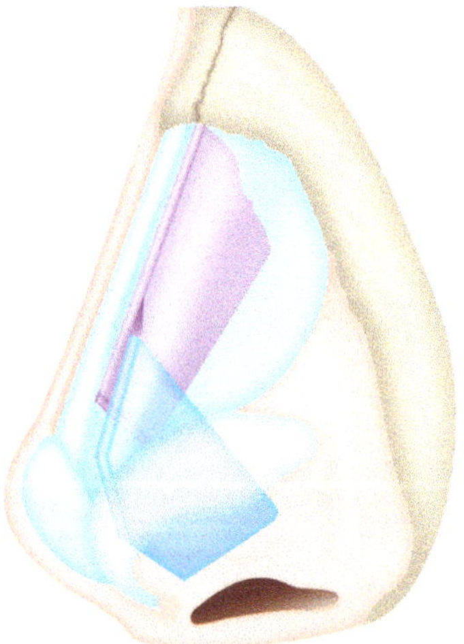

Fig. 2: Anterior septal reconstruction (ASR) with the residual dorsal septum in purple and ASR graft in blue.

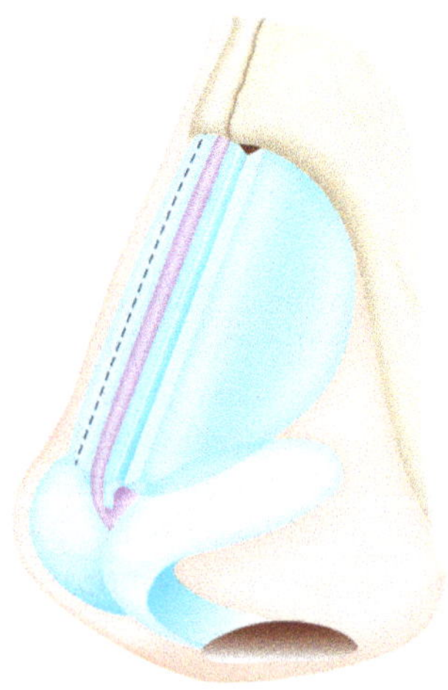

Fig. 4: Turn-in flaps (blue) on each side of the dorsal septum (purple).

preserve the INV area and prevent postoperative collapse.[9] The spreader flap is usually best performed at the time of primary rhinoplasty.

During secondary rhinoplasty, the excess ULC used for autospreader grafts is typically unavailable, necessitating the use of spreader grafts, which can be created from autologous cartilage donor sites such as septum, rib, or ear.[10] They are usually 1–2 mm thick, 3–6 mm wide, and 10–15 mm long, and are placed in a submucosal pocket between the ULC and the septum.[10]

DYNAMIC NASAL VALVE COLLAPSE/ LATERAL WALL INSUFFICIENCY

Internal Valve/Zone 1

Several technique to correct dynamic LWI in zone 1 can be used, such as lateral crural strut grafts (LCSG), bone-anchored sutures, radiofrequency thermotherapy, and butterfly grafting.

The *LCSGs* are autologous strips of cartilage—harvested either from the septum, rib, or concha—which are sutured to the deep lateral crura in an undermined pocket and sutured in place (Fig. 5). LCSGs are also used in the boxy nasal tip, malpositioned lateral crura, alar rim retraction, alar rim collapse, and concave lateral crura.

Bone-anchored sutures are used to suspend the area of maximal collapse to the infraorbital rim using an open rhinoplasty approach or a transconjunctival incision, creating a force vector that leads to stabilization of the ala that resist negative inspiratory forces.[11]

Radiofrequency (RF) thermotherapy is an effective and safe alternative. Low-energy radiofrequency, applied via a submucosally placed probe extending from the intermediate crust toward the pyriform aperture, results in tissue fibrosis and retraction that decreases lateral nasal collapse.[12]

The *butterfly graft* is an only graft harvested from conchal cartilage in the shape of a "V" and is then placed midline on the nasal dorsum with the vertex of the "V" pointing caudally.[13]

External Valve/Zone 2

Dynamic LWI in Zone 2 can be corrected using alar rim grafts or alar batten grafts.

Alar rim grafts (Fig. 6) are small struts of cartilage placed along the alar rim.[14] The major indications for alar rim graft placements are Zone 2 LWI (external nasal valve collapse), prevention or correction of the alar concavity, advancing the ala caudally, widening the nostril, and elongation of the short nostril.[14]

Batten grafts are pieces of autologous curvilinear cartilage placed in a pocket created at the point of maximal collapse

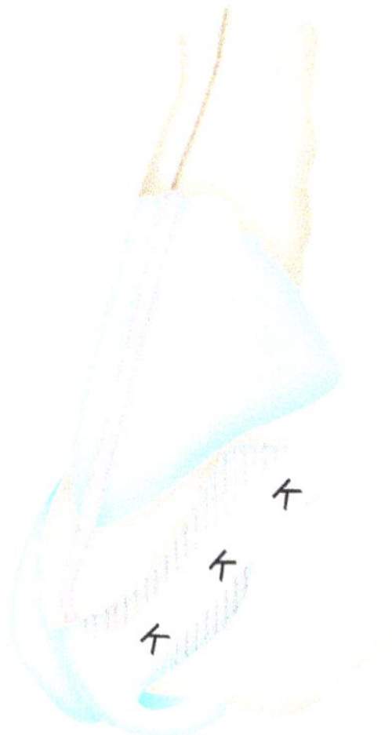

Fig. 5: Lateral crural strut graft (LCSG) placement (green) underneath the lateral crus (crosshatched).

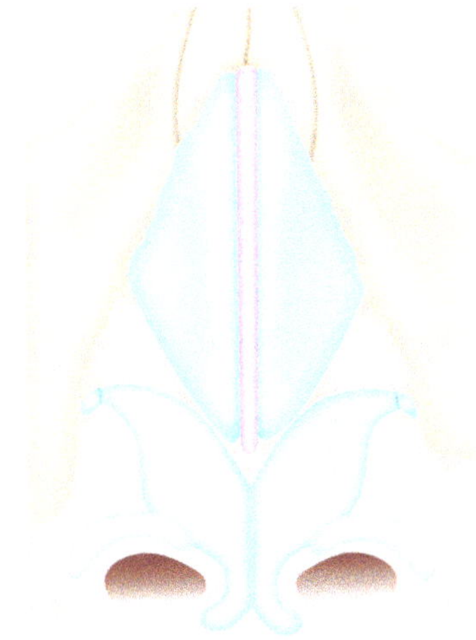

Fig. 6: Alar rim grafts (light blue) placed in precise pockets at the alar rims bilaterally.

and extending from the pyriform aperture to just below the dorsum.[15]

REFERENCES

1. Cobo R. Correction of dorsal abnormalities in revision rhinoplasty. Facial Plast Surg. 2008;24(3):327-38.
2. Paun SH, Nolst Trenite GJ. Revision rhinoplasty: an overview of deformities and techniques. Facial Plast Surg. 2008;24(3):271-87.
3. Most SP. Trends in functional rhinoplasty. Arch Facial Plast Surg. 2008;10(6):410-13.
4. Tsao GJ, Fijalkowski N, Most SP. Validation of a grading system for lateral nasal wall insufficiency. Allergy Rhinol (Providence). 2013;4(2):e66-68.
5. Most SP. Comparing methods f or repair of the external valve: one more step toward a unified view of lateral wall insufficiency. JAMA Facial Plast Surg. 2015;17(5):345-6.

6. Most SP. Anterior septal reconstruction: outcomes after a modified extracorporeal septoplasty technique. Arch Facial Plast Surg. 2006;8(3):202-7.

7. Gubisch W. Treatment of the scoliotic nose with extracorporeal septoplasty. Facial Plast Surg Clin North Am. 2015;23(1): 11-22.

8. Moubayed SP, Most SP. The autospreader flap for midvault reconstruction following dorsal hump resection. Facial Plast Surg. 2016;32(1):36-41.

9. Loh KT, Chua JJ, Lee HM, et al. Prevention and management of vision loss relating to facial filler injections. Singapore Med J. 2016;57(8):438-43.

10. Wittkopf M, Wittkopf J, Ries WR. The diagnosis and treatment of nasal valve collapse. Curr Opin Otolaryngol Head Neck Surg. 2008;16(1):10-3.

11. Lieberman DM, Most SP. Lateral nasal wall suspension using a bone-anchored suture technique. Arch Facial Plast Surg. 2010;12(2):113.

12. Weissman JD, Most SP. Radiofrequency thermotherapy vs bone-anchored suspension for treatment of lateral nasal wall insufficiency: a randomized clinical trial. JAMA Facial Plast Surg. 2015;17(2):84-9.

13. Barrett DM, Casanueva FJ, Cook TA. Management of the nasal valve. Facial Plast Surg Clin North Am. 2016;24(3): 219-34.

14. Unger JG, Roostaeian J, Small KH, et al. Alar contour grafts in rhinoplasty: a safe and reproducible way to refine alar contour aesthetics. Plast Reconstr Surg. 2016;137(1):52-61.

15. Cervelli V, Spallone D, Bottini JD, et al. Alar batten cartilage graft: treatment of internal and external nasal valve collapse. Aesthetic Plast Surg. 2009;33(4):625-34.

Multiple Choice Questions

Q 1. Which of the following surgical techniques will NOT improve an upper lateral cartilage nasal valve collapse?

A. Flaring suture placement
B. Splay graft placement
C. Columellar graft placement
D. Butterfly graft placement

Ans: C. Columellar graft placement

Q 2. Which of the following anatomic REGIONS is bounded by the nasal septum, the caudal margin of the upper lateral cartilage and the floor of the nose?

A. Rhinion
B. Nasal valve
C. Sellion
D. Scroll region

Ans: B. Nasal valve

Q 3. Which of the following statements regarding "tip recoil phenomenon" is TRUE?

A. It is related to the maximum degree of possible tip rotation
B. It is related to the upper lateral cartilage
C. It is related to the distance between domes in tip bifidity
D. It is related to a weak lower lateral cartilage

Ans: D. It is related to a weak lower lateral cartilage

Q 4. Which of the following is a major tip support mechanism in rhinoplasty?

A. Attachment of the upper lateral cartilage (ULC) to the lower lateral cartilage (LLC)
B. Anterior and posterior nasal spine
C. Attachment of the sesamoid cartilage complex to the pyriform aperture
D. Attachment of lower lateral cartilage (LLC) to skin-soft tissue envelope (S-STE)

Ans: A. Attachment of the upper lateral cartilage (ULC) to the lower lateral cartilage (LLC)

Q 5. Which of the following operative techniques is NOT useful in order to correct nasal valve collapse (widen the valve angle)?

A. Spreader grafts
B. Flaring sutures
C. Butterfly grafts
D. Internal dermal grafts

Ans: D. Internal dermal grafts

Q 6. A 21-year-old male patient has a significant "S" shaped nasoseptal deformity due to a motor vehicle accident. There is displacement of nasal bones, upper lateral cartilages and septum. Which of the following is the LEAST useful in order to correct the problem?

A. Septoplasty technique using the external approach
B. Use of bilateral spreader cartilage grafts
C. Killian, hemitransfixion and closed approach
D. Evaluation of the internal nasal valve preoperatively

Ans: C. Killian, hemitransfixion and closed approach

Q 7. Which of the following statements about Rhinoplasty is TRUE?

A. The internal nasal valve is bounded by the cephalic margin of the lower lateral cartilages and the septum
B. Rocker deformity is due to lateral osteotomy done too low into the thick ascending process of the maxilla
C. Inadequate support of the lower lateral cartilages after dorsal hump removal can result in an inverted-V deformity
D. It is standard to resect less hump at the rhinion in order to avoid over-resection at this level

Ans: D. It is standard to resect less hump at the rhinion in order to avoid over-resection at this level

Q 8. Which of the following REVISION RHINOPLASTY techniques is INCORRECTLY applied?

A. Midnasal asymmetry and narrowing ----- spreader grafts
B. Alar retraction ----- composite grafts
C. Ptotic nose ----- domal truncation
D. Inadequate tip projection ------ tip grafts

Ans: C. Ptotic nose ----- domal truncation

Q 9. Which of the following lines in the drawing represents a Killian incision?

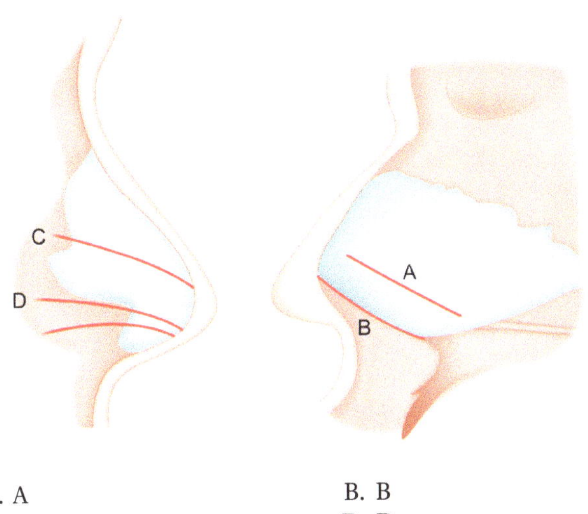

A. A
B. B
C. C
D. D

Ans: A. A

Q 10. Which of the following deformities will be corrected by the use of a composite skin-cartilage graft placed into the pocket shown in the picture?

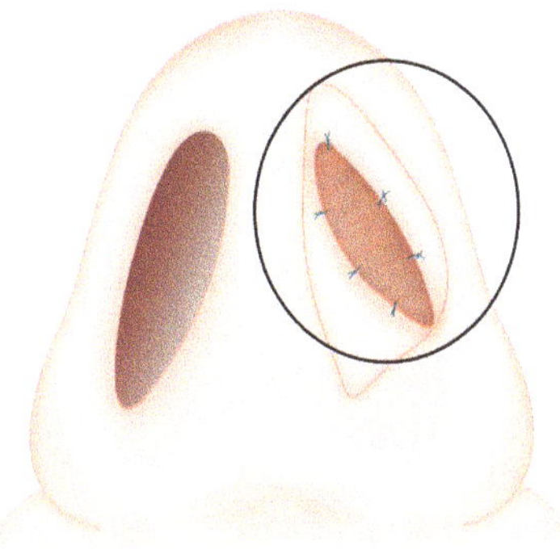

A. Alar margin retraction
B. Bossa formation
C. Alar pinching with tip narrowing
D. Alar stenosis

Ans: A. Alar margin retraction

Q 11. Which of the following statements is FALSE about surgical correction of a deviated septum?

A. Killian-type and hemitransfixion incisions are best performed in the concave side of the septal deviation
B. Hemitransfixion incision is ideal for caudal septal deviation
C. Hemitransfixion incision will not affect significantly the nasal tip support
D. Killian-type of incision will affect significantly the nasal tip

Ans: D. Killian-type of incision will affect significantly the nasal tip

Q 12. Which of the following etiologies is MOST COMMONLY associated with external nasal valve dysfunction?

A. Congenital
B. Traumatic
C. Iatrogenic
D. Senescent (aging)

Ans: C. Iatrogenic

Q 13. Which of the following minor nasal tip support mechanisms has been recently considered a CRITICAL AND A MAJOR support mechanism?

A. Intercrural ligament
B. Cartilaginous septal dosum
C. Membranous septum
D. Alar cartilages attachment to the overlying skin and musculature

Ans: D. Alar cartilages attachment to the overlying skin and musculature

Q 14. Which of the following etiologies is MOST COMMON in twisted noses?

A. Trauma
B. Iatrogenic
C. Inflammatory
D. Congenital

Ans: A. Trauma

Q 15. Which of the following surgical techniques is the MOST effective in opening the internal nasal valve?

A. Spreader grafts
B. Flaring sutures
C. Splay grafts
D. Butterfly grafts

Ans: A. Spreader grafts

Q 16. Which of the following statements is TRUE about the external nasal valve dysfunction?

A. The most common etiology of External Nasal Valve dysfunction is aging.
B. The incidence of external nasal valve collapse will be minimized by preserving the upper lateral cartilage
C. The diagnosis of dysfunction can be made by stabilizing the alar rim to see, if nasal airflow improves
D. The diagnosis of dysfunction can be made by the Cottle maneuver

Ans: C. The diagnosis of dysfunction can be made by stabilizing the alar rim to see if nasal airflow improves

Q 17. Which of the following statements about "Spreader Grafts" used in Rhinoplasty is FALSE?

A. Spreader grafts should span from the caudal border of the nasal bone to the anterior septal angle.
B. Nasal septal cartilage is the ideal spreader graft material.
C. Conchal cartilage is not used as spreader graft material due to the intrinsic bowing.
D. Horizontal mattress sutures are the ideal sutures for use with spreader grafts

Ans: C. Conchal cartilage is not used as spreader graft material due to the intrinsic bowing

Q 18. Which of the following operatives maneuvers will DECREASE projection?

A. Lateral crural steal
B. Columellar strut
C. Lateral crural overlay
D. Septocolumellar suture

Ans: C. Lateral crural overlay

Q 19. Which of the following surgical maneuvers in rhinoplasty WILL NOT IMPROVE PROJECTION?

A. Excision of the cephalic lower lateral cartilage
B. Transdomal sutures
C. Lateral crural steal
D. Columellar strut

Ans: A. Excision of the cephalic lower lateral cartilage

Q 20. Which of the following statements is related to the tip recoil phenomenon?

A. Rotation
B. Projection
C. Tip support
D. Width to the lower lateral cartilage

Ans: C. Tip support

Q 21. Which of the following surgical techniques used in rhinoplasty is the one represented in the drawing below?

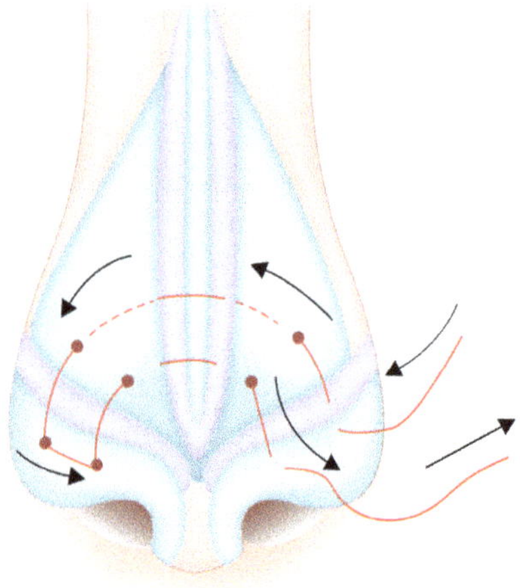

A. Flaring suture
B. Interdomal sutures
C. Septo-columellar suture
D. Tip Suspension suture

Ans: A. Flaring suture

Q 22. Which of the following statements is FALSE regarding use of the endonasal spreader graft for management of internal nasal valve insufficiency?

A. Autogenous materials are used for grafting
B. The upper lateral cartilage should be divided from the septum
C. Grafts are placed between the nasal septum and the upper lateral cartilage
D. Grafts are placed subperichondrally

Ans: B. The upper lateral cartilage should be divided from the septum

Q 23. Stem: Which of the following deformities is related to the bilateral disarticulation of upper lateral cartilages?

A. "Rocker" deformity
B. "Inverted V" deformity
C. "Open" roof deformity
D. "V" deformity

Ans: B. "Inverted V" deformity

Q 24. Which of the following incision/approach in rhinoplasty is FALSE?

A. Transcartilaginous/anterograde
B. Intercartilaginous/retrograde
C. Intercartilaginous/delivery
D. Intercartilaginous and marginal/delivery

Ans: C. Intercartilaginous/delivery

Q 25. Which of the following is considered a MINOR TIP SUPPORT mechanism of the nose?

A. Nasal septum
B. Nasal spine
C. Medial crural footplate attachment to the caudal septum
D. Attachment of the caudal border of the upper lateral cartilages to the cephalic border of the lower lateral cartilages

Ans: B. Nasal spine

Q 26. Which of the following anatomical term is defined by "the most anterior and caudal point of the cartilaginous septum"?

A. The rhinion
B. The tip defining point
C. The anterior septal angle
D. The posterior septal angle

Ans: C. The anterior septal angle

Q 27. Which of the following is considered a MAJOR TIP support of the nose?

A. Interdomal ligament
B. Cartilaginous dorsum
C. Alar cartilage attachment to the skin
D. Medial crural footplate attachments to caudal septum

Ans: D. Medial crural footplate attachments to caudal septum

Q 28. Which of the following nasal abnormalities is corrected by using "flaring sutures"?

A. The nasal rotation
B. The nasal projection
C. The nasal alar flare
D. The nasal valve angle

Ans: D. The nasal valve angle

Q 29. Which of the following nasal surgeries will NOT improved overprojection?

A. Delivery approach
B. Lateral crural steal
C. Alar cartilage reduction
D. Septal cartilage reduction

Ans: B. Lateral crural steal

Q 30. Which of the following statements is true regarding the cartilage graft - yellow color - used in the drawing below?

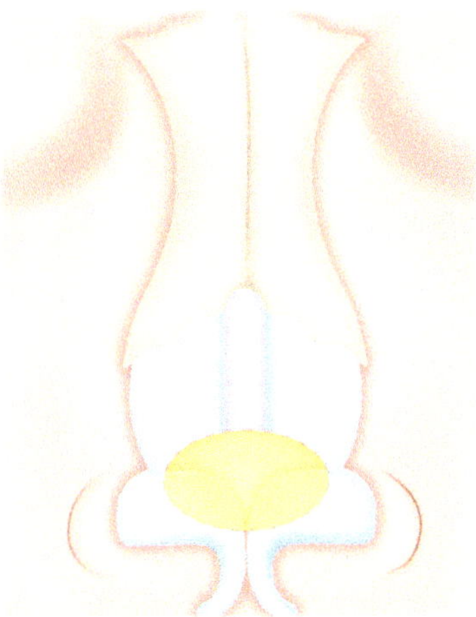

A. Improve the valve angle
B. Decrease the valve angle
C. Increase the nasal length
D. Decrease the nasal length

Ans: A. Improve the valve angle

Q 31. Which of the following regarding the "butterfly grafts" is FALSE?

A. Conchal cartilage is an ideal donor area for "butterfly grafts"
B. "Butterfly grafts" are used to widen the valve angle
C. "Butterfly grafts" are placed at the scroll area
D. The caudal border of the "butterfly graft" is placed superficial to the cephalic border of the lateral crura

Ans: D. The caudal border of the "butterfly graft" is placed superficial to the cephalic border of the lateral crura

Q 32. Which of the following surgical techniques in rhinoplasty is NOT related with the management of an obstructed cartilage vault?

A. Spreader cartilage grafts
B. Butterfly cartilage grafts
C. Cephalic resection of the lower lateral cartilage
D. Flaring sutures

Ans: C. Cephalic resection of the lower lateral cartilage

Q 33. Which of the following statements related to rhinoplasty is FALSE?

A. Most of the septorhinoplasties can be performed under local anesthesia and IV sedation
B. Uncomplicated septorhinoplasty usually take about 1 hour.
C. The nose is usually packed after septorhinoplasty
D. The protective splint and nasal dressings are removed 7 days after surgery

Ans: C. The nose is usually packed after septorhinoplasty

Q 34. In revision rhinoplasty, which of the following managements is BEST in the treatment of excessive narrowing of the alar base?

A. M-plasty
B. O-T plasty
C. Z-plasty
D. V-Y plasty

Ans: C. Z-Plasty

Q 35. Which of the following statements about nasal anatomy is FALSE?

A. The arterial supply to the external structures of the nose is derived from the ophthalmic, facial and internal maxillary
B. The sensibility of the external nose is through branches of the ophthalmic and maxillary divisions of the fifth cranial nerve
C. The narrowest part of the bony vault is at the level of the rhinion
D. The supratip defines the cephalic limit of the nasal tip

Ans: C. The narrowest part of the bony vault is at the level of the rhinion

Q 36. Which of the following nerves is the external nasal nerve a terminal branch of?

A. The anterior ethmoidal nerve
B. The posterior ethmoidal nerve
C. The supratrochlear nerve
D. The supraorbital nerve

Ans: A. The anterior ethmoidal nerve

Q 37. Which of the following branches supply the sensory innervation of the tip of the nose?

A. Infraorbital nerve
B. Supratrochlear branch of the ophthalmic nerve
C. Infratrochlear branch of the ophthalmic nerve
D. External nasal branch of the anterior ethmoidal nerve

Ans: D. External nasal branch of the anterior ethmoidal nerve

Chapter 8

Cosmetic Rhinoplasty

Gregory S Dibelius, Kirkland N Lozada

■ BASIC OVERVIEW

Functional Considerations

Minimal functional considerations in esthetic rhinoplasty:
- *Tip support*: All major and minor tip support structures must be respected. See Table 1
- *Internal nasal valve*:
  - Caudal upper lateral cartilage (ULC), septum, inferior turbinate
  - Normal angle is 10–15°
  - Comprises 50% of nasal airway resistance.
  - Spreader grafts, spreader flaps (autospreader), batten grafts can be used to preserve or augment internal nasal valve.
  - *Narrow nose syndrome*: Short nasal bones, long and weak ULC, thin skin. At risk for collapse of ULC and internal nasal valve.
- *External nasal valve*: Caudal border of lower lateral cartilage (LLC), columella, and nasal floor. Dynamic collapse is often seen.

Incisions and Approaches

Approaches are generally classified as closed (endonasal) or open (external).

Closed approaches are classified as nondelivery or delivery approaches.

Table 1: Tip support mechanisms.	
Major	**Minor**
1. Lower lateral cartilage (shape, strength, and size)	1. Cartilaginous dorsal septum
2. Scroll region (connection between upper and lower lateral cartilages)	2. Interdomal ligaments
3. Attachment of the medial crural footplates to the caudal septum	3. Fibrous attachment of the sesamoid cartilages with the piriform aperture
	4. Nasal spine
	5. Membranous septum
	6. Attachment of lower lateral cartilages to overlying skin/soft tissue envelope

Closed Approach: Nondelivery Technique

Nondelivery approaches provide the least surgical exposure of the tip cartilages and are appropriate in patients with minimal bulbosity of the nasal tip, without any significant tip deformities, and favorable triangularity on base view. They are comprised of cartilage-splitting and retrograde approaches.
- *Cartilage splitting*: A transcartilaginous (through the cartilage of the lateral crus) incision is placed 5–8 mm cephalic to the caudal margin of the lateral crus. The cephalic margin of the lateral crus is resected.
- *Retrograde*: An intercartilaginous incision (between the ULC and LLC) is made in the vestibular skin with retrograde dissection (cephalic to caudal) of the lateral crus. The cephalic margin of the lateral crus is resected.

Closed Approach: Delivery Technique

This approach provides greater exposure of the alar cartilages. The LLCs are delivered into the nasal vestibule as bipedicled chondrocutaneous flaps. This is accomplished by creating intercartilaginous and marginal incisions (along caudal margin of LLC). *The intercartilaginous incision is connected to the hemitransfixion incision bilaterally.* More extensive nasal tip maneuvers (transdomal sutures, interrupted strip techniques) can be executed with this greater exposure.

Due to decreased surgical exposure, closed approaches require manipulation of cartilage under tension and/or in nonanatomic position and can limit the accuracy and precision of a given surgical maneuver.

Open or External Approach

This approach provides the greatest exposure of the nasal framework. Marginal incisions are combined with a transcolumellar incision to reflect the skin-soft tissue envelope from the nasal framework in a sub-SMAS plane. The nasal tip cartilages can be viewed completely and manipulated in anatomic position without tension. Disadvantages include a columellar scar and prolonged postoperative edema. A distinct advantage of this approach is in teaching rhinoplasty to trainees.

Table 2: Common maneuvers to modify tip rotation and projection.		
	Projection	*Rotation*
Cephalic trim		↑
Lateral crural steal	↑	↑
Tongue-in groove	↑ or ↓	↑ or ↓
Lateral crural overlay	↓	↑
Medial crural overlay	↓	↓
Columellar strut	↑	↑
Cap graft	↑	
Shield graft	↑	
Plumping graft	↑	↑
Full transfixion incision	↓	↓
Nasal spine reduction	↓	

Surgical Correction and Esthetic Contouring

Sequence of Rhinoplasty

There is non-specific sequence that must be followed. A generalized "top-down" approach allows the upper and middle vaults to determine the appropriate position of the tip, and all fine tip work is done after more aggressive maneuvers (osteotomies, rasping, excessive retraction) are performed that would otherwise disrupt delicate tip work.

The following is an open approach sequence proposed by JR Tebbetts: Exposure → initial tip → initial dorsum → septum → osteotomies → final dorsum → final tip → tip-lip complex → alar base.

Tip modifications
- Tip modifications include rotation, projection, and contour (Table 2).
- *Tripod theory*: Simplified model of tip dynamics.
  - Two superolateral legs = bilateral lateral crura
  - One inferomedial leg = paired medial crura
- *Lateral crural steal*: Suture recruitment of lateral crus into intermediate crus
- *Lateral crural overlay*: Division of lateral crus with overlapping and suture reconstitution
- *Medial crural overlay*: Division of medial crus with overlapping and suture reconstitution
- *Plumping graft*: Premaxillary graft at columellar-labial angle.

Tip maneuvers to improve contour
- *Cephalic margin resection of lateral crus*: Preserve 6–8 mm of lateral crus strip.
  - Interrupted versus complete strip techniques.
- *Dome division with suture reconstitution*: Greater risk of asymmetry
- *Dome defining suture*: Horizontal mattress placed at tip defining point
- *Interdomal suture*: Placed between tip defining points

- *Lateral crural spanning sutures*: Suture between LLCs cephalic to tip defining points. Can correct convexities of LLCs that contribute to a boxy tip configuration.
- *Tip grafting*:
  - *Cap graft (Peck graft)*: Horizontal graft over alar domes, increases tip projection
  - *Shield graft (Sheen graft, infratip graft)*: Shield-shaped graft over caudal edge of medial crura into tip, increases projection, definition
- *Lateral crural strut graft*:
  - Placed under lateral crus with lateral end of graft over piriform aperture
  - correct alar retraction, rim collapse, malpositioned lateral crura
  - lateral crural can be repositioned with strut grafts to more drastically control tip esthetics.

Alar-columellar relationship
A 2–4 mm of columellar show on lateral view is normal. Alar-columellar relationship can be considered by constructing a line between the most posterior and anterior points of the nostril on lateral view (Fig. 1). It is described in terms of the contribution of each component:
- Rohrich and Gunter classification of alar-columellar disproportion.
- Alar retraction is corrected using skin or composite grafting intranasally.
- Hanging columella is corrected by mucosal resection.

Alar base
Alar reduction procedures are performed mainly to correct alar flaring (Weir excision) or nostril size (nasal sill excision), or a combination of both.

Premaxillary augmentation is performed using grafting (bone, cartilage, fat, or alloplastic material) to correct tissue deficiency.

Dorsum
Hump: Overprominence of dorsum. Cartilage is sharply resected, while bone is reduced with osteotome or rasp. Resection is incremental. Open roof created can be closed with lateral osteotomies. Do not violate vestibular mucosa. Must account for thinner skin over the midvault.

Nasion: Radix should start at level of supratarsal crease and be 8-9 mm to the corneal plane. Radix grafting used to augment a low radix. Lowering of high radix can be performed with a glabellar push rasp. *A low nasion gives the illusion of a widened nose on frontal view.*

Dorsal lines: Dorsal onlay or lateral nasal wall grafts. Camouflage can be attained with soft tissue grafting.

Osteotomies: Most controlled method is a medial to lateral sequence. Medial osteotomies mobilize the internasal suture area and allow for full mobilization of the nasal bones. Intermediate osteotomies are used to correct asymmetries/deformities of the body of the nasal bones and can be performed either unilaterally or bilaterally. Lateral

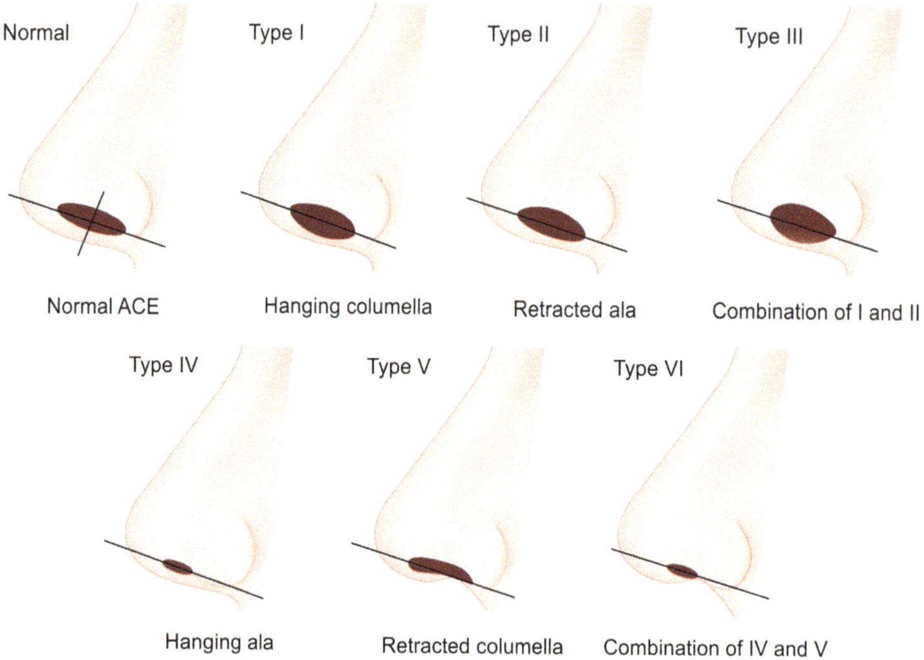

Fig. 1: Types of alar-columellar relationship.

osteotomies are typically performed in a "high-low-high" fashion to preserve support at the inferior pyriform aperture. "Low-low-high" may be preferable, if bony vault is overwide at the pyriform aperture. "High-low-low" is performed, if the bony nasal width is overly wide at the intercanthal level.

Dorsal grafting options: Autologous cartilage (septum, ear, rib), diced cartilage wrapped in temporalis fascia, split calvarial bone, homografts, alloplastic grafts.

Specific Deformities

Aging nose: Multilevel changes in nasal tissues.
- *Soft tissue*: Loss of support, thickness, elasticity, actinic changes. Drooping, ptotic tip
- *Bone*: Become brittle
- Cartilage calcification
- *Midface changes*: Bony resorption
- Airway obstruction

Tension nose: Excessive growth of quadrilateral cartilage. High dorsum, anterior/inferior displacement of tip cartilages, blunting of nasolabial angle, shortening of upper lip. Soft tissue/skin is *stretched* over overdeveloped caudal septum. Corrected using the deprojection-reprojection operation.

Cleft Lip Nose

Unilateral cleft: Alar base posterior/lateral/inferior due to maxillary deficiency. Lateral crus is long while medial crus is short on cleft side. Septum caudally deviated to noncleft side.

Bilateral cleft: Both alar bases are posterior/lateral/inferior due to maxillary deficiency. Longer LLCs with short medial crura. Broad, flat tip with poor projection.

Noncaucasian Rhinoplasty

Asian: Low/concave dorsum, low starting point, thick sebaceous skin, shortened nose, weak cartilages, poor projection, retracted columella, hanging alar lobule.

African American: Thick sebaceous skin, short nose, decreased projection, acute nasolabial angle, concave dorsum, broad tip, flared ala.

Latino: Thick sebaceous skin, bulbous poorly defined tip, decreased projection and rotation, acute nasolabial angle, small nasal bones, relatively weaker framework.

Middle Eastern: Prominent, convex dorsum, wide bony vault, long nose, tip ptosis, acute nasolabial angle, bulbous tip, asymmetries.

Most Common Complications

Pollybeak: Supratip fullness.

Etiologies:
- Under-resection of cartilaginous dorsum
- Loss of nasal tip support
- Edema/scarring of the supratip region.

Open roof: Must be closed after hump reduction with smooth edges, can lead to dorsal irregularities.

Bossae: "Bump" deformity.

Saddle nose: Loss of dorsal and/or caudal support. Scooped appearance, apparent widening on frontal view, loss of tip projection. Reconstructive options range from dorsal onlay grafting to complete reconstruction of L-strut and tip support.

Inverted V: Inferomedial collapse of the ULC showing an inverted V on anteroposterior view.

Rocker deformity-osteotomies taken superiorly into the frontal bone.

■ BIBLIOGRAPHY

1. Cobo R. Rhinoplasty in Latino patients. Clin Plastic Surg. 2016;43:237-54.
2. Gunter JP, Friedman RM. Lateral crural strut graft: technique and clinical applications in rhinoplasty. Plast Reconstr Surg. 1997;99:943-55.
3. Gunter JP, Landecker A, Cochran CS. Frequently used grafts in rhinoplasty: nomenclature and analysis. Plast Reconstr Surg. 2006;118(1):14e-29e.
4. Gunter JP, Rohrich, RJ, Friedman RM. Classification of alarcolumellar discrepancies in rhinoplasty. Plast Reconstr Surg. 1996;97(3):643-8.
5. Guyuron B. The aging nose. Dermatologic Clin. 1997;15(4):659-64.
6. Johnson CM, Godin MS. The tension nose: open structure rhinoplasty approach. Plast Reconstr Surg. 1995;95(1):43-51.
7. Kim DW, Toriumi DM. Management of posttraumatic nasal deformities: the crooked nose and the saddle nose. Facial Plast Surg Clin North Am. 2004;12:111-32.
8. Kridel RWH, Scott BA, Foda HMT. The tongue-in-groove technique in septorhinoplasty. Arch Facial Plast Surg. 1999;1:246-56.
9. Peng GL, Nassif PS. Rhinoplasty in the African American patient anatomic considerations and technical pearls. Clin Plastic Surg. 2016;43:255-64.
10. Sajjadian A. Rhinoplasty in Middle Eastern patients. Clin Plastic Surg. 2016;43:281-94.
11. Sykes JM, Tasman A, Suarez, GA. Cleft lip nose. Clin Plastic Surg. 2016;43:223-35.
12. Tardy ME, Toriumi DM, Hecht DA. Philosophy and principles of rhinoplasty. In: Papel ID, Frodel JL, Holt GR, Larrabee WF, Nachlas NE, Park SS, Sykes JM, Toriumi DM (Eds). Facial Plastic and Reconstructive Surgery, 3rd edition. New York: Thieme Medical Publishers, Inc.; 2009. pp. 207-528.
13. Tebbetts JB. The Next Dimension: Rethinking the Logic, Sequence, and Techniques of Rhinoplasty. In: Gunter JP, Rohrich RJ, Adams WP (Eds). Dallas Rhinoplasty: Nasal Surgery by the Masters. 1st edition. St. Louis: Quality Medical Publishing, Inc.; 2002. pp. 219-53.
14. Toriumi DM, Becker DG. Rhinoplasty Dissection Manual. Philadelphia: Lippincott Williams & Wilkins; 1999.
15. Toriumi DM, Checcone, MA. New concepts in nasal tip contouring. Facial Plast Surg Clin North Am. 2009;17:55-90.
16. Toriumi DM, Swartout B. Asian rhinoplasty. Facial Plast Surg Clin North Am. 2007;15:293-307.

Multiple Choice Questions

Q 1. On the lateral view the columellar show or alar/columellar relationship SHOULD BE how many mm?

A. 0 mm

B. 1 mm

C. 3 mm

D. 5 mm

Ans: C. 3 mm

Q 2. Which of the following statements ABOUT THE NOSE describe the drawing below? Please note distance from the subnasale to tip-defining point (B-A) and length of the upper lip (B-C).

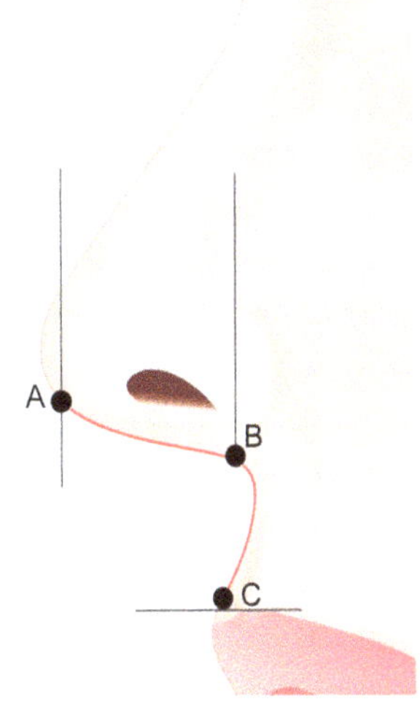

A. Projection/Goode method

B. Projection/Simons method

C. Rotation/Goode method

D. Rotation/Simons method

Ans: B. Projection/Simons method

Q 3. Which of the following sequences is the one which defines the PROPER order in which to perform the different types of rhinoplasty osteotomies?

A. Intermediate, lateral, medial

B. Medial, lateral, intermediate

C. Intermediate, medial, lateral

D. Medial, intermediate, lateral

Ans: D. Medial, intermediate, lateral.

Q 4. Which of the following statements about the African American nose is FALSE?

A. The nose is flat, broad and short

B. The nose has an overdevelopment of the anterior nasal spine

C. The nose has an acute nasolabial angle

D. The nose has a short, thick and hidden columella

Ans: B. The nose has an overdevelopment of the anterior nasal spine.

Q 5. Which of the following group/patients is NOT usually predisposed to the tip bossae formation?

A. Patients with thin skin and nasal tip bifidity

B. Patients with thick skin and normal interdomal width

C. Patients with over-resection of the lateral crura

D. Patients with thin skin, strong cartilages and excessive interdomal width

Ans: B. Patients with thick skin and normal interdomal width

Q 6. A wide, flat and broad nose is MOST likely a:

A. Leptorhine nose

B. Platyrhine nose

C. Middle Eastern nose

D. Latino nose

Ans: B. Platyrhine nose.

Q 7. Which of the following operative maneuvers will DECREASE projection in rhinoplastic surgery?

A. Lateral crural steal

B. Plumping grafts

C. Premaxillary grafts

D. Nasal spine reduction

Ans: D. Nasal spine reduction

Q 8. Which of the following methods involves the measure of TIP PROJECTION in relation to the length of the upper lip?

A. Simons

B. Gonzalez-Ulloa

C. Byrd

D. Crumley

Ans: A. Simons

Q 9. Which of the following operative maneuvers will DECREASE ROTATION?

A. Full-transfixion incision

B. Plumping grafts

C. Columellar strut

D. Lateral crura steal

Ans: A. Full-transfixion incision

Q 10. Which of the following combination of incisions is used in the delivery approach in rhinoplasty?

A. Intercartilaginous and transcolumellar

B. Intercartilaginous and marginal

C. Transcartilaginous and marginal

D. Transcartilaginous and transcolumellar

Answer: B. Intercartilaginous and marginal

Q 11. Which of the following statements regarding the OPEN approach in rhinoplasty is FALSE?

A. Combines bilateral marginal incisions and a transcolumellar incision

B. Compromises a major support mechanism for the tip of the nose

C. Compromises a minor support mechanism for the tip of the nose

D. Fosters prolonged nasal tip postoperative edema

Ans: B. Compromises a major support mechanism for the tip of the nose

Q 12. The distance from the nasal tip to the alar line measures 0.55-0.60 of the distance from the nasion to the tip of the nose. To WHOM do we attribute this rule?

A. Goode

B. Crumley

C. Byrd

D. Simmons

Ans: A. Goode

Q 13. Which of the following with reference to rhinoplasty is NOT considered an incision?

A. Intercartilaginous

B. Transcartilaginous

C. Transcolumellar

D. Cartilage-splitting

Ans: D. Cartilage-splitting

Q 14. Which of the following with reference to rhinoplasty is NOT considered an approach?

A. Complete strip

B. Retrograde

C. Delivery

D. External

Ans: A. Complete strip

Q 15. Which of the following statements is FALSE regarding the delivery approach in rhinoplasty?

A. Combines intercartilaginous and marginal incisions to create bilateral chondrocutaneous flaps

B. Good access to the tip and nasal dome

C. Minimal disturbance of the nasal tissues

D. Involves the separation of a major tip support of the nose and disruption of the upper and lower lateral cartilages

Ans: C. Minimal disturbance of the nasal tissues

Q 16. Which of the following operative maneuvers will DECREASE PROJECTION?

A. Cephalic resection

B. Columellar strut

C. Lateral crura steal

D. Full-transfixion incision

Ans: D. Full-transfixion incision

Q 17. Which of the following statements regarding nasal tip asymmetries is FALSE?

A. The lower third of the nose is infrequently a source of dissatisfaction in rhinoplasty revision.

B. Concavity of the lateral crura can be treated with lateral crura turnover.

C. Lateral alar asymmetries can be corrected with curved auricular cartilage from the ear concha.

D. Infralobular septal tip grafts are useful in order to increase projection.

Ans: A. The lower third of the nose is infrequently a source of dissatisfaction in rhinoplasty revision.

Q 18. Which of the following statements regarding Polly Beak deformity is FALSE?

A. It occurs due to over-resection of the bony hump

B. It occurs due to under-resection of the cartilaginous pyramid at the anterior septal angle

C. It occurs due to fullness of the middle third of the nose

D. It occurs due to poor supratip redrapage with a thick skin

Ans: C. It occurs due to fullness of the middle third of the nose

Q 19. Which of the following describes the DEFORMITY produced when rhinoplastic osteotomies are done too high reaching the frontal bone?

A. Open-roof deformity

B. Rocker deformity

C. Inverted-V deformity

D. Step deformity

Ans: B. Rocker deformity

Q 20. Which of the following statements about rhinoplasty is TRUE?

A. The best visualization of the tip structures is accomplished by the bipedicle approach.

B. The nasal skin is thicker at the mid-dorsum.

C. The nasal skin thinnest superiorly and inferiorly

D. The medial osteotomy is performed before the lateral osteotomy

Ans: D. The medial osteotomy is performed before the lateral osteotomy

Q 21. Which of the following statements about the external rhinoplasty approach is TRUE?

A. The external rhinoplasty approach divides only one major support mechanism of the nose

B. The external rhinoplasty approach divides the minor support mechanism of the nasal skin attachment

C. A bilateral rim incision produces a well camouflaged scar

D. There is no contraindication for use of a shield tip graft

Ans: B. The external rhinoplasty approach divides the minor support mechanism of the nasal skin attachment

Q 22. Which of the following statements is FALSE regarding complications in rhinoplasty?

A. Open-roof deformity is due to an inadequate lateral osteotomy

B. Excessive cephalic resection of the lateral crus of the lower lateral cartilage is usually the cause of alar retraction

C. The columellar incision in the external rhinoplasty should be beveled to avoid trapdoor deformity

D. Osteotomies done too high reaching the frontal bone can cause the rocker deformity

Ans: C. The columellar incision in the external rhinoplasty should be beveled to avoid trapdoor deformity

Q 23. Which of the following RELATES to "polly beak" deformity?

A. Inadequate resection of the upper third of the nose

B. Inadequate resection of the dorsal septal cartilage

C. Excessive resection of the upper lateral cartilage

D. Inadequate removal of the lower lateral cartilage

Ans: B. Inadequate resection of the dorsal septal cartilage

Q 24. Which of the following surgical maneuvers is INCORRECT in open structure rhinoplasty technique?

A. Mandatory incision-separation of the upper and lower alar cartilage

B. Tip projection preservation with use of transfixion incision and the standard septocolumellar suture

C. Columellar strut sutured in place

D. Shield shaped tip graft sutured in place

Ans: A. Mandatory incision-separation of the upper and lower alar cartilage

Q 25. Which of the following statements is FALSE regarding open rhinoplasty technique?

A. Osteotome or rasp can be used to reduce a dorsal hump

B. A single cut linear technique or a perforating technique are adequate for lateral osteotomies

C. Lateral osteotomy begins at the anterior turbinate

D. Lateral osteotomy follows a low, high, low pathway

Ans: D. Lateral osteotomy follows a low, high, low pathway

Q 26. Which of the following statements regarding rhinoplasty osteotomies is TRUE?

A. Lateral osteotomy is done before the intermediate

B. Medial osteotomy is done after the lateral osteotomy

C. Lateral osteotomy follows a high, low, high pathway

D. Perforating osteotomy is mandatory in all cases of rhinoplasty revision

Ans: C. Lateral osteotomy follows a high, low, high pathway.

Q 27. Which of the following statements regarding open structure rhinoplasty is FALSE?

A. The marginal incision is made along the caudal margin of the intermediate and medial cruras

B. The skin-soft tissue envelope is dissected from the lower lateral cartilages

C. The columellar strut is placed between the medial crura and extended to the nasal spine

D. The leading edge of the tip graft is placed to 2 mm above the existing domes

Ans: C. The columellar strut is placed between the medial crura and extended to the nasal spine

Q 28. Which area of the nose is IDEAL for alloplastic implant placement?

A. Tip

B. Dorsum

C. Ala

D. Sill

Ans: B. Dorsum

Q 29. Which of the following incisions employed in rhinoplasty is INCORRECT in order to gain access to the tip and dorsum?

A. Transcartilaginous incision

B. Intercartilaginous incision

C. Transcolumellar incision

D. Rim incision

Ans: D. Rim incision

Q 30. Which of the following represents a marginal incision?

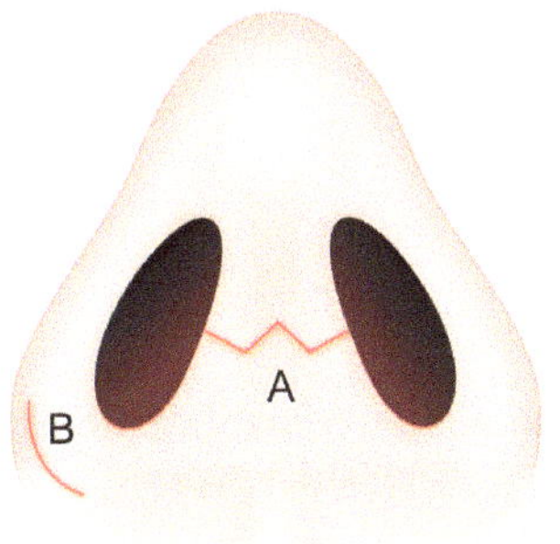

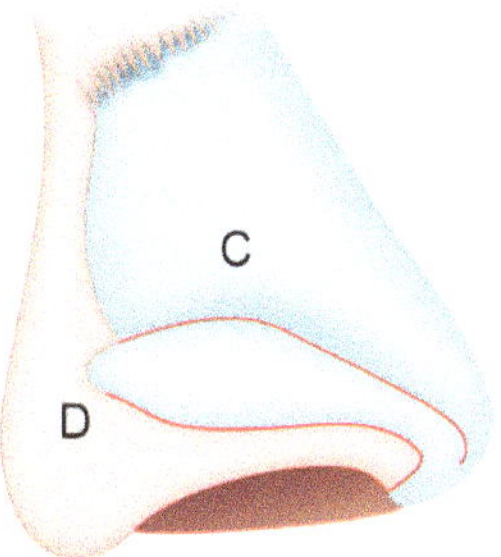

A. A

B. B

C. C

D. D

Ans: D. D

Q 31. Which of the following about the African American nose is FALSE?

A. The nasal tip is flat and bulbous
B. There is flaring of the lateral ala
C. The columella is short with poor tip projection
D. The skin is thin secondary to decreased subcutaneous fibro-fatty tissue

Ans: D. The skin is thin secondary to decreased subcutaneous fibro-fatty tissue

Q 32. Which of the following statements is FALSE regarding the surgical technique represented in the drawing below?

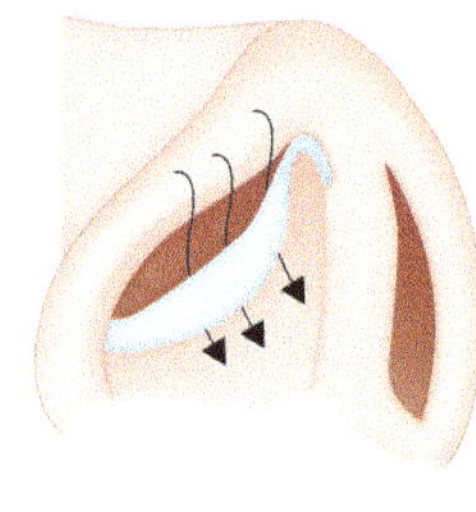

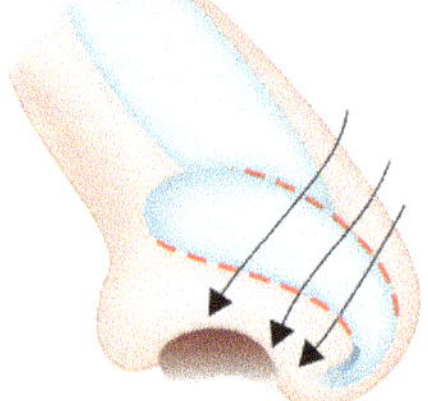

A. The lower lateral cartilage is exposed through intercartilaginous and marginal incisions
B. A bipedicle condrocutaneous flap is surgically created
C. Conservative reduction of the caudal margin of the lower lateral cartilage is recommended
D. Preservation of 6 mm of the complete strip of residual lower lateral cartilage is preferred

Ans: C. Conservative reduction of the caudal margin of the lower lateral cartilage is recommended

Q 33. Which of the following is the IDEAL incision to be used in a non delivery approach for conservative tip refinement in the presence of medium skin thickness and adequate tip cartilage symmetry?

A. Transcartilaginous
B. Marginal
C. Transcolumellar
D. Retrograde-eversion incision

Ans: A. Transcartilaginous

Q 34. Which of the following statements regarding the tip graft in rhinoplasty is FALSE?

A. A shield-shaped tip graft can be sculpted from the auricular cartilage
B. Tip grafts are sutured to the caudal margin of the medial or intermediate crura
C. Medium skin thickness is conducive to better camouflage
D. Cyanoacrylate tissue adhesives are ideal for reinforcing tip sutures

Ans: D. Cyanoacrylate tissue adhesives are ideal for reinforcing tip sutures

Q 35. Which of the following statements regarding aesthetic nasal proportions is INCORRECT?

A. Male noses tend to be longer and have a dorsal hump
B. The projection is measured in the lateral view using a 3-4-5 triangle
C. The lobule comprises one third of the nasal height and the columella the remaining two thirds
D. The upper lateral cartilages are a pair of triangular cartilages that are attached situated over the caudal surface of the nasal bone

Ans: D. The upper lateral cartilages are a pair of triangular cartilages that are attached situated over the caudal surface of the nasal bone

Q 36. Which of the following is the MOST important factor in DECREASING the incidence of nasal alar retraction during rhinoplasty?

A. The incidence of alar retraction will decrease by using a nondelivery approach and transcartilaginous incisions during surgery
B. Alar retraction will decrease by avoiding trauma to the caudal septal area
C. The incidence of alar retraction will decrease by gentle care of the lower lateral cartilage and soft-tissue envelope during surgery
D. The incidence of alar retraction will decrease by conservative resection of the alar cartilage during surgery

Ans: D. The incidence of alar retraction will decrease by conservative resection of the alar cartilage during surgery

Q 37. Which of the following statements regarding "pinching" of the nose is TRUE?

A. Pinching is due to overexcision of the lower lateral cartilages
B. Pinching is due to overexcision of the upper lateral cartilages
C. Pinching is increased with open rhinoplasty
D. Pinching is increased with exposure and delivery of the lower lateral cartilages

Ans: A. Pinching is due to overexcision of the lower lateral cartilages

Q 38. Which of the following statements regarding the use of irradiated homograft costal cartilage in revision rhinoplasty is TRUE?

A. Irradiated homograft costal cartilage is a poor material alternative for revision rhinoplasty
B. Before using the implant it must be soaked in gentamicin sulfate solution
C. The use of this material implies a very high rate of infection
D. The use of this material implies a very high rate of extrusion

Ans: B. Before using the implant it must be soaked in gentamicin sulfate solution

Q 39. Which of the following statements is TRUE regarding the use of irradiated costal cartilage in augmentation rhinoplasty?

A. Warping is quite common; 20%
B. Significant resorption is also common; 25%
C. All perichondrium should be removed from the rib graft
D. The most medial portion of the rib donor is the ideal for grafting

Ans: C. All perichondrium should be removed from the rib graft

Q 40. Which of the following statements regarding rhinoplasty is TRUE?

A. The best visualization is achieved by a bipedicle (bucket-handle) approach
B. The nasal skin is thinner superiorly and inferiorly
C. Medial osteotomies are performed before lateral
D. Lateral osteotomies start at the level of the floor of the nose

Ans: C. Medial osteotomies are performed before lateral

Q 41. Which of the following nasal aesthethic is NOT characteristic of a man?

A. Strong nasal dorsum with no supratip break
B. Strong nasal dorsum and a clearly defined supratip break
C. Nasolabial angle of 90 degrees
D. Dorsal line either straight or with a small bony hump

Ans: B. Strong nasal dorsum and a clearly defined supratip break

Q 42. Area A in the drawing below represents the resected area of the cephalic margin of the lower lateral cartilage (LLC) and area B represents the residual lower lateral cartilage (LCC). Which of the following statements is TRUE?

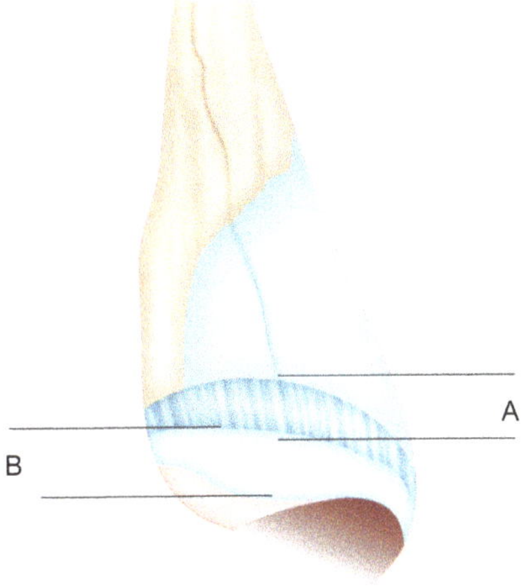

A. The area of cephalic resection of the LLC (A) should not be more than 4 mm
B. The residual LLC (B) should not be more than 2 mm
C. The residual LLC (B) should not be more than 4 mm
D. The residual LLC (B) should be at least 6 mm

Ans: D. The residual LLC (B) should be at least 6 mm

Q 43. The distance represented between the arrows is:

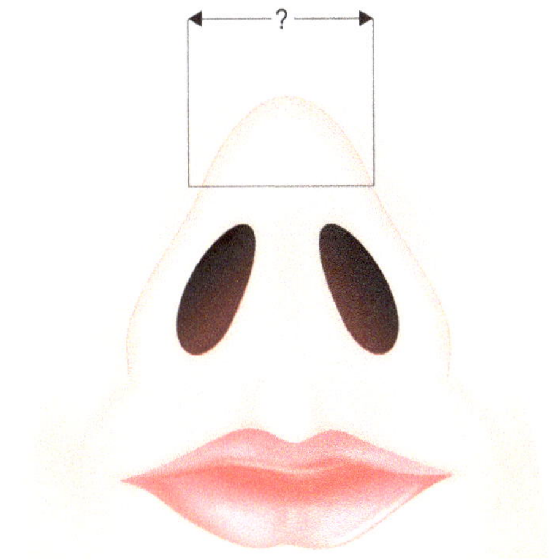

A. 30% of the width of the nasal base
B. 50% of the width of the nasal base
C. 75% of the width of the nasal base
D. 1/3 of the width of the nasal ala

Ans: C. 75% of the width of the nasal base

Q 44. Which of the following statements about rhinoplasty is TRUE?

A. Straight-line removal of a nasal hump can result in an over-reduced profile
B. The mimetic muscle most important in influencing the position of the nasal tip is the levator labii superioris
C. Lateral osteotomies should be "angle cut" to avoid collapse of the nasal vault
D. The membranous septum is a major tip support mechanism of the nose

Ans: A. Straight-line removal of a nasal hump can result in an overreduced profile

Q 45. Which of the following statements about External Rhinoplasty is TRUE?

A. The major vasculature of the nasal tip is located below the musculoaponeurotic layer of the nose
B. The most common complications of the transcolumellar incision is necrosis
C. The proper dissection plane is above the cartilages and bone and above the musculoaponeurotic layer of the nose
D. External rhinoplasty divides a minor support mechanism of the nose

Ans: D. External rhinoplasty divides a minor support mechanism of the nose

Q 46. Which of the following is NOT an approach in rhinoplasty?

A. Intercartilaginous
B. Delivery, bipedicle chondrocutaneous
C. Nondelivery, cartilage splitting
D. Nondelivery, retrograde eversion

Ans: A. Intercartilaginous

Q 47. Which of the following will NOT preserve or enhance tip projection in rhinoplasty?

A. Autogenous cartilage tip grafts
B. Complete transfixion incision
C. Transdomal sutures
D. Complete strip technique

Ans: B. Complete transfixion incision

Q 48. Which of the following is BEST served by a nonopen approach?

A. Cleft-lip nose deformity
B. Conservative tip refinement and rotation
C. Marked underprojection
D. Nasal tip rhinoplasty revision

Ans: B. Conservative tip refinement and rotation

Q 49. Which of the following is the MOST difficult to correct with a revision rhinoplasty?

A. Excess tissue in the bony pyramid
B. Excess of tissue in the upper cartilaginous vault
C. Excess in reduction of the both lower lateral cartilages
D. Excess of tissue in the caudal septum and lower cartilaginous vault

Ans: C. Excess in reduction of the both lower lateral cartilages

Q 50. Which of the following acquired nasal deformities is due to the EXCESSIVE EXCISION of lower lateral cartilage and vestibular skin?

A. Bosselation
B. Pinching
C. Alar retraction
D. Columellar retraction

Ans: C. Alar retraction

Q 51. Which of the following acquired nasal deformities is MOST likely the result of OVERRESECTION of the lateral crus of the lower lateral cartilage?

A. Bosselation
B. Pinching
C. Short nose
D. Polly-beak formation

Ans: B. Pinching

Q 52. Which of the following is TRUE about the African American nose?

A. Thin nasal tip skin
B. Thin or insignificant subcutaneous adipose tissue in the nasal
C. Nasal bone is usually small in both length and height
D. The nasal spine is overdeveloped

Ans: C. Nasal bone is usually small in both length and height

Q 53. Which of the following represents the VENTRAL position applied to the nose?

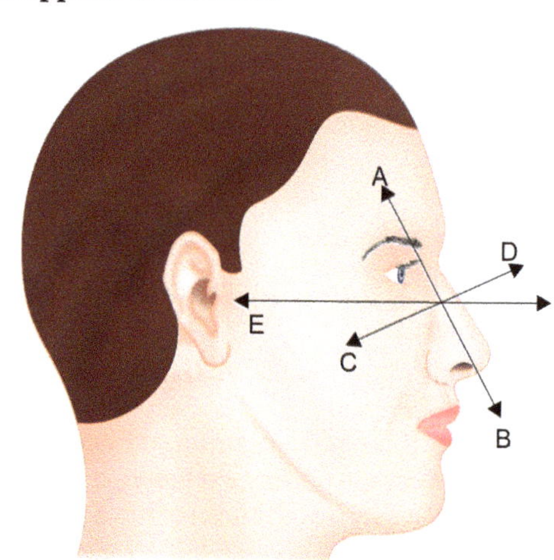

A. A
B. B
C. C
D. D

Ans: C. C

Q 54. Which of the following statements is FALSE regarding open rhinoplasty?

A. A high transverse transcolumellar incision is recommended
B. The Gull Wing Incision heals with a more favorable scar than the V-shaped Incision
C. It provides better surgical exposure
D. 5-0 prolene sutures are used to close the columellar incision

Ans: A. A high transverse transcolumellar incision is recommended

Q 55. Which of the following statements about facial analysis for rhinoplasty is CORRECT?

A. The nasofrontal angle connects the nasion to the trichion and the nasion to the nasal tip
B. The ideal nasolabial angle in men is 110 degrees
C. Adequate projection of the nose is present when 60% of the horizontal nasal projection lies anterior to the upper lip
D. Columellar show measures 6 mm in the male patient

Ans: C. Adequate projection of the nose is present when 60% of the horizontal nasal projection lies anterior to the upper lip

Q 56. Which of the following statements regarding base view analysis in rhinoplasty is FALSE?

A. The nostrils should have, in the leptorrhine nose, their long axis oriented at a 30 degree-angle to the columella
B. The lobule is one third of the height of an isosceles triangle and the columella two thirds the height

C. The width or the nostril should be about the same length as the width of the columella

D. The nostrils should be symmetrical and pear shaped

Ans: A. The nostrils should have, in the leptorrhine nose, their long axis oriented at a 30 degree-angle to the columella

Q 57. With reference to the drawing below the width of the base of the bony sidewall of the nose is approximately what percent of the width of the alar base?

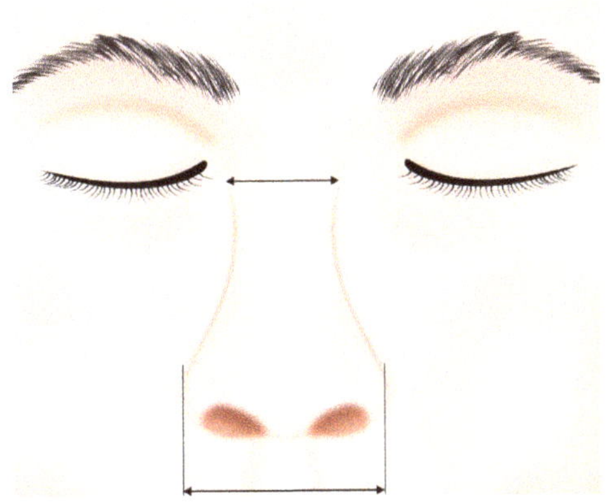

A. 40%

B. 50%

C. 60%

D. 75%

Ans: D. 75%

Q 58. Which of the following statements about rhinoplasty complications is FALSE?

A. The incidence of postoperative rhinoplasty complications is about 12%

B. There are complications related to under-resection

C. There are complications related to over-resection, usually associated with scarring

D. Complications related to excessive reduction are usually the easiest to correct

Ans: D. Complications related to excessive reduction are usually the easiest to correct

Q 59. Which of the following statements about a ptotic and underrotated tip is FALSE?

A. Lack of tip support will lead to a tip ptosis with an overly obtuse nasolabial angle

B. A lateral crural steal will increase rotation and projection

C. A full-transfixion incision will decrease rotation and projection

D. Columellar strut will increase rotation and projection

Ans: A. Lack of tip support will lead to a tip ptosis with an overly obtuse nasolabial angle

Q 60. Which of the following statements about alar retraction is FALSE?

A. The vestibular mucosa should always be preserved in order to avoid scar contracture

B. In minor cases of alar retraction, cartilage grafts can be used for the repair

C. In severe cases of alar retraction, composite auricular grafts are used for the repair

D. The cymba concha of the ipsilateral ear provides the best contour for composite grafting

Ans: D. The cymba concha of the ipsilateral ear provides the best contour for composite grafting

Q 61. Which of the following statements is TRUE regarding rhinoplastic surgical maneuvers?

A. Lateral crural steal will decrease rotation

B. Full-transfixion incision will increase rotation

C. Plumping grafts will increase projection

D. A deep nasofrontal angle will increase nasal length

Ans: C. Plumping grafts will increase projection

Q 62. Which of the following statements related to rhinoplasty is FALSE?

A. In the basal view, the tip lobule represents the upper third and the columella represents the lower two thirds

B. A dorsal hump is usually comprises of cartilage and bone

C. Older, thick-skinned patients with a widened interdomal distance are prone to bossae

D. Saddle nose deformity is usually associated with obstruction of the internal valve

Ans: C. Older, thick-skinned patients with a widened interdomal distance are prone to bossae

Q 63. Which of the following statements is FALSE about the African American nose?

A. The middle third of the nose is usually short

B. Narrowing of the wide dorsum is best achieved by osteotomies

C. Nasal base is usually wider than the intercanthal distance.

D. The nasolabial angle is usually acute

Ans: B. Narrowing of the wide dorsum is best achieved by osteotomies.

Q 64. The term "angle of domal divergence" signifies a measurement of

A. Rotation

B. Projection

C. Definition

D. Interdomal distance

Ans: D. Interdomal distance

Q 65. Which of the following statements is UNCHARACTER-ISTIC of the African American nose?

A. Acute nasolabial angle
B. Acute alar dome angle
C. Underrotated nasal tip
D. Broad and flattened dorsum

Ans: B. Acute alar dome angle

Q 66. Which of the following statements is TRUE about the African American nose?

A. The nasolabial angle is usually 90 degrees
B. The ratio of columella to nasal tip lobule is 1:1 or 1.5: 1
C. The nasal tip projection is usually adequate
D. Alar hooding is extremely rare

Ans: B. The ratio of columella to nasal tip lobule is 1:1 or 1.5: 1

Q 67. Which of the following is DESCRIBED as that part of the nose above the nostrils as viewed from the below?

A. Tip of the nose
B. Tip defining point
C. Lobule
D. Scroll

Ans: C. Lobule

Q 68. Which of the following with respect to the African American nose is TRUE?

A. Nasolabial angle approximately 90 degrees
B. Thin skin and subcutaneous fibro fatty tissue
C. Absent anterior nasal spine
D. Convex nasal bones

Ans: C. Absent anterior nasal spine

Q 69. Which of the following statements regarding nasal osteotomies is FALSE?

A. They are used to straighten an asymmetrical nasal pyramid
B. Medial osteotomies are usually done first
C. Intermediate osteotomies are done after the lateral osteotomies
D. Lateral osteotomies are done through an stab incision at the level of the attachment of the inferior turbinate

Ans: C. Intermediate osteotomies are done after the lateral osteotomies

Q 70. Which of the following INCISIONS is the one recommended for the retrograde approach in rhinoplasty?

A. Transcartilaginous
B. Intercartilaginous
C. Transcolumellar and marginal
D. Rim

Ans: B. Intercartilaginous

Q 71. Which of the following percentage represents the 20 year survival rate of nasal tip grafts from autogenous septal cartilage?

A. 65%
B. 75%
C. 85%
D. 95%

Ans: D. 95%

Q 72. Which of the following statements is related to the sutures used in the drawing below?

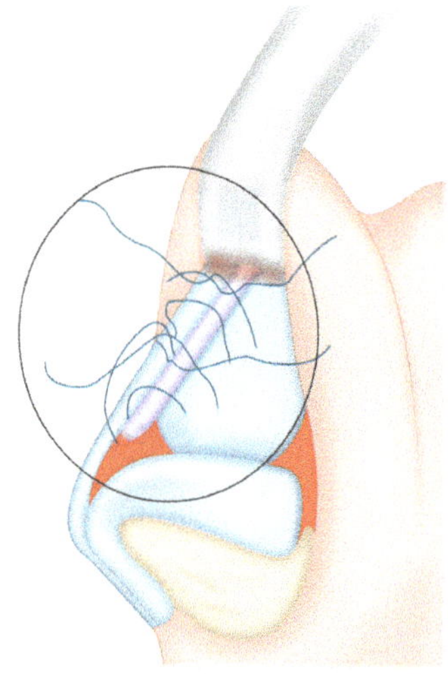

A. Transdomal sutures
B. Interdomal sutures
C. Flaring sutures
D. Dome-binding sutures

Ans: C. Flaring sutures

Q 73. Which of the following statements regarding percutaneous lateral osteotomies is FALSE?

A. The percutaneous incision should be made with the flat edge of a 2 mm straight chisel
B. Percutaneous osteotomies produce an imperceptible scar 100% of the time
C. The percutaneous entry site is not closed with sutures
D. The chisel should be cleansed of any foreign body matter or material

Ans: B. Percutaneous osteotomies produce an imperceptible scar 100% of the time

Q 74. Which of the following WILL NOT increase nasal tip projection?

A. Onlay tip graft
B. Columella strut
C. Approximation of medial crura footplates
D. Reduction of alar base

Ans: D. Reduction of alar base

Q 75. Which is of the following statements about the Mestizo nose is FALSE?

A. The radix is low
B. The dorsum is slightly concave
C. The columella is short
D. The tip is rotated caudally

Ans: B. The dorsum is slightly concave

Q 76. Which of the following is a CONTRAINDICATION for use of the lateral crura overlay tip technique?

A. Acute nasolabial angle associated with tip ptosis
B. Overprojection associated with tip ptosis
C. Underprojection associated with tip ptosis
D. Long, inferiorly oriented lateral crura with tip ptosis

Ans: C. Underprojection associated with tip ptosis

Q 77. Which of the following is NOT RELATED to the aging nose?

A. Increased length
B. Dorsal concavity
C. Tip drop
D. Subcutaneous fat atrophy

Ans: B. Dorsal concavity

Q 78. Which of the following statements about a "SHORT NOSE" is FALSE?

A. There is decreased distance from the nasion to the tip defining point
B. There is a low ratio of tip projection to nasal length
C. There is a nasolabial angle greater than expected
D. There is a overprojection of nasal tip

Ans: D. There is a overprojection of nasal tip

Q 79. Which of the following is the BEST management for a dorsal nasal cyst noted one year postrhinoplasty?

A. Needle aspiration
B. Incision and drainage
C. Corticoid injections
D. Surgical excision

Ans: D. Surgical excision

Q 80. Which of the following is NOT a characteristic of the Asian nose?

A. Wide and strong nasal bones
B. Broad and flat nasal dorsum
C. Wide and flat tip cartilages
D. Limited tip projection

Ans: A. Wide and strong nasal bones

Q 81. Which of the following nasal features is the one characterizing a Pinocchio tip deformity?

A. Long nose
B. Supratip deformity
C. Hanging columella
D. Excessive nasal tip projection

Ans: D. Excessive nasal tip projection

Q 82. Which of the following columellar incisions is NOT used in open rhinoplasty?

A. Z-shape incision
B. Inverted V-shape incision
C. Stair-step incision
D. Slightly curvilinear insicion

Ans: A. Z-shape incision

Q 83. Postrhinoplasty, when should the protective splint of the nose be removed?

A. 2 days
B. 4 days
C. 7 days
D. 10 days

Ans: C. 7 days

Q 84. Which of the following complications is the one created by combining large excisions of lateral crura with vertical dome divisions (Goldman technique)?

A. Tent-pole appearance
B. Alar retraction
C. Bossa deformity
D. Tip ptosis

Ans: A. Tent-pole appearance

Q 85. For which of the following nasal deformities is the TONGUE-IN-GROOVE technique indicated?

A. Nasal valve collapse
B. Hanging ala
C. Hanging columella
D. Retracted ala

Ans: C. Hanging columella

Q 86. Which of the following facial analysis is related to a female rather than a male patient?

A. Wider, straighter and less concave dorsal aesthetic lines
B. Dorsum 2 mm behind a line drawn from the radix to the tip-defining points
C. Decreased tip rotation
D. Chin tangential to a plumb line from the lower lip

Ans: B. Dorsum 2 mm behind a line drawn from the radix to the tip-defining points

Q 87. Which of the following nasal types LESS FREQUENTLY requires nasal alar modifications?

A. Asian
B. African American
C. Caucasian
D. Oriental

Ans: C. Caucasian

Q 88. Which of the following nasal inadequacies is BEST corrected with an umbrella graft?

A. Saddle nose
B. Inadequate tip rotation
C. Inadequate tip projection
D. Inadequate internal nasal valve

Ans: C. Inadequate tip projection

Q 89. Which of the following will NOT predispose to nasal tip bossa formation secondary to rhinoplasty?

A. Open approach
B. Asymmetric dome cartilages
C. Presence of sharp edges
D. Wide separation of the domes

Ans: A. Open approach

Q 90. Which of the following statements about a pinched nasal tip is INCORRECT?

A. It is usually iatrogenic
B. It is caused by excision resection of the lower lateral cartilage
C. It is involved collapse of the internal nasal valve
D. Autogenous nasal septal cartilage is used for correction

Ans: C. It is involved in collapse of the internal nasal valve

Q 91. In face-nasal analysis, in profile view, the nose should project from the face, with a right angle triangle (according to Crumley and Lancer). Which of the following is the adequate proportion?

A. 2-3-4 triangle
B. 3-4-5 triangle
C. 4-5-6 triangle
D. 5-6-7 triangle

Ans: B. 3-4-5 triangle

Q 92. Which of the following is NOT a feature of the African American nose?

A. Bulbous nasal tip
B. Thin alar skin
C. Short columella
D. Poor tip projection

Ans: B. Thin alar skin

Q 93. Which of the following nasal parameters is measured by the "Goode's method"?

A. The nasal length
B. The nasal rotation
C. The nasal projection
D. The nasal alar flare

Ans: C. The nasal projection

Q 94. The ideal nasofacial angle SHOULD BE:

A. 35 degrees
B. 90 degrees
C. 100 degrees
D. 120 degrees

Ans: A. 35 degrees

Q 95. Which of the following nasal topographic analysis is FALSE?

A. The narrowest part of the bony vault is at the level of the rhinion
B. The lobule is divided into the tip, supratip and infratip
C. The nasal skin is thinner and more mobile in the upper half of the nose
D. The nasal skin thickness is the thinnest at the rhinion

Ans: A. The narrowest part of the bony vault is at the level of the rhinion

Q 96. Which of the following is considered an adequate NASOLABIAL angle in a male?

A. 30 degrees
B. 50 degrees
C. 90 degrees
D. 110 degrees

Ans: C. 90 degrees

Q 97. The SIMON's nasal projection in relation to the upper lip should have a ratio of:

A. 1:1
B. 1:1.5
C. 1:2
D. 1:2.5

Ans: A. 1:1

Q 98. Which of the following statements in rhinoplasty is FALSE?

A. The intercartilaginous incision is made between the cephalic margin of the lower lateral cartilage and the caudal margin of the upper lateral cartilage
B. The intracartilaginous incision is made transversely through the upper lateral cartilage
C. The intracartilaginous incision is also called transcartilaginous incision
D. The bipedicled flap involves an intercartilaginous incision and another incision placed in the caudal margin of the lower lateral cartilage

Ans: B. The intracartilaginous incision is made transversely through the upper lateral cartilage

Q 99. Which of the following statements is TRUE regarding the thickness of the soft tissue of the nasal dorsum?

A. The soft tissues of the nasal dorsum are thinner in the upper aspect of the nose
B. The soft tissue of the nasal dorsum are thinner in the lower aspect of the nose
C. The soft tissue of the nasal dorsum are thinner in the midnasal aspect of the nose
D. The soft tissue of the nasal dorsum are thinner in the area just lateral to the midline

Ans: C. The soft tissue of the nasal dorsum are thinner in the midnasal aspect of the nose

Q 100. Which of the following statements is FALSE regarding rhinoplasty?

A. Reduction of a dorsal nasal hump should be conservative.
B. A dorsal nasal hump usually has both bone and cartilage components
C. Intermediate osteotomies, if necessary, should be done last
D. Medial osteotomies should be done first

Ans: C. Intermediate osteotomies, if necessary, should be done last

Q 101. What is the name of the incision demonstrated in the drawing below?

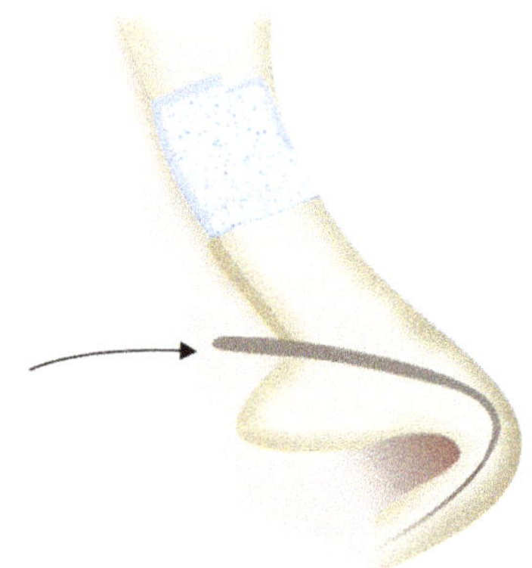

A. Intercartilaginous
B. Transcartilaginous
C. Marginal
D. Cephalic

Ans: A. Intercartilaginous

Q 102. Which of the following grafts are used to increase an inadequate nasofrontal angle?

A. Dorsal onlay grafts
B. Spreader grafts
C. Radix grafts
D. Dorsal sidewall onlay grafts

Ans: C. Radix grafts

Q 103. Which of the following nasal areas IS NOT indicated to implant GORE-TEX in rhinoplasty?

A. Nasal dorsum
B. Supratip dorsum
C. Nasal tip
D. Lateral nasal wall

Ans: C. Nasal tip

Q 104. Which of the following statement is FALSE regarding the drawing presented below?. A forceps elevates the alar complex and a transdomal suture is placed. The alar complex is excised.

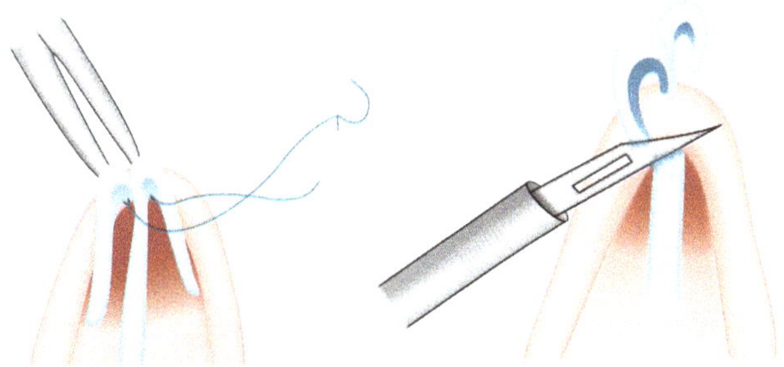

A. The delivery approach is used in conjunction with a transfixion incision
B. The excision involves the resection of the dome and the adjacent lateral crura
C. The presented resection will deproject the nasal profile
D. Alar base reduction is contraindicated associated with this technique

Ans: D. Alar base reduction is contraindicated associated with this technique

Q 105. Which of the following statements regarding GORE-TEX is TRUE?

A. Gore-Tex is a Porous high-density Polyethylene
B. Gore-Tex has pore sizes ranging from 125-250 μm
C. Gore-Tex can be used for columellar graft augmentation
D. Gore-Tex most common complication is infection

Ans: D. Gore-Tex most common complication is infection

Q 106. Which of the following is NOT a typical characteristic of the Asian nose?

A. Tip: bulbous, poor defined, underprojected
B. Ala: flared with a short columella
C. Skin: thin
D. Nasal septum: small anterior nasal spine

Ans: C. Skin: thin

Q 107. Which of following statements is TRUE regarding the INCISION/APPROACH represented in the picture?

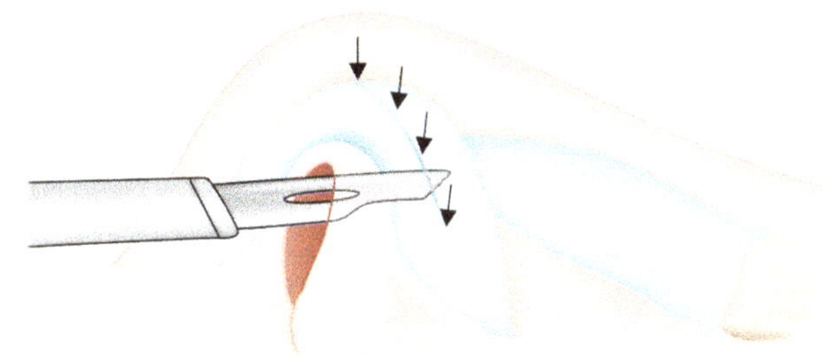

A. It is a transcartilaginous incision
B. It is used as a delivery approach
C. It is commonly used in nasal dome division
D. It is an ideal incision/approach to treat major nasal tip

Ans: A. It is a transcartilaginous incision

Q 108. Which of following statements regarding the graft used in the picture is TRUE?

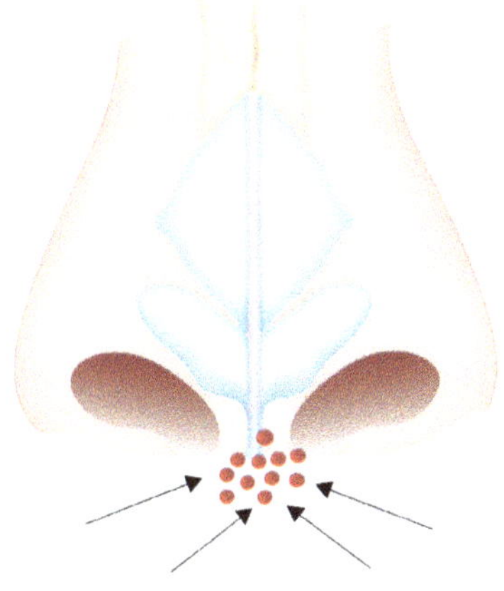

A. It is a caudal septal graft
B. It is placed in the anterior aspect of the columella
C. It is used to decrease the columellar-labial angle
D. It is used to create the appearance of nasal tip rotation

Ans: D. It is used to create the appearance of nasal tip rotation

Q 109. Which of the following rhinoplasty postoperative statements is FALSE?

A. The protective splint and dressing are removed in one week
B. 90% of the postoperative nasal swelling disappear by 7 days
C. Make up can be used after 7 days
D. A rhinoplasty final result is seen in 3 months

Ans: D. A rhinoplasty final result is seen in 3 months

Q 110. What is the proper time to see the rhinoplasty patient for his/her first postoperative clinic visit?

A. 24 hours
B. 48 hours
C. 3 days
D. 7 days

Ans: D. 7 days

Q 111. Which of the following surgical technique will repair the alar-columellar deformity shown below?

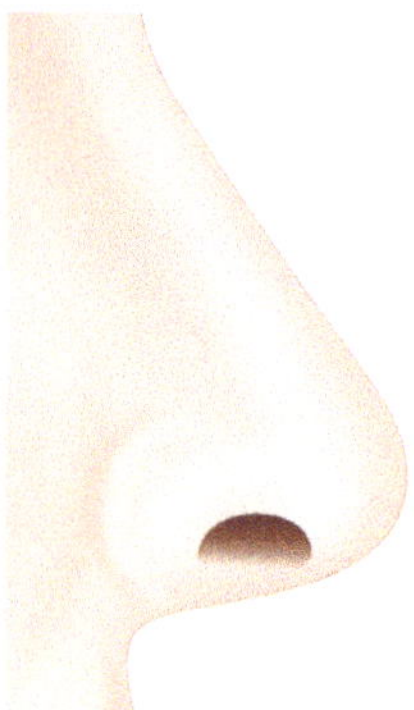

A. Local flap (skin and soft tissue)
B. Cartilage graft, septal
C. Composite graft, cymba concha of the left ear
D. Composite graft, cymba concha of the right ear

Ans: C. Composite graft, cymba concha of the left ear

Q 112. Which of the following nasal muscles is the one that can DEPRESS THE NASAL TIP caudally and "round up" the supratip area?

A. Dilator naris anterior
B. Depressor septi nasi
C. Transverse nasalis
D. Levator labii-superioris alae nasi

Ans: B. Depressor septi nasi

Q 113. Which of the following sensory nerve is the ONE that will produce tip numbness after rhinoplasty?

A. Supratrochlear branch of the ophthalmic nerve
B. Infratrochlear branch of the ophthalmic nerve
C. Supratrochlear and infratrochlear branches of the ophthalmic nerve
D. External nasal branch of the anterior ethmoidal nerve

Ans: D. External nasal branch of the anterior ethmoidal nerve

Q 114. Which of the following complications is MOST commonly seen after using costal cartilage for nasal dorsal augmentation?

A. Infection
B. Extrusion
C. Warping
D. Resorption

Ans: C. Warping

Q 115. Which of the following statements regarding irradiated rib homograft cartilage is FALSE?

A. The cartilage is sterilized by exposure to 30.000 Gy
B. Before using the implant should be soak in gentamicin sulfate solution
C. It is easily carved
D. It is less resistant to infection compared with most alloplasts

Ans: D. It is less resistant to infection compared with most alloplasts

Chapter 9

Genioplasty and Mandibular Procedures

Michael G Roskies

INTRODUCTION

Chin augmentation is the most commonly performed adjunctive procedure to rhinoplasty,[1] and evaluation of chin position during rhinoplasty is necessary to achieve an aesthetic facial profile. It is important to recognize that patients wishing to reduce a perceived nasal prominence may benefit instead from an augmentation genioplasty serving to establish facial harmony.

RELEVANT ANATOMY

The chin (or mentum) is formed by the paired mentalis, depressor anguli oris, and depressor labii inferioris muscles and their overlying soft tissue. The mentalis originates from the mentum and inserts into the chin soft tissue. When contracted, it causes inward movement of the chin and subsequent raising of the central portion of the lower lips. It is the only elevator of the lower lip. In combination with the orbicularis oris, the mentalis allows the lips to "pout". Both the depressor labii inferioris and depressor anguli oris originate from the oblique line of the mandible; the former inserts on the skin of the lower lip and the latter on the angle of the mouth. When contracted, they help depress the lower lip. The three muscles are innervated by the marginal mandibular branch of the facial nerve (CN VII). The blood supply to the chin is via the facial artery. Sensation to the lower lip and chin is provided by the mental nerve, a branch of the inferior alveolar nerve (CN V3). The mental nerve travels through the mandibular canal and exits the mental foramen below the second mandibular premolar, halfway between the alveolar ridge and inferior border of the mandible. The second premolar lies on the same vertical line defined by the pupil and infraorbital foramen (Fig. 1). As the mandibular canal is located 2–3 mm below the mental foramen, osteotomies should be made 5 mm below the latter to avoid injury.

The effects of aging on chin position are a result of bone resorption that occurs in several key areas. In children, the mental foramen lies closer to the inferior border of the mandible and slightly more anteriorly; however, atrophy of the alveolar ridge during aging or in toothless individuals

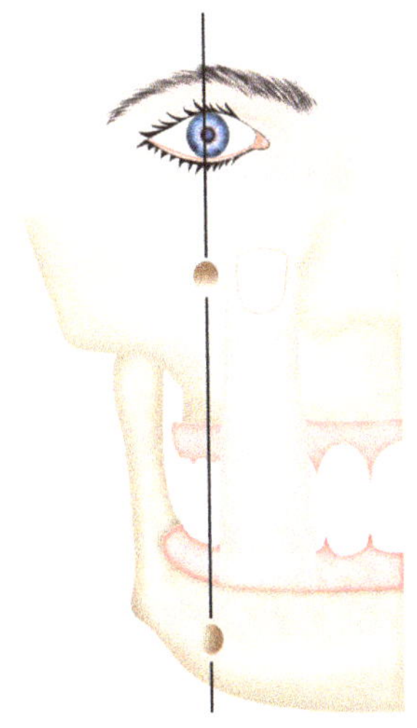

Fig. 1: Location of mental nerve within mid pupillary line.

causes the foramen to lie more superiorly. Additionally, the prejowl sulcus forms along the inferior edge of the mandible anterior to the jowls as a result of the gradual resorption of bone laterally. This sulcus contributes to the commissure-mandibular groove, creating marionette lines within the soft tissues of the aging face.[2] Finally, bone resorption in the anterior region of the mandible leads to an insufficient projection of the chin that contributes to a blunted cervicomental angle.[3]

Mandibular maldevelopment can be classified into micrognathia or retrognathia. Whereas micrognathia refers to size and retrognathia refers to position in relation to the maxilla, in most cases, the two abnormalities codevelop. Micrognathia is a common feature to congenital syndromes like Treacher-Collins and the Pierre-Robin sequence and the surgeon should be aware of concomitant anomalies and complications (e.g. glossoptosis and airway obstruction during anesthesia).[4]

PREOPERATIVE ASSESSMENT

A relevant patient history should include age, history of facial trauma, and previous surgeries. Smoking or other conditions predisposing to improper healing or implant infection (such as diabetes mellitus, hypothyroidism, or autoimmune diseases) should be elicited. A focused history on previous dental surgeries (correcting malocclusion without addressing the facial skeleton) and significant temporomandibular joint disorders should be obtained.

The general facial assessment should include observation and palpation with the patient at rest and during animation. Methods to evaluate chin position are listed in Table 1. Briefly divide the face into horizontal thirds and vertical fifths. The distance between the glabella and subnasale should be equal to the distance between the subnasale and menton. When focusing on the lower portion of the face, the chin as it relates to the lips should be analyzed. Riedel's line (Fig. 2) connects the most prominent portions of the upper to the lower lips and should extend to touch the most prominent portion of the menton. On profile view, if the chin falls behind this line, the patient is micrognathic. Additionally, the Gonzales-Ulloa technique can be used. Two imaginary lines are drawn: (1) the Frankfurt horizontal line from the upper margin of the external auditory canal to the lower orbital rim and (2) a perpendicular line running through the soft tissue nasion. Ideally, this perpendicular line should transect both lips and the pogonion (anteriormost portion of the chin) in men and should lie 1–2 mm anterior to the pogonion in women (Fig. 3).[2]

The soft tissue of the chin should be assessed. "Mentalis strain" is a result of muscular hypertrophy in an attempt to create lower lip competence in the context of microgenia. The labiomental groove is influenced by chin pad projection and lower lip procumbency (seen in class II malocclusion). Chin ptosis ("witch's chin") is caused by a weakening of the muscular attachments to the soft tissues that then fall below the mandibular line and accentuates the submental crease.[5]

Evaluating for malocclusion will determine the need for orthognathic surgery. The Angle classification describes the relationship between the mesial buccal cusp of the maxillary first molar and the buccal groove of the mandibular first molar. Class I is "normal occlusion" as the cusp fits directly into the buccal groove. In class II occlusion, the cusp lies anterior to the buccal groove (seen in retrognathia and resulting in overbite). In class III occlusion, the cusp lies posterior to the buccal groove (seen in prognathia and resulting in underbite). A patient in normal class I occlusion may only need an isolated genioplasty, whereas those in class II or class III will likely need mandibular body work.

Temporomandibular joint should be assessed preoperatively and can be described according to the Wilkes classification of internal derangement which factors in degree of disk displacement, pain and functional disturbance (Table 2).

Table 1: Other methods to evaluate chin position are listed below.	
Method	*Definition*
Gonzales-Ulloa zero meridian	Perpendicular line to Frankfort horizontal line drawn from nasion, and should hit the pogonion in men
Legan angle	Angle between glabella, subnasale, and pogonion should equal 12° ± 4°
Merrifield Z angle	Angle between the Frankfort plane, and a line between the anterior lips and pogonion should equal 80° ± 5°
Mentolabial sulcus	A line is drawn from nasion to pogonion. The mentolabial sulcus should be 4 mm behind this line.
Vertical line from inferior vermilion	A vertical line perpendicular to the Frankfort plan is dropped from the inferior vermilion border. Male pogonion should be tangential to this line, and female pogonion should be 2–3 mm behind this line.

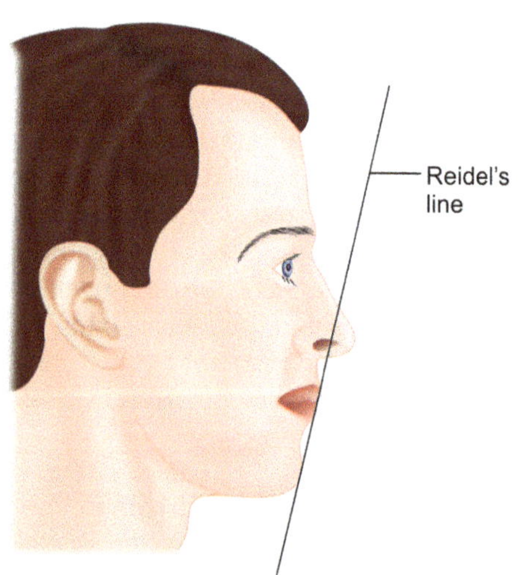

Fig. 2: Reidel's line.

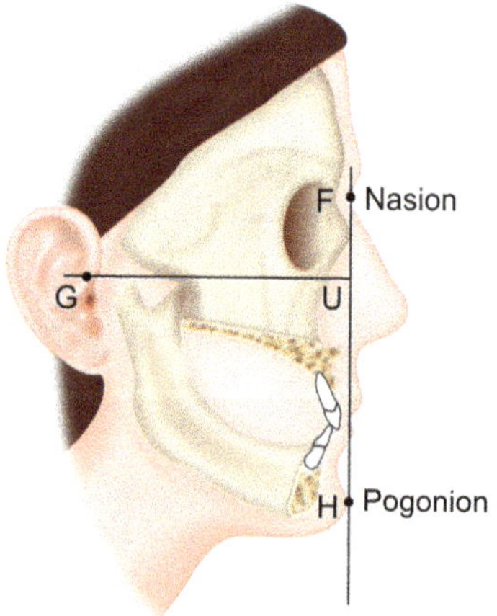

Fig. 3: Gonzales-Ulloa line.

Table 2: Wilkes classification of internal derangement.		
Stage	*Disk displacement*	*Pain, limitation, clicks*
Stage I	Early, reducing	No pain or limitation Early opening click
Stage II	Late, reducing	≥1 episode of pain Mid-late opening click
Stage III	Nonreducing (acute)	Multiple painful episodes Locking, restricted mobility
Stage IV	Nonreducing (chronic)	Increasing functional disturbance
Stage V	Nonreducing (chronic)	Osteoarthritis, crepitus, grinding Difficult function

Photodocumentation in the frontal, profile, and oblique views should be obtained. With patients positioned in the Frankfort plane, assess the face, lip, chin pad, labiomental fold, and prejowl region. Cephalometric radiography relates the position of the dentition and skull base to the position of the soft tissues of the face.[6] AP views will show any horizontal asymmetries of the facial skeleton that may be magnified with a simple symmetric implant. The Steiner method in lateral view helps determine whether orthognathic surgery is necessary. Briefly, three lines are made between the sella (S), nasion (N), maxilla (A), and mandible (B). From these, the SNA (skull base to midface), SNB (skull base to mandible), and ANB (midface to mandible) angles are created and compared to norms. Figure labeled "Steiner" has been shown in Figure 4.

DECISION MAKING

The initial decision in surgical planning should address the underlying chin deficiency and corresponding treatment

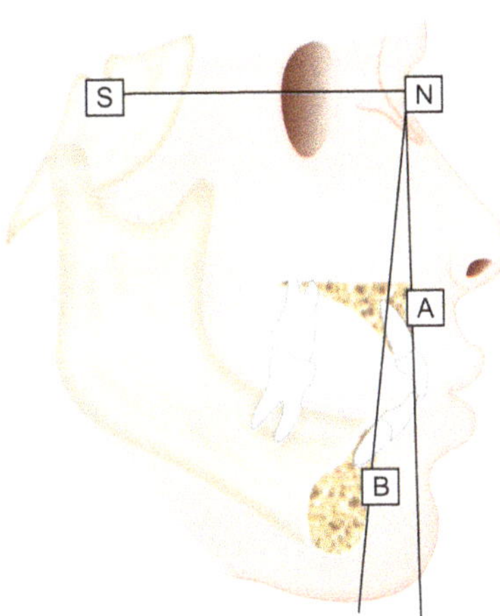

Fig. 4: Steiner method.

options including alloplasts, osseous genioplasty, or fillers. Alloplastic implants address modest symmetric hypoplasia in the sagittal plane, but an osseous genioplasty is best suited for complex three-dimensional deformities requiring additional vertical manipulation. Genioplasty is recommended in revision and asymmetric cases.[7] Fillers can be used to address rhytids and provide soft tissue augmentation in the prejowl region. Orthognathic surgery may be used in conjunction with genioplasty in patients with accompanying malocclusion. These patients often demonstrate lower lip retrusion, an exaggerated labiomental fold, and a decreased height of the lower face.[8]

SURGICAL APPROACHES

Surgical approaches include both intraoral and extraoral (submental). The intraoral incision is made on the labial side of the gingivolabial sulcus from one canine to the other. Advantages of the intraoral incision include avoidance of an external scar. The disadvantages are imprecise reattachment of the mentalis muscle (can cause increase lower lip position and dental show), inability to internally stabilize implant and suture line irritation.[6] The 2 cm extraoral skin incision can be made inferior to the submental crease. Sharp dissection is carried to the periosteum. Subperiosteal placement of implants has been shown to cause bone erosion in ~50% of patients;[9] therefore, anteriorly, the periosteum must be preserved. Advantages of the submental approach for implants include a more precise placement, decreased cephalad migration, avoidance of oral contamination, and prevention of lip ptosis.[10] Additionally, it allows for simultaneous access to the submental area when cervical facial rhytidectomy is being performed.[3] The main disadvantage is external scarring, although scarring is inconspicuous with proper incision placement and closure.

GENIOPLASTY

Genioplasty is performed through an intraoral approach in a subperiosteal plane laterally. A horizontal osteotomy allows for AP advancement (Fig. 5). To create vertical shortening, an oblique osteotomy with distal segment advancement can be used.

For more significant reduction, two oblique osteotomies with ostectomy are used. Lower lip position is not addressed by osseous genioplasty. The major complications specific to genioplasty are sensory loss (occurring from damage to the inferior alveolar nerve), intraoral wound dehiscence and plate exposure. Lip paresthesia is most commonly transient, but can be permanent (defined as persisting at 1 year) in 0.2% of cases. The risk increases to 15% when combined with orthognathic surgery.[6] Dyskinesis of the mentalis has been reported as high as 10% and is managed with injection of botulinum toxin.

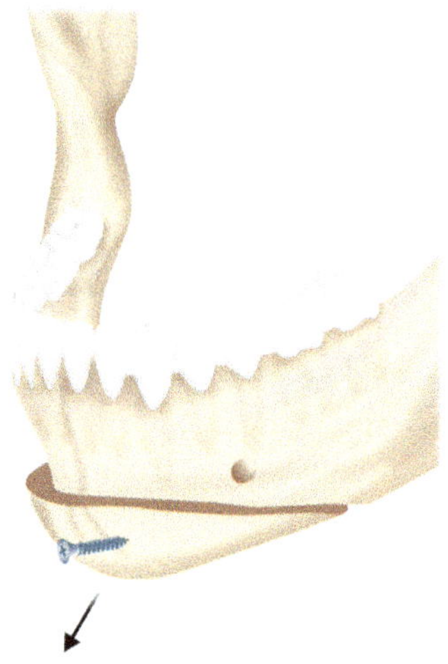

Fig. 5: AP advancement in sliding genioplasty.

MANDIBULAR IMPLANTS

A variety of biocompatible alloplastic implants are used. Solid implants like Silastic (silicone) are easier to manipulate and prevent tissue ingrowth; however; fibrous encapsulation occurs. Porous implants like polytetrafluoroethylene (PTFE or Gore-Tex) and polyethylene (Medpor) lack encapsulation, resist degradation, and provide tissue ingrowth potential (provides stabilization). Disadvantages to all include infection and displacement, although this is rare. To secure the implants, some authors advocate for a periosteal suture through a submental approach and some propose using no sutures at all.

Complications specific to mandibular implants include mucosal dehiscence and exposure of underlying bone chin ptosis, displacement, and bone resorption.[6] Mucosal dehiscence has been reported as high as 8.5%. Management includes daily irrigations and antibiotics. Chin ptosis can be avoided with appropriate closure of the mentalis muscle. Bone resorption can be avoided with dissection in a supraperiosteal layer over the anterior aspect of the mandible. If displaced, the implant is at risk of extrusion and should be removed/replaced. Infection with implants is exceedingly rare (0/125 in one series[7]) and is usually prevented by soaking the implant in an antibiotic solution preoperatively.

FILLER GENIOPLASTY

Filler materials are used for soft tissue augmentation. Calcium hydroxyapatite and hyaluronic acid (HA) are FDA-approved for the correction of moderate to deep facial wrinkles and, when injected supraperiosteally, can address the prejowl sulcus and marionette lines. Please refer to the fillers section for specific properties of each filler. Immediate complications include hypersensitivity and pain. Early complications include bruising, edema, infection, and vascular compromise. Late complications include HSV activation, visible irregularities, granuloma, and product migration. Untoward effects of HA can be treated with massage, warm compresses, and hyaluronidase.

REFERENCES

1. Glasgold AI, Glasgold MJ. Intraoperative custom contouring of the mandible. Arch Otolaryngol Head Neck Surg. 1994;120(2):180-4.
2. Mittelman H, Spencer JR, Chrzanowski DS. Chin region: management of grooves and mandibular hypoplasia with alloplastic implants. Facial Plast Surg Clin North Am. 2007;15(4):445-60, vi.
3. Romo T, Yalamanchili H, Sclafani AP. Chin and prejowl augmentation in the management of the aging jawline. Facial Plast Surg. 2005;21(1):38-46.
4. Shah FA, Ramakrishna S, Ingle V, et al. Treacher Collins syndrome with acute airway obstruction. Int J Pediat Otorhinolaryngol. 2000;54(1):41-3.
5. Zide BM, Pfeifer TM, Longaker MT. Chin surgery: I. Augmentation—the allures and the alerts. Plast Reconstr Surg. 1999;104(6):1843-53; discussion 61-2.
6. Sati S, Havlik RJ. An evidence-based approach to genioplasty. Plast Reconstr Surg. 2011;127(2):898-904.
7. Gui L, Huang L, Zhang Z. Genioplasty and chin augmentation with Medpore implants: a report of 650 cases. Aesthet Plast Surg. 2008;32(2):220-6.
8. Rosen HM. Aesthetic guidelines in genioplasty: the role of facial disproportion. Plast Reconstr Surg. 1995;95(3):463-9; discussion 70-2.
9. Saleh HA, Lohuis PJ, Vuyk HD. Bone resorption after alloplastic augmentation of the mandible. Clin Otolaryngol Allied Sci. 2002;27(2):129-32.
10. Guyuron B. MOC-PS(SM) CME article: genioplasty. Plast Reconstr Surg. 2008;121(4 suppl):1-7.

Self-Assessment Exercise

Q 1. Name four procedures used to address microgenia.
Ans:

A. Implants

B. Osseous genioplasty

C. Orthognathic surgery

D. Fillers

Q 2. What are the three paired muscles that make up the chin? What is their blood supply and innervation?
Ans:

A. Mentalis

B. Depressor labii inferioris

C. Depressor anguli oris

D. Innervation: motor—marginal branch of CNVII, sensory—inferior alveolar branch of CNV3

E. Blood supply—facial artery

Q 3. Osteotomies during genioplasty should be made where in relation to the mental foramen? Why?

Ans:

- At least a 5 mm distance inferiorly
- To avoid injury to the inferior alveolar nerve running through the mandibular canal 2–3 mm below the mental foramen.

Q 4. State three effects of aging on chin position.

Ans:

- Atrophy of alveolar ridge causes mental foramen to lie more superiorly
- Prejowl sulcus created from bone resorption laterally
- Decreased chin projection from bone resorption anteriorly.

Q 5. Name two congenital syndromes associated with microgenia.

Ans:

- Treacher-Collins syndrome
- Pierre Robin sequence.

Q 6. Describe two methods of assessing the chin in lateral view.

Ans:

- *Riedel's line:* A line drawn connecting the prominent portions of the upper and lower lips, extending to the most prominent portion of the menton
- *Gonzalez-Ulloa line:* A line drawn perpendicular to the Frankfort horizontal should transect the lips and pogonion.

Q 7. Describe the classification used for malocclusion.

Ans:

Angle classification:

- Class I: normal
- Class II: overbite—cusp lies anterior to buccal groove
- Class III: underbite—cusp lies posterior to buccal groove.

Q 8. Name the advantages and disadvantages of the intraoral approach.

Ans:

- Advantages: avoidance of external scar
- Disadvantages: imprecise reattachment of muscle (dental show), inability to stabilize implant and suture line irritation.

Q 9. Implants should be placed in what plane and why?

Ans: Supraperiosteal. Subperiosteal implant placement causes bone erosion in 50% of patients.

Q 10. What is the risk of permanent lip paresthesia after genioplasty? What procedures increase this risk?

Ans:

- 0.2% risk with isolated genioplasty
- Increases to 15% when combined with orthognathic surgery.

Multiple Choice Questions

Q 1. Which of the following statements defines the POGONION?

A. Anterior hairline at the midline
B. Lowest contour point of the chin
C. Anterior most point of the chin
D. Point of deepest depression at the root of the nose

Ans: C. Anterior most point of the chin

Q 2. The GNATHION is:

A. The depression at the root of the nose
B. The most prominent anterior projection of the chin
C. The lower border of the soft-tissue contour of the chin
D. The junction of the line tangential to the pogonion and the line tangential to the menton

Ans: D. The junction of the line tangential to the pogonion and the line tangential to the menton

Q 3. In a preoperative computer analysis a patient has a LEGAN angle of 20 degrees. Which of the following statements is TRUE?

A. There is poor nasal tip projection
B. There is adequate nasal tip projection
C. There is poor chin projection
D. There is adequate chin projection

Ans: C. There is poor chin projection

Q 4. Which of the following is REPRESENTED by the two lines in the drawing below?

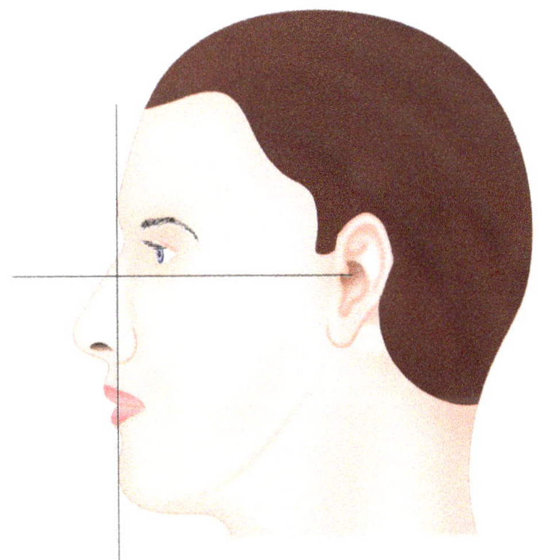

A. Appropriate chin position
B. Appropriate nose rotation
C. Appropriate nose projection
D. Appropriate nasion position

Ans: A. Appropriate chin position

Q 5. The drawing below represents a plane from the subnasale to the pogonium. Which of the following is the proper position of the lower lip and upper lip in relation to the mentioned plane?

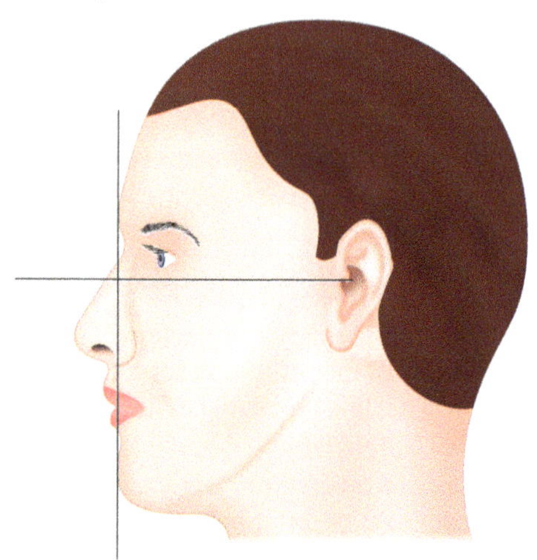

A. Upper lip 3.5 mm, lower lip 2.2 mm, both anteriorly
B. Upper lip 2.2 mm, lower lip 3.5 mm, both anteriorly
C. Upper lip 4.5 mm, lower lip 3.5 mm, both anteriorly
D. Upper lip 3.5 mm, lower lip 4.5 mm, both anteriorly

Ans: A. Upper lip 3.5 mm, lower lip 2.2 mm, both anteriorly

Q 6. Which of the following statement defines the "most anterior point of the chin soft tissue"?

A. Menton
B. Subnasale
C. Pogonion
D. Cervical point

Ans: C. Pogonion

Q 7. What is the following PERCENTAGE of patients will usually benefit from chin augmentation for better facial balance?

A. 1%
B. 5%
C. 10%
D. 20%

Ans: D. 20%

Q 8. Which of the following chin augmentation implants DOES NOT allow any fibrovascular in-growth?

A. Expanded polytetrafluoroethylene (ePTFE)
B. Polyamide mesh
C. Solid silicone rubber
D. Polyamide nylon mesh

Ans: C. Solid silicone rubber

Q 9. Which of the following areas represented in the drawing of the MOUTH below indicates the MESIAL side of the tooth?

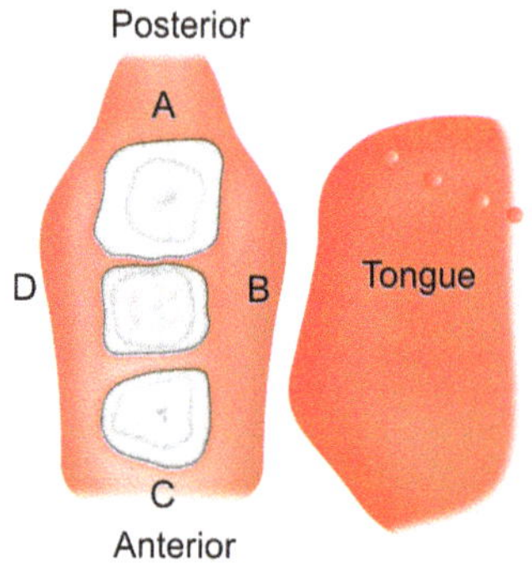

A. A
B. B
C. C
D. D

Ans: C.

Esthetic Facial Surgery

SECTION OUTLINES

Chapter 10

Rhytidectomy

Marie-Renee Atallah, Sami P Moubayed

■ INTRODUCTION

Rhytidectomy techniques have greatly evolved over the past hundred years. The following section reviews the basic principles behind each type of facelift.

■ RELEVANT ANATOMY[1-3]

Aging is influenced by various factors that cause characteristic features (Box 1): Gravity, heredity, malnutrition, sun exposure, and exposure to environmental toxins, such as smoking.[4,5] On the microscopic level, aging is associated with changes in all tissue layers. The skin loses its thickness and elasticity as the results of fragmentation of the dermal collagen matrix.[4] The youthful face is formed by several fat compartments, which are separated by septal barriers (Fig. 1). With aging, there is loss of volume and ptosis of fat compartments. Each independent fat compartment does not age at the same rate, thus altering its relation to the others and leading to the development of folds in the adjacent regions.[6] Change in facial shape and configuration is also associated with an increase in the tone of the facial mimetic muscles, causing rhytids. Finally, bone resorption participates in the remodeling of facial morphology.

Superficial Musculoaponeurotic System

To plan and perform rhytidectomy, rigorous knowledge of the facial anatomy is essential. The description of the superficial musculoaponeurotic system (SMAS) has led to the development of the current facelift techniques.[8,11] The SMAS is the third anatomic layer of the face, following skin and subcutaneous tissue. Facial muscles of expression form the muscular component of this layer. In the parotid region, the SMAS fuses with the zygomaticus major and buccinator muscles at the level of the modiolius. It also forms a connection with the levator labii superioris alaeque nasi muscle. In the neck, it is in continuity with the platysma muscle. Superiorly, at the level of the zygomatic arch, the SMAS become more fibrous in its consistency and adheres to the periosteum. Above this level, it is in the uninterrupted plane with the temporoparietal fascia, which joins the galea at the level of the scalp. In the cheek area, the SMAS is also fibrous in consistency and is thinner. It is discontinuous and has multiple attachments to the dermis. The SMAS is superficial to the parotidomasseteric fascia in the region of the cheek. In the temporal region, the deep temporal fascia lies underneath the temporoparietal fascia. This layer separates in two sheets at the level of the superior orbital margin,[9] forming an intermediate temporalis fascia. An intermediate temporal fat pad is located between the two sheets (Fig. 2).

Nerve Supply to the Face

The facial nerve innervates the facial muscles through their deep surfaces, except for the mentalis, buccinators, and levator anguli oris. The temporal branch provides the motor innervation to the forehead. It travels in the plane of the temporoparietal fascia. It can be visualized in the line extending from 0.5 cm below the tragus to 1.5 cm above the lateral brow. The zygomatic and buccal branches supply innervation to the midface muscles. The middle division branches of the facial nerve run 2.3 mm from the Zuker's

---

Box 1: Features of the aging patient

- Glabella frown lines
- Transverse forehead creases
- Temporal wasting
- Crow's feet
- Descent of lateral eyebrow
- Rounding of the palpebral fissure
- Elongation of the vertical aperture of the eye and scleral show
- Increased length of lower eyelid
- Laxity of the orbicularis retaining ligament, allowing pseudo-herniation of orbicular fat through orbital septum and causing double contour deformity
- Midface flattening
- Descent of malar fat pad
- Prominence of the nasolabial folds
- Melolabial fold
- Obtuse cervicomental angle
- Jowling
- Platysmal banding
- Skin laxity of the submental and neck region

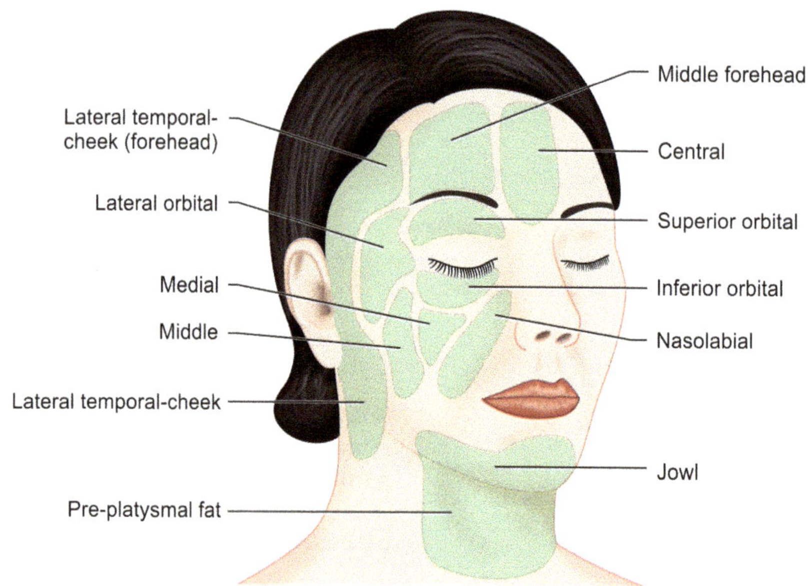

Fig. 1: Subcutaneous compartments of the face.

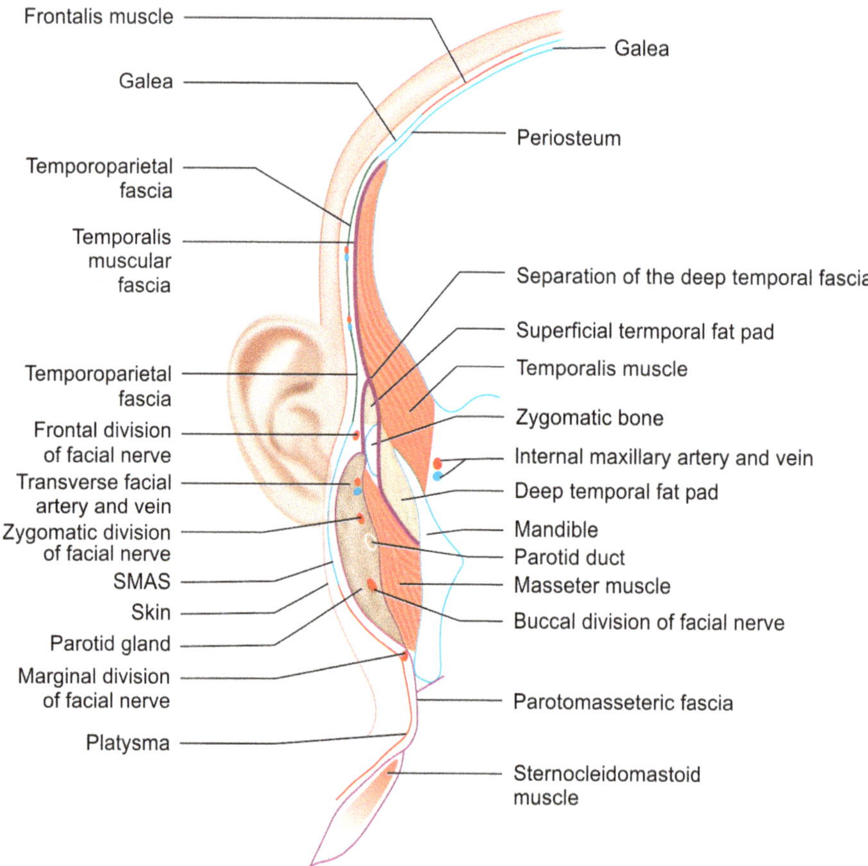

Fig. 2: Various factors of the fragmentation of dermal collagen matrix: septal barriers.

point, which is a surface landmark located midway between the root of the helix and the commissure of the mouth.[10] The zygomatic branch runs 1 cm below the zygomatic arch in the sub-SMAS plane toward the cheek. The buccal branch is also in this plane during its course toward the muscle of the lips. The marginal mandibular branch provides innervation to the lower face. After its exit from the parotid gland, it runs in the parotidomasseteric fascia until the angle of the mandible, where it continues its course in the subplatysmal plane. It curves to travel 1–2 cm below the body of the mandible and heads toward the chin,[11] but it has been described up to 4 cm to the lower angle of the mandible in some cases.[12,13]

The sensory innervation of the forehead is supplied by the terminal branches of the ophthalmic nerve (V_1), the supratrochlear nerve and the supraorbital nerves, which exit the skull by the foramen of the same name. The maxillary nerve (V_2) provides sensory innervation to the midface. Its terminal branches are the infraorbital nerve, which exit the skull by its own foramen in the maxilla, and the zygomaticotemporal branch, which comes out of the zygoma. The latter contributes to the innervation of the temporal region. The sensory innervation of the external ear is composed of the great auricular (C2-C3), lesser occipital (C2-C3), auriculotemporal (V_3) and Arnold's nerve (X).

Preoperative Assessment

Past medical history should be questioned for any conditions that could increase the operative risk or prolong the healing process. It includes screening for hypertension, smoking and any uncontrolled systemic disease. Medications and supplements that could impair blood clotting should be identified. The physician should then explore patient's motivation for facelift surgery. The objective is to identify which patients will most likely benefit from the surgery. A good candidate is a patient in a stable physical, psychological and emotional state.

Physical examination should start with the identification of the facial anatomic landmarks (Fig. 3). The height of face is divided in three-thirds, separated at the level of the glabella and the subnasale. Facial width is divided into five segments, separated by the lateral and medial canthus on both sides. Dedo's classification (Table 1) is used to describe the aging neck.

Skin should be evaluated in terms of skin-type, according to Fitzpatrick classification (Table 2) and photoaging, according to Glogau classification (Table 3). Photography is an essential tool in the preoperative assessment. It is helpful for surgical planning, but is also a powerful tool for patient education regarding what can be realistically expected considering his anatomy. The photographs should include a full-face frontal, right and left oblique, right and left lateral views and a close-up on each ear.[5]

Decision Making

Facelift is a procedure aiming to correct downward slope of facial structures. Good candidates for facelift include patients in their 40s with good skeletal structure and mild aging, primarily facial. However, facelift does not address changes in the skin, such as rhytids, and does not compensate for loss of volume. Combining rhytidectomy

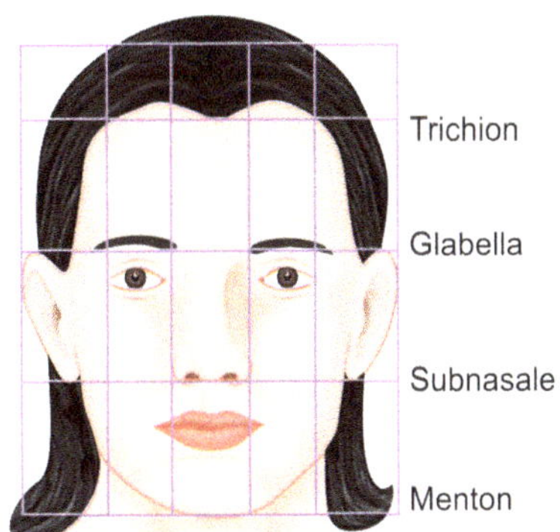

Fig. 3: Facial thirds and fifths

Table 1: Dedo classification[30]

Type	Characteristics
I	Minimal cosmetic deformity
II	Only skin laxity
III	Excessive cervical adipose tissue accumulation
IV	Platysmal banding
V	Microgenia or retrognathia
VI	Low positioned hyoid bone and obtuse cervicomental angle

Table 2: Fitzpatrick classification of skin type[31]

Skin type	Skin color	Characteristics
I	White	Always burns and severely, never tans
II	White	Usually burns, tans minimally with difficulty
III	White	Sometimes burns, tans moderately
IV	White	Rarely burns and minimally, tans very easily
V	Brown	Very rarely burns, tans very easily
VI	Dark brown or black	Never burns, always tans

Table 3: Glogau classification of photoaging[31]

Type	Age	Characteristics
I	20–30	No keratosis, few wrinkles, require no makeup
II	30–40	Early keratose, wrinkles on animation, requires little makeup
III	50–60	Advanced photoaging, wrinkles at rest, always require makeup
IV	60–70	Severe photoaging, severe wrinkles, poor benefits with makeup

with adjunctive procedures can contribute to achieve a more complete and satisfying facial rejuvenation.[17,31]

First of all, procedures such as chemical peel and laser resurfacing can be beneficial for treatment of the appearance of the skin. Secondly, utilization of fillers and autologous lipotransfer can address the issue of loss volume in the midface. Implants can be used for correction of loss of volume due to bone resorption and need for skeletal augmentation. They can be used for malar or chin augmentation. Finally, liposuction is used as adjunctive procedures to facelift in most patients in order to address excess of adipose tissue in the submental and neck region. Please refer to the specific sections of this book for the indications, contraindications, advantages, and disadvantages of each adjunctive procedure.

In adjunction to the procedures described in the next section, additional procedures can be done to improve the rejuvenation of the forehead and the neck regions.[18] The ptosis of the forehead can be addressed either by a subperiosteal or a subgaleal approach. The subperiosteal approach provides better long-term results.[19] Corset platysmaplasty is a procedure indicated for redundancy in the neck. The procedure starts with placement of an incision in the submental crease. Then, the subplatysmal fat is removed. The medial edges of the two platysma are sutured together from the level of the chin to the cricoid with an uninterrupted suture. This procedure achieves optimal contouring of the neck.

Surgical Approaches

Incision placement is different in male and female because of anatomic differences in the hair distribution. Incisions should always be placed in the axis of hair follicles to diminish risk of alopecia. Also, preauricular incision in female should be posttragal as it provides better camouflage of the scar. In males this portion of the incision is in the preauricular crease, with a small strip of preauricular hairless skin preserved. This prevents the displacement of hair in the external auditory canal postoperatively.

Skin Only

The first facelift technique consisted in subcutaneous undermining only. However, this technique is never indicated, because its results are limited, is associated with a high risk of skin slough, and high relapse rate.

Superficial Musculoaponeurotic System-lift

Patients with mild-to-moderate jowls and submental fat are ideal patients for SMAS-lift, combined with closed liposuction and wide subcutaneous undermining.[20] If platysmal bands are present, the procedure can be combined with anterior platysmaplasty.

The incision starts in the temporal area, posterior to the temporal hairline, heading toward the helix. The degree of angulation depends on the amount of planned lift. The incision is then extended anteriorly around the helix, following a natural skin crease. The preauricular incision is carried as described above. For patients with mild signs of aging, no retroauricular incision is needed and the incision ends at the base of the earlobe (mini-facelift). If a more significant lift is desired, the incision can be continued around the earlobe toward the postauricular sulcus. At the upper third of the auricle, the incision is curved posteroinferiorly, traversing the mastoid and continued in the occipital hairline. A subcutaneous skin flap is then elevated, by undermining in the temporal, cheek and jaw region. It is important in the temporal dissection to stay superficial to the superficial temporal fascia to avoid injury to the frontal branch of facial nerve.

The next step is lateral SMASectomy. The SMAS is incised from over the malar eminence to the angle of the mandible, parallel to the nasolabial fold, and the platysma is incised in continuity over a few centimeters until the anterior portion of the sternocleidomastoid muscle. In SMAS plication, the SMAS is folded on itself and sutured posteriorly without elevation of a sub-SMAS flap. In SMAS imbrication, a segment is resected depending of the degree of laxity and an undermining of the SMAS is done. It is then repositioned in a superoposterior vector and sutured, which achieve improvement of the neck, cervicomental angle, jowls and nasolabial fold.[21] Skin redraping is then performed, also superoposteriorly, which accomplishes correction of the midface and jowls.[22] The pre- and retroauricular skin is close with 5-0 nylon sutures, while the temporal and occipital incisions are closed with staples. A compressive dressing is made. The dressing and drains should be removed on postoperative day 1. Sutures are removed of postoperative day 5 and staples day 10.

Disadvantages of this technique include its longevity and a possible "operated appearance" following the procedure.

Deep Plane Lift

Hamra first described the deep plane lift in 1990. This type of lift confers a greater improvement of the melolabial fold and the midface.

The incision for deep plane lift is the same as for SMAS-lift, although the retroauricular incision is always performed.[1] There is significantly less elevation of the subcutaneous flap—it is elevated only the necessary distance required for skin resection. The SMAS is incised in a line parallel to the skin incision, starting from lateral canthus downward to the angle of the mandible. The sub-SMAS dissection is more extensive. In the parotid area, it is important to stay superficial to the parotidomasseteric fascia to avoid injury to the facial nerve. In the cheek area, the plane of dissection is superficial to the zygomatic muscles, which achieves the release of the dermal attachments of the malar eminence. The sub-SMAS dissection is then continued inferiorly, connecting with the subplatysmal plane. No dissection below the angle of the mandible is necessary. The flap is then suspended and mobilized as needed and closure is executed as above. This technique should be performed by an experienced surgeon, because it carries a higher risk to the facial nerve.

Composite Lift

Hamra further introduced the composite rhytidectomy. Its purpose is to correct three ptotic areas: (1) the SMAS, (2) jugal fat and (3) orbicularis oculi muscle. This technique allows mobilization of these deep structures of the face, while maintaining their anatomic relationship, thus resulting in a more natural appearance. The composite rhytidectomy is a bipedicled flap based of the angular, infraorbital and facial arteries.[24] The first step of the procedure consists of a lower lid blepharoplasty incision, elevation of orbicularis oris muscle flap and advancement in superomedial direction. The next steps are the same as in deep plane technique. The deep dissection is carried with the formation of a communication between the facelift and blepharoplasty dissection. The principal disadvantages of this procedure are the risk for lid malposition, ectropion and prolonged edema.

Periosteal Lift

The subperiosteal lift is used to address ptosis of the superior and middle third of the face. It can be carried out with open (modification of craniofacial approach) or endoscopic techniques. The dissection is in the subperiosteal plane over the scalp and the midface. In the temporal area, the dissection is in the plane of the deep temporal fascia. The advantage of this plane of dissection is that it is avascular and far from the plane of the facial nerve.[19] The flap is then repositioned in a superolateral fashion.

■ COMPLICATIONS

Hematoma

Hematoma is a dreaded complication that can lead to slough and prolonged recovery. The incidence of postoperative hematoma varies between 1% and 15%[26] and the rate of large, expending hematomas requiring surgical intervention varies between 25% and 7%.[27] Most postoperative hematomas develop within 24 hours of the surgery. Expanding and large hematomas should be promptly recognized, and require surgical reintervention for clot evacuation and control of bleeding. Minor collections can be managed with aspiration or by milking of the hematoma.

Perioperative high blood pressure, especially systolic, is a major risk factor for the formation of hematoma. Control of hypertension should be obtained prior to the surgery. Perioperative monitoring of blood pressure is crucial. Efforts should be made to reduce contribution factors, such as retching, vomiting, pain, cough, and agitation.

Male gender is also another important risk factor for hematoma, increasing the risk by twofold.[28] It is believed that males have thicker dermis, containing more hair follicles and sebaceous glands, thus having greater vascularization.[26,29]

In comparing surgical techniques, a meta-analysis including 41 studies concluded that limited facelift procedures are significantly less prone to formation of expanding hematoma compared to extended procedures.[30] However, there was no statistical difference in the rate of expanding hematoma between the techniques (SMAS flap, SMAS plication, and deep-plane). A retrospective study on 1,078 patients showed increased hematoma risk with anterior platysmaplasty.[28,30] Use of aspirin, NSAIDs or LMWH and smoking are other risk factors. Drains and tissue adhesives do not decrease risk of hematoma.[30]

Infections

Wound infection occurs in less than 1% of cases[26,28] and result in delayed healing. Unilateral erythema, edema and pain should raise the suspicion of an infection. Cellulitis should be treated with antibiotics, with coverage for *Staphyloccocus* and *Steptococcus*. Abscesses should be incised and drained. There is no consistent evidence regarding the role of perioperative antibiotics.[28]

Sensory Nerve Damage

Most sensory nerve injuries are associated with terminal branches, causing transient numbness. They last 8–12 weeks, but in some cases can persist until 1 year following the operation.

Damage to the great auricular nerve during rhytidectomy occurs between 1% and 7%,[26] making it the most commonly injured nerve during facelift. Its injury causes paresthesia or anesthesia in the lower half of the ear. Care should be taken when dissecting in the subplatysmal plane over the sternocleidomastoid muscle to avoid injury to the great auricular nerve.

Motor Nerve Damage

Injury to the facial nerve is the most serious complication of facelift, with an incidence of 0.3%–2.6%.[26,11] The associated paresis of the facial expression muscles is most often temporary resulting from neuropraxia, although permanent paralysis can occur following transection of the nerve. To avoid injury to the marginal mandibular branch, care should be taken when dissecting in the subplatysmal plane below the angle of the mandible, as it is located just beneath the platysma in this area. The limits of the danger zone for marginal mandibular nerve injury are: the angle of the mandible laterally, the oral commissure medially and from the mandible border to a parallel line three centimeters below. Injury to the temporal branch occurs primarily when facelift is combined with a forehead procedure. Injury to the buccal branch can occur with sub-SMAS dissection of the cheek during midface-lift.[26]

Seroma and Prolonged Edema

Seromas have an incidence of 2%[5] and usually occur between the 5th and the 7th postoperative day. They should be treated with aspiration to avoid prolongation of the healing process, and application of a pressure dressing. Utilization of drains and fibrin glue can help decrease their formation. Prolonged edema can result from subperiosteal dissection, thus is often associated with endoscopic technique. It can last up to 4–6 weeks. It can also occur following evacuation of a hematoma.

Skin Slough

Skin slough is a dreaded complication, because it leads to unfavorable scarring. The most frequent location is the retroauricular area. Its incidence is 1–3%.[26] The most important risk factor for skin slough is smoking, with an incidence in smokers up to 19.4%.[32] Smoking causes irreversible occlusive changes in the microcirculation of the dermis, thus leading to skin necrosis. All patients should be advised to stop all nicotine products at least 2 weeks before the surgery for better results. Other important risk factors for skin slough include extensive undermining and wound closure with excessive tension. Prompt management of hematomas can also help reduce the occurrence of skin slough. Almost all cases can be managed conservatively, with reepithelialization by secondary intention.

Pigment Changes

Skin hypopigmentation can result from skin necrosis, excessive tension on wound closure and electrocauterization of the dermis. Hyperpigmentation results from the inflammatory process. It can last several months, but is always a temporary. Risk factors include Fitzpatrick skin type IV to VI and postoperative sun exposure. When rhytidectomy is combined with laser skin resurfacing, incidence of hyperpigmentation is 6–30%.[33]

■ DISSATISFIED PATIENT

It is crucial to build a strong patient-relationship in order to earn each patient's trust. The most effective way to do so is to listen to the patient and be attentive to her or his concerns. It is essential to seek patient motivation for surgery, which will help to identify which patient will most likely benefit from the surgery. Patient education is also necessary in order to establish realistic postoperative goals. Procedures and expected results should be properly explained to the patients to diminish the risk of dissatisfaction. Also, patients with specific risk factors for complications should be warned of its increased risk and management in such case should be explained. Longevity of the expected results should be addressed. Choice of procedures should be based on patient anatomy and surgeon preference.

■ REFERENCES

1. Adamson PA, Litner JA. Evolution of rhytidectomy techniques. Facial Plast Surg Clin North Am. 2005;13:383-91.

2. Pasha R, Golub JS. Otolaryngology Head and Neck Surgery: Clinical Reference Guide, 4th edition. San Diego: Plural Publishing Inc; 2013.

3. Janfaza P, Nadol JB Jr, Galla RJ, et al. Surgical Anatomy of the Head and Neck. United Kingdom: Harvard University Press; 2011.

4. Fitzgerald R, Graivier MH, Kane M, et al. Update on facial aging. Aesthet Surg J. 2010;30 Suppl:11S-24S.

5. Cheng ET, Perkins SW. Rhytidectomy analysis: twenty years of experience. Facial Plast Surg Clin North Am. 2005;13:15-31.

6. Rohrich RJ, Pessa JE. The fat compartments of the face: anatomy and clinical implications for cosmetic surgery. Plast Reconstr Surg. 2007;119:2219-27.

7. Gassner HG, Rafil A, Young A, et al. Surgical anatomy of the face: implications for modern face-lift techniques. Arch Facial Plast Surg. 2008;10:9-19.

8. Owsley JQ. Face lift. Plast Reconstr Surg. 1997;100:514-9.

9. Quatela VC, Onley DR. Management of the midface. Facial Plast Surg Clin North Am. 2006;14:213-20.

10. Dorafshar AH, Borsuk DE, Bojovic B, et al. Surface anatomy of the middle division of the facial nerve: Zuker's point. Plast Reconstr Surg. 2013;131:253-7.

11. Shadfar S, Perkins SW. Anatomy and physiology of the aging neck. Facial Plast Surg Clin North Am. 2014;22:161-70.

12. Wang TM, Lin CL, Kuo KJ, et al. Surgical anatomy of the mandibular ramus of the facial nerve in Chinese adults. Acta Anat (Basel). 1991;142:126-31.

13. Baker DC, Conley J. Avoiding facial nerve injuries in rhytidectomy. Anatomical variations and pitfalls. Plast Reconstr Surg. 1979;64:781-95.

14. Johnson JT, Rosen CA. Bailey's Head and Neck Surgery Otolaryngology, 5th edition. Philadelphia: Wolters Kluwer; 2014.

15. Flint PW, Haughey BH, Lund VJ, et al. Cummings Otolaryngology Head and Neck surgery, 6th edition. Philadelphia: Saunders Elsevier; 2015.

16. Chung KC, Gosain Ak, Gurtner GC, et al. Grabb and Smith's Plastic Surgery, 7th edition. Philadelphia: Wolters Kluwer; 2014.

17. DeFatta RJ, Williams EF 3rd. Evolution of midface rejuvenation. Arch Facial Plast Surg. 2009;11:6-12.

18. Hudson DA. An Analysis of unsolved problems of face-lift procedures. Ann Plast Surg. 2010;65:266-9.

19. Baker DC. Lateral SMASectomy, plication and short scar facelifts: indications and techniques. Clin Plast Surg. 2008;35:533-50.

20. Henderson J, O'Neill T, Logan A. Direct anterior neck skin excision for cervicomental laxity. Aesthetic Plast Surg. 2010;34:299-305.

21. Stallworth CL, Wang TD. Fat grafting of the midface. Facial Plast Surg. 2010;26:369-75.

22. Moyer JS, Baker SR. Complications of rhytidectomy. Facial Plast Surg Clin North Am. 2005;13:469-78.

23. Beer GM, Goldscheider E, Weber A, et al. Prevention of acute hematoma after face-lifts. Aesthetic Plast Surg. 2010;34:502-7.

24. Chang S, Pusic A, Rohrich RJ. A systematic review of comparison of efficacy and complication rates among face-lift techniques. Plast Reconstr Surg. 2011;127:423-33.

25. Lawson W, Naidu RK. The male facelift: an analysis of 115 cases. Arch Otolaryngol Head Neck Surg. 1993;119:535-9.

26. Mustoe TA, Park E. Evidence-based medicine: face lift. Plast Reconstr Surg. 2014;133:1206-13.
27. DeFatta RJ, Williams EF 3rd. Midface lifting: current standards. Facial Plast Surg. 2011;27:77-85.
28. Guyuron B. An evidenced-based approach to face lift. Plast Reconstr Surg. 2010;126:2230-3.
29. Brackup AB. Combined cervicofacial rhytidectomy and laser skin resurfacing. Ophthal Plast Reconstr Surg. 2002; 18:24-39.
30. Dedo DD. "How I do it"—plastic surgery. Practical suggestions on facialplastic surgery. A preoperative classification of the neck for cervicofacial rhytidectomy . Laryngoscope. 1980;90(11 Pt 1):1894-6
31. Fitzpatrick TB. The validity and practicality of sun-reactive skin types Ithrough VI. Arch Dermatol. 1988;124(6):869-71.

Self-Assessment Exercise

Q 1. Aging affects what tissue layers?

Ans: All tissue layers: skin, fat, muscle and bone.

Q 2. Which facelift types carry the highest risk for facial nerve injury?

Ans: Deep plane and composite rhytidectomy.

Q 3. Name three characteristic features in the midface of the aging patient.

Ans:
Elongation of vertical aperture of the eye and scleral show
Increased length of the lower eyelid
Pseudoherniation of orbital fat
Descent of malar fat pad
Midface flattening
Prominence of the nasolabial folds

Q 4. What are the limits of the danger zone for injury of the marginal mandibular nerve (VII)?

Ans:
Lateral: angle of the mandible
Medial: oral commissure
Superior: Body of mandible
Inferior: Line 3 cm parallel and below mandible

Q 5. What are the two most important risk factors for acute hematomas?

Ans: Hypertension and male gender.

Multiple Choice Questions

Q 1. The Satyr's ear (Devil's ear) deformity is BEST treated with:

A. Excision and primary closure   B. Transposition flap
C. V-Y plasty   D. Z-plasty

Ans: C. V-Y plasty

Q 2. A-50-year-old female underwent rhytidectomy and blepharoplasty procedures with local anesthesia and I.V. sedation. The next day postoperative, less than 24 hours after the surgical procedure, the patients have noted to have a right-sided paralysis of the temporal branch of the facial nerve. The BEST immediate treatment is:

A. Reassurance
B. Corticosteroids
C. Immediate exploration and direct anastomosis with microscope assistance
D. Immediate exploration and direct anastomosis without microscope assistance

Ans: A. Reassurance

Q 3. Which of the following statements regarding the indications for rhytidectomy is FALSE?

A. Rhytidectomy will correct ptosis of the jowl
B. Rhytidectomy will correct blunting of the cervicomental angle
C. Rhytidectomy will correct the wrinkles and creases of facial skin
D. Rhytidectomy will be most helpful in patients with a high posterior hyoid bone

Ans: C. Rhytidectomy will correct the wrinkles and creases of facial skin

Q 4. Which of the following statements about rhytidectomy is TRUE?

A. In men the posttragal incision is preferable
B. In women the pretragal incision is preferable
C. A well executed standard rhytidectomy will correct nasolabial folds
D. A strong jawline and cheek bones and a high posterior hyoid bone are the ideal

Ans: D. A strong jawline and cheek bones and a high posterior hyoid bone are the ideal

Q 5. Which of the following is MOST commonly associated with flap necrosis in rhytidectomy?

A. Smoking history
B. SMAS rhytidectomy
C. SMAS rhytidectomy with plication technique
D. Excessive pressure applied by postoperative facial bandage

Ans: A. Smoking history

Q 6. Which of the following IS INCORRECT postoperative rhytidectomy procedure?

A. The surgeon checks on the patient the night of the surgery
B. Unilateral facial pain is considered a warning sign
C. The first visit with the patient is on the second postoperative day
D. The preauricular sutures are removed on the fifth day postoperative day

Ans: C. The first visit with the patient is on the second postoperative day

Q 7. Which of the following features indicate POOR candidacy for rhytidectomy?

A. Minimal photoaging
B. Shallow cheek-lip grooves
C. Acute cervicomental angle
D. Shallow cheek bones

Ans: D. Shallow cheek bones

Q 8. Which of the following statements about complications after facelift is FALSE?

A. Male patients have a higher incidence of hematoma
B. Deep plane facelift has a higher incidence of hematoma formation
C. Infection is most commonly associated with hematoma
D. Infection is most commonly related to *Staphylococus aureus*

Ans: B. Deep plane facelift has a higher incidence of hematoma formation

Q 9. The MAJORITY of hematomas after rhytidectomy presents WITHIN:

A. The first 4 hours
B. The first 6 hours
C. The first 12 hours
D. The first 24 hours

Ans: D. The first 24 hours

Q 10. Which of the following conditions is BEST improved by Rhytidectomy?

A. Ptosis of the jowl
B. Fine creases and deep rhytids of the skin
C. Malar ptosis
D. Wrinkles related to facial expressions

Ans: A. Ptosis of the jowl

Q 11. Which of the following measures or drugs should NOT be discontinued prior to rhytidectomy?

A. Statins
B. Aspirin
C. Steroids
D. Vitamin E

Ans: A. Statins

Q 12. Which of the following statements regarding rhytidectomy is TRUE?

A. Imbrication involves folding the SMAS fascia on itself and securing it with a permanent buried suture.
B. Plication involves incision, resection of the SMAS fascia and reapproximation of the cut SMAS fascia edges with a permanent buried suture.
C. Imbrication offers better and longer lasting results than plication
D. Imbrication carries a greater chance for surgical morbidity than plication

Ans: D. Imbrication carries a greater chance for surgical morbidity than plication

Q 13. A patient has a pathologic platysma muscle accentuation with banding noted in repose. Which of the following is the proper classification of these cervical abnormalities?

A. Class II
B. Class III
C. Class IV
D. Class V

Ans: C. Class IV

Q 14. In which of the following areas will DEEP PLANE RHYTIDECTOMY address PRIMARILY THE LAXITY problem?

A. Submental area
B. Platysma area
C. Buccolabial area
D. Submandibular area

Ans: C. Buccolabial area

Q 15. Which of the following statements about cervicofacial rhytidectomy is FALSE?

A. Flap elevation is done in the superficial subcutaneous plane
B. Plication and Imbrication will decrease closing tension on the skin flap
C. Skin redraping has a superior-posterior component
D. Suctioning has proven better than penrose drains with compression dressings

Ans: D. Suction drainage has been proven better than penrose drains with compression dressings

Q 16. Which of the following anatomical areas is the most common place in which minor skin sloughing occurring after facelift procedure and not related to an unrecognized hematoma?

A. Temporal area
B. Preauricular area
C. Lobule area
D. Mastoid area

Ans: D. Mastoid area

Q 17. Which of the following measurements can reduce the incidence of hematoma formation in male rhytidectomy?

A. Use of vasoconstriction infiltration in the surgical wound
B. Use of suctioning systems rather than penrose drains
C. Meticulous perioperative blood pressure control and monitoring
D. Heavy smoking history

Ans: C. Meticulous perioperative blood pressure control and monitoring

Q 18. Which of the following factors is the GREATEST contributor to skin necrosis after facelift surgery?

A. Smoking
B. Diabetes mellitus
C. Arteriosclerosis
D. Previous radiation therapy to the head and neck

Ans: A. Smoking

Q 19. Which one of the following complications related to the Deep-Plane Rhytidectomy has been found in higher frequency than that found with more superficial Rhytidectomy?

A. Hematoma
B. Infection
C. Skin necrosis
D. Facial nerve injury

Ans: D. Facial nerve injury

Q 20. Which of the following sutures is related "to sutures that cause a flap or edge of SMAS tissues to overlap deeper structures and even other SMAS elements" and are used in Facelift Procedures?

A. Plicating sutures
B. Imbricating sutures
C. Suspending sutures
D. Gilles sutures

Ans: B. Imbricating sutures

Q 21. Which of the following is related to Composite Rhytidectomy?

A. Musculocutaneous flap containing both platysma muscle and cheek fat

B. Musculocutaneous flap containing both platysma muscle and oris muscle

C. Musculocutaneous flap contains both orbicularis oculi and oris muscle

D. Musculocutenous flap containing orbicularis oculi, cheek fat, and platysma muscle

Ans: D. Musculocutenous flap containing orbicularis oculi, cheek fat, and platysma muscle

Q 22. In performing a composite rhytidectomy the proper plane of dissection will be ON TOP of which of the following anatomical structures?

A. Masseter muscle

B. Orbicularis oculi muscle

C. Orbicularis oris muscle

D. Zygomatic major and minor muscles

Ans: D. Zygomatic major and minor muscles

Q 23. Which of the following areas is MOST commonly complicated by skin flap necrosis in rhytectomy?

A. Temporal

B. Preauricular

C. Postauricular

D. Midcheek

Ans: C. Postauricular

Q 24. Which of the following in NOT considered a favorable characteristic in a female facelift candidate?

A. Strong forward chin

B. Minimal photo-aging

C. Low hyoid bone

D. Prominent cheek structure

Ans: C. Low hyoid bone

Q 25. A 51-year-old female actress in good general health is requesting a rhytidectomy. She has a strong jawline, well defined cheek bones, low seated submandibular glands, a high posterior hyoid bone and a thin neck skin with the expected photoaging for her age. Which of the following is NOT considered IDEAL in this patient?

A. High posterior hyoid bone

B. Low seated submandibular glands

C. Shape of the cheek bone

D. Thickness of skin

Ans: B. Low seated submandibular glands

Q 26. Which of the following face and neck abnormalities of aging is BEST corrected by the Rhytidectomy?

A. Cervico-mental angle

B. Deep nasolabial folds

C. Lateral perioral jowling

D. Orbicularis oculi muscle ptosis

Ans: A. Cervico-mental angle

Q 27. Which of the following statements is NOT improved by a facelift procedure?

A. Ptosis of the jowl

B. Cervicomental angle

C. Malar fat pad ptosis

D. Turkey gobbler deformity

Ans: C. Malar fat pad ptosis

Q 28. Which of the following complications in rhytidectomy and its incidence is TRUE?

A. Facial nerve palsy (0.8%)

B. Hematoma (1%)

C. Skin slough (15%)

D. Alopecia (10%)

Ans: A. Facial nerve palsy (0.8%)

Q 29. If you compare the classic rhytidectomy procedure versus the deep plane rhytidectomy, the DEEP PLANE rhytidectomy will have a lower incidence of:

A. Deformity of the ear lobe

B. Nerve paresis

C. Hematoma

D. Infection

Ans: C. Hematoma

Q 30. Which of the following statements is FALSE in rhytidectomy?

A. Rhytidectomy mainly corrects ptosis of the jowl

B. Pretragal location of the incision is preferable in women

C. Rhytidectomy will not decrease prominent nasolabial folds

D. Preserving the anterior hair tuft is fundamental in women

Ans: B. Pretragal location of the incision is preferable in women

Q 31. A 47-year-old woman is complaining of the gradual onset of bilateral facial masses, left greater than right, over several years. No other complaints are reported. The physical examination revealed bilateral, well-demarcated, walnut-sized masses located in the lower cheek area above the jowl. The most common successful management of this condition is:

A. Deep plane face lift

B. Excision of the enlarged nasolabial folds

C. Intraoral buccal lipectomy

D. Midface lift

Ans: C. Intraoral buccal lipectomy

Q 32. Which of the following midface muscles is critical in the effective rejuvenation/reposition of the mid-face?

A. Orbicularis oculi muscle

B. Zygomatic major muscle

C. Levator labii superioris muscle

D. Masseter muscle

Ans: A. Orbicularis oculi muscle

Chapter 11

Blepharoplasty

Angelique P Berens, Sapna A Patel, Grace Wandell

■ ANATOMY

Musculature (Figures 1A and B)

- *Frontalis* brow elevator.
- *Procerus:* Inferior brown displacement. Horizontal glabellar wrinkles.
- *Corrugator supercilii:* Inferior-medial brow movement. Vertical glabellar wrinkles.
- *Orbicularis oculi:* Pretarsal (controls blink), preseptal, and orbital (voluntary closure).
  - Lateral control tendon: Attaches lateral orbicularis to tubercle of Whitnall
  - Medial canthal tendon: Pretarsal orbicularis tendon attachment anteriorly to anterior lacrimal crest and posteriorly to posterior lacrimal crest.

Orbital Septum

Originates at arcus marginalis, fuses with levator aponeurosis (upper) or capsulopalpebral fascia (lower) to insert on tarsal plate. Separates anterior and posterior lamella.
- Anterior lamella: Skin and orbicularis
- Posterior lamella: Tarsus and conjunctiva

Fat Compartments and Lacrimal Gland (Fig. 2)

Fat pads lie deep to orbital septum.
- *Upper lid (two fat pads):*
  - Lateral compartment occupied by lacrimal gland
  - Medial and central fat pads separated by trochlea
- *Lower lid (three fat pads):*
  - Medial, central, and lateral
  - Inferior oblique separates medial and central
  - Arcuate expansion of Lockwood's ligament separates central and lateral fat pads.
- *Lacrimal gland:* Superolateral in upper lid; pink and firm.
- *Accessory fat pad:* Variably found behind the orbital septum. May contribute to a lateral bulge.
- *Midface fat:*
  - *Subcutaneous malar fat pad:* Superficial to orbicularis.
  - *Suborbicularis oculi fat (SOOF):* Deep to orbicularis.

Eyelid

- *Upper eyelid retractors (Figure 3A):*
  - *Levator palpebrae superioris:* Splits into levator aponeurosis anteriorly and Müller's muscle posteriorly

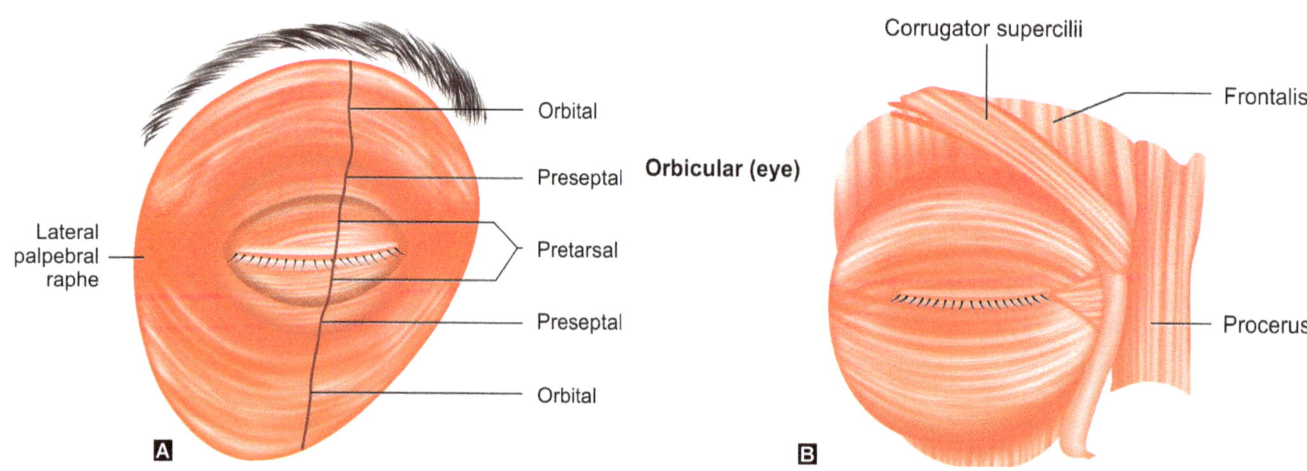

Figs. 1A and B: Ocular musculature

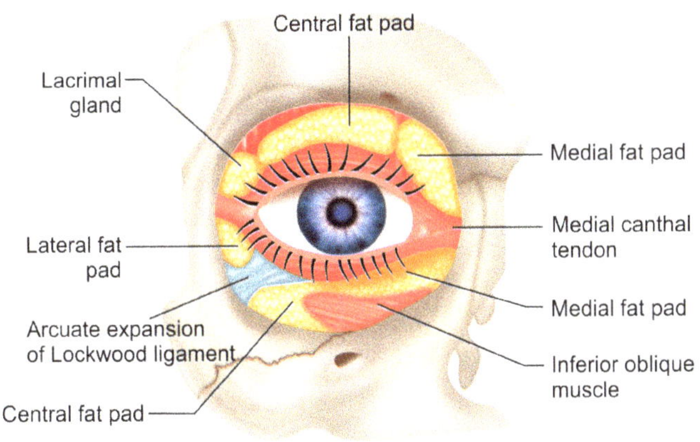

Fig. 2: Fat compartments

– *Whitnall ligament*: Refers to levator aponeurosis superior to tarsus and serves to support levator muscle.
– *Müller muscle's*: Attaches to the superior tarsal plate. Sympathetic innervation. Retracts lid 2 mm.
– Levator aponeurosis: Fuses with orbital septum and dermis to define upper-eyelid crease, also attaches to canthal tendons, orbicularis oculi and tarsal plate.
– Upper lid crease: Formed by insertion of levator aponeurosis into dermis (after traveling through orbicularis oculi). 8–10 mm above lash margin in Caucasians and 4–6 mm in Asians. Absence of crease in Asians due to levator insertion onto septum and not into dermis, which allows orbital fat to travel anteriorly.
- *Lower eyelid retractors*:
  – *Capsulopalpebral fascia* (Figure 3B) Inferior rectus fascia to the inferior tarsal border. Similar to levator aponeurosis of upper lid.
  – *Inferior tarsal muscle*: Undersurface of capsulopalpebral fascia to the lower lid conjunctiva. Sympathetic innervation.

– *Arcuate expansion (Lockwood's ligament)*: Fascial band extending from the capsulopalpebral fascia to the inferolateral orbital rim. Suspensory ligament of eyeball.
- *Tarsal plates*:
  – *Superior tarsus*: 10 mm in Caucasians; 4 mm in Asians.
  – *Lower tarsus*: 4–6 mm.
- *Lateral canthus*: Retinaculum of the levator aponeurosis, lateral orbicularis oculi, Lockwood's ligament, and the check ligament of the lateral rectus.

Innervation

- *Sensory*:
  – *Ophthalmic division (CNV)*: Splits into lacrimal and frontal nerves.
  – *Lacrimal nerve*: Conjunctivae and upper eyelid.
  – *Frontal nerve*: Further divides to supratrochlear nerve and supraorbital nerve.
    » Supratrochlear nerve: Conjunctivae, upper eyelids, and inferomedial forehead.
    » Supraorbital nerve: Upper lid, forehead, and anterior scalp.
- *Motor*:
  – *CNIII*: Levator palpebrae superioris.
  – *Temporal division of CNVII*: Supplies orbicularis oculi and frontalis along their deep surfaces. Over the zygomatic arch, commonly lies within or just deep to the superficial musculoaponeurotic system (SMAS).

Blood Supply

- *Ophthalmic artery [internal carotid artery (ICA)]*: Branches into frontal, supraorbital and supratrochlear arteries.

■ PERIORBITAL CHANGES WITH AGING

- *Features of youthful periorbita*: High volume, crisp upper eyelid crease in a low position, higher eyebrows

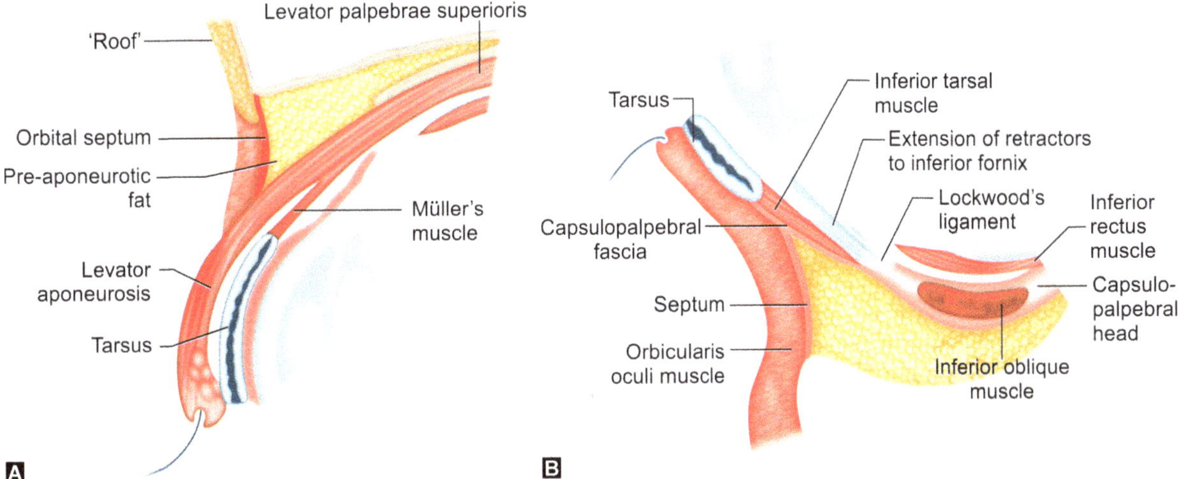

Figs. 3A and B: (A) Upper lip cross-sectional anatomy; (B) lower lip cross-sectional anatomy

typically at the level of the orbital rim for males and above the orbital rim for females.

- *Festoons*: Lower lid orbicularis oculi folds create a hammock-like bag due to weak orbital septum.
- *Malar bags*: Folds of soft tissue only (vs festoons).
- *Tear trough triad*:
  1. *Lower fat herniation (steatoblepharon)*: Due to weakening of orbital septum and Lockwood's suspensory ligament.
  2. *Orbital rim depression*: Due to arcus marginalis fusion.
  3. *Malar retrusion causing orbital rim depression*: Deficit of tissue below the orbital rim.
- *Double contour*: Due to juxtaposition of prolapsed lower lid orbital fat and fallen malar fat pad with orbital rim in between.
- *Brow descent*
- *Crease changes*: Elevated upper eyelid crease due degenerating tarsal-levator sling. Deep, hollow upper eyelid sulcus. Crease obscured by redundant tissue.
- *Dermatochalasis*: Loss of skin elasticity with prolapsed orbital fat.

■ ASSOCIATED CONDITIONS

- *Collagen vascular disease*: Interferes with glandular lubrication (Ehlers-Danlos syndrome, Sjogren's syndrome, lupus, scleroderma, etc.).
- *Myxedema and hypothyroidism*: Mimics dermatochalasis and baggy eye; need to rule out prior to blepharoplasty.
- *Graves' disease*: Infiltrative ophthalmopathy results in vertical eyelid retraction and inadequate corneal protection after surgery.
- *Blepharochalasis*: Younger-middle aged females. Recurrent attacks of painless unilateral or bilateral lid edema. Approach blepharoplasty with caution.

■ PREOPERATIVE ASSESSMENT

A complete medical history with special attention to a history of ocular disease, glaucoma, glasses contacts, ophthalmic drops should be discussed and documented.

- *Schirmer test*: Assesses dry eyes. Filter paper positioned over lateral lid margin and the distance between wet line of strip and lid is measured after 5 minutes. Abnormal (tear deficiency) is less than 5 mm. 10 mm of wet line on the paper is considered the minimal value for this test.
- *Bell's phenomenon:* While holding lids open assess.
- *Lagophthalmos:* Inability to close the eyelids (see complication below)
- *Brow position*: Palpate to determine location. If the central brow is at or below the orbital rim suggests need for browlift prior to blepharoplasty.
- *Ptosis*:
  - *Margin-reflex distance (MRD-1):* Distance between corneal light reflex and upper lid margin (normal is between 3 mm and 4.5 mm).
  - *Levator function:* Distance of upper lid movement during upward and downward gaze (normal > 12 mm).
- *Skin type*:
  - *Thin skin*: Conservative removal of fat.
  - *Thick skin*: More fat/muscle excision to improve definition of superior orbital sulcus.
- *Pinch test*: Grasp redundant skin with forceps. With the lower blade of the forceps on the mark of the natural skin crease, ensure the lid does not open to determine skin excision.
- *Distraction (snap) test* : Pull lower lid out. Abnormal is more than 10 mm of displacement. Release lid and should "snap" back in less than 2 seconds. Risk of ectropion or scleral show. May benefit from lid tightening.
- *Retraction test*: Pull lower lid down and observe recoil. Tests lax canthal tendon.
- *Abnormal test*: Little or no recoil, puncta displacement of more than 3 mm. Patient may benefit from a tendoplication to prevent ectropion.
- *Scleral show*: May indicate need for lid tightening or tendoplication procedure.
- *Eye prominence*: Measured via exophthalmometry.
- *Negative vector*: Anterior portion of globe protrudes past malar eminence predicts a high risk for complications in lower lid blepharoplasty.
- Standard preoperative photos: Close up frontal with eyes open, closed and looking up, close up oblique, and close up lateral right and left.

■ SURGICAL TECHNIQUES

Upper Lid Blepharoplasty

- *Indications*: Improve appearance and/or peripheral vision. Address before lower lid to avoid lagophthalmos.
- *Disadvantages*:
  - Deep or hollow upper eyelid sulci may be worsened with brow ptosis.
  - Hypopigmented upper crease scar, especially if globe is prominent.

Surgical Technique

- Mark supratarsal crease as the inferior incision in an awake patient (8–12 mm from lid margin) and extend from orbital rim and just lateral to puncta. Use green forceps for pinch test to estimate how much skin can be removed without causing lid eversion.
  - In general maintain 10–12 mm from brow. The medial and lateral ends should form a roughly 30° angle.
- Inject local anesthesia (Wydase + 1–2 mL local) to the subcutaneous space to create a plane of dissection and decrease bruising.
- Excision can be skin alone or minimal excision of orbicularis oculi inferiorly to recreate a distinct upper eyelid. Fat typically protrudes in medial pocket and a

small amount of medial orbicularis oculi is resected. Gentle pressure is applied superior to incision to determine how much fat needs to be excised. A small amount of fat is clamped and snipped with the stub cauterized. Avoid the lacrimal gland.

- Hemostasis using bipolar electrocautery.
- Approximate skin with 6-0 prolene in subcuticular fashion and 3 simple interrupted. Remove sutures in 5–7 days to avoid track marks.

Eyelid Ptosis repair: *Performed during upper eyelid blepharoplasty if indicated.*

Technique:

- Grasp lower edge of incision with Castroviejo forceps. Dissect pretarsal orbicularis to expose tarsal plate and remove strip of orbicularis.
- Open orbital septum medially and laterally.
- Identify levator aponeurosis via gentle cotton tip dissection by first visualizing the preaponeurotic fat pad (posterior to septum and anterior to levator).
- Insert a Desmarres retractor to expose the levator aponeurosis. To confirm finding the levator, if the patient is awake, the surgeon can have them look up while grasping it. Detach at tarsus and from underlying Müller's muscle.
- Use a 6-0 silk suture to pass a half thickness horizontal mattress slip knot through the tarsal plate 5 mm from the lashes and the cut edge of the aponeurosis.
- Add additional stitches to adjust lid contour and secure knots.

Lower Lid Blepharoplasty: Skin or Skin-Muscle Flap Approach

- *Indications*:
  - Significant bony rim visibility.
  - Suborbicularis orbital fat or malar fat pad ptosis.
  - Underdeveloped infraorbital bony rims.
  - Prominent nasojugal groove.
  - Deep-set eyes with fat protrusion.
- *Advantages*:
  - Excises excess lower lid skin.
- *Disadvantages*:
  - Higher risk of ectropion.
  - Visible scar.
  - Sunken eye appearance if excessive infraorbital fat is removed.
  - Risk of scleral show with over aggressive skin resection.
  - Skin only flap causes significant ecchymosis.

Surgical Technique

- Inject lower eyelid with anesthetic containing hyaluronidase.
- Create and excise a standing ridge of skin through orbicularis, 2 mm inferior to the lower lid margin from the lower punctum medially to a 6–10 mm lateral to the lateral canthus.
- Elevate skin-muscle flap by incising pretarsal muscle (bevel to preserve small amount of pretarsal muscle) and dissect muscle flap inferiorly to 1.5 cm below the bony orbital rim.
- Dissect below orbital rim blunt with cotton-tip applicator. Avoid infraorbital nerve.
- Incise orbital septum using electroautery to identify the prolapsed fat.
- Gently palpate globe to herniate orbital fat.
  - May resect or reposition fat with conservation to avoid sunken appearance.
  - Prolapsed fat may be draped over the orbital rim and sutured to the anterior malar skin.
- Skin-muscle flap advanced in superior/lateral direction to determine where to suspend along the orbital rim (5-0 PDS) for optimal lower lid contour. Excess skin/muscle resected.
- Close subciliary incision with 7-0 blue polypropylene at the lateral canthus and 6-0 chromic for the rest of the incision.

Lower Lid Blepharoplasty: Transconjunctival Approach

- *Indications*:
  - Isolated fat herniation
  - No/minimal skin excess.
- *Advantages*:
  - Hidden incision
  - Reduced postoperative ectropion because it does not disturb orbicularis oculi.
- *Disadvantages*:
  - Does not reduce lower eyelid skin or improve eyelid laxity

Surgical Technique

Incision through the conjunctival sac:

- Inject local anesthetic
- Incise 3–4 mm below tarsal plate with microcautery electrodissection
- Suspend proximal conjunctival flap (posterior lamella) over cornea with suture
- Dissect preseptal plane down to the inferior orbital rim
- Insert Desmarres retractor to expose the bony orbital rim, this prevents excising fat below the orbital rim
- Incise orbital septum to release intraorbital fat from medial to lateral canthi
- Mobilize fat: Identity fat pockets based on the color and division of the central and medial compartments by the inferior oblique.
  - Prior to any fat resection, use a Q-tip to gently tease through it to ensure there is no muscle

- – Clamp fat with a hemostat, cut it, and cauterize the remaining stump
  - – Any fat is saved for potential replacement in case of asymmetries or over-resection resulting in hollowing
- Close incision with 6-0 absorbable sutures. This incision can also be left often, but a simple single interrupted stitch is often placed if fat is replaced.
- For excess skin consider Pinch-incision, 35% trichloroacetic acid (TCA) peel or laser resurfacing.

Lateral Canthopexy

- *Indications*:
  - – Scleral show
  - – Flaccidity of the lower eyelid
  - – Ectropion, paralysis, and lid retraction
  - – *Lateral canthal tendon laxity*: Leads to lower lid laxity and descent of the lateral canthus and lower eyelid.
- *Surgical technique:*
  - – Incise laterally to expose orbital rim.
  - – Place a 5-0 Vicryl through anterior lamella of lateral canthus to the inside of the lateral orbital rim to the periosteum.

ASIAN EYELID

Refer to "upper eyelid retractors" for more details of anatomy of Asian upper eye lid. Table 1 summarizes considerations for blepharoplasty.

Supratarsal Fold Creation in the Asian Eyelid

Surgical Technique

- Mark incision 7–9 mm above ciliary margin to remove skin of 3–4 mm
- *Medial extent of incision*: Medial to medial canthus for outside fold or lateral to medial canthus for an inside fold

Table 1: Considerations for Asian versus non-Asian blepharoplasty

	Asian	non-Asian
Levator aponeurosis insertion	Partial to full adhesion in the orbital septum → variable crease presence	Inserts into supratarsal crease dermis
Preaponeurotic fat in inferior upper eyelid	More preaponeurotic fat	Less preaponeurotic fat
Superior tarsus	~4 mm	~10 mm
Epicanthal fold	Persistent	Disappears by birth or adolescence
Deep set eyes	Rare to perform surgery for deep set eyes	Deep set eyes common

- Incise skin, bipolar vascular arcade, and remove a strip of orbicularis oculi and preseptal tissue at inferior edge to debulk pretarsal tissue and access the postseptal fat pad
- Assistant will push postseptal fat pad forward; gently incise laterally along preseptal tissue to herniate fat
- Elevate preseptal tissue upward with a mosquito to protect levator
- Sweep fat superior with Q-tip until levator identified. Levator to be detached from tarsus
- *Creases fixation sutures with 5-0 nylon starting at mid-pupil*: Inferior skin edge, horizontal through levator, superior skin edge—tie down and notice 90-degree eversion of the eyelashes.
- Exact fixation on opposite eye; alternate back and forth to ensure symmetry.

COMPLICATIONS

- *Blindness* caused by retrobulbar hemorrhage, globe perforation (especially during infiltration with local anesthetic), or closed-angle glaucoma attack
- *Retrobulbar hemorrhage* results in increased intraocular pressure (IOP) (30–40), proptosis, severe pain, and/or visual changes. To prevent irreversible blindness immediate treatment is required. Lateral canthotomy/cantholysis, mannitol (20% 1.5–2 g/kg with first 12.5 g in 3 minutes), and acetazolamide (500 mg IV)
- *Hematoma* most commonly from orbicularis *muscle* can be treated conservatively with ice, head elevation, blood pressure (BP) control. Open wound when clinically indicated
- *Unfavorable scar* and retraction. Common complication of lower lid blepharoplasty leading to *scleral show* or *ectropion* due to failure to address lower lid laxity or excess excision. Treat with steroids and squinting exercises
- *Lagophthalmos* can occur due to over-resection, orbicularis paresis, and levator spasm. Can be treated with massage, taping, and nocturnal lubrication
- *Infection* uncommon secondary to high vascularity
- *Chemosis* course can be shortened by blephamide ophthalmic drops
- *Corneal injury (abrasion):* It is usually iatrogenic at the time of the surgery. Pain, eye discomfort and blurring vision are usually reported by the patient. Fluorescein eyedrops and slit-lamp examination can confirm the corneal trauma. Treatment is eye closure for 2-3 days with an antibiotic ophthalmic solution.
- *Ptosis* from unrecognized brow/lid ptosis or unintentional levator detachment
- *Milia* can be treated in clinic, by simply unroofing with an 18-gauge needle
- *Diplopia* often caused by irritation or damage of inferior oblique

- *Epiphora* due to lacrimal apparatus disruption due to punctal eversion, wound contracture, edema, orbicularis oculi dysfunction, or canaliculus obstruction/laceration. If lacerated, place a silastic stent.
- Persistent herniated fat due to inadequate resection.

■ BIBLIOGRAPHY

1. Baker SR. Orbital fat preservation in lower-lid blepharoplasty. Arch Facial Plast Surg. 1999;1:33-7.
2. De Castro CC. A critical analysis of the current surgical concepts for lower blepharoplasty. Plast Reconstr Surg. 2004;114:785-93.
3. Fagien S. Advanced rejuvenation upper blepharoplasty: enhancing aesthetics of the upper periorbita. Plast Reconstr Surg. 2002;11:278-92.
4. Friedman O, Zaldivar RA, Wang TD. Blepharoplasty. In: Flint PW, Haughey BH, Lund VJ (Eds). Cummings Otolaryngology Head and Neck Surgery, 6th edition. Philadelphia: Saunders Elsevier; 2015. pp. 439-52.
5. Glat PM, Jelks GW, Jelks EB, et al. Evolution of the lateral canthoplasty: techniques and indications. Plast Reconstr Surg. 1997;100:1396-405.
6. Kamer FM, Mingrone MD. Experiences with transconjunctival upper blepharoplasty. Arch Facial Plast Surg. 2000;2:213-6.
7. Patipa M. Evaluation and management of lower eyelid retraction following cosmetic surgery. Plast Reconstr Surg. 2000;106:438-59.
8. Perkins SW, Batniji RK. Rejuvenation of the lower eyelid complex. Facial Plast Surg. 2005;21:279-85.
9. Persichetti P, DiLella F, Delfino S et al. Adipose compartments of the upper eyelid: anatomy applied to blepharoplasty. Plast Reconstr Surg. 2004;113:379-80.
10. Prado A, Andrades P, Danilla S, et al. Nonresective shrinkage of the septum and fat compartments of the upper and lower eyelids: a comparative study with carbon dioxide laser and Colorado needle. Plast Reconstr Surg. 2006;117:1725-35.
11. Rohrich RJ, Coberly DM, Fagien S, et al. Current concepts in aesthetic upper blepharoplasty. Plast Reconstr Surg. 2004;113:32e-42e.
12. Thorne CH, Chung KC, Gosain AK, et al. Grabb and Smith's Plastic Surgery, 7th edition. Philadelphia: Wolters Kluwer Health/Lippincott Williams & Wilkins; 2013.
13. Yousif NF, Sonderman P, Dzwierzynski WW, et al Anatomic considerations in transconjunctival blepharoplasty. Plast Reconstr Surg. 1995;96:1271-8.

Multiple Choice Questions

Q 1. The "pinch technique" in blepharoplasty is MOST commonly used with which technique?

A. Lower eyelid blepharoplasty, SOOF (suborbicularis oculi fat) technique
B. Transconjuntival lower lid blepharoplasty.
C. Subciliary transcutaneous lower eyelid blepharoplasty, skin technique
D. Subciliary transcutaneous lower eyelid blepharoplasty, skin-muscle technique.

Ans: B. Transconjuntival lower lid blepharoplasty.

Q 2. A webbed scar resulting as a complication of upper eyelid blephroplasty is BEST corrected by which technique?

A. Single excision
B. Serial excision
C. Z-plasty repair
D. Geometric broken line closure repair

Ans: C. Z-plasty repair

Q 3. Which statement is TRUE about the NORMAL ANATOMY of the lower eyelid?

A. The lateral canthal angle is 2 mm inferior to the medial canthal angle
B. The lateral canthal angle is 2 mm superior to the medial canthal angle
C. The lower eyelid margin is 2 mm above the inferior corneal limbus
D. The lower eyelid margin is 5 mm below the inferior corneal limbus

Ans: B. The lateral canthal angle is 2 mm superior to the medial canthal angle.

Q 4. Which of the following is NOT a treatment for retrobulbar hematoma occurring as a complication of blepharoplasty?

A. Diamox, 500 mg, slow IV push
B. Decadron, 10 mg IV push
C. Medial canthotomy with inferior cantholysis
D. Opening suture lines

Ans: C. Medial canthotomy with inferior cantholysis

Q 5. The MOST common complication of transconjunctival lower blepharoplasty is:

A. Bleeding
B. Eyelid malposition
C. Inadequate fat excision
D. Inferior oblique muscle injury

Ans: C. Inadequate fat excision

Q 6. Which of the following is the MOST common complication of transcutaneous blepharoplasty?

A. Ectropion
B. Entropion
C. Epiphora
D. Eyelid malposition

Ans: D. Eyelid malposition

Q 7. The transconjunctival blepharoplasty is BEST indicated for addressing one of the following anatomic abnormalities:

A. Pseudoherniated orbital fat
B. Lower eyelid rhytids
C. Lower eyelid skin laxity
D. Hypertrophied orbicularis oculi muscle

Ans: A. Pseudoherniated orbital fat

Q 8. The drawing below represents the upper and lower eyelid skin incisions planned in a blepharoplasty procedure. What is the MINIMAL DISTANCE that should remain between both incisions at their lateral aspect? (Indicated by the arrows).

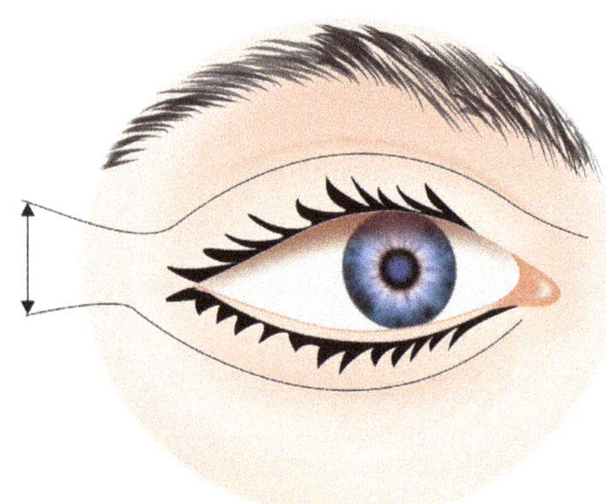

A. 3 mm   B. 5 mm
C. 10 mm   D. 15 mm

Ans: B. 5 mm

Q 9. Which of the following statements regarding cosmetic surgery of the Asian Face is TRUE?

A. 90% of Asian faces exhibit a "single eyelid"
B. In the Asian eye, filaments of the levator penetrate the orbital septum, and the orbicularis muscle and attach to the overlying dermis
C. Hypertrophic scarring of the face is more common in Asians than Caucasians
D. Skin malignancies are more common among Asians than Caucasians

Ans: C. Hypertrophic scarring of the face is more common in Asians than Caucasians

Q 10. Which of the following conditions is BEST improved by subciliary blepharoplasty?

A. Fine wrinkles of the lowert eyelids
B. Crow's feet
C. Malar bags
D. Hypertrophied orbicularis muscle

Ans: D. Hypertrophied orbicularis muscle

Q 11. Which of the following blepharoplastic surgical techniques is the MOST appropriate for a 53-year-old male patient with severe skin abundance of the lower eyelid, almost no fat pocket redundancy and no evidence of lower eyelid laxity?

A. Transcutaneous blepharoplasty with skin-muscle flap
B. Transcutaneous blepharoplasty with skin flap

C. Transconjunctival blepharoplasty with repositioning of orbital
D. No surgical blepharoplastic operation is indicated

Ans: B. Transcutaneous blepharoplasty with skin flap

Q 12. Which of the following complications is NOT commonly seen in cosmetic blepharoplasty?

A. Lower lid malposition
B. Scleral show
C. Change in shape of the medial canthal region
D. Lateral canthal dystopia

Ans: C. Change in shape of the medial canthal region

Q 13. Which of the following quantitative measures represents a MINIMAL NORMAL Schirmer's test value?

A. 6 mm   B. 8 mm
C. 10 mm   D. 15 mm

Ans: C. 10 mm

Q 14. Which of the following photographic views is UNNECESSARY in the preoperative evaluation for blepharoplasty?

A. Frontal close up of the eyes with eyes open and closed
B. Frontal close up of the eyes with upward gaze
C. Close up of the eyes, right and left lateral
D. Basal (full face)

Ans: D. Basal (full face)

Q 15. You are called to see one of your patients in the recovery room, 4 hours after a blepharoplasty procedure. After evaluation you suspect an orbital hematoma. Which of the following is the FIRST STEP in the treatment of this condition?

A. Open the surgical wound   B. Lateral canthotomy
C. Steroids and diuretics IV   D. Orbital decompression

Ans: A. Open the surgical wound

Q 16. The MOST common complication of upper blepharoplasty in persons of Asian ethnicity is:

A. Asymmetry
B. Unsatisfactory scar formation
C. Infection
D. Bleeding

Ans: A. Asymmetry

Q 17. The MOST common complication of the aponeurotic repair of blepharoptosis is?

A. Overcorrection
B. Undercorrection
C. Recurrence of ptosis
D. Notching of the eyelid margin

Ans: B. Undercorrection

Q 18. In the emergency treatment of retrobulbar hematoma, which of the following is INCORRECT?

A. Opening the suture lines
B. Mannitol IV
C. Diamox IV
D. Lidocaine IV

Ans: D. Lidocaine IV

Q 19. Which of the following chemical peeling agents is RECOMMENDED for use in conjunction with transcutaneous skin flap Lower Eyelid Blepharoplasty?

A. Tricloroacetic acid 25%
B. Jessner's solution
C. Phenol 88%
D. None

Ans: D. None

Q 20. Injury to the superior oblique muscle is MOST commonly seen during surgery related to the:

A. Medial upper eyelid fat pocket
B. Central upper eyelid fat pocket
C. Medial lower lid fat pocket
D. Lateral upper eyelid fat pocket

Ans: A. Medial upper eyelid fat pocket

Q 21. Which of following statements is FALSE regarding the lateral canthus in cosmetic blepharoplasty?

A. The lateral canthal tendon becomes attenuated (lax) with age
B. In cases of lateral canthal tendon laxity the canthus can be pulled to the lateral limbus of the eye
C. Lateral tarsal strip is effective in the treatment of mild degrees of eyelid laxity
D. Lateral canthal plication is effective in the treatment of mild, moderate and severe degrees of laxity

Ans: D. Lateral canthal plication is effective in the treatment of mild, moderate and severe degrees of laxity

Q 22. Which fat pocket is MOST commonly involved postsurgically in the persistence of fat pseudoherniation?

A. Lateral lower eyelid fat pocket
B. Medial lower eyelid fat pocket
C. Central upper eyelid fat pocket
D. Medial upper eyelid fat pocket

Ans: A. Lateral lower eyelid fat pocket

Q 23. Which of the following statements regarding blepharoplasty is TRUE?

A. Direct access to the fat pads is achieved by the transconjunctival postseptal approach
B. In the transconjunctival preseptal approach an incision is made 5 mm below the inferior border of the inferior tarsal
C. The medial and central fat compartments of the lower eyelid are separated by the inferior rectus muscle
D. The lateral fat pad is whiter than the medial fat pad

Ans: A. Direct access to the fat pads is achieved by the transconjunctival postseptal approach

Q 24. The drawing below REPRESENTS the:

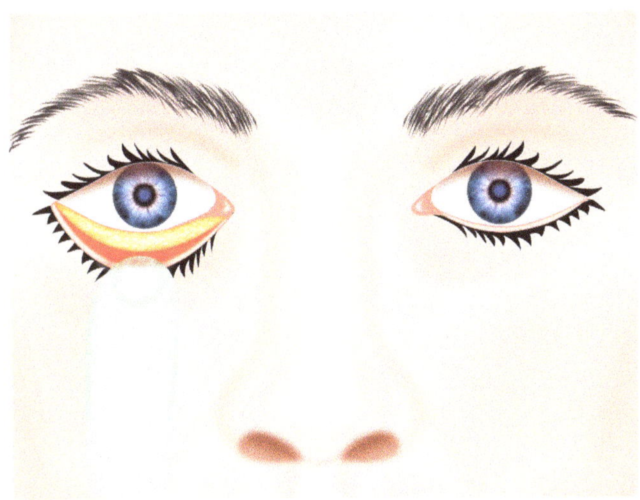

A. Distraction test
B. Snap test
C. Pinch test
D. Retraction test

Ans: D. Retraction test

Q 25. Your patient, is a 40-year-old female who has just had an inferior subciliary blepharoplasty and is complaining of a severe left eye pain immediately after her arrival to the recovery room. Both vision and intraocular pressure are normal. There is mild bruising around both eyes but no evidence of gross hematoma. The next step in the management of the patient is:

A. Close observation with visual check up
B. Open the surgical wound
C. Fluorescein test
D. Lateral canthotomy

Ans: C. Fluorescein test

Q 26. Which of the following COMPLICATIONS can most likely be prevented by identifying the lacrimal gland and avoiding fat removal from the lateral area of the upper eyelids during the performance of blepharoplasty?

A. Hooding of the lateral canthus
B. Tear deficiency
C. Persistent fat bulging
D. Blepharoptosis

Ans: B. Tear deficiency

Q 27. Which of the following measures is NOT INDICATED in the management of postoperative orbital hemorrhage after blepharoplasty?

A. Elevate the head of the patient's bed
B. Ice pack compresses
C. Lateral canthotomy and inferior cantholysis
D. Mannitol

Ans: B. Ice pack compresses

Q 28. Which of the following eyelid types is represented in the drawing below?

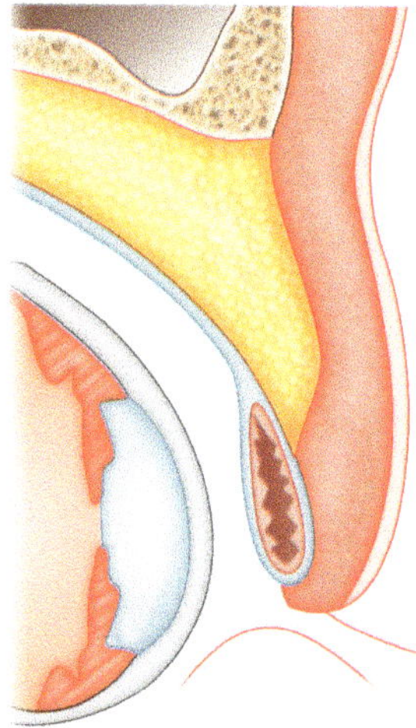

A. The Caucasian	B. The African American
C. The Asian	D. The Latino

Ans: C. The Asian

Q 29. Which of the following measurements represents NORMAL levator function?

A. 5 mm	B. 10 mm
C. 2 mm	D. 20 mm

Ans: B. 10 mm

Q 30. Which of the following statements regarding normal periocular anatomic relationships is FALSE?

A. Vertical palpebral aperture (10 mm)
B. Horizontal palpebral aperture (34 mm)
C. Lateral canthal angle (Acute)
D. Lower lid margin (Below inferior limbus)

Ans: D. Lower lid margin (Below inferior limbus)

Q 31. Which of the following statements about eyelid ptosis evaluation is TRUE?

A. The normal measurement of palpebral fissure is usually less than 10 mm
B. Normal levator function is usually greater than 11 mm
C. Margin reflex distance-1 (MRD1), is the distance between the center of the pupil in primary position and the central margin of the lower eyelid
D. Margin reflex distance-2 (MRD2), which is the distance between the center of the pupil in primary position and the central margin of the upper eyelid

Ans: B. Normal levator function is usually greater than 11 mm

Q 32. Which of the following is THE MOST RELIABLE indicator for identifying a patient at risk of developing postblepharoplasty Dry Eye Syndrome?

A. History
B. Schirmer's test
C. Tear film break-up time
D. Quantitative tear lysozyme level

Ans: A. History

Q 33. Which of the following statements about Corneal Abrasion postblepharoplasty is FALSE?

A. A temporary Frost traction suture can help to protect the eye during lower lid blepharoplasty
B. The use of ophthalmologic ointment is helpful to avoid drying and corneal ulcer formation
C. Rose Bengal solution staining and slit lamp will made the diagnosis
D. The treatment of corneal abrasion is to close the eye, use antibacterial ointment and patched for 48 hours.

Ans: C. Rose Bengal solution staining and slit lamp will made the diagnosis

Q 34. Which of the following is the MOST COMMON cause of permanent Lagophthalmos?

A. Eyelid laxity not corrected
B. Excessive resection of the upper eyelid skin
C. Orbital septum trauma with scarring
D. Eyelid incision healing with scarring and contracture

Ans: B. Excessive resection of the upper eyelid skin

Q 35. Which of the following statements about superficial eyelid topography is FALSE?

A. Mean Reflex Distance-1 (MRD-1) is the distance from the center of the pupil up to the inferior edge of the upper eyelid
B. Mean Reflex Distance-2 (MRD-2) is the distance from the center of the pupil down to the superior edge of the lower eyelid
C. Eyelid ptosis will decrease the MRD-1 measurement
D. Ectropion of the lower lid will decrease the MRD-2

Ans: D. Ectropion of the lower lid will decrease the MRD-2 measurement

Q 36. According to female esthetics, what is the ideal pretarsal eyelid/eyebrow ratio?. Refer to the drawing of the Female Eye below.

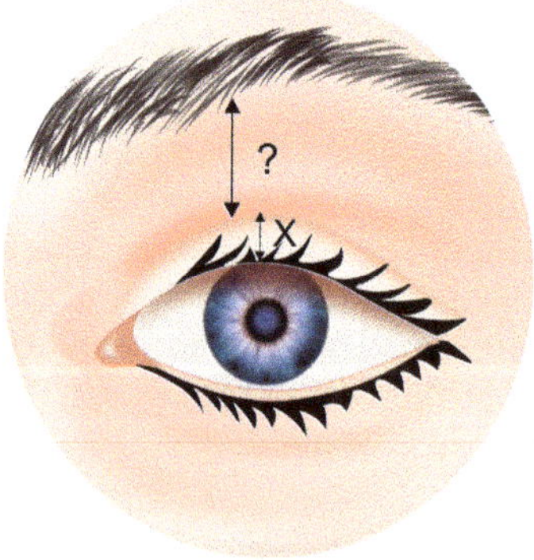

A. 2.5X	B. 3.0X
C. 3.5X	D. 4.0X

Ans: C. 3.5X

Q 37. Which of the following complications is the MOST COMMON after Epicanthoplasty in the Asian patient?

A. Keloid formation
B. Hypertrophic scar
C. Skin necrosis
D. Asymmetry

Ans: B. Hypertrophic scar

Q 38. Which of the following statements about the "Pinch" blepharoplasty technique is FALSE?

A. It is usually performed for the transconjunctival removal of fat in lower eyelid blepharoplasty
B. The removal of transconjunctival fat is done after the "Pinch" skin excision.
C. The line of incision is 5 mm below the lateral margin of the eyelid, leaving an island of intact skin of 5 mm height
D. Straight scissors are used to excise the "wall" of skin, leaving the Orbicularis Muscle intact

Ans: B. The removal of transconjunctival fat is done after the "Pinch" skin excision

Q 39. Which of the following periocular anatomic relationships is NOT ideal or normal?

A. The brow is Located at or above the superior orbital rim
B. The vertical palpebral aperture is approximately 10 mm
C. The horizontal palpebral aperture is approximately 34 mm
D. The lateral canthal angle is obtuse

Ans: D. The lateral canthal angle is obtuse

Q 40. Which of the following statements is FALSE regarding the surface eyelid anatomy?

A. The upper eyelid skin crease is approximately 10 mm superior to the eyelid margin
B. The upper eyelid skin crease is formed by the attachment of the Müller's muscle
C. The lateral canthal angle is 2 mm higher than the medial canthal angle
D. The distance from the medial canthus to the midline of the nose is approximately 15 mm

Ans: B. The upper eyelid skin crease is formed by the attachment of the Müller's muscle

Q 41. The hollowed-out appearance following cosmetic blepharoplasty is MOST commonly associated with:

A. Excessive of skin resection
B. Excessive of muscle resection
C. Excessive fat resection
D. Damage to the lacrimal gland

Ans: C. Excessive fat resection

Q 42. The prevalence of orbital hemorrhage associated with cosmetic blepharoplasty is approximately:

A. 1 case in 500
B. 1 case in 1000
C. 1 case in 1500
D. 1 case in 2000

Ans: D. 1 case in 2000

Q 43. The prevalence of blindness associated with cosmetic blepharoplasty is approximately:

A. 1 case in 500
B. 1 case in 1000
C. 1 case in 10,000
D. 1 case in 20,000

Ans: D. 1 case in 20,000

Q 44. Which of the following features is NOT associated with an ideal or beautiful youthful eye?

A. No scleral show
B. Palpebral aperture has an almond shape
C. Upper eyelid covers 1 mm of the superior limbus
D. Negative lateral canthal tilt

Ans: D. Negative lateral canthal tilt

Q 45. A 55-year-old woman is consulting you for a possible blepharoplasty. She has had a recent LASIK surgery. What is the proper timing to perform a blepharoplasty in this patient?

A. There is no time contraindication for blepharoplasty and LASIK surgery
B. The patient should wait 2 months after her LASIK surgery
C. The patient should wait 4 months after her LASIK surgery
D. The patient should wait 6 months after her LASIK surgery

Ans: D. The patient should wait 6 months after her LASIK surgery

Q 46. Which of the following medical conditions is NOT related to an increased risk for lower eyelid retraction in the execution of a lower eyelid blepharoplasty?

A. Globe proptosis
B. High myopia
C. Diabetes
D. Thyroid ophthalmopathy

Ans: C. Diabetes

Q 47. Several hours after a four-quadrant blepharoplasty (Subciliary approach) you are called by the patient's husband and explains to you that his wife has a severe pain into the left eye of 1-2 hours duration. You have just seen the patient. The physical examination does not reveal evidence of gross bleeding or hematoma. The eye is mildly swollen but not proptotic. The fluorescein test is negative. Which of the following diagnostic possibilities is the MOST likely?

A. Orbital hematoma
B. Corneal abrasion
C. Herpes virus conjunctivitis
D. Angle-closure glaucoma

Ans: D. Angle-closure glaucoma

Q 48. Which of the following is CRITICAL to the safety of blepharoplasty patients with preoperative dry eyes?

A. No excision of eyelid skin
B. "Pinch" Technique for excision of skin redundancy
C. Preservation of orbicularis muscle and its function
D. Fat removal through a buttonhole incision in the orbicularis muscle

Ans: C. Preservation of orbicularis muscle and its function

Q 49. The snap test is useful for determining what in blepharoplasty?

A. Lower lid skin elasticity
B. If eye ptosis is present
C. Extent of skin excision
D. Risk of ectropion

Ans: D. Risk of ectropion

Q 50. What is the distance from lid margin to the inferior extent of your incision in upper transcutaneous blepharoplasty?

A. 6 mm above lid crease for males, 7 mm for women
B. The transition from thin eyelid skin to thick brown skin
C. At the level of the existing supratarsal crease
D. 8-12 mm above eyelid margin

Ans: D. 8-12 mm above eyelid margin

Q 51. All of the following below are true *except* for which answer?

A. The procerus creates horizontal glabellar wrinkles while the corrugator creates vertical glabellar wrinkles
B. Lockwood's ligament is found in the upper lid and Whitnall's ligament is in the lower lid
C. Müller's muscle retracts the upper lid 2-3 mm
D. The supratrochlear and lacrimal nerves provide sensory innervation to the conjunctivae

Ans: B. Lockwood's ligament is found in the upper lid and Whitnall's ligament is in the lower lid

Q 52. All of the following *except* which answer form the "tear trough deformity triad" of aging periorbita?

A. Lower lid skin redundancy
B. Inferiorly displaced orbital rim
C. Malar retrusion due loss of soft tissue below the orbital rim
D. Steatoblepharon due to orbital septum weakening

Ans: A. Lower lid skin redundancy

Q 53. All of the below *except* which answer are true of the Asian eyelid and blepharoplasty for this population.

A. The superior tarsus is typically shorter in the Asian population
B. Asians typically have less preaponeurotic fat in the inferior eyelid
C. Non-Asians typically have a supratarsal crease because the levator aponeurosis inserts into the dermis, while Asians' aponeurosis usually is adhesive to the orbital septum
D. The lower tarsus is usually shorter in Asians compared to Caucasians

Ans: B. Asians typically have less preaponeurotic fat in the inferior eyelid

Q 54. Which of the following statements regarding eyelid anatomy is FALSE?

A. The posterior lamella is composed by the tarsus, the lower lid retractors and the conjuntiva
B. The lower lid margin should be tangential to the inferior limbus of the iris

C. The lateral canthus is approximately 2 mm higher than the medial canthus
D. The shape and the position of the upper eyelid is the primary determinant of the general eye shape

Ans: D. The shape and the position of the upper eyelid is the primary determinant of the general eye shape.

Q 55. Which of the following eyelid anatomical structures does NOT function as a "retractor"?

A. Whitnall's ligament
B. Levator aponeurosis
C. Müller's muscle
D. Capsulopalpebral fascia

Ans: A. Whitnall's ligament

Q 56. Which of the following eyelid structures (cross-sectioned drawing below) is the ONE represented by the arrow?

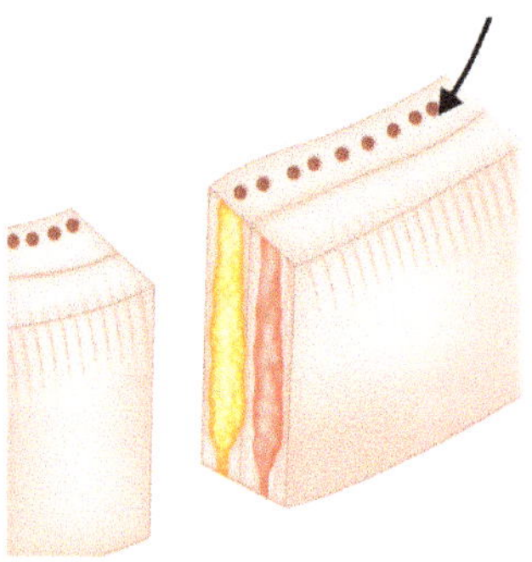

A. Meibomian glands
B. Sweat glands
C. Gray line
D. Tarsus

Ans: A. Meibomian glands

Q 57. Which of the following anatomic statements regarding anatomy of the eyelids is TRUE?

A. The Müller muscle is innervated by the third cranial nerve
B. The capsulopalpebral fascia is a primary retractor of the lower eyelid
C. The levator palpebrae superioris is innervated by the sympathetic nervous system
D. The arterial supply to the eyelids comes totally from branches of the external carotid artery system

Ans: B. The capsulopalpebral fascia is a primary retractor of the lower eyelid

Q 58. Which of the following eyelid topography is related to the orbicularis oculi muscle of Riolan?

A. Meibomian gland orifices
B. Gray line
C. Tarsus
D. Eyelash follicles

Ans: B. Gray line

Q 59. Which is the proper sensory innervation of the eyelids?

A. CN V1
B. CN V2
C. CN V3
D. CN V1 and CN V2

Ans: D. CN V1 and CN V2

Q 60. Which of the following statements in eyelid anatomy is FALSE?

A. All of the eyelid fat pads lie deep to the orbital septum
B. The lower eyelid contains three fat pads: medial, central, and lateral
C. The capsulopalpebral fascia is one of the lower eyelid
D. The eyelid retractors are superficial to the fat pads

Ans: D. The eyelid retractors are superficial to the fat pads

Q 61. It is a connective tissue structure that attaches peripherally at the periosteum of the orbital margin, lies just deep to the orbicularis oculi muscle and centrally fuses with the lid retractor structures near the lid margins. Which of the following best described the eyelid structure presented previously?

A. The lateral palpebral ligament
B. The medial palpebral ligament
C. The orbicularis retaining ligament
D. The orbital septum

Ans: D. The orbital septum

Q 62. Which of the following statements related to brow/upper lid anatomy is FALSE?

A. The Müller muscle is innervated by the cranial nerve III
B. The highest point of the brow is at the lateral limbus
C. The lateral canthus of eyelid is located 2 mm higher than the medial canthus
D. The lacrimal sac drains into the nasal cavity as the nasolacrimal duct located in the inferior meatus

Ans: A. The Müller muscle is innervated by the cranial nerve III

Q 63. Which of the following anatomical structures is RELATED to the posterior lamella of the eyelid?

A. The grey line
B. The orbital septum
C. The tarsal plate
D. The pretarsal orbicularis oculi muscle

Ans: C. The tarsal plate

Q 64. Which of the following anatomic structures represented in the drawing below is the ONE INDICATED BETWEEN THE TWO ARROWS?

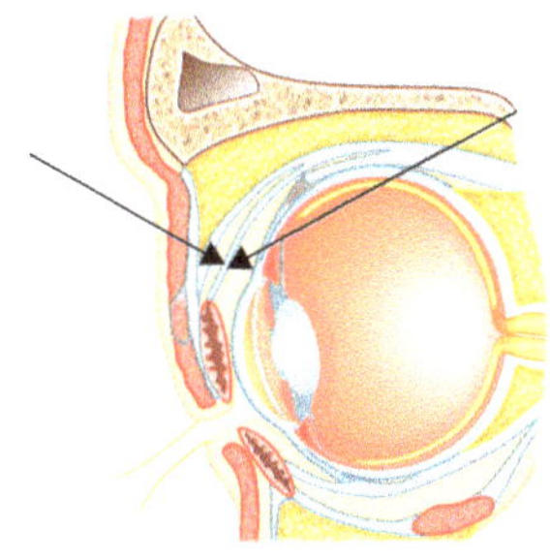

A. Levator palpebrae superioris
B. Müller muscle
C. Orbital septum
D. Superior rectus muscle

Ans: B. Müller muscle

Q 65. Which of the following represents the distance between the upper lid margin and the inferior limbus?

A. MRD-1
B. MRD-2
C. MLD-3
D. FRD-1

Ans: C. MLD-3

Chapter 12

Browplasty

Elizabeth Jasso-Ramírez, José Juan Montes-Bracchini

■ INTRODUCTION

Facial aging gives the impression of a tired and angry look in the upper face.[1,2] In the treatment of the aging upper face is important to consider the upper eyelid and brow as a unit assessing brow ptosis and blepharochalasis. The upper third of the face ages in a unique pattern, and there are four main features: (1) glabellar, (2) lateral canthal rhytids, (3) forehead rhytids, and (4) ptosis of the lateral brow.[3]

Etiology

Glabellar rhytids as well as lateral canthal rhytids are dynamic, which means that they are hyperfunctional lines resulting from the pulling on the skin by the musculature beneath.

The glabellar rhytids may be seen in younger patients, aged 20–50 years, in contrast to other wrinkles in the face that are caused by aging with changes in the collagen and elastin in the dermis.[3,4] Transverse deep forehead creases appear due to the action of the paired frontalis muscles.[5]

According to Knize there are three forces that act to cause lateral brow ptosis:[6]
1. Frontalis muscle resting tone
2. Gravity, loss of skin tone
3. Corrugator supercilii muscle hyperactivity + the action of the lateral orbicularis oculi muscle.

Summary of Blood Supply, Motor and Sensory Innervation of Forehead and Periorbital Structures

In order to understand the etiology of the forehead and lateral canthal rhytids is important to remember the muscles that elevate and depress the eyebrow (Table 1 and Fig. 1):[7,8]

- *Frontalis muscle*:[6,7,9]
  - The paired frontalis muscles are large, vertically oriented muscles that cover almost all the forehead. They are continuous with the galea and the occipitalis muscle
  - *Motor innervation*: Temporal branch of the facial nerve.
- *Corrugator supercilii*:[6,7,9]
  - Obliquely oriented, located in the inferomedial brow deep to the frontalis muscle in its inferior portion
  - The paired corrugator supercilii muscles are the only periorbital muscles with a bony origin → medial head originating from the frontal bone and insertion into the skin of the middle portion of the brow
  - *Motor innervation*: It is innervated by two different branches of the facial nerve
    1. Medial portion of the muscle innervated by the "zygomatic branch of the facial nerve"

Table 1: Etiology of the forehead and lateral canthal rhytids.

Function	Muscle	Muscle action	Rhytids
Levators of the eyebrow	The paired frontalis muscle	Superior portion contraction causes descent of the anterior hairline Inferior portion contraction causes elevation of the brow	Horizontal creases of the forehead
Depressors of the eyebrow	Midline procerus muscle	Descent of medial brow Creation of transverse midline nasal rhytids	Horizontal glabellar rhytids
	The paired corrugator muscle	Inferomedial descent of the medial head of the brow	Vertical rhytids of the glabellar region Gives the angry expression
	Orbicularis oculi muscles	Descent of the lateral brow	Dynamic lateral canthal rythids Ptosis of the lateral brow

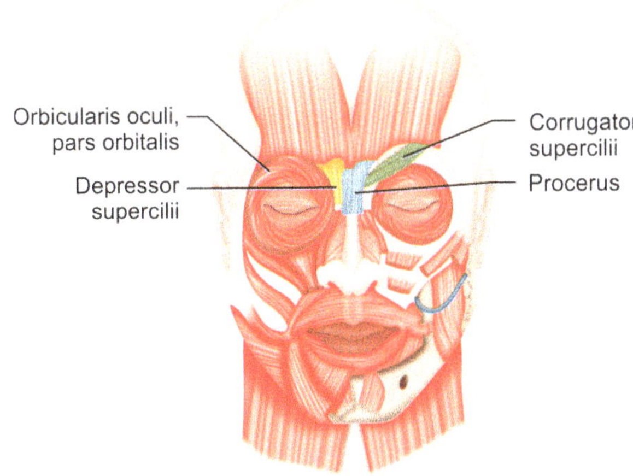

Fig.1: Elevator and depressor muscles of the upper third of the face

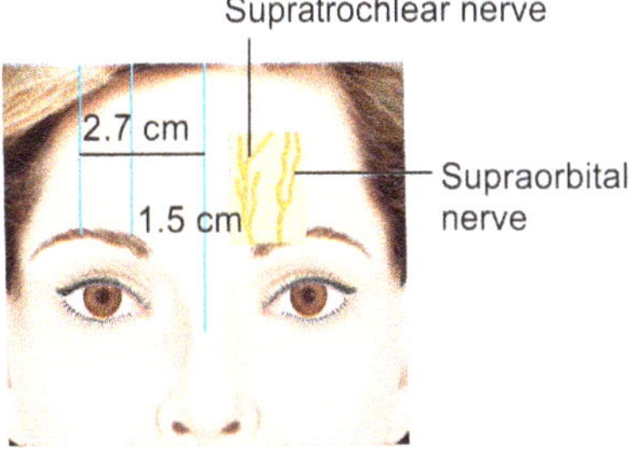

Fig. 2: Supratrochlear and supraorbital bundles

2. Lateral portion is innervated by the "temporal branch of the facial nerve".
   i. The supraorbital and supratrochlear neurovascular bundles exit a foramen in the supraorbital rim, pierce the corrugator muscles and then go through the frontalis muscles, the branches of the nerves travel on the superficial aspect of the frontalis muscle.

- *Procerus:*[6,7,9]
  - The procerus muscle is located in the midline at the root of the nose, with a pyramidal shape
  - It originates from periosteum and perichondrium of the nasal bones and upper lateral cartilages, and the fascia of the nasal superficial musculoaponeurotic system
  - It interdigitates with:
    » Frontalis muscle (superiorly)
    » Nasalis muscle (inferiorly)
    » Depressor supercilii, orbicularis oculi and deeper corrugator muscle (laterally).
  - *Motor innervation:*
    » Zygomatic branch of the facial nerve.
- *Orbicularis oculi:*[6,7,9]
  - Paired sphincteric muscles, thin, lying superficial to the corrugators
  - Separated into pretarsal (superficial to the tarsal plates), preseptal (superficial to the orbital septum) and orbital
  - The orbicularis interdigitate with the corrugator and frontalis muscles superiorly
  - It travels superficial to the temporal fascia (laterally), medially covers the depressor supercilii, inferiorly the muscle travel between the superficial and deep fat pads of the cheek

- *Motor innervation:*
  - » Medial and inferior portions are innervated by the "zygomatic branch of the facial nerve"
  - » Lateral and central portions are innervated by the "anterior portion of the temporal branch of the facial nerve".
- *Sensory innervation:*[10]
  - The sensory innervation of the brow and anterior scalp region is provided by the ophthalmic division of the trigeminal nerve (V_1)
  - *V_1 divides into:*
    » Lacrimal nerve→ sensation to skin and conjunctiva and upper eyelid
    » Frontal nerve → divides into supraorbital and supratrochlear nerves.
    - Supratrochlear nerve → innervates the conjunctiva, upper eyelids, and inferomedial aspect of the forehead. Located 1.5–1.7 mm from the midline
    - Supraorbital nerve → innervates the upper lid skin, forehead and anterior scalp. Located 1 mm lateral to the supratrochlear nerve (Fig. 2).
- *Blood supply:*[11]
  - The blood supply of the forehead originates from the internal and external carotid artery systems
  - Internal carotid artery (ICA) → ophthalmic artery → branches to form the frontal, supraorbital and supratrochlear arteries
  - External carotid artery (ECA) → supplies the scalp via the superficial temporal artery
  - The middle temporal artery (branch of the superficial temporal artery) runs in the temporal fascia at or below the zygomatic arch, several branches of this artery from the deep temporal fascia penetrate the underlying temporalis muscle.

▌PATIENT EVALUATION

Relevant Elements on Patient History

A complete patient history must be obtained with attention to:[12]

- Psychiatric history, previous facial surgeries and patient expectations for surgery.

- Ophthalmic history including dry eye symptoms (blurred vision, burning eyes, foreign body sensation, and need of lubricating ophthalmic drops)
- Thyroid disease
- Personal or family history of coagulopathies, history of bleeding problems in prior surgeries
- Use of herbal supplements, blood thinners, and vitamins.

Relevant Elements of Physical Examination

The physical examination should be performed with the patient looking in a mirror,[9] the examination of the position of the patient's brow and its comparison with the ideal brow position is the most critical point during the evaluation of the upper third of the face.[13]

Resting brow position can be evaluated by asking the patient close his or her eyes and then opening them. Identification of orbital and brow asymmetries is important as well as examination of upper and lower eyelids.

The distance between the midpupil and the upper edge of the eyebrow is ideally 2.5 cm, we should obtain measures from the lateral and medial canthus, and the distance from the brow to the hairline.

The eyebrow can be digitally elevated by the surgeon to the level desired, while keeping in mind that it should be at the level of the supraorbital rim or above it.

The ideal brow position is different in females and males (Table 2 and Fig. 3):[2,13,14]
- Evaluation of the hairline: ideal distance is 5 cm from the upper edge of the brow to the hairline
- This distance will influence in the approach chosen
- Assess the presence of glabellar and forehead rythids (dynamic and static).

■ TREATMENT

The description, indications, contraindications, advantages, and disadvantages of each procedure are described in Table 3.

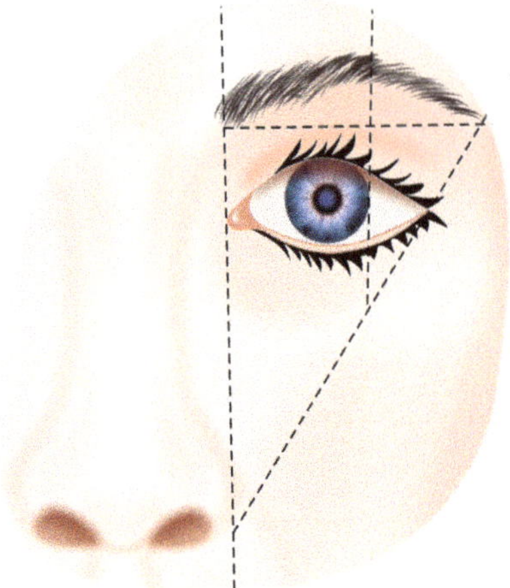

Fig. 3: Brow characteristics

Cosmetic

Cosmetic treatment has been shown in Table 3.[15]

Reconstruction of Brow Defects

The hairline and the eyebrows are natural boundaries on the upper third of the face on which to hide incisions, although hair-bearing areas limit flap designs to those that are not distorting the shape of the brow or the hair-bearing sites.

The lateral forehead, or temple region, constitutes a subunit that can affect the lateral aspect of the eyebrow, although the brow itself is a separate subunit. The skin of the lateral forehead is more elastic and can act as a reservoir site for tissue when undergoing reconstruction.

The relaxed skin tension lines, while running horizontally at the central forehead, curve upon reaching the temporal scalp.[16]

Table 2: Ideal brow position is different in females and males	
Brow characteristics by gender	
Female brow	*Male brow*
• Ideal brow position: Above the supraorbital rim • Gently curved shape • Thicker medially and thinner laterally • The medial end of the brow should begin at a vertical line through the ala of the nose • The lateral end of the brow should lie on an oblique line drawn through the ala of the nose and the lateral canthus • The highest point of the brow should lie along a vertical line of the lateral limbus.[13] • Y-shaped configuration between the brow, medial orbital rim and nasal bones	• Ideal brow position: At the level of the supraorbital rim • Horizontal shape • Thicker • T-shape configuration between the brow, medial orbital rim and nasal bones.

Table 3: The treatment procedure in browplasty.

Type of lift	Advantages	Disadvantages	Indication	Contraindication	Incision	Dissection	Suspension
Direct browplasty	Precise brow elevation Less dissection, less edema and less ecchymosis	Visible scar above the eyebrow Difficulty in contouring the medial brow	Facial paralysis (unilateral brow ptosis) Deep forehead furrows over the brows		Skin excision just above the brows	Subcutaneous	Transverse suspension of the orbicularis muscle to subgaleal tissue (periosteum) above the brow
Coronal forehead lift	Incision hidden behind the hairline Good exposure of the forehead musculature	Elevation of the frontal hairline Scalp anesthesia in periincisional area	Female with low frontal hairline Female who wears hair over the frontal hairline	Females with high frontal hairline Male pattern baldness	5–7 cm back from frontal hairline Always beveled parallel to hair follicles	Subgaleal	No
Midforehead	Close proximity to the brow Precise contouring of the brow Access to the corrugator supercilii muscle	May leave a visible scar	Significant forehead rhytids with male with baldness Older females with thin hair	Hypertrophic scarring or keloid	In a forehead crease Not s traight line shape Is closed in two layers: 1. Dermis 2. Everting stitch to close skin	Subcutaneous	Suture from the upper orbicularis muscle to periosteum at the upper margin of skin incision
Prehairline/pretrichial lift	No elevation of hairline Direct access to forehead muscles	Increased risk of scalp anesthesia Visible scar if not well executed Difficult technique	When wishes to decrease the height of forehead	Hypertrophic scars healing	Anterior to the frontal hairline Beveled	Subgaleal	No
Endoscopic approach	Decreased incidence of scarring, alopecia, and numbness of the scalp	Equipment required	Short foreheads (less than 6 cm from brow to hairline)		A temporal incision is made approximately 12 mm long. The authors make the incision parallel to the hair follicles	Subperiosteal	Multiple techniques, most commonly endotine

■ COMPLICATIONS

It is important to realize that any complication can be avoided or minimized by a complete preoperative patient history and physical examination, however, every surgical or non-surgical procedure is in risk to present one.[2,13,17] Complication rates are low for any brow lift approach.

- *Bleeding*: It may be arterial, venous or from skin edges.
  - Superficial temporal or zygomaticotemporal arteries
  - Supraorbital or supratrochlear vascular bundles
  - Sentinel vein.
- *Nerve injury*: Temporary or permanent (1%).[9,11]
  - Supraorbital or supratrochlear → should be identified and preserved to avoid injury → "hypoesthesia of the midforehead to the vertex". Up to 8 weeks

- Zygomaticotemporal and auriculotemporal branches (V_2 trigeminal nerve) → dissection in a plane directly superficial to the deep temporal fascia to avoid injury → "temporal and lateral paresthesia"
- Traction neuropraxia secondary to suspension
- Temporal branch of the facial nerve → be careful while dissecting the temporal area, identifying the sentinel vein will help to protect the nerve → "paralysis of the forehead".

- *Alopecia and scarring*: It seems to be more common in the frontal than the temporal areas, and could be due to poor incision and closure technique. Avoided by beveling incisions to avoid follicular injury.

  Ramirez treats these areas with a topical mixture of tretinoin 0.1% and minoxidil 5% on equal volume, applied to the affected areas twice daily.[11]

- *Brow asymmetry*:
  - *Preexisting brow asymmetries or blepharoptosis*: Preoperative evaluation is essential to detect them
  - *Iatrogenic causes*: Asymmetric muscle resection or suspension → full bilateral release of the conjoined tendon and arcus marginalis.
  - *Over elevation*: Over resection of the skin in coronal lift or excessive suspension.
    » Lagophthalmos can occur, may be temporary or more uncommonly permanent → can cause dry eye syndrome symptoms.
    » Increased risk of lagophthalmos with concomitant upper blepharoplasty.
  - *Under elevation*: Secondary to insufficient release, suspension or fixation.[18]
  - *Over-resection of the corrugator and procerus muscles*: Permanent "surprised" appearance (excessive medial brow elevation).

- *Flap necrosis*: It can be present when excessive pressure is applied to the flap or with undrained hematoma.[2]
- *Brow or eyelid ptosis (from botulinum toxin injections)*:[3,7,8,19,20]

■ REFERENCES

1. Wysong A, Joseph T, Kim D, et al. Quantifying soft tissue loss in facial aging: a study in women using magnetic resonance imaging. Dermatol Surg. 2013;39:1895-902.
2. Cook TA, Brownrigg PJ, Wang TM, et al. The versatile midforehead browlift. Arch Otolaryngol Head Neck Surg. 1989;115:163-8.
3. MacDonald MR, Spiegel JH, Raven RB, et al. An anatomical approach to glabellar rhytids. Arch Otolaryngol Head Neck Surg. 1998;124:1315-20.
4. Paul MD. (2001). The evolution of the brow lift in aesthetic plastic surgery. Plast Reconstr Surg. 2001;208:1409-24.
5. Koch RJ, Troell RJ, Goode RL. Contemporary management of the aging brow and forehead. Laryngoscope. 1997;107:710-5.
6. Knize DM. An anatomically based study of the mechanism of eyebrow ptosis. Plast Reconstr Surg. 1996;97:1321-33.
7. Stupak HD, Maas CS. New procedures in facial plastic surgery using botulinum toxin A. Facial Plast Surg Clin North Am. 2003;11:515-20.
8. Sykes JM, Trevidic P, Suárez GA, et al. Newer understanding of specific anatomic targets in the aging face as applied to injectables: facial muscles—identifying optimal targets of neuromodulators. Plast Reconstr Surg. 2015;136: (5 Suppl):56S-61S.
9. Ramirez O, Robertson KM. Update in endoscopic forehead rejuvenation. Facial Plast Surg Clin North Am. 2002;10:37-51.
10. Webster RC, Gaunt JM, Hamdan US, et al. Supraorbital and supratrochlear notches and foramina: anatomical variations and surgical relevance. Laryngoscope. 1986;96:311-5.
11. Frodel JL, Marentette LJ. The coronal approach: anatomic and technical considerations and morbidity. Arch Otolaryngol Head Neck Surg. 1993;119:201-7.
12. Lighthall JG, Wang TD. Complications of forehead lift. Facial Plast Surg Clin North Am. 2013;21:619-24.
13. Kerth TA, Toriumi DM. Management of the aging forehead. Arch Otolaryngol Head Neck Surg. 1990;116:1137-42.
14. Keen M, Blitzer A, Aviv J, et al. Botulinum toxin A for hyperkinetic facial lines: results of a double-blind, placebo-controlled study. Plast Reconstr Surg. 1994;94:94-9.
15. Putterman Am Evaluation of the cosmetic oculoplastic surgery, 2nd edition. Philadelphia: WB Saunders 1993. pp. 12-26.
16. Larrabee W, Sherris D. Principles of Facial Reconstruction: A Subunit Approach to Cutaneous Repair, 2nd edition. New York: Thieme Medical Publishers; 2009.
17. Knize DM. Limited incision forehead plasty. Plast Reconstr Surg. 1999;103:271-84.
18. Nassif PS. Evolution in techniques for endosocpic brow lift with deep temporal fixation only and lower blepharoplasty—transconjunctival fat repositioning. Facial Plast Surg. 2007;23:27-4.
19. Carruthers J, Fagien S, Matarasso S, et al. Consensus recommendations on the use of botulinum toxin type a in facial aesthetics. Plast Reconstr Surg. 2004;114(6 Suppl):1S-22S.
20. Maas CS. Botulinum neurotoxins and injectable fillers: minimally invasive management of the aging upper face. Facial Plast Surg Clin North Am. 2006;14:241-5.

Multiple Choice Questions

Q 1. Which of following statements is TRUE about brow position?

A. In men, the brow should be well above the orbital rim

B. In women, the brow is more horizontal and is positioned more inferiorly than the male eyebrow

C. The medial end of the brow is located along a vertical line drawn through the ala of the nose

D. The lateral end of the eyebrow is located 2 mm above an horizontal line passing through the medial end of the eyebrow

Ans: C. The medial end of the brow is located along a vertical line drawn through the ala of the nose

Q 2. Which of the following statements is TRUE regarding the Tricophytic Approach to brow and forehead elevation?

A. There is increased risk of brow malposition
B. There is limited access to the corrugator musculature
C. It is indicated in patients who have a high frontal hairline
D. The incision should be beveled with a curvilinear regular line pattern

Ans: C. It is indicated in patients who have a high frontal hairline

Q 3. A 57-year-old man has a asymmetric brow ptosis, deep static forehead rhytids and a high frontal hairline. Which of the following surgical managements is the MOST appropriate in this case?

A. Midforehead rhytidectomy
B. Midforehead browplasty
C. Prethichial forehead lift
D. Endoscopic forehead lift

Ans: B. Midforehead browplasty

Q 4. Which of the following statements regarding Endoscopic Forehead Lift is FALSE?

A. Subgaleal plane dissection is most commonly used
B. Three small vertical incisions of 2 cm each just behind the hairline are commonly used
C. Is indicated in patients with brow ptosis, horizontal and vertical forehead and glabellar rhytids
D. There is no scalp excision but there is fixation with screws or sutures

Ans: A. Subgaleal plane dissection is most commonly used

Q 5. A middle age attractive female, has a normal frontal hairline, minimal forehead wrinkles and an asymmetrical moderate brow ptosis with minimal upper eyelid skin excess. Which of the following surgical techniques is the BEST for this particular patient?

A. Endoscopic forehead-brow lift
B. Trichophytic forehead-brow lift
C. Direct brow lift
D. Midforehead lift

Ans: A. Endoscopic forehead-brow lift

Q 6. Which of the following statements is FALSE regarding the brow and forehead endoscopic lifting?

A. The indications are the same as those for a coronal open approach

B. It will improve horizontal forehead rhytids
C. It will improve vertical glabellar rhytids
D. Patients with facial nerve paralysis on one or both sides are excellent candidates

Ans: D. Patients with facial nerve paralysis on one or both sides are excellent candidates

Q 7. Which of the following brow lift techniques is performed in the subcutaneous plane?

A. Coronal
B. Petrichial
C. Midforehead
D. Lateral endoscopic forehead approach

Ans: C. Midforehead

Q 8. What is the appropriate plane of dissection in the CORONAL FOREHEAD LIFT?

A. Subcutaneous
B. Subgaleal
C. Subperiosteal
D. Above the frontalis muscle

Ans: B. Subgaleal

Q 9. What is the appropriate plane of dissection in the ENDOSCOPIC FOREHEAD LIFT?

A. Subcutaneous
B. Subgaleal
C. Subperiosteal
D. Posteriorly above the frontalis muscle, anteriorly subperiostealy

Ans: C. Subperiosteal

Q 10. A 51-year-old patient is requesting an improving of his aging upper third of the face. Which of the following surgical techniques in forehead lifting is the BEST for this patient, taking into the consideration that has male pattern baldness and a high clearly defined frontal hairline?

A. Thichophytic forehead lift   B. Endoscopic forehead lift
C. Midforehead lift   D. Pretrichial forehead lift

Ans: C. Midforehead lift

Q 11. A 46-year-old patient requests correction of his asymmetric brow ptosis. Which of the following surgical techniques is the BEST for this purpose?

A. Coronal lift   B. Endoscopic lift
C. Direct brow lift   D. Temporal lift

Ans: C. Direct brow lift

Q 12. Which of the following dissections is RECOMMENDED for protection of the facial nerve in the temporal approach for endoscopic brow elevation?

A. Dissection in the areolar tissue plane (innominate fascia)
B. Dissection in the supraperiosteal plane
C. Dissection medial and inferior to a branch of the zygomaticotemporal vein

D. Dissection lateral and superior to a branch of the zygomaticotemporal vein

Ans: C. Dissection medial and inferior to a branch of the zygomaticotemporal vein

Q 13. **Which of the following forehead and eyebrow lifting procedures will afford THE MOST ACCURATE AND THE GREATEST ELEVATION per millimeter of tissue excised?**
A. Direct eyebrow lift
B. Midforehead lift
C. Temporal eyebrow lift
D. Pretichial open forehead lift

Ans: A. Direct eyebrow lift

Q 14. **Which of the following anatomical landmarks identified more precisely the location of the frontal branch of the facial nerve in temporal endoscopic forehead dissection?**
A. The zygomatic arch
B. The temporal sentinel vein
C. Superficial fat pad
D. The arc marginalis

Ans: B. The temporal sentinel vein

Q 15. **Which of the following is the proper and the safest plane of dissection in endoscopic midface lift ?**
A. Above the superficial temporal fascia
B. Below the superficial temporal fascia
C. Above the deep temporal fascia
D. Below the deep temporal fat pad

Ans: C. Above the deep temporal fascia

Q 16. **Which of the following statements regarding midforehead browlift is FALSE?**
A. It is a desirable procedure for the man with a receding hairline
B. No hairline distortion is produced and no undermining is performed above the incision
C. The browlift is always done prior to the upper lid blepharoplasty
D. The incisions on either side of the forehead should be always at the same level

Ans: D. The incisions on either side of the forehead should be always at the same level

Q 17. **With respect to corrective surgery of the upper third of the aging face, which of the following approaches involve dissection at the subcutaneous level?**
A. Pre-trichial
B. Post-trichial
C. Midforehead
D. Endoscopic

Ans: C. Midforehead

Q 18. **Which of the following anatomical structures is localized between the deep temporal fascia and the temporalis muscle?**
A. Superficial fat pad
B. Intermediate fat pad
C. Deep temporal fat pad
D. Temporal fascia proper

Ans: C. Deep temporal fat pad

Q 19. **Which of the following is the CORRECT plane of elevation for the forehead flap?**
A. Subgaleal
B. Subperiosteal
C. Between the frontalis muscle and the subcutaneous layer
D. Between the frontalis muscle and the galea aponeurosis

Ans: A. Subgaleal

Q 20. **Which of the following is the MOST commonly used plane of dissection in coronal brow lift?**
A. Subcutaneous
B. Subgaleal
C. Subperiosteal
D. Combination of subcutaneous/Subperiosteal

Ans: B. Subgaleal

Q 21. **Which of the following muscles is considered the MAIN elevator of the brow?**
A. Corrugator
B. Procerus
C. Frontalis
D. Lateral orbicularis oculi

Ans: C. Frontalis

Q 22. **The insertion of the corrugator supercilli occurs at:**
A. Midbrow
B. Midline
C. Nasal bone
D. Orbital rim

Ans: A. Midbrow

Q 23. **Insertion of the procerus muscle is located at:**
A. Nasal bone
B. Nasal cartilage
C. Galea of the glabella
D. Medial canthus

Ans: A. Nasal bone

Q 24. **The nerve providing sensation to the medial forehead is:**
A. Trigeminal
B. Ophthalmic
C. Supratrochlear
D. Temporal facial branch

Ans: C. Supratrochlear

Q 25. **The main difference, between men and women regarding eyebrows is:**
A. Men brow is below the orbital rim
B. Women brow is flat above the orbital rim

C. Women brow is arched shaped
D. Men brow is above the orbital rim

Ans: C. Women brow is arched shaped

Q 26. Palpebral ptosis is defined as:

A. Less than 8 mm width of palpebral fissure
B. Less than 10 mm width of palpebral fissure
C. Less than 6 mm width of palpebral fissure
D. More than 8 mm of palpebral fissure

Ans: B. Less than 10 mm width of palpebral fissure

Q 27. Which of the following facial muscles will raise the eyebrows?

A. The frontalis
B. The procerus
C. The orbicularis
D. Temporoparietalis

Ans: A. The frontalis

Q 28. Which of following statements about the anatomy in the temporal region is FALSE?

A. The superficial temporalis fascia and the temporoparietal fascia are synonymous terms for the same fascia
B. The temporal artery and vein travel inferiorly to the tempoparietal fascia
C. The termpoparietal fascia is continuous with the SMAS in the lower face
D. The deep temporal fascia is considered the true temporalis

Ans: B. The temporal artery and vein travel inferiorly to the tempoparietal fascia

Q 29. Which of the following measurements noted below represents the distance indicated by the "X" in the drawing?

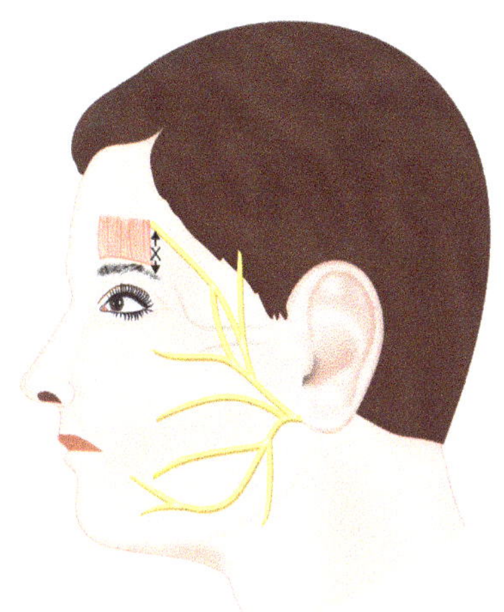

A. 1.0 cm
B. 1.5 cm
C. 2.5 cm
D. 3.0 cm

Ans: B. 1.5 cm

Q 30. Which of the following statements about the Coronal/ Hairline Forehead Lift is FALSE?

A. It cannot be applied to male patients with male-pattern
B. Subperiosteal plane dissection is used
C. Scoring-resection of frontal and corrugator muscles is done
D. Numbness in the forehead flap and beyond the incision line

Ans: B. Subperiosteal plane dissection is used

Chapter 13

Cheiloplasty

Amani Ben Moussa, Badr Ibrahim

■ INTRODUCTION

Gross Anatomy

The lips extend vertically from the subnasale to the mental crease and horizontally between each melolabial crease and each labiomental crease. The main muscle of the lips is orbicularis oris.

The lip is separated in white and red lip (vermillion). The red lip is formed by a dry and wet segment. The vermillion border is a thin cutaneous portion on the edge of the red lip demarcating the transition to the white line. The raised cutaneous area of white lip at the vermillion border is called the "white roll". The white line is a cutaneous transition between the vermillion and the white lip. The philtrum represents the compact decussating fibers of the orbicularis oris muscle at the central portion of the upper lip. Cupid's bow is formed by elevations in the vermillion due to the philtral ridges connected by a depression in between them in the central lip. The upper lip is separated in one central philtrum subunit and two lateral subunits. The lower lip is one single subunit.

The upper lip forms one-third of the lower face. The lower lip and chin forms two-thirds of the lower face. Lip shape is directly influenced by the underlying hard tissue support of the lower facial one-third and dental occlusion planes. The maxilla and mandible are the bony support of the soft tissue of the lips. Vertical maxillary/chin excess or deficiency may lead to decreased or increased lip showing. Changes in lip size and shape may at times be best achieved with orthodontic treatments and maxillofacial surgery rather than by surgery to the lips. The upper lip and lower lips are positioned 3.5 mm and 2.2 mm anterior to the subnasale-pogonion line.

Motor, Sensory and Blood Supply

- *Upper lip sensory*: Infraorbital nerve (CN V_2)
- *Lower lip sensory*: Inferior alveolar nerve (CN V_3)
- *Motor supply of the lips*: Buccal and marginal mandibular branches of the facial nerve (CN VII).

- The facial artery's superior (SLA) and inferior (ILA) labial branches provide the vascular supply of the lips. They are branches of the facial artery.
  - SLA branches into:
    - » Angular artery
    - » Septal artery
  - ILA branches into:
    - » Horizontal mental branch
  - In the central portion, the SLA and ILA are at 10 mm of depth from the free margin of the lip.

Normal Microanatomy of the Lips

The white lip is made of hair bearing skin. The vermillion is made of thin keratinized stratified squamous epithelium. The red lip does not contain hair follicles, sweat glands and sebaceous glands except at the vermillion border. The red lip has a rich vascular plexus below its dermis giving its red color. The wet portion of the red lip is lined by a thicker stratified squamous non-keratinized epithelium that becomes oral mucosa. The lip contains numerous accessory salivary glands in submucosa (serous, mucous and mixed glands).

Effects of Aging on the Perioral Complex

- Appearance of vertical wrinkles
- Marionettes lines
- Redistribution in length and form of the lips without total volume loss:
  - Flattening of the upper lip due to its elongation and convexity
  - Thinning of the red lips
  - Flattening of the white roll resulting in an entropion and ectropion of the upper and lower lip respectively
  - Increased area of white lip (skin around the mouth).
- Decrease in structural components of the lips:
  - Ptosis of the oral commissure
  - Loss of definition and reduced height of the vermillion
  - Loss of definition of cupid's bow.

LIP RECONSTRUCTION

Trauma or Cancer

- Skin-only defect
  - Local advancement flaps
  - Skin grafting
  - Healing by secondary intention
- Mucosa-only defect
  - Mucosal advancement flap
  - Healing by secondary intention
- Through-and-through defect
  - Up to one half
    » Primary closure
  - One half to two-thirds
    » Abbe flap (if involving commissure, two stages)
    » Estlander flap
    » Karapandzic flap (if Abbe or Estlander are unavailable)
  - Two-thirds to complete lip
    » Bernard-Burow flap (and Webster modification)
    » Gate flap
    » Dieffenbach advancement flap.

Congenital Reconstruction

- Please refer chapter "Cleft Lip and Palate".

COSMETIC REJUVENATION OPTIONS OF THE AGING LIP AND PERIORAL COMPLEX

- Perioral rhytid treatment
  - Botulinum toxin, fillers, lasers, and peels (please see respective chapters).
- Lip augmentation with fillers
  - Hyaluronic acid (Juvederm, and Restylane)
  - Other fillers are not recommended for lip augmentation (see fillers chapter for more details).
- Lip augmentation with implants
  - *Autologous*: Dermis-fat, superficial musculoaponeurotic system (SMAS), temporalis fascia, palmaris longus
  - *Implants*: Acellular dermal matrix (AlloDerm), ePTFE (Gore-Tex), silicone (silastic).
- Surgical lip augmentation
  - *Direct lip lift (DLL)*: Also known as vermillion lip lift or the gull wing lip lift
    » Incisions along new and old vermillion borders of upper and lower lip are made to remove white lip surrounding them
    » An overcorrection of 1 mm can be performed because the new vermillion tends to drop 1–1.5 mm 6 months postoperative.

- Indirect lip lift
  - » Incisions at the base of the nose, with multiple variations that can include columella, orbicularis oris, and philtral incisions (Fig. 1)
  - » Examples: Bullhorn lip lift, philtrum stretching, philtrum lift, extended, Greenwald, double-duck, and Italian technique.
  - Suture suspension
  - Corner of the mouth lift (CML)
    » Achieves lifting of the commissures using excisions of the white lip adjacent to the upper oral commissures
    » Examples: Greenwald lentoid excision, triangular incision, rhomboidal incision, Valentine anguloplasty, extended.
  - V-Y lip augmentation (VYLA)
    » Performed in the vestibular mucosa of the lip
    » Examples:
      - Transverse Y-V: Bulge of the central vermillion with decreased horizontal length
      - Double V-Y: Protrusion of the central and lateral vermillion
      - V-Y in V-Y: Significant vermillion protrusion and lip augmentation.
- Surgical lip reduction (reduction cheiloplasty)
  - Removal of a fusiform or elliptical segment of the lips and closing to reposition the lips. Always orbicularis-sparing.
    » Elliptical excision
    » Brazilian bikini lip reduction (Fig. 2)

COMPLICATIONS

- Fillers and implants
  - Edema and erythema
  - Lumpiness
  - Granulomas
  - Allergic reactions
  - Ecchymosis
  - Residual pain during smiling or opening of the mouth
  - Hypoesthesia
  - Tight and stiff lip
  - Asymmetry
  - Malposition
  - Extrusion
- Surgical lip augmentation
  - Asymmetry
  - Edema
  - Hypertrophic scars
  - Undercorrection
  - Infection and suture abscess
  - Hypoesthesia and paresthesia
  - Lip dryness.

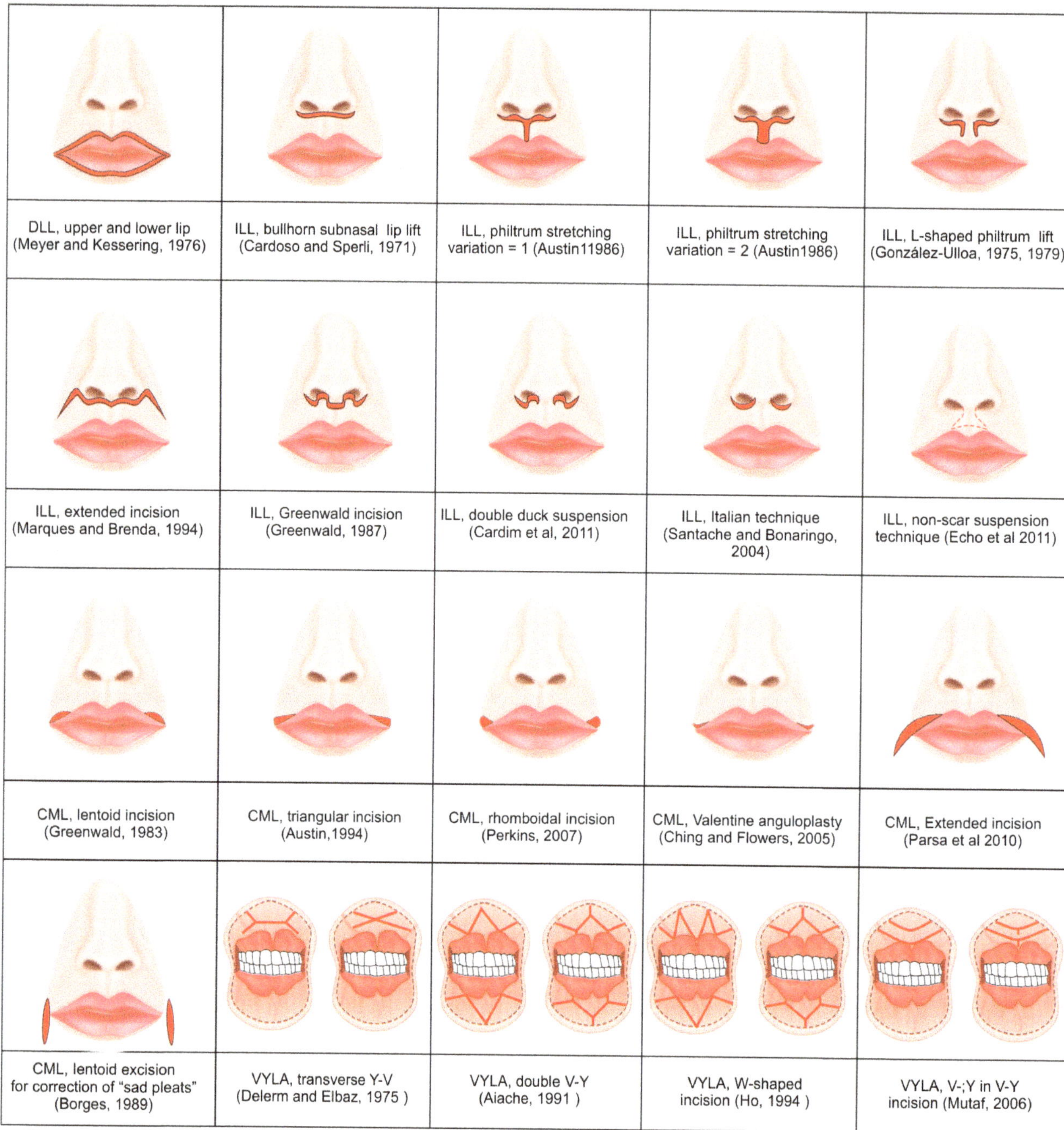

Fig. 1: Red compact lines: line of incision. Each type of VYLA surgery includes two images, which correspond to before and after the plasties are performed. Red dotted lines: trajectory of suspension thread (Echo et al. 2011). Red compact areas: areas of skin excision.

Abbreviations: DLL, direct lip lift; ILL, indirect lip lift; CML, corner of the mouth lift; Y-V, Y-V plasty; V-Y, V-Y plasty; VYLA, V-Y lip augmentation.

Source: Adapted from Moragas JS, Vercruysse HJ, Mommaerts MY. "Non-filling" procedures for lip augmentation: a systematic review of contemporary techniques and their outcomes. J Craniomaxillofac Surg. 2014;42:943-52.

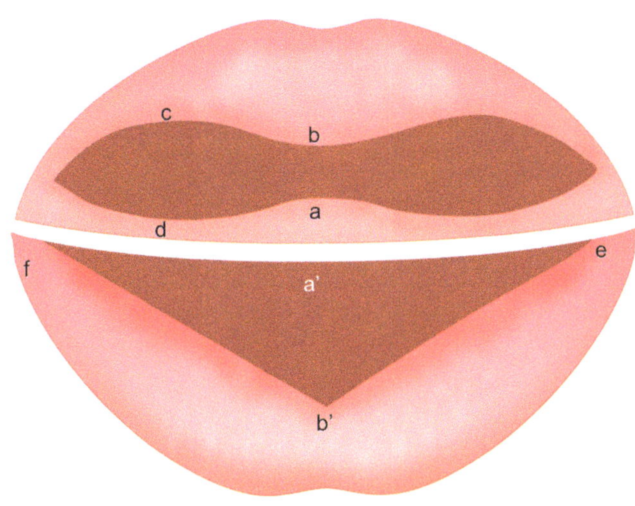

Fig. 2: "Brazilian" bikini lip reduction.

- Reduction cheiloplasty
  - Under-reduction
  - Over-reduction (can need re-operation and oral mucosal grafting)
  - Edema
  - Mucous retention cyst.

■ BIBLIOGRAPHY

1. Al-Hoqail RA, Abdel Meguid EM. The lip: A histologic and analytical approach of relevance to esthetic plastic surgery. J Craniofac Surg. 2009;20:726-32.
2. Byrne PJ, Hilger HP. Lip augmentation. Facial Plast Surg. 2004;20:31-8.
3. Cupp CL, Larrabee WF Jr. Reconstruction of the lips. Operative Techniques in Otolaryngology-Head and Neck Surgery. 1993;4:46-53.
4. Fanous N, Brousseau VJ, Yoskovitch A. The 'bikini lip reduction': A detailed approach to hypertrophic lips. Can J Plast Surg. 2007;15:205-10.
5. Guerrissi JO. Surgical treatment of the senile upper lip. Plast Reconstr Surg. 2000;106:938-40.
6. Langstein HN, Robb GL. Lip and perioral reconstruction. Clin Plast Surg. 2005;32:431-5.
7. Moragas JS, Vercruysse HJ, Mommaerts MY. "Non-filling" procedures for lip augmentation: a systematic review of contemporary techniques and their outcomes. J Craniomaxillofac Surg. 2014;42:943-52.
8. Niamtu J 3rd. Lip reduction surgery (reduction cheiloplasty). Facial Plast Surg Clin North Am. 2010;18:79-97.
9. Pepper JP, Baker SR. Local flaps: cheek and lip reconstruction. JAMA Facial Plast Surg. 2013;15:374-82.
10. San Miguel Moragas J, Reddy RR, Hernández Alfaro F, et al. Systematic review of "filling" procedures for lip augmentation regarding types of material, outcomes and complications. J Craniomaxillofac Surg. 2015;43:883-906.
11. Schulte DL, Sherris DA, Kasperbauer JL. The anatomical basis of the Abbé flap. Laryngoscope. 2001;111:382-6.

Multiple Choice Questions

Q 1. Which of the following statements about lip esthetics is FALSE?

A. The distance from the menton to the subnasale should be one third of the distance from the menton to the hairline

B. The distance from the subnasale to the stomion is one third of the distance comprising the lower third of the face

C. The lower lip and chin constitute one half of the distance comprising the lower third of the face

D. The upper lip should lie 3.5 mm anterior to the line formed by the subnasale to the pogonion

Ans: C. The lower lip and chin constitute one half of the distance comprising the lower third of the face

Q 2. Which of the following relationships of the lips to the nasomental line is CORRECT?

A. Upper lip is 4 mm anterior; lower lip 2 mm anterior

B. Upper lip is 4 mm posterior, lower lip 2 mm posterior

C. Upper lip is 2 mm anterior, lower lip 4 mm posterior

D. Upper lip is 4 mm posterior, lower lip 4 mm posterior

Ans: B. Upper lip is 4 mm posterior, lower lip 2 mm posterior

Q 3. Which of the following measurements is the DISTANCE, represented in the drawing below, between the upper lip and the nasomental line?

A. 0 mm, tangential to the nasomental line

B. 2 mm, posterior to the nasomental line

C. 4 mm, posterior to the nasomental line

D. 6 mm, posterior to the nasomental line

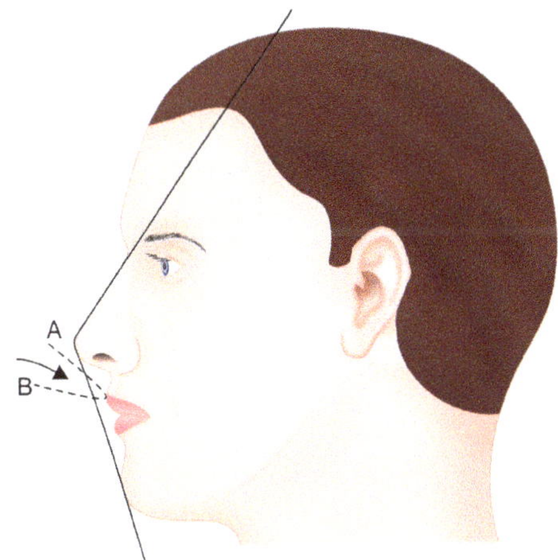

Ans: C. 4 mm, posterior to the nasomental line

Q 4. Which of the following perioral age related changes is FALSE?

A. The upper lip lengthens
B. The philtrum flattens
C. The vermillion has a flat and thin profile
D. The upper incisors are visible in repose

Ans: D. The upper incisors are visible in repose

Q 5. Which of the following statements about the characteristic of normal perioral findings in young individuals is TRUE?

A. The interface of the upper and lower lips forms a W
B. The lower lip should be more anterior than the upper lip on profile view
C. Both lips should protrude beyond a vertical line drawn from the subnasale to the pogonium
D. The upper and lower lips meet in the midline

Ans: C. Both lips should protrude beyond a vertical line drawn from the subnasale to the pogonium

Q 6. Which of the following statements is NOT characteristic of aging lips?

A. Blunting of the philtrum
B. Flattening of the white roll of the upper and lower lips
C. Lip projection is unchanged
D. Decreased vermillion show

Ans: C. Lip projection is unchanged

Q 7. Which of the following statements related to the perioral region is FALSE?

A. The oral commisure should be within a vertical line drawn from the medial limbus of the iris
B. The lips may have an inter-labial gap of 3 mm on repose
C. The lower lip, on profile, is more anteriorly positioned than the upper lip
D. The white roll of the lip separates the vermillion from the skin

Ans: C. The lower lip, on profile, is more anteriorly positioned than the upper lip

Q 8. Which of the lip esthetic subunits is the one indicated by the arrow?

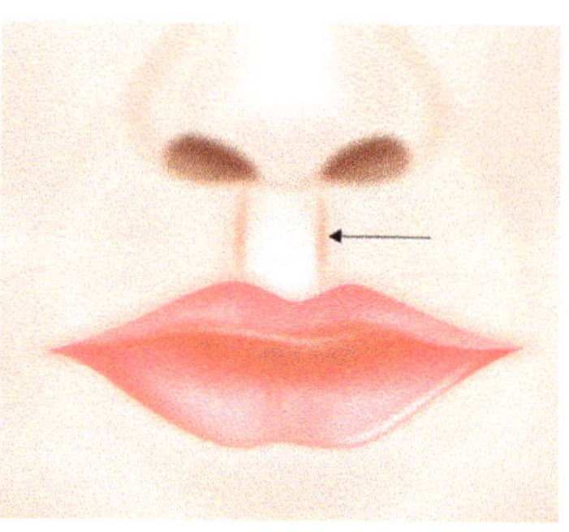

A. Philtrum dimple   B. Philtrum column
C. Cupid's bow   D. Vermillion border

Ans: B. Philtrum column

Q 9. Which of the following statements regarding the buccal fat pad is FALSE?

A. The normal buccal fat pad has four extensions from its body
B. The antero-inferior displacement of the pterygoid extension is the cause of the "pseudoherniation" of the buccal fat pad
C. "Pseudoherniation" of the buccal fat pad presents clinically as a soft, nontender, walnut-sized, lower cheek subcutaneous
D. The "pseudoherniation" of the buccal fat pad is reduced temporarily by pushing it in and upward toward the zygoma

Ans: B. The antero-inferior displacement of the pterygoid extension is the cause of the "pseudoherniation" of the buccal fat pad

Q 10. Which of the following statements about Lip Advancement is FALSE?

A. Lip advancement is ideal in patients with significant vermillion roll
B. Lip advancement is preferred in cases of undefined Cupid's Bow
C. The upper lip is outlined 0.5 cm above the vermillion border at the level of philtral colums
D. The upper lip is outlined with 0.3 cm above at the central upper lip

Ans: A. Lip advancement is ideal in patients with significant vermillion roll

Chapter 14

Liposuction

Sarah M Kidwai, Ketan Mehta

BACKGROUND

The practice of removing fat from regions of the body, including the face and neck, has been performed as early as 1932.[1] Illouz introduced the technique of blunt suction to remove fat, or liposuction, in the late 1970s.[2] Within just a few years, liposuction for the face and neck was introduced as an alternative to the traditional lipectomy.[3] Before the advent of liposuction, the excision of facial and neck fat was performed via sharp direct excision of fat via a skin incision.[1,4,5] Unfortunately, these procedures led to many complications, including scarring, excessive skin excision leading to contractures, depression or dimpling of the skin, nerve paresis, or bunching deformities of the neck.[6-9] Liposuction allows for avoidance of postoperative skin depression and scarring as well as decreased incidence of nerve injury and hematoma.[3,10]

AGING OF THE FACE AND NECK

- Liposuction is commonly performed in conjunction with rhytidectomy, which is performed most commonly to address complaints related to aging of the face and neck (Table 1).

ANATOMY OF THE CERVICOFACIAL FAT

- Describe anatomical boundaries of each region that can be liposuctioned (submental, jowls, cervical, and facial). Anatomical boundaries of the neck:
  - Inferior border of the neck superiorly
  - Supraclavicular area inferiorly
  - Anterior borders of the trapezius muscles laterally.

Table 1: Aging of the face and neck.

Intrinsic aging factors	Extrinsic aging factors
Thinning of epidermis	Sun exposure
Loss of subcutaneous fat	Gravity
Effacement of dermal epidermal junction	Nicotine
Loss and disorganization of elastic fibers and collagen (elastosis)	

- Platsyma
  - *Origin*: Fascia overlying the pectoralis and deltoid muscles
  - *Insertion*: Multiple points above the angle of the mandible
    - » Posterior fibers combine with the depressor anguli oris, mentalis, risorius, and orbicularis oris before insertion at level of commissure
    - » Central fibers insert directly into the periosteum of the mandible
  - Decussation of muscle fibers (Fig. 1):
    - » Type I (75%): Limited decussation of fibers extending 1–2 cm below mandibular symphysis.
    - » Type II (15%): Decussation of fibers from mandibular symphysis to thyroid cartilage.
    - » Type III (10%): No decussation. Superficial cervical fascia.
  - Continuation of the superficial musculoaponeurotic system (SMAS)
  - Divides to envelope the platysma
- Cervicofacial fat
  - Superficial layer of fat lateral to platysma, which is continuous with cheeks and nasolabial folds. Anteriorly and medially, this forms the submental fat
  - *Submental fat*: It is anterior and medial continuation of submental fat located within submental triangle
    - » Subcutaneous fat
    - » Thin layer of fascia due to absence of platysma at the midline
    - » Deep subplatysmal fat
    - » Considerations:
      - Excess removal can result in sunken "cobra deformity" because of adherence of submental skin to mylohyoid
      - Laterally, damage to marginal mandibular nerve or grater auricular nerve.
  - Areas that can be considered for liposuction
    - » Jowls
    - » Nasolabial region

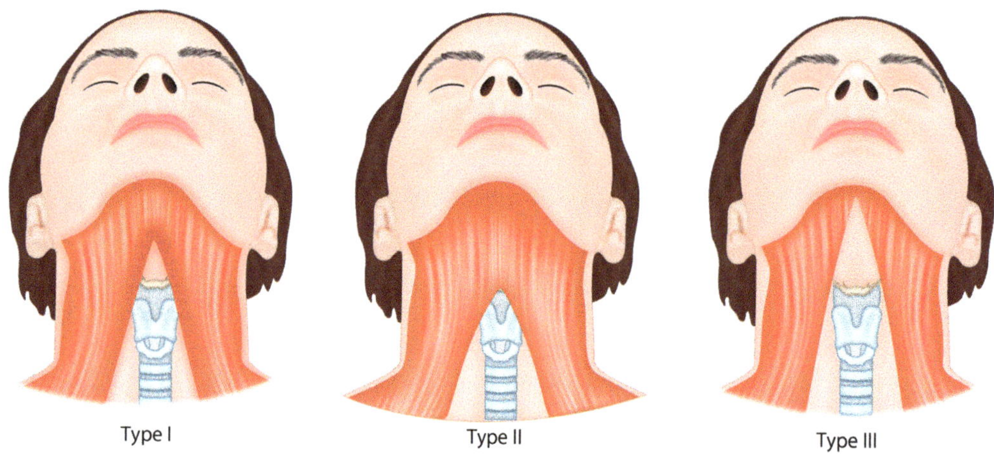

Fig. 1: Decussation of platysmal fibers. Type I (75%): Limited decussation of fibers extending 1–2 cm below mandibular symphysis. Type II (15%): Decussation of fibers from mandibular symphysis to thyroid cartilage. Type III (10%): No decussation

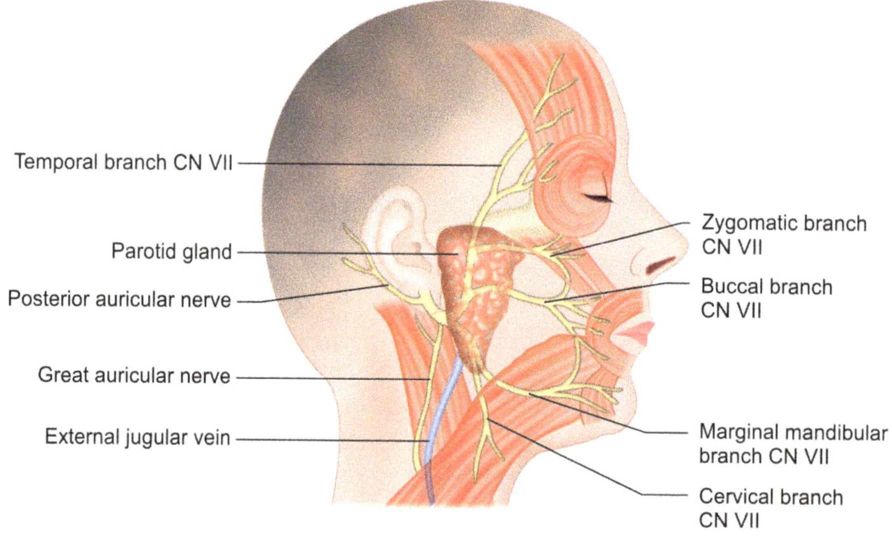

Fig. 2: Major nerves encountered during cervicofacial liposuction

- » Submental region
- » Buccal area
- » Lateral neck.
- Neurovascular structures (Fig. 2)
  - *Marginal mandibular branch of the facial nerve* along the inferior border of the mandible. Anterior to the facial artery, the nerve is superior to mandibular border.
    - » Injury: It is weakness of lower lip depression but preservation of lower lip eversion.
  - *Cervical branch of the facial nerve* enters the deep surface of the platysma superolaterally.
    - » Injury: It is weakness of lower lip depression and lower lip eversion.
  - *Great auricular nerve* deep to the platysma inferiorly and covered by SMAS superiorly as it travels along lateral border of sternocleidomastoid muscle.
    - » Approximately 6.5 cm inferior to the body external auditory canal in midtransverse belly of the sternocleidomastoid

  - » Injury: Numbness of the lower two-thirds of the ear and preauricular and postauricular skin.
- Skeletal structures
  - Size and position of mandible
    - » Retrognathia versus prognathia or microgenia
  - Facial convexity
    - » Increased mandibular plane angle associated with obtuse chin-neck angle
  - Hyoid position
    - » Inferior position may exacerbate effects of aging process
- Theory of finite number of fat cells
  - During the fourth month of gestation, adipocytes develop from early fibroblasts. The number of these cells triples during the first year of life, then increases at puberty.[11]
  - Adipocyte precursor cells remain throughout adulthood, and can be stimulated to become mature adipocytes with weight gain.[12]

– When mature adipocytes are formed because of weight gain, they are relatively resistant to diet and exercise.[12]
- Lipolysis
  – Biochemical pathway involving enzymes and precursors that occurs most prominently in white and brown adipose tissue for the catabolism triacylgylcerol within adipocytes.
  – Nonsurgical methods for fat reduction utilize energy devices, like external lasers, radiofrequency, cryolipolysis, and ultrasound, to similarly breakdown adipocytes. Injectable pharmacologic agents have been recently introduced.[13]

■ PREOPERATIVE ASSESSMENT

- Relevant history
  – Sun exposure
  – Medical history
  – Diet
  – Previous weight gain and loss
  – Inherited skin tone and thickness
  – Weight loss
    » Past weight loss and current attempts at weight loss
    » Massive weight loss may lead to large amount of redundant skin and soft tissue, which may be amenable to other facial rejuvenation techniques like rhytidectomy without liposuction.[14]
- Relevant physical examination
  – Facial regions considered for liposuction:
    » Submentum, lateral neck, jowls, nasolabial fold, and buccal areas
    » Areas of excess tissue or laxity should be avoided.
  – Skin elasticity: Skin that rebounds well, good candidate for liposculpture because it can conform to underlying bony structures after fat removal
  – Analysis of the submentum
    » Note ptosis of submandibular glands
    » Pinch test—evaluate submental fat thickness
      - Fat superficial to platysmal easily grasped compared to fat deep to platysma
      - Minimum thickness is 0.3–0.5 inch[15]
  – Analysis of the neck: Ask the patient to grimace, whistle, and smile
    » Presence and degree of platysmal banding can be appreciated when patient is grimacing
      - Flat, broad, even platysma → liposuction for smooth rejuvenated appearance
      - Platysmal banding→ skin tightening techniques.
    » Evaluate musculature of perioral area when patient is grimacing, whistling, or smiling
    » Ideal cervical mental angle: 105–120° (Fig. 3)
      - Low set hyoid bone can create obtuse angle.

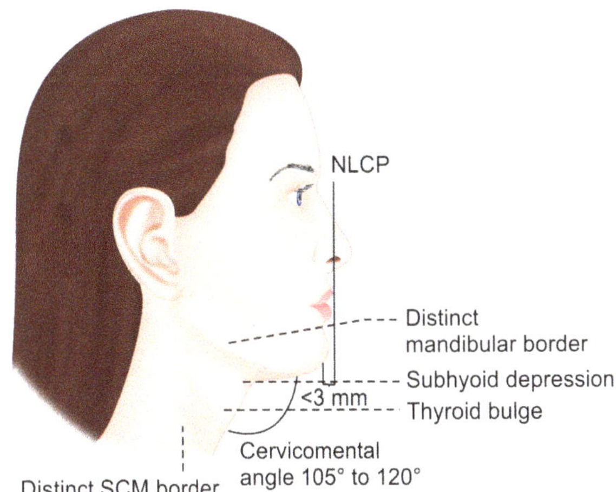

Fig. 3: Ideal cervicofacial measurements
NLCP: Nose-Lip-chin-Plane; SCM: Sternocleidomastoid

  – Analysis of the jowls
    » Palpation and oblique traction of the cheek to help define this area
    » Fat and round with a definite bulge, lipoplasty is an option.
  – Analysis of the nasolabial folds
    » Using simple upward traction
    » If improved with elevation, liposuction unlikely to yield long-lasting results
    » If noticeable bulges with elevation, liposuction is an option.[15]
  – Analysis of buccal area
    » Bulging midcheek may benefit from excision of buccal fat bad (Bichat's pad)
    » Liposuction of preparotid fat to decrease full face.
    » Note size and position of mandible and hyoid bone.
- Liposuction can be performed in conjunction with:
  – Chin implants
  – Rhytidectomy
  – Malar implants.

■ SURGICAL TECHNIQUE

- Instruments required
  – Traditional liposuction system (Fig. 4): Five major components: (1) cannula, (2) handle, (3) suction tubing, (4) collection canister, and (5) vacuum pump
  – Low pressure in canister allows aspirate to flow through system as a result of difference in pressures
  – Rate of aspiration is inversely proportional to cannula length, directly proportional to cannula and suction-tubing diameter, and greatly reduced with a cannula diameter less than 4 mm.[16]
  – Pressures for effective liposuction are 300–600 mm Hg, with a loss of approximately 25 mm Hg per 1,000 feet of altitude.[17,18]
  – Cannula types:[18]

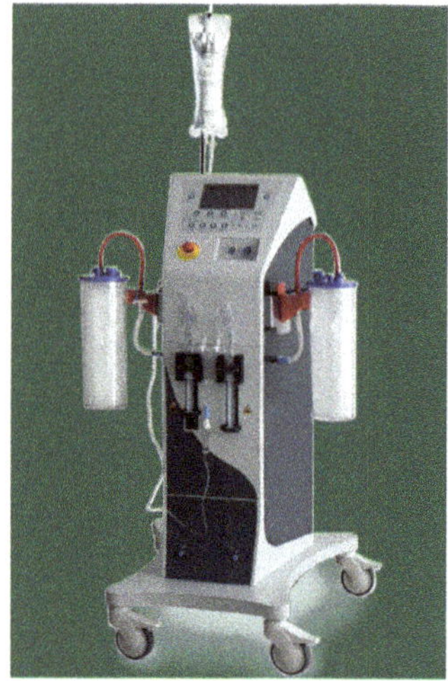

Fig. 4: Traditional liposuction system

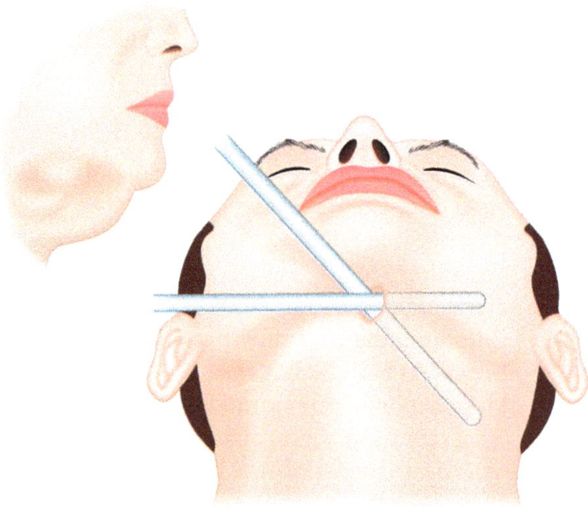

Fig. 5: Submental incision for liposuction

» Standard: Blunt tips, no ports at tips, and no sharp edges
» Cannula diameter ranges from 2 to 6 mm
» Cannula length ranges from 16 to 34 cm
» Vented cannula—small continuous leak in cannula at the shaft to reduce viscosity of tissue in suction tubing in order to improve flow
» Suction-assisted lipoplasty (SAL): Surgeon's arm provides back and forth motion of cannula to allow mechanical disruption of fat cells
» Power-assisted lipoplasty (PAL): Augmented form of SAL where a rapidly reciprocating cannula provides the back and forth motion in place of surgeon's arm

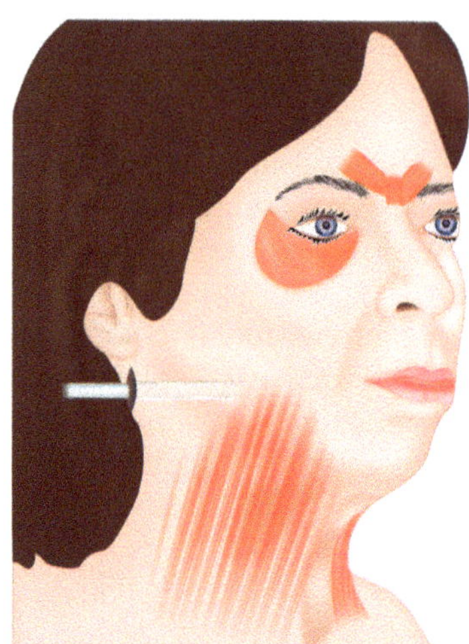

Fig. 6: Incision anterior and inferior to lobule for jowl liposuction

» Ultrasound-assisted lipoplasty (UAL), laser-assisted lipolysis (LAL), water-assisted liposuction (WAL), and radiofrequency-assisted liposuction (RFAL) are some other types of liposuction that utilize different energy forms for disruption and suctioning of fat cells.
- Brief summary of surgical technique
  - Incisions (2–4 mm):
    » Submental liposuction (Fig. 5): Behind submental crease
    » Jowl liposuction (Fig. 6): Anterior and inferior to ear lobule, postauricular, or submental incision
    » Melolabial liposuction: Pyriform recess in nasal antrum, lower lateral vestibule of nostril, or sublabial incision.
  - Area usually injected with local anesthetic and epinephrine for local vasoconstriction
  - After insertion into correct plane, gentle pushing and pulling motions.
    » *Crisscross technique* to create smooth appearance of skin
    » *Pinch and roll technique* to determine the degree and extent of liposuction needed
    » *Spoke-wheel pattern* while is often avoided outside of the head and neck because of poor postoperatively results, is used for facial liposuction.[19] The tunneling motion back and forth is performed radially, or in a spoke-wheel pattern, from the incision for a smooth, even appearance.[5]
    » Considerations:
      - Fenestra of the cannula should be away from the skin flap to maintain a subdermal layer of fat to prevent subdermal vasculature injury and skin dimpling (Fig. 7).
      - The areas of fat can be approached from different directions to achieve a thorough removal of fat.

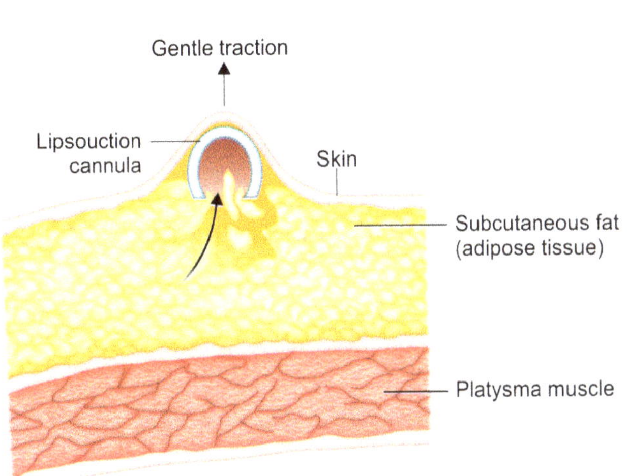

Fig. 7: Liposuction cannula with fenestration facing down within the subcutaneous fat layer above platysma

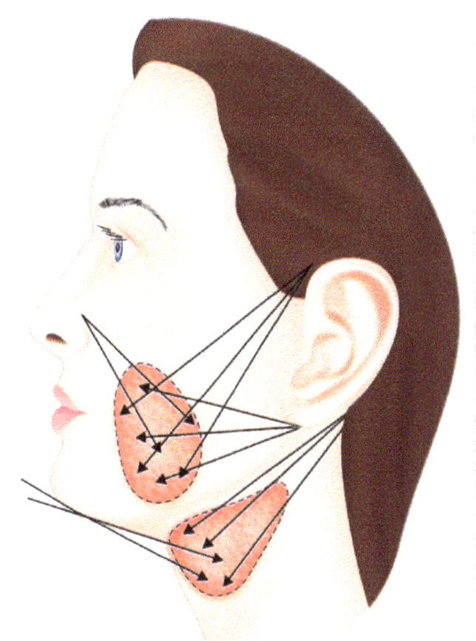

Fig. 8: Jowl suctioning from three different directions for optimal results

Suctioning of the jowls from different directions is shown in Figure 8.[15]
- Near the inferior border of the mandible, care should be taken to avoid excessive pressure against the mandible to avoid injury to marginal mandibular nerve
- Area usually injected with local anesthetic and epinephrine for local vasoconstriction.

■ COMPLICATIONS

Complications of liposuction have been described in Table 2.[5,11,20-23]

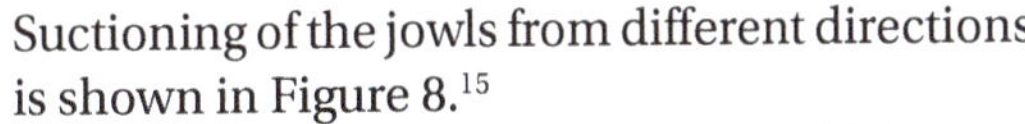

Table 2: Complications, etiology, treatment, and prevention of liposuction.			
Complications	*Etiology*	*Treatment*	*Prevention*
Hematoma and seroma formation (1–10%)	• Subdermal vessel injury and dependent collection of fluid • Major: Within 24 hours, increasing facial edema and pain • Minor: May not be detected until after dressing change	• Incision and drainage • Needle drainage • Elastic pressure dressing	• Avoidance of vascular arcades intraoperatively • Postoperative elastic pressure dressing • Placement of suction drains
Skin dimpling	• Lack of an even subdermal layer of fat • Initial presentation of fat pad caused skin stretching	• Skin tightening procedure • Fat transfer injections	• Maintain a layer of subcutaneous fat during liposuction • Incision to include skin resection[11]
Complications	*Etiology*	*Treatment*	*Prevention*
Nerve injury	• Subplatysmal liposuctioning[5] • Intra-oral or sublabial or approach[5] • Greater auricular nerve, facial nerve branches, trigeminal nerve branches	• Usually self-limited and transient • Electrical muscle exerciser or stimulator if delayed return	• Avoidance of pressure near areas of important nerves
Platysmal band deformity (6.6%)	• Prominence of platysma fibers that is apparent on the skin • More common in patients with undecussated platysma fibers (Fig. 1) • Usually occurs when rhytidectomy performed[20]	• Surgical correction[20] • Botulinum toxin A injection[21]	• Identify patients at risk: Redundant cervical skin, mild preoperative bands, submental obesity[20]

Contd...

Contd...

Scar hypertrophy or contracture	• Keloid tendency • Poor wound healing • Improper suture technique • Excessive wound tension	• Responds well to intralesional injection of triamcinolone acetonide[22]	• Use of small horizontal incision in submental area • Proper wound closure and care
Hypoesthesia	• Cutaneous nerve injury in subdermal layer • More common in periauricular and submental regions	• Usually self-limited and returns in few weeks to several months[23]	• Difficult to avoid
Skin sloughing (1–6%)	• Superficial skin necrosis in areas of suture • Risk factors: Smoking history, systemic medical conditions, superficial skin dissection, excessive skin tension	• Smaller areas will epithelize • Larger areas may require scar revision[23]	• Avoid superficial dissection and excessive skin tension

■ REFERENCES

1. Maliniak JW. Is the surgical restoration of the aged face justified? Indications, method of repair, end result. Med J Rec. 1932;135:321-4.
2. Illouz YG. Body contouring by lipolysis: a 5-year experiences with over 3,000 cases. Plast Reconstr Surg. 1983;72:591-7.
3. Teimourian B. Face and neck suction-assisted lipectomy associated with rhytidectomy. Plast Reconstr Surg. 1983;72:627-33.
4. Davis AD. Obligations in the consideration of meloplasties. J Int Coll Surg. 1955;24:567-71.
5. Adamson JE, Horton CE, Crawford HH. The surgical correction of the "turkey gobbler" deformity. Plast Reconstr Surg. 1964;34:598-605.
6. Guerrerosantos J, Sandoval M, Salazar J. Long-term study of complications of neck lift. Clin Plast Surg. 1983;10:563-72.
7. Vistnes LM, Souther SG. The platysma muscle: anatomic considerations for aesthetic surgery of the anterior neck. Clin Plast Surg. 1983;10:441-8.
8. Weisman PA. One surgeon's experience with surgical contouring of the neck. Clin Plast Surg. 1983;10:521-41.
9. Kamer FM, Binder WJ. Avoiding depressions in submental lipectomy. Laryngoscope. 1980;90:1396-400.
10. Wilkinson TS. The repair of submental depression occurring after rhytidectomy. Plast Reconstr Surg. 1976;57:33-5.
11. Markman B. Anatomy and physiology of adipose tissue. Clin Plast Surg. 1989;16:235-44.
12. Van R, Bayliss C, Roncari D. Complete differentiation of adipocyte precursors: a culture system for studying the cellular nature of adipose tissue. Cell Tissue Res. 1978;195:317-29.
13. McDiarmid J, Ruiz JB, Lee D, et al. Results from a pooled analysis of two European randomized, placebo-controlled, phase 3 studies of ATX-101 for the pharmacologic reduction of excess submental fat. Aesthetic Plast Surg. 2014;38:849-60.
14. Narasimhan K, Ramanadham S, Rohrich RJ. Face lifting in the massive weight loss patient: modifications of our technique for this population. Plast Reconstr Surg. 2015;135:397-405.
15. Mladick RA. Lipoplasty: an ideal adjunctive procedure for the face lift. Clin Plast Surg. 1989;16:333-41.
16. Young VL, Brandon HJ. The physics of suction-assisted lipoplasty. Aesthet Surg J. 2004;24:206-10.
17. Hetter GP. Optimum vacuum pressures for lipolysis. Aesthetic Plast Surg.1984;8:23-6.
18. Fodor PB, Cimino WW, Watson JP, et al. Suction-assisted lipoplasty: physics, optimization, and clinical verification. Aesthet Surg J. 2005;25:234-46.
19. Fischer G. Liposculpture. 3. Surgical technique in liposculpture. J Dermatol Surg Oncol. 1991;17:964-6.
20. Kamer FM, Minoli JJ. Postoperative platysmal band deformity. A pitfall of submental liposuction. Arch Otolaryngol Head Neck Surg. 1993;119:193-6.
21. Kane MA. Nonsurgical treatment of platysmal bands with injection of botulinum toxin A. Plast Reconstr Surg. 1999;103:656-63.
22. Kamer FM, Pieper PG. Surgical treatment of the aging neck. Facial Plast Surg. 2001;17:123-8.
23. Spira M, Gerow FJ, Hardy B. Cervicofacial rhytidectomy. Plast Reconstr Surg.1967;40:551-61.

Multiple Choice Questions

Q 1. Which of the following statements is TRUE regarding facial liposuction?

A. The cannula should be directed under the SMAS
B. The lumen of the cannula should be close to the skin
C. The procedure will correct fine rhytids and redundant lax skin
D. The areas of greatest effectiveness are submental, submandibular and jowl

Ans: D. The areas of greatest effectiveness are submental, submandibular and jowl

Q 2. Which of the following criteria allows THE BEST POSSIBLE results in a Closed Suction Lipectomy?

A. Generalized facial accumulations (non-obese patient)
B. Ptosis and excess skin folds
C. Good laxity of the skin
D. Good bony contour

Ans: C. Good laxity of the skin

Q 3. Which of the following statements in cervicofacial liposuction is FALSE?

A. The patient surgical area is marked while sitting upright
B. 4 mm blunt-tipped suction cannula can be used

C. 2 atm negative pressure is usually applied for suctioning

D. The cannula openings is always directed away from the skin

Ans: C. 2 atm negative pressure is usually applied for suctioning

Q 4. Which of the following is the MOST common complication of suction-assisted lipectomy in the Head and Neck?

A. Hematoma

B. Infection

C. Skin irregularities

D. Nerve paresia

Ans: C. Skin irregularities

Q 5. Which of the following statements regarding Suction-assisted Lipectomy in the head and neck is FALSE?

A. Local anesthesia with IV sedation is ideal in this surgical procedure

B. Lipectomy in the lower aspect of the neck is done utilizing an incision behind the ear lobule

C. Lipectomy dissection should be done deep to the platysma muscle

D. The surgeon should never turn the opening of the cannula toward the skin

Ans: C. Lipectomy dissection should be done deep to the platysma muscle

Q 6. Which of the following statements regarding Suction-assisted Liposuction in the face and neck is FALSE?

A. Good elasticity in the skin is ideal for the efficacy of lipectomy

B. Platysmal banding can be significant improved by neck liposuction

C. Dimpling, depressions, or scarring will not be improved by neck liposuction

D. A high, posteriorly placed hyoid bone will produce a more favorable cosmetic result.

Ans: B. Platysmal banding can be significant improved by neck liposuction

Q 7. What is the approximately recommended NEGATIVE pressure necessary for the proper execution of neck and face liposuction?

A. 1 atm of negative pressure

B. 2 atm of negative pressure

C. 3 atm of negative pressure

D. 4 atm of negative pressure

Ans: A. 1 atm of negative pressure

Note: *(suction at -700 mm Hg - approximately 1 atm negative pressure)*

Chapter 15

Otoplasty

Beatrice Voizard, Anastasios Maniakas

■ EMBRYOLOGY AND ANATOMY

The six pharyngeal arches develop during the fourth week of gestation. The mesenchyme of the first arch (or mandibular arch) and second arch (or hyoid arch) guides the outer ear development. The six auricular hillocks (or hillocks of His) located on the arches will each contribute to a specific component of the pinna (or auricular cartilage). The antihelix furls during weeks 12–16 and the helix furls much later during the 6 months of gestation. The ectoderm of the first branchial groove will form the conchal cavity, with its upper, middle and lower portions forming the cymba concha, cavum concha, and intertragal incisura, respectively.[1] Most of the ear structure (the tragus, helical crus, helix, antihelix, the antitragus, and the lobule) comes from the hyoid arch. The auditory canal and tympanic membrane are derived from an invagination of the ectoderm of the first pharyngeal cleft, which separates the mandibular and hyoid arches. This invagination is guided by the tympanic ring, a C-shaped bony structure derived from the first arch that will fuse with the temporal bone when the external auditory meatus is flattened down and opposed to the endoderm of the middle ear cavity (Fig. 1).

The pinna is a single piece of yellow elastic fibrocartilage covered by firm perichondrium on both faces. On its anterior and lateral surfaces, subcutaneous adipose tissue is minimal, and the skin adheres firmly to the cartilage. The posterior surface is covered with two layers of fat and looser skin, with a larger subdermal arteriovenous plexus in the areolar connective tissue.[2]

- *Lobule*: Composed of firm trabecular subcutaneous tissue.
- Ligaments:
  - *Anterior ligament*: Tragus and helical root to the zygomatic process
  - *Posterior ligament*: Posterior wall of the concha to the mastoid.
- *Muscles*: Auricularis superior, obliquus auriculae, transversus auriculae, auricularis posterior, tragicus, helicis minor, helicis major, and auricularis anterior (Fig. 2).

Arterial Supply (Fig. 3)

- *Anterior and anterolateral surface*: The superficial temporal artery, a branch of the external carotid artery, emerges from the parotid capsule, deep to the veins, deep to the anterior auricular muscle and 10 mm in front of the ear and gives off three branches—(1) superior, (2) medial and (3) lateral. Since there is no significant subcutaneous adipose tissue separating this surface of auricular cartilage from the overlying skin, the perichondrium supplies the nutrients to the auricular cartilage. The subdermal vascular plane allows for flap viability.[2]
- *Posterior surface*: The posterior auricular artery travels in the posteroauricular crease and crosses below the great auricular nerve and under the posterior auricular muscle.[2]

Venous Drainage

Complimentary veins drain into the external jugular vein.

Lymphatic Drainage

The anterior region drains into the preauricular lymph node and superior, middle and inferior branches drain into the infra-auricular lymph node (Fig. 4).[3]

Innervation of External Ear

Contribution of both Cranial and Spinal Nerves (Fig. 5)

The great auricular nerve originates from C2-C3 and gives anterior and posterior branches at the base of the auricle. The anterior branch supplies the inferior half on the lateral surface of the auricle. The posterior branch supplies the

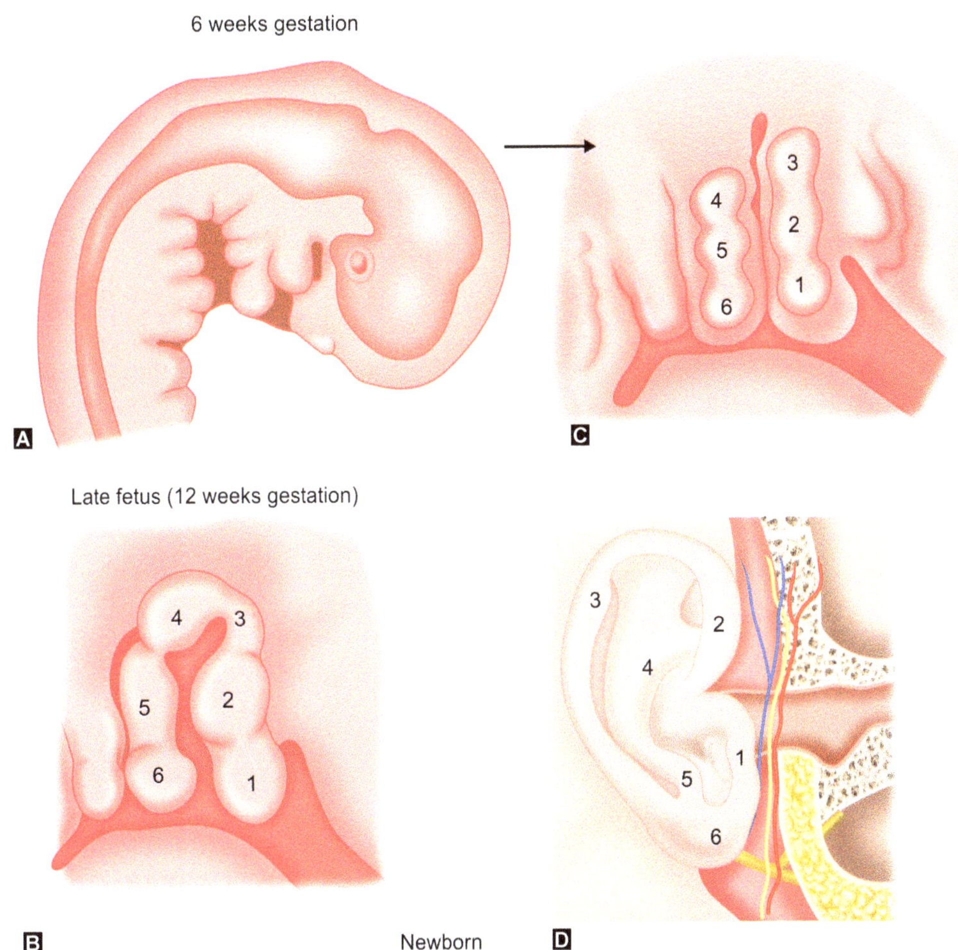

Figs. 1A to D: (A) Fetal shape at 6 weeks gestation; (B) Close-up view of the hillocks of His on the hyoid and mandibular arches; (C) Position of the hillocks at 12 weeks gestation; (D) Anatomy of the normal auricle at birth.

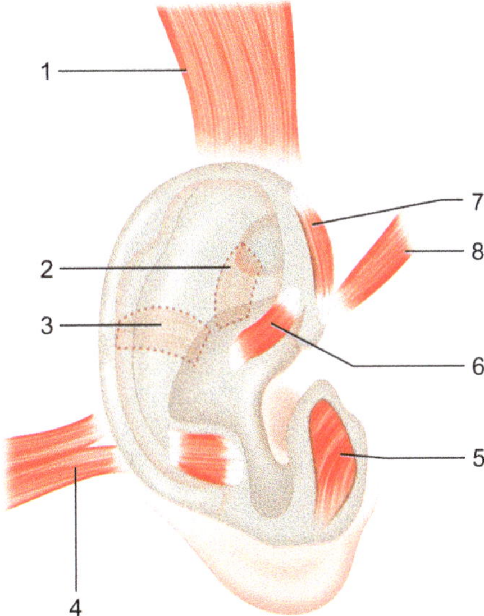

Fig. 2: Internal and external auricular muscles: 1: Auricularis superior; 2: Obliquus auriculae; 3: Transversus auriculae; 4: Auricularis posterior; 5: Tragicus; 6: Helicis minor; 7: Helicis major; 8: Auricularis anterior

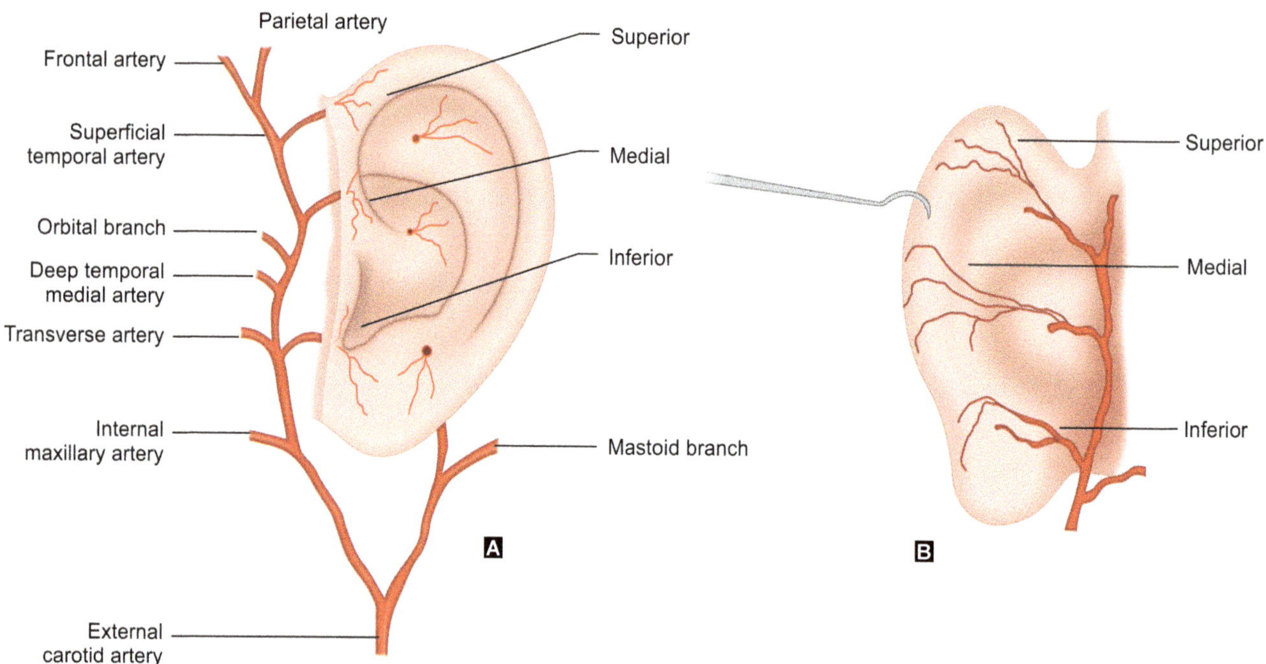

Figs. 3A and B: Arterial blood supply (Owsley 2004): (A) Anterior auricular arteries; (B) Posterior auricular arteries

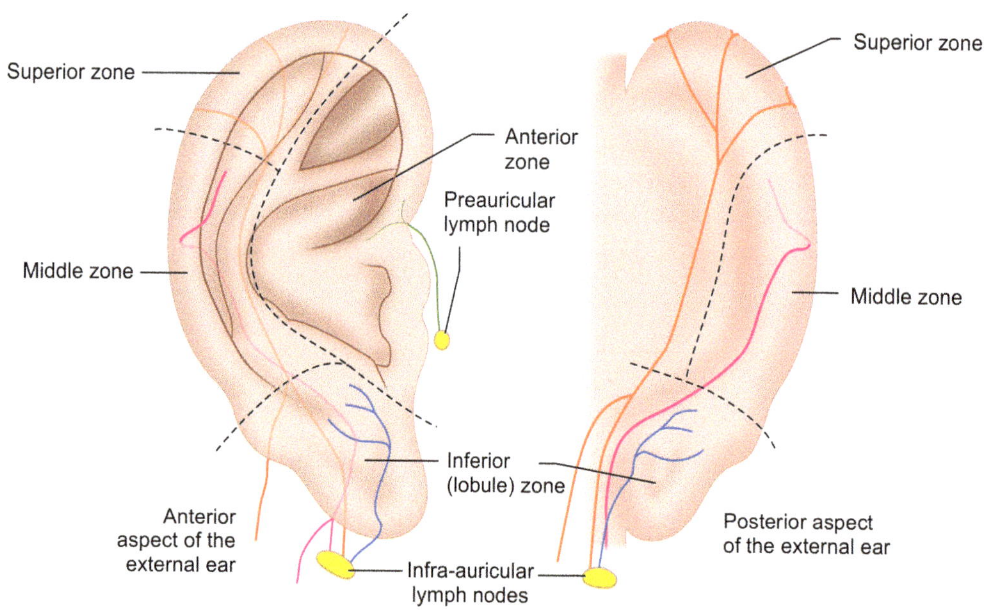

Fig. 4: Lymphatic drainage (Pan, le Roux et al. 2011)

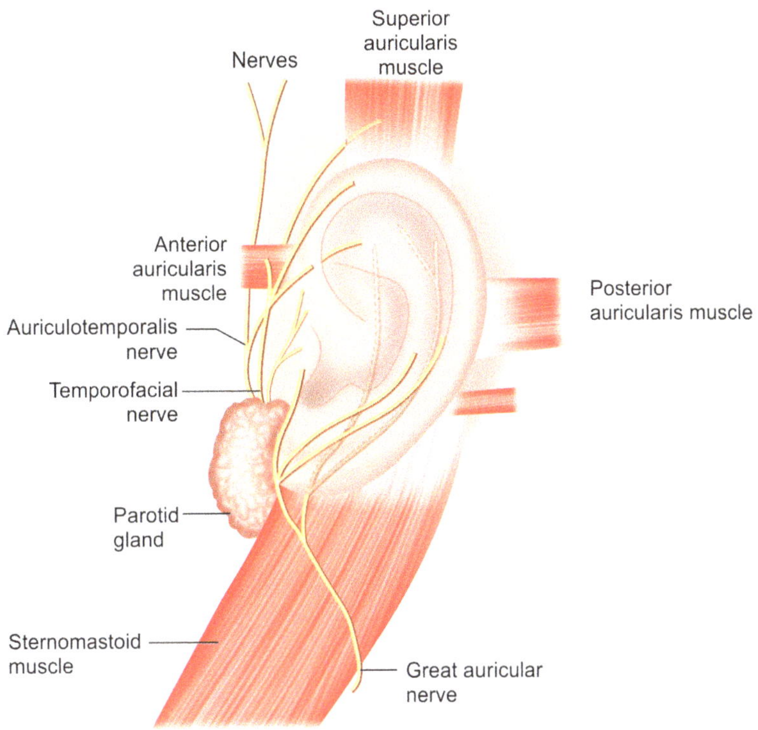

Fig. 5: Auricle innervation (Owsley 2004)

equivalent area on the medial side and travels 8 mm posterior to the posteroauricular crease.[2] Great auricular nerve dissection will lead to permanent lobule anesthesia and may additionally lead to transient auricular anesthesia. *The auriculotemporal nerve*, a branch of V3, supplies the anterosuperior surface and the adjacent temporal skin, and *the lesser occipital nerve* supplies the posterosuperior surface. *The auricular branch of vagus nerve (nerve of Arnold)* supplies the conchal bowl and the posterior wall of the external auditory meatus.[2]

■ PATHOPHYSIOLOGY

Prominent Ears, Protruding Ears and Bat Ears

- *Definition*: A 20 mm helix-mastoid distance at the upper third of the auricle or an oculocephalic angle greater than 40° (see aesthetic analysis section for details).
- Incidence = 5% in white population. Genetic predisposition: autosomal dominant with variable penetrance.[1]
- Unfurled margin of the helical rim is the most common abnormality.[1]

- Deeply cupped concha,[4] resulting from excessive conchal cartilage most commonly on the posterior conchal wall[2] and frequently present with deformity of the antihelix, is the second most common abnormality.[1]
- Poorly developed or absent antihelical fold, either involving the superior or anterior crus, will diminish the definition between the scapha and concha.[2]
- An anteromedially displaced insertion of the postero-auricular muscle may contribute to auriculocephalic angle widening.[5]
- Protruding earlobes.

Other Common Ear Deformities (Fig. 6)

- *Lop*: Overfolding of the upper portion of the ear, that results in the obliteration of the scapha. In some cases, the overfolding extends to the anterior crus and results in the obliteration of the triangular fossa (Fig. 6A).
- *Satyr*: Variable degree of overfolding of the helical rim resulting in a pointed and sharp upper portion of the pinna (Fig. 6B).
- *Shell*: Absence of the superior antihelical crus, with variable degree of broadening of the inferior antihelical crus, with possible helix folding abnormalities (Fig. 6C).[6]

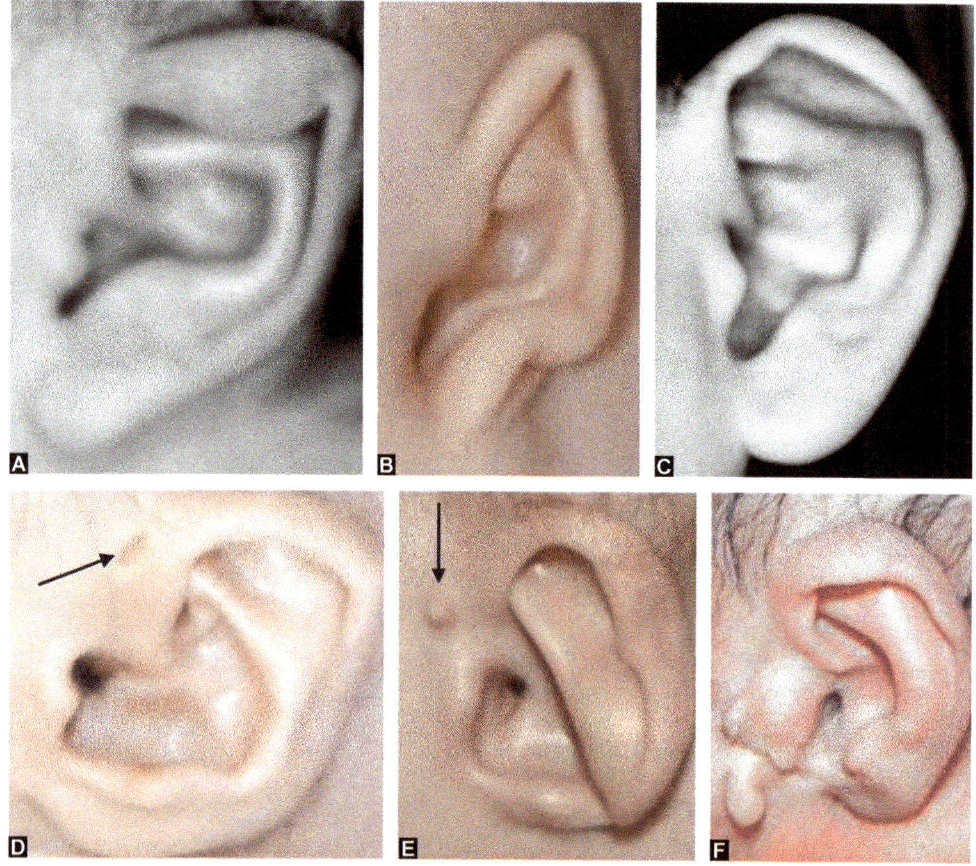

Figs. 6A to F: Common ear deformities: (A) Lop ear; (B) Satyr ear; (C) Shell ear; (D) Preauricular pit; (E) Preauricular tag; (F) Pretragal ectopias (Humter, fries et al. 2009)

- *Preauricular pit*: Indentation anterior to the insertion of the ear, superior to the tragus, resulting from a hillock fusion abnormality.[6] Prevalence = 0.9–5% (Fig. 6D).[7]
- *Tag*: Protrusion of skin and fat with or without cartilage that can be either auricular (located anteriorly or posteriorly on the pinna), preauricular (anterior to the insertion of the ear) or that can appear anywhere along the anterior border of the sternocleidomastoid.[6] Prevalence of preauricular tags less than 1% (Fig. 6E).[7]
- *Pretragal ectopia*: Complex preauricular ectopic cartilaginous tissue, which may have a helix-like shape and should be distinguished from tags (Fig. 6F).[6]

Microtias

Microtia is defined as longitudinal length more than 2 SD below the mean ear length. Prevalence ranges from 1 in 20,000 to 1 in 4,000 births. Microtias are divided into four categories (Table 1).[6,8-10]

- *Associated syndromes*: Microtia is associated with other anomalies or syndromes in 20–60% of cases, the most common of which are craniofacial microsomia, Townes-Brocks, Treacher-Collins and Nager syndromes (the latter two are known as mandibulofacial dysostoses).[11.]

Although oculo-auriculo-vertebral spectrum (OAVS) and microsomia have overlapping clinical expressions, the suggested idea that all microsomia are a milder form of OAVS remains controversial. The shared characteristics of OAVS and microsomia are notably right-side preponderance and male predilection.[11]

- *Genetics*: Different single gene mutations are associated with microtia in familial and syndromic cases, whereas polygenic or multifactorial causes are more likely responsible for the sporadic cases.

There are three major hypotheses regarding the pathogenesis of microsomia: (1) neural crest cell (NCC) disturbance may result in craniofacial malformations

Table 1: Different types of microtia

Deformity	Ear components	Surgical implications
First-degree microtia	All present	Reconstruction possible without the use of extra skin or cartilage
Second-degree microtia	Some absent, but not all	Some skin and cartilage required for partial reconstruction
Third-degree microtia	Some present, but none conform to recognized ear components	Skin and cartilage are needed for total reconstruction
Anotia	Total absence of auricular structures	Skin and cartilage are needed for total reconstruction

(e.g. the TCOF1 mutation causes neural crest cells (NCC) disturbance leading to Treacher-Collins syndrome), (2) vascular disruption leading to transient focal tissue ischemia and increased fragility, (3) altitude and the resulting chronic hypoxia are suspected to play a role (prevalence of microtia has been reported up to five times higher in regions of high altitude such as Quito, Ecuador).

Cauliflower Ear (Otohematoma)

When subperichondrial hematoma secondary to a trauma of the ear is not properly drained in the acute phase of the injury, the accumulation of blood acts as a barrier between the cartilage and its perichondrial blood supply. This results in cartilage necrosis, fibrosis and formation of neocartilage that deforms the auricle.[12]

■ HISTORY AND PHYSICAL EXAMINATION

Patients' goals and expectations should be discussed to select the most effective technique and appropriate timing for surgery. *The main goal of surgery is to produce a natural appearance with symmetry and proper position.*

- *On history*: Tics such as pulling on the auricle or scratching the helical rim can compromise surgical results and should be evaluated. Physical activities associated with repetitive ear manipulation (notably sports helmets) need to be interrupted in the postoperative period.
- *Photographs* (frontal, oblique, lateral and posterior views) and *measurements* (height, width, distance from the scalp, and auculocephalic angle) should be obtained to compare symmetry and evaluate the cause of prominence or deformity.[13]
- *Functional examination (audiometry)*: Ear malformations may be the first indications of hearing impairment in children. Hearing impairment was found to be 4–7 times more prevalent in children with preauricular skin tags and ear pits, therefore audiometry is recommended in the preoperative investigation of these patients.[7] As any ear surgery may comprise a certain risk to the patient's hearing, preoperative audiometry may be routine practice in certain centers.

Aesthetic Ear Analysis (Fig. 7)

- *Normal relationship of ears to the head* should be evaluated carefully with the patient's head held in the Frankfurt horizontal plane, with observer's eyes at the level of the patient ears.[6] Many positional factors will affect the evaluation: a hyperextended neck will make ears appear low-set and a head tilt will make ears appear unevenly set. The evaluator should remember that posteriorly inclined ears will appear low-set and small ears will appear high-set. Ear position is described by four characteristics:
  - *Location or horizontal position*: The horizontal position is measured from the subnasal to the tragus if the meatus is preserved, or to the base of the lobule if the meatus is atrophic.[14] Normal ear positioning is about one ear length posterolaterally to orbital rim.
  - *Level or vertical position*: Many methods have been used to study the preferred vertical position, including measuring the distance between the ear and the ghation and the distance between the tragus and the vertex of the head. These measurements can be obviated by the variability of the facial landmarks (e.g. unilateral microsomia, micrognathia, skull deformities, etc.).[14] The simplest rule to remember is that the preferred auricle position is between two horizontal lines: one drawn from the lateral eyebrow to the uppermost portion of the auricle, and one drawn from the nasal ala to the lowermost portion of the earlobe.[2,14]
  - *Inclination*: Inclination is the angle formed between the longitudinal and vertical axes of the ear.[14] The preferred angle ranges from 22 to 26°,[14] which is a greater posterior inclination than the line parallel to the bridge of the nose, used as a landmark in many reference books.
  - *Protrusion*: Protrusion is determined by three important angles. The cephaloconchal angle is a 90° angle formed by the posterior wall of the conchal bowl and the mastoid. The scaphaconchal angle is another 90° angle, formed by the antihelical fold. Combined with the curvature of the helix, these two angles set

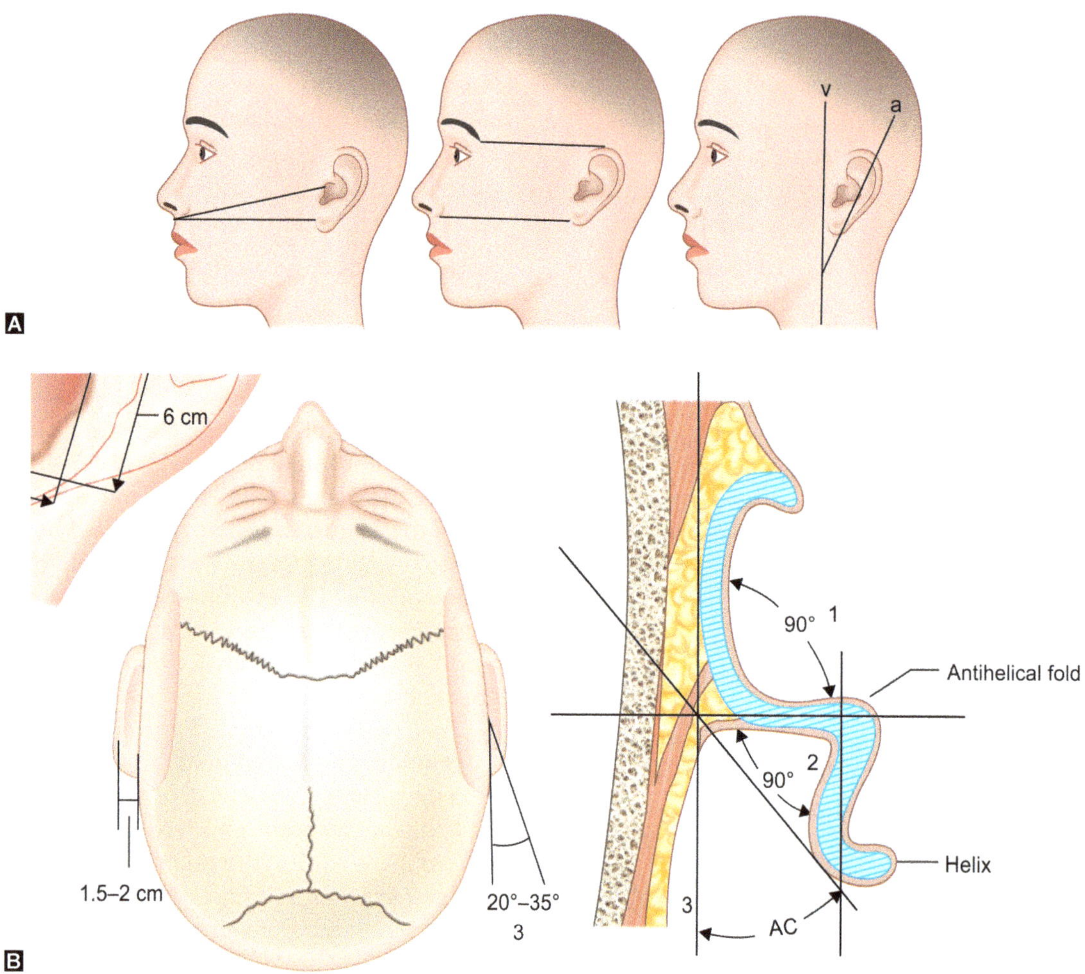

Figs. 7A and B: Aesthetic ear analysis: (A) Location, level and inclination are evaluated with the head in the Frankfurt horizontal, from the lateral view. (B) Auricular protrusion 1: cephaloconchal angle, 2: scaphaconchal angle, 3: auriculocephalic angle

the auricle at a 25–30° angle from the surface of the mastoid area, named the auriculocephalic angle.[2] Ears that protrude 40–45° generally appear abnormal.[1] There are simpler landmarks used to evaluate protrusion. First, from the frontal view, the helical rim should be just lateral to the most lateral aspect of the antihelix. Second, at the level of the mastoid area, the maximal distance between the helical rim and the scalp should be 20 mm. Third, the uppermost aspect of the helix should be no further than 10 mm lateral to the scalp.[2] Lastly, the difference in lateral protrusion of both auricles should be no more than 3 mm.

- *Size*:
  » The width of the auricle should be 60% of its height
  » The average adult lobule measured from the base of the antitragus to the lowest dependent edge is 15–20 mm.[15]

INDICATIONS AND PATIENT SELECTION

Indications

- Patients' perception of their ears will often diverge from an experts' point of view and the social impacts of ear protrusion or deformity will vary greatly from one patient to another. Therefore, indication for aesthetic correction is subjective.
- In some cases, protrusion should be corrected because it causes safety issues (for US army soldiers, helmets would cause skin lacerations on protruding ears).[16]
- The inability or noncompliance of the patient to care for their dressing may be considered as a contraindication. Young children should be informed that deformities can be corrected at a later point in life without any major consequences.

Patient Selection

Otoplasty

- *Ideal age for otoplasty*: The preferred age for correction of prominent ears has long been 5 years old, since teasing and its psychosocial effects begin during preschool years. It is becoming more common to operate younger patients because the excessive worry of caregivers regarding appearance is thought to have an impact earlier on in the psychosocial development of the child. Eighty-five percent of ear development is complete by the age of 3 years. Otoplasty does not impair further ear growth, as patients undergoing unilateral otoplasty before 3 years old do not show any asymmetry late in life. Furthermore, Gosain et al. noted that the cartilage is more malleable in children less than 3 years old, which reduces the overall need for scoring, rasping or burring.[17]
- In patients requiring reconstructive surgeries for other malformations, otoplasty should be performed concurrently, reducing costs and risks associated with anesthesia.[17]
- Patients with posteroauricular eczema or otitis externa should be treated preoperatively and the operation should be delayed until the eczema or otitis resolves.[5]

Reconstruction with Autogenous Graft

It is the preferred technique for the vast majority of pediatric patients with microtia. Some patients have such severe soft tissue hypoplasia that there is insufficient skin to coat the cartilaginous framework. In other cases, severe skeletal hypoplasia may prevent adequate projection. Orthognathic surgery and microvascular soft tissue augmentation need to be performed prior to auricular reconstruction.[9] The earliest age to proceed is 4 or 5 years old, allowing time for adequate mastoid pneumatization. The prime time is 6 years old, as there is enough costal cartilage by this age.[10]

Prosthetic Implants and Prosthetic Auricles

Prosthetic implants and prosthetic auricles are considered best for patients in whom autogenous reconstruction has failed or who have a low or unfavorable hairline. Even after hair ablation, the scalp's thicker skin would leave the auricular framework inadequately covered, blunting aesthetic results.[11]

Molding Techniques

Otoplasty using retention stiches in infants whose cartilage is very soft may cause accordion-like folding.[18] If started during the first weeks of life, taping a bendable splint along the helical rim, antihelix and concha for 2–12 weeks can correct up to 90% of deformities. After the age of 3 weeks, molding is less successful.[19,20]

■ SURGICAL PRINCIPLES

The ideal measurements are subject to controversy and should be used as guidelines in the visual assessment of ear morphology, but symmetry and aesthetic harmony is the ultimate goal of otoplastic surgery.

- *Otoplasty*: More than 170 surgical techniques have been described in the literature.[2] The main goals of otoplasty are to reduce the auriculocephalic angle, to create an antihelical fold and to correct any residual lateral protrusion of the helical root and lobule.
  - *Preoperative antibiotics* are not routinely given, except in the case of a simultaneous preauricular sinus excision.[21]
  - *Anesthesia* can be either regional or general. Regional anesthesia is contraindicated for children under age 3 or 4, and for patients undergoing simultaneous surgical correction of other deformities. Anesthetic solution should be instilled at the base of the auricle for regional anesthesia. It may also be needed at the posterior wall of the external auditory meatus. Infiltrating the regional anesthetic solution beneath the skin will facilitate hydrodissection of the planes and help in avoiding violation of the anterior skin during cartilage suture placement.[2,13]
  - *The sterile preparation should include* the external auditory meatus and external ear, and extend to the hair around the ear.[5]
  - *Drapes* should allow visibility of the entire face and both ears.[4,21]

■ COMMON APPROACHES

Cartilage Shaping Techniques

Mustardé Mattress Sutures (Fig. 8)

Squeezing or holding back the ear gently will recreate a natural looking antihelical fold and allow the surgeon to draw 3–4 Mustardé-type mattress sutures on the anterior surface of the pinna. A posterior incision is made and converse scissors serve to undermine the posterior skin of the superior half of the ear in the supraperichondrial plane. Some authors will suggest passing a 27-gauge needle through the conchal cartilage from the anterior skin markings and using a surgical pen to mark the posterior side of the cartilage,[13] whereas others will dip a hypodermic needle in methylene blue to tag the cartilage directly by

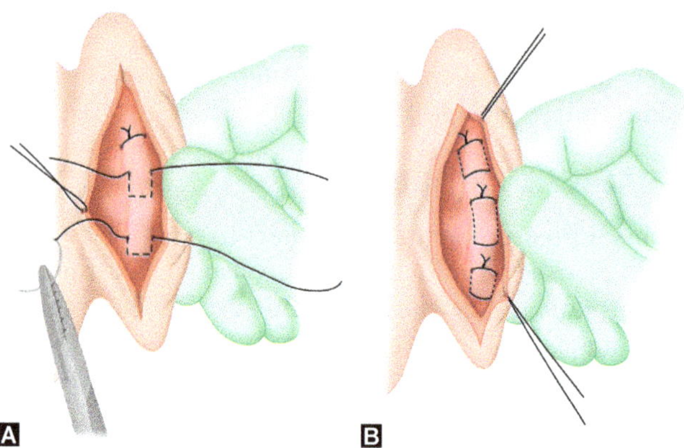

Figs 8A and B: Mustardé mattress sutures. A line is drawn on the crest of the antihelix and the mattress sutures are parallel to the line, at least 7 mm apart, to make sure the fold will not be too narrow (Owsley 2004)

transfixion tattooing.[2] Nonresorbable mattress sutures are passed through full thickness of the cartilage without violating the anterior skin, and are initially left untied to be tied one after the other at the end, either from superior to inferior or inversely as the assistant gently pinches the edge of the new antihelical fold to preserve its shape.

Furnas Conchal Setback Technique (Fig. 9)

If excessive cupping of the concha is the only cause of prominence, concha-mastoid setback sutures alone are sometimes sufficient to correct the defect.[4] To mark the incision site, the surgeon presses the conchal posterior wall and floor against the mastoid until the desired position is achieved. Markings are then made on the anterior surface of the auricle, at the line of junction between the auricular cartilage and the mastoid. An ellipse of posteroauricular skin is excised to expose the cartilage. The dissection stops at the ponticulus (the conchal ridge where the auricularis posterior muscle is attached). The fibers of the posteroauricular muscle are gently dissected, and care is taken here to preserve the branch of the posteroauricular nerve. The recipient site is prepared by undermining a posteroauricular skin flap leaving a thin layer of tissue over the mastoid periosteum, on a surface of 10 × 20 mm.[4] The conchal cartilage is sutured in a backhanded motion to facilitate suturing the periosteum with a forehanded movement.[13] A minimum of 3 concha-mastoid sutures are recommended: these are to be placed at the fossa triangularis, cavum concha and cymba concha.[1] A protrusion of the angular ledge of the auditory canal may result from sutures placed too far back on the concha and too far forward on the mastoid, reducing the diameter of the auditory canal, which must therefore be examined while suturing.[4] Some authors have proposed removing the outer

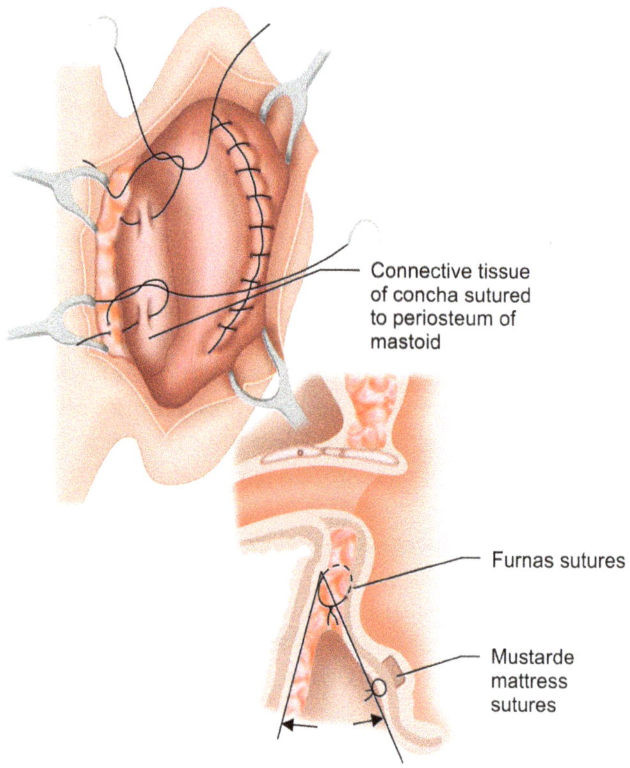

Figs. 9A and B: (A) Concha mastoid sutures; (B) Axial view showing the location of the combined Furnas and Mustardé sutures.

plate of the mastoid bone or thinning the cartilage when one or the other is too prominent.

Cartilage Cutting Techniques

Davis Conchal Setback Technique

A bean-shaped piece of conchal bowl cartilage is excised, sparing the helical crux and leaving an 8 mm posterior conchal wall ridge at the conchal-scaphal junction. The posteroauricular muscle and connective tissue is removed, since the anterior auricular skin of the conchal floor will be draped onto the mastoid surface.

Farior and Converse Techniques

Both techniques rely on longitudinal incisions at the antihelical fold to create an island of cartilage protruding anterior to the concha.

Anterior Scoring Technique (Fig. 10)

A 35 mm posteroauricular incision is made 10 mm proximal to the helical rim, falling into the concavity of the antihelical fold, remaining hidden. A transcartilaginous incision is made, starting from the cauda helicis along the helix and

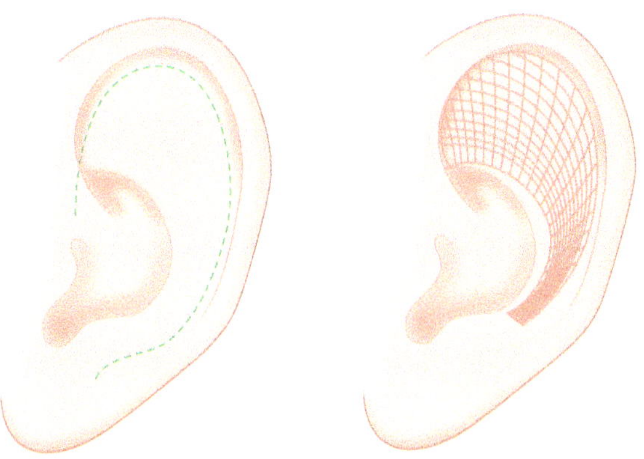

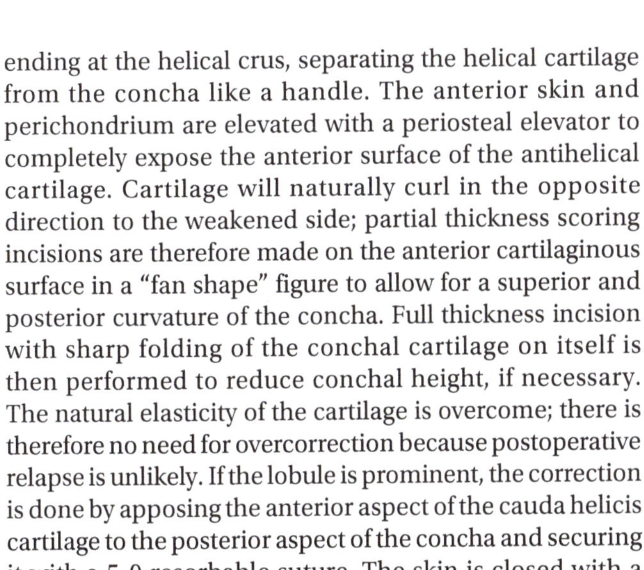

Fig. 10: The transcartilaginous incision showed in green runs parallel to the helical rim. The fan-shaped scoring incisions gather at the middle third of the ear and will curve the conchal cartilage superiorly and posteriorly.

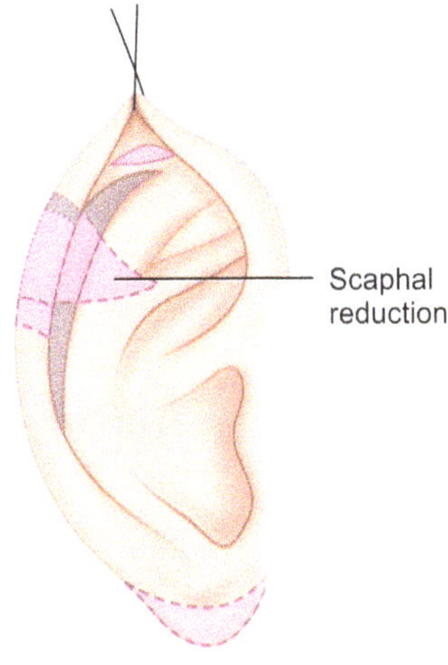

Fig. 11: Scaphal reduction

ending at the helical crus, separating the helical cartilage from the concha like a handle. The anterior skin and perichondrium are elevated with a periosteal elevator to completely expose the anterior surface of the antihelical cartilage. Cartilage will naturally curl in the opposite direction to the weakened side; partial thickness scoring incisions are therefore made on the anterior cartilaginous surface in a "fan shape" figure to allow for a superior and posterior curvature of the concha. Full thickness incision with sharp folding of the conchal cartilage on itself is then performed to reduce conchal height, if necessary. The natural elasticity of the cartilage is overcome; there is therefore no need for overcorrection because postoperative relapse is unlikely. If the lobule is prominent, the correction is done by apposing the anterior aspect of the cauda helicis cartilage to the posterior aspect of the concha and securing it with a 5-0 resorbable suture. The skin is closed with a running horizontal mattress with 5-0 catgut suture.[21]

Many surgeons will combine two techniques. Owsley described a Mustardé-type mattress suture combined to anterior scoring of the antihelical fold to weaken the cartilage and facilitate folding.[2] Fritsch described incisionless otoplasty using a 27-gauge phlebotomy needle as a microknife to perform anterior scoring of the antihelix, followed by incisionless suture loop placement along the antihelix and incisionless Furnas-type retention sutures pulling the conchal bowl close to the mastoid.[18]

Skin excision: The need for posteroauricular skin excision is a controversial matter. Some authors recommend it while others argue that putting the skin under tension will predispose to hypertrophic or keloidal scarring,[2] or that it will result in recurrence if tension alone is relied on to correct the protrusion.[21]

Scaphal Reduction

Scaphal reduction can be achieved by full thickness excision of a wedge of cartilage if required (Fig. 11).[1]

Reduction of Hypertrophic Earlobes

- For a minor reduction, many authors will choose an elliptical partial thickness soft tissue excision on the posterior surface of the lobule. The amount of tissue that needs to be removed is evaluated by pinching the posterior surface.
- Full thickness excisions are required for more prominent earlobes. Simple wedge incisions can result in notching. Hochman and Thomas propose a square excision and superior rotation of the lobule to avoid inferior lobule edge incision, and therefore, notching (Fig. 12).[15]

Microtia Reconstruction

Brent Technique (Three to Four Stage Techniques)

1. The ear base is carved in the synchondrosis of the 6th and 7th rib cartilages. The helix is carved in the 8ht rib cartilage. In adult patients whose rib cartilages are often fused, the entire framework can be carved in one single piece. One option for the creation of the antitragus, intertragal groove and tragus is to fasten a piece of cartilage to the inferior aspect of the framework to form the antitragus, curve it to form the groove and suture it to the helical crus with a bridging mattress suture to form the tragus. A piece of cartilage is excised and banked underneath the chest incision or underneath

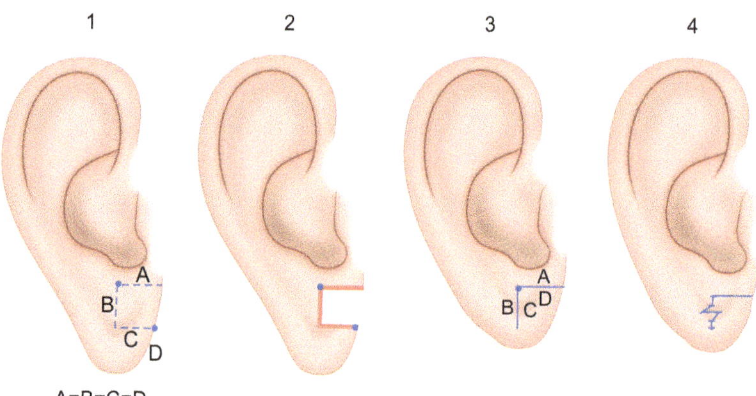

Fig. 12: The anteroinferior edge (D) is deepithelialized. A Z-plasty is done on the vertical portion of the scar.

the scalp posterior to where the framework is placed. The vestigial remnant is removed. The framework is placed in a subcutaneous pocket. Two small drains are left in place for 5 days with vacuum chest tubes. This allows for the overlying skin to coat the cartilaginous structure.[22]

2. The second stage is earlobe transposition. In stage 3 microtia, the framework is truncated in stage 1 to transpose the existing earlobe, whereas in anotia, the lobule is carved into the framework.[21] A thin inferiorly based pedicle flap can also be used to create the lobule in case of complete anotia.[10]

   If an auditory canal is to be drilled by the otologist for atresia repair, it should be done after the two first stages of reconstruction.[10] This is not always done, and the feasibility of the procedure depends on the degree of skeletal hypoplasia and the location of the remnant.[9]

3. The banked piece of cartilage elevates the auricle from the mastoid as it wedged under the framework and is covered with an occipitalis fascia turnover "book flap". A split thickness skin graft covers the posterior surface of the elevated framework.[22]

4. The tragus is constructed with a skin and cartilage graft form the anterolateral concha of the contralateral ear if it had not been carved into the original framework in stage 1.[22]

Nagata Technique (Two-Stage Technique)

1. The first stage combines rib cage harvesting and shaping, tragus construction and earlobe transposition. The auricular framework is shaped differently: the 9th rib cartilage is used to create the antihelix and its two cruxes, which are attached to the framework with stainless steel wire sutures. The framework is then placed in a subcutaneous pocket, as it is for the Brent technique.

2. The auricular framework is raised with a wedged piece of cartilage harvested at the donor site. Second rib cartilage harvesting implies more donor site morbidity. The elevation is covered by a temporoparietal fascia flap, which requires additional scalp incisions.[22]

Modified Nagata Technique (Firmin Modification)

The auricular framework is raised with the posterior surface of the base exposed allowing for additional mobilization of the entire base all the way to the concha.

Alloplastic Reconstruction

- Silicone frameworks have been abandoned since they tend to extrude and do not withstand trauma, resulting in a high failure rate. More recently, *porous polyethylene implants* covered by a temporoparietal flap have been used but long-term outcome has not been sufficiently studied to assess failure rate.
- Alloplastic grafts do not allow for framework growth after reconstruction, which is considered to be an important advantage of autografts.[22]

Prosthetic Reconstruction

Anaplastologists can produce prosthetic auricles that are osseointegrated, fixed on transcutaneous abutments directly connected to the living bone. The degree of detail and projection of the prosthetic auricle is often superior to that of an autogenous reconstruction. The temperature, texture, and color of normal skin remain hard to match, making it a less favorable option in most patients. Notably, in patients who do not have a tragus, the anterior border of the prosthetic auricle will show more than in patients who have a tragus or a sufficient preservable cartilaginous remnant.[9]

Local and Distant Flap Reconstructive Techniques

The temporoparietal is a fascial flap that can be transposed to the head on its vascular pedicle. Its rich vascular supply, provided by the superficial temporal artery and vein, allows for a reliable transfer to a hostile recipient bed such as bone and cartilage and renders it capable of receiving a skin graft. Being pliable and very thin, the flap is an excellent choice to cover a traumatic or excisional deficit reconstructed with a partial autogenous graft with good cosmetic results.[23.]

■ COMPLICATIONS

Early (<14 Days)

- Allergic reaction to material or anesthetic.
- Hematoma.
  - Can be a consequence of either an occult coagulopathy, overuse of epinephrine leading to a rebound effect, dissection in inappropriate planes, insufficient electrocautery hemostasis, and postoperative trauma.
  - Incidence = 2–3.5% after otoplasty.[5]
  - Manifests as excessive pain, bluish swelling of the posteroauricular region, and blood-soaked dressing within 24 hours.[5]
  - May be avoided by leaving three 4 mm gaps in the posteroauricular closure (at 5 mm from the incision's apex, at its midpoint and at the end of the suture).[13] An adequately positioned dressing that obliterates dead space will help prevent hematoma formation and recurrence.[2]
  - Is treated by removal of clot, drainage and antibiotics to prevent infection.[6]
  - If untreated, it may result in infection, skin necrosis or it may produce a cauliflower ear deformity, as discussed here.

Infection/Perichondritis

- Species most often identified: *Staphylococcus, Streptococcus, Pseudomonas aeruginosa,* and *Escherichia coli.*[5]
- Incidence = 2.4–2.5%.[5]
- Manifests as erythema, discharge, edema and pain, usually more than 5 days postoperatively.[5]
- Wound culture and sensitivity should be obtained to select the appropriate antibiotics. Purulent abscesses should be drained and debrided of necrotic tissue completed by removal of suture material.[5]
- If untreated, can lead to perichondritis with residual deformity due to loss of cartilage.[5]

Pressure Necrosis

It has been reported with alloplastic reconstruction and can occur following the significant soft tissue manipulation during the first stage of the Nagata autologous technique.[22]

Paresthesia, Pain and Hypersensitivity

It can result following the intraoperative manipulations of the auricular nerves and may be a permanent complication if the nerves are completely severed. Early rib cartilage harvest complications: the most common complication is atelectasis, but other complications range from pneumonia, pneumothorax, pneumomediastinum and chest wall abrasion and pleural tear.[10]

Late

Relapse can result from the use of resorbable sutures, or of loosening of permanent sutures. Some authors overcorrect prominent ears at time of surgery to avoid these complications.[5]

Asymmetry

Asymmetry can be avoided by positioning the patient in a way that allows for a good frontal view preperatively. Cartilage irregularity is often present before surgery, though, and patients should be informed that achieving perfect symmetry is rarely possible.

Telephone Ear (Overcorrection)

Correction of the ear with a combined Mustardé and Furnas technique will frequently result in lateral protrusion of the helical root and of the lobule.[10] If the middle Furnas suture is placed too far back on the mastoid, this same deformity may arise[1] because of overcorrection of the middle third of the auricle.[5]

Cartilaginous Irregularity

It results more commonly from cartilage cutting techniques, as rough edges of cartilage incisions can be visible through the anterior surface's skin.[5]

Hypertrophic Scaring and Keloids

- Consequence of an imbalance between tissue repair and tissue regeneration mechanisms.
- A hypertrophic scar is typically raised, fibrotic and erythematous. It results from closure under tension

secondary to excessive posteroauricular skin excision, and may regress over time.[5] It can be avoided, as discussed above, by limiting or avoiding skin excision.

- Keloid scarring extends beyond the original incision line, and may be symptomatic (pain and/or paresthesia). Darker pigmented patients and patients who have a positive family history for keloids are at greater risk. They can be avoided by closing the incision passively, and treated with steroids or special pressure dressings.[5]

Late Rib Cartilage Harvest Complications

A visible chest wall deformity is a direct consequence of rib cartilage harvesting in most patients, but it can be reduced either by preserving a small cartilage rim on the superior margin of the 6th rib, or by leaving most of the perichondrium *in situ* to promote cartilage regeneration.[22]

■ REFERENCES

1. Adamson PA, Doud Galli SK, Chen T. Otoplasty. In: Flint PW, Haughey BH, Lund VJ (Eds). Cummings Otolaryngology Head and Neck, 6th edition. Philadelphia, PA: Elsevier; 2015. pp. 468-73.
2. Owsley TG. Otoplastic surgery for the protruding ear. Atlas Oral Maxillofac Surg Clin North Am. 2004;12:131-9.
3. Pan WR, le Roux CM, Levy SM, et al. Lymphatic drainage of the external ear. Head Neck. 2011;33:60-4.
4. Furnas DW. Correction of prominent ears by conchamastoid sutures. Plast Reconstr Surg. 1968;42:189-93.
5. Owsley TG, Biggerstaff TG. Otoplasty complications. Oral Maxillofac Surg Clin North Am. 2009;21:105-18.
6. Hunter A, Frias JL, Gillessen-Kaesbach G, et al. Elements of morphology: standard terminology for the ear. Am J Med Genet A. 2009;149A:40-60.
7. Roth DA, Hildesheimer M, Bardenstein S, et al. Preauricular skin tags and ear pits are associated with permanent hearing impairment in newborns. Pediatrics. 2008;122:e884-90.
8. Weerda H. Classification of congenital deformities of the auricle. Facial Plast Surg. 1988;5:385-8.
9. Thorne CH, Brecht LE, Bradley JP, et al. Auricular reconstruction: indications for autogenous and prosthetic techniques. Plast Reconstr Surg. 2001;107:1241-52.
10. Aguilar EA III, Echo A. Congenital auricular malformation. In: Johnson JT, Rosen CA, (Eds). Bailey's Head and Neck Surgery—Otolaryngology, 5th edition. Philadelphia: Wolters Kluwer Lippincott Williams & Wilkins; 2013. pp. 3161-75.
11. Luquetti DV, Heike CL, Hing AV, et al. Microtia: epidemiology and genetics. Am J Med Genet A. 2012;158A:124-39.
12. Hosmer K. Ear disorders. In: Tintinalli JE, Stapczynski JS, John Ma O, (Eds). Tintinalli's Emergency Medicine, 8th edition. New York: McGraw-Hill Education; 2016. pp. 1583-4.
13. Mobley SR, Nelson Schreiber NT. Otoplasty: anatomy, embryology, and technique. In: Johnson JT, Rosen CA, (Eds). Bailey's Head and Neck Surgery—Otolaryngology, 5th edition. Philadelphia: Wolters Kluwer Lippincott Williams & Wilkins; 2013. pp. 3142-59.
14. Posnick JC, al-Qattan MM, Whitaker LA. Assessment of the preferred vertical position of the ear. Plast Reconstr Surg. 1993;91:1198-203.
15. Hochman M, Thomas JR. Reduction of hypertrophic earlobes. Laryngoscope. 1992;102:827-8.
16. Salgado CJ, Mardini S. Corrective otoplasty for symptomatic prominent ears in U.S. soldiers. Mil Med. 2006;171:128-30.
17. Gosain AK, Kumar A, Huang G. Prominent ears in children younger than 4 years of age: what is the appropriate timing for otoplasty? Plast Reconstr Surg. 2004;114:1042-54.
18. Fritsch MH. Incisionless otoplasty. Facial Plast Surg. 2004;20:267-70.
19. Ullmann Y, Blazer S, Ramon Y, et al. Early nonsurgical correction of congenital auricular deformities. Plast Reconstr Surg. 2002;109:907-13.
20. Byrd HS, Langevin CJ, Ghidoni LA. Ear molding in newborn infants with auricular deformities. Plast Reconstr Surg. 2010;126:1191-200.
21. Caouette-Laberge L, Guay N, Bortoluzzi P, et al. Otoplasty: anterior scoring technique and results in 500 cases. Plast Reconstr Surg. 2000;105:504-15.
22. Zim SA. Microtia reconstruction: an update. Curr Opin Otolaryngol Head Neck Surg. 2003;11:275-81.
23. Cheney ML, Varvares MA, Nadol JB Jr. The temporoparietal fascial flap in head and neck reconstruction. Arch Otolaryngol Head Neck Surg. 1993;119:618-23.

Self-assessment Exercise

Q 1. Which are the two most common abnormalities underlying ear prominence?

Ans:
- Deeply cupped concha
- Unrolled margin of the helical rim.

Q 2. Which are the two conditions that need to be treated before performing otoplasty?

Ans:
- Posteroauricular eczema
- Otitis externa.

Q 3. Cite two reasons that would justify the use of a prosthetic auricle rather than autologous grafting for microtia reconstruction.

Ans:
- Significant hypoplasia
- Low or unfavorable hairline
- Patients in whom autogenous reconstruction has failed.

Q 4. Describe the ideal location of the three concha-mastoid Furnas-type sutures.

Ans:

- Fossa triangularis
- Cymba concha
- Cavum concha.

Q 5. Give two reasons why posteroauricular skin incisions should not be closed under tension?

Ans:

- Hypertrophic scarring
- Keloids
- Relapse, if the tension is relied on to further correct the position of the auricle.

Q 6. At which stage should the auditory canal be drilled during microtia reconstruction using the Brent technique?

Ans: After earlobe transposition (stage 2), and before auricle elevation (stage 3).

Q 7. Explain the two tragus construction options of the Brent technique for microtia reconstruction.

Ans:

- Fastening a piece of cartilage to the inferior aspect of the framework, curving it and suturing it to the helical crus with a bridging mattress suture.
- Transposing a skin and cartilage graft form the anterolateral concha of the contralateral ear.

Q 8. What are the two most useful characteristics of the temporoparietal flap?

Ans:

- Reliable transfer to a hostile recipient bed
- Can receive a skin graft immediately.

Q 9. Which species should be covered by antibiotics in the case of postoperative infection after otoplasty?

Ans: *Staphylococcus, Streptococcus, Pseudomonas aeruginosa,* and *Escherichia coli.*

Q 10. Explain the cause of the telephone ear deformity.

Ans: When the middle Furnas conchal setback suture is placed too far back on the mastoid, the overcorrection of the middle third of the ear may result in lateral protrusion of the helical root and the lobule.

Multiple Choice Questions

Q 1. An aggressive helical rim setback will PRODUCE which of the following occurrences?

A. Protrusion of the lobule

B. Reverse telephone ear deformity

C. Telephone ear deformity

D. Vertical post deformity

Ans: B. Reverse telephone ear deformity

Q 2. A patient is complaining of ear pain on the third postoperative day after an otoplastic procedure. Which of the following conditions is MOST likely the cause of the ear pain?

A. Hematoma

B. Infection

C. Granuloma

D. Wound dehiscence

Ans: B. Infection

Q 3. Which of the following statements defines the "FURNAS" technique for correcting the protruding ear?

A. Permanent sutures through the conchal cartilage to the mastoid periosteum

B. Permanent mattress sutures placed along the cartilage and anterior perichondrium through a posterior incision

C. Reshaping or splitting the auricular cartilage to weaken its resistance which will allow the creation of the proper configuration

D. Combination of sculpting and suturing techniques to create the proper shape configuration

Ans: A. Permanent sutures through the conchal cartilage to the mastoid periosteum

Q 4. A 6 year-old patient is complaining of ear pain 10 hours after the otoplasty surgery. What is the MOST likely diagnosis?

A. Skin necrosis

B. Herpes infection

C. Hematoma

D. Would dehiscence

Ans: C. Hematoma

Q 5. In which part of the ear anatomy is the FURNAS SUTURE technique applied?

A. Scapha

B. Antihelix

C. Concha

D. Triangular fossa

Ans: C. Concha

Q 6. When an elective otoplasty is MOST commonly performed?

A. At 4 years of age

B. At 6 years of age

C. At 9 years of age

D. At 12 years of age

Ans: B. At 6 years of age

Q 7. When is it USUALLY recommended to remove the auricle dressing after otoplastic surgery?

A. 1 day

B. 2 days

C. 3 days

D. 4 days

Ans: A. 1 day

Q 8. Which of the following ear structures in the drawing below will be modified by the represented tissue excision?

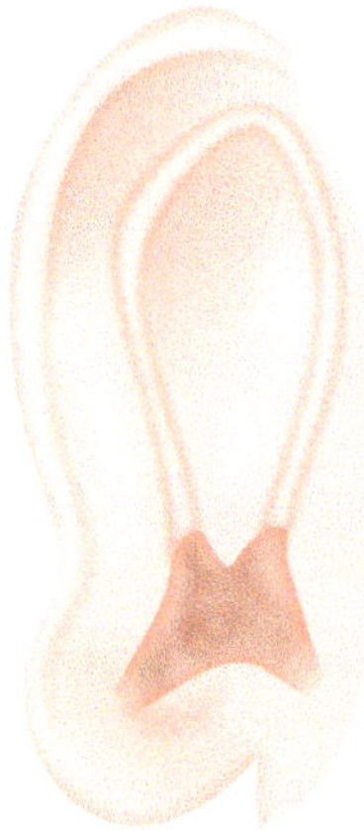

A. Lobule
B. Inferior aspect of the concha
C. Inferior aspect of the helix
D. Inferior aspect of the antihelix.

Ans: A. Lobule

Q 9. Which is of the following is the MOST common cause of PROTRUDING EARS?

A. Lack of antihelical fold
B. Prominent concha
C. Prominent cauda helicis and lobule
D. Superior aspect of the helix folded downward

Ans: A. Lack of antihelical fold

Q 10. Which of the following aesthetic complications is related to postsurgical otoplasty and is defined by excessive conchal setback with protrusion of the upper and lower poles of the auricle?

A. Overcorrection
B. Prominent lobule
C. Telephone
D. Reverse telephone

Ans: C. Telephone

Q 11. Which of the following otoplasty technique is related to traditional conchal setback?

A. The Becker technique
B. The Ely technique
C. The Furnas technique
D. The Nachlas technique

Ans: C. The Furnas technique

Q 12. Which of the following statements is TRUE about the scapha?

A. It is the fossa located between the concha cymba and the concha cavum
B. It is the fossa located between the helix and the antihelix
C. It is the fossa located between the superior and inferior crus of antihelix

D. It is the fossa located between the tragus and antitragus

Ans: B. It is the fossa located between the helix and the antihelix

Q 13. What area of the auricle will improve the Gosain's technique in otoplastic surgery?

A. The helix
B. The antihelix
C. The earlobe
D. The concha

Ans: C. The earlobe

Q 14. Which of the following DESCRIBES the cymba?

A. A fossa between the superior and inferior crus of the antihelix
B. A fossa between the helix and antihelix
C. A portion of the concha located superiorly to the crus of the helix
D. A portion of the concha located inferiorly to the crus of the helix

Ans: C. A portion of the concha located superiorly to the crus of the helix

Q 15. Which of the following describes the FRANKFORT LINE in aesthetic facial surgery?

A. Superior margin of the tragus to the infraorbital rim (lateral plane)
B. Line connecting the ear lobule to the subnasale (lateral plane)
C. A line parallel to the Gonzales-Ulloa line (lateral plane)
D. A line connecting both infraorbital rims (frontal plane)

Ans: A. Superior margin of the tragus to the infraorbital rim (lateral plane)

Q 16. Which of the following auricular anatomy WILL CONTINUE TO CHANGE IN APPEARANCE throughout lifetime?

A. Antihelix
B. Concha
C. Helix
D. Lobule

Ans: D. Lobule

Q 17. Which of the following statement is related to a "Vertical Post Deformity"?

A. An overly corrected superior antihelix
B. An overly corrected inferior antihelix
C. An overly corrected concha cavum
D. An overly corrected concha cymba

Ans: A. An overly corrected superior antihelix

Q 18. Which of the following areas of the auricle will be anesthetized by the injection of local anesthesia into the LESSER OCCIPITAL NERVE?

A. Posterior surface of the auricle
B. Inferior auricle and skin over the mastoid
C. Superior half of the auricle
D. Inferior half of the auricle

Ans: A. Posterior surface of the auricle

Q 19. Which of the following indicates the SENSORY INNERVATION of the areas represented by the TWO ARROWS?

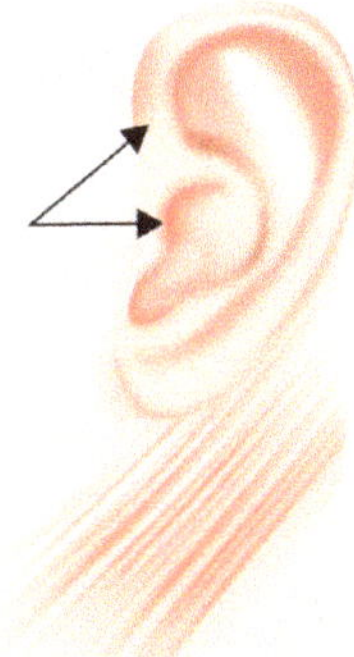

A. Auriculotemporal nerve
B. Auricular nerve
C. Greater auricular nerve
D. Lesser occipital nerve

Ans: A. Auriculotemporal nerve

Q 20. Which of the following ear structures give sensory innervation the auriculotemporal nerve (V)?

A. Lobule
B. Conchal bowl
C. Inferior aspect of auricle
D. Anterior aspect of the helix and tragus

Ans: D. Anterior aspect of the helix and tragus

Q 21. Which of following region of the auricle should remain after ear resection, if oncolagically feasible, from the prosthetic standpoint of view?

A. Tragus
B. Upper portion of the auricle
C. Lower portion of the auricle
D. Concha

Ans: A. Tragus

Chapter 16

Scar Revision and Dermabrasion

Érika Mercier, Sami P Moubayed

■ INTRODUCTION

All healing wounds go through the stages of inflammation, proliferation and remodeling. The latter stage can last for over a year, during which wound maturation occurs, resulting in the final appearance and size of the scar, and reaching up to 80% of the tensile strength of normal skin. The progression through these stages can be altered by external processes described in Chapter 1 (Basic Techniques).

■ MAIN SCAR REVISION INDICATIONS

- Malpositioned
- Hypertrophic
- Deformed (widened, depressed, webbed, and trap-door)
- Discolored
- Deforming a facial landmark (brows and vermilion)
- Interfering with facial function.

Malpositioned Scar

When planning the positioning of an incision, taking into consideration the relaxed skin tension lines (RSTLs) and Langer's lines will help create most inconspicuous scar. The RSTLs are fine lines on the facial skin that are formed by the action of the underlying muscles and as a result, are perpendicular to them (Fig. 1). Langer's lines are topological lines formed by the natural orientation of collagen in the dermis. These lines are parallel to underlying muscle fibers (Fig. 2). When possible, planned incisions should be placed either parallel to or within a 30–40° angle of RSTLs to give the most pleasing results. If an incision does not respect these principles, it will create an unaesthetic and more obvious scar. Scar revision for the malpositioned scar should aim to surgically reposition the wound to respect the previously mentioned anatomic landmarks.[1] It is also crucial to consider anatomic subunits when planning the positioning of a scar. Facial anatomic subunits include the forehead, eyelids, nose, cheeks, lips and chin (Fig. 3). The aesthetic borders between or around these units generally make good locations for scar placement, such as the hairline, infraorbital rims,

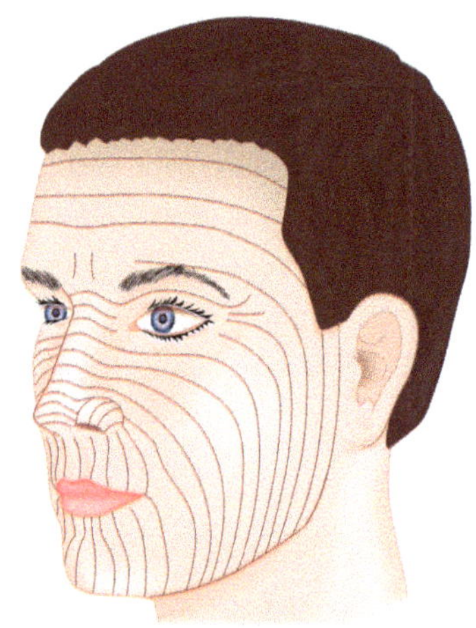

Fig. 1: Relaxed skin tension lines (RSTL).[3]

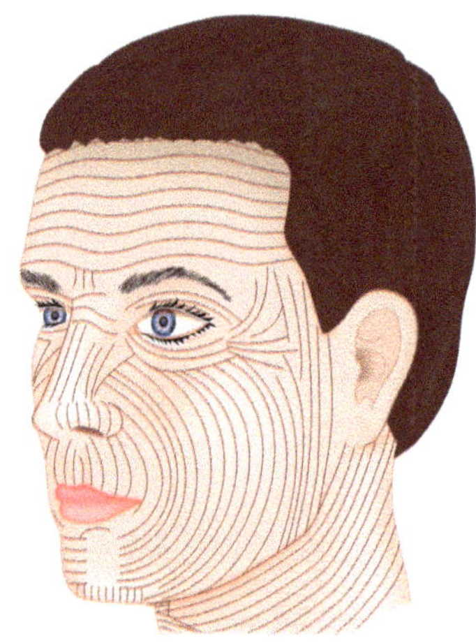

Fig. 2: Langer's lines.[4]

nasofacial grooves, melolabial folds, vermilion borders, and preauricular sulci.[2-4]

Hypertrophic Scar and Keloid

The distinction between hypertrophic scars and keloids must be made clinically by the physician in order to

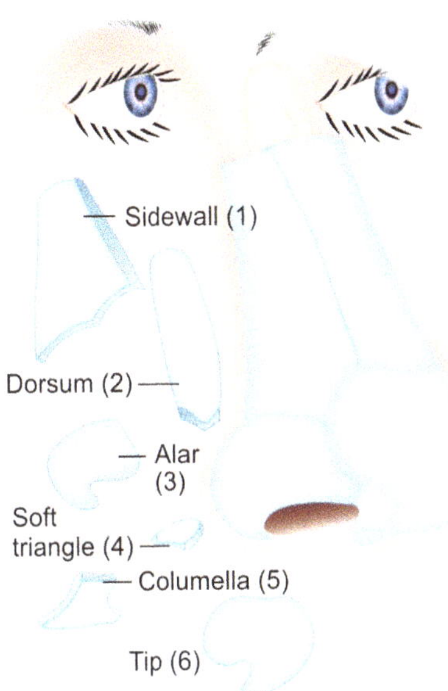

Fig. 3: Anatomic subunits[2]

prescribe the appropriate treatment. Table 1 summarizes the main defining characteristic of hypertrophic scars and keloids, and highlights the major differences between them.[5-8] Table 2 classifies ways to prevent and minimize the development of hypertrophic scars and keloids, at different stages of progression.[7,9,10]

Treatment Options

The algorithm in Flowchart 1 can help orient the treatment of hypertrophic scars.[8]

- *Pressure dressing and silicone*: The mechanism by which silicone gel sheets and pressure dressings exert their action is by occluding the wound, increasing temperature and hydration in keratinocytes[2] and reducing hemostasis, hyperemia and fibrosis in the wound.[11] Silicone gel sheets can be used either as a monotherapy to soften an existing scar, or as an adjunct to surgical scar excision to prevent hypertrophic or keloid recurrence. They must be applied 12 hours a day (or 24 hours ideally) for 2 to 6 months to be effective.[8] They are painless, give earlier symptomatic relief than Kenalog injections and create a more pleasing result on hypertrophic scars than injections.[11] One Canadian randomized controlled study by Sproat et al. found that symptomatic poststernotomy scars treated with silicone gel sheets yielded better subjective and objective results when compared with scars treated by Kenalog injections, and thus support their use.[9] Silicone gel sheets are also less costly than many other treatment options. However, they may not be suitable for open wounds or irregular surfaces as their adherence may be compromised. Their main limitation is patient compliance. For earlobe keloids, pressure earrings are available.

Table 1: Comparison of hypertrophic scars and keloids.[5-8]

	Hypertrophic scar	Keloid
Extension	Remain in the original injury field	Extend beyond the original injury field
Natural evolution	May involute within 12–18 months	Do not regress
Response to treatment	Does not tend to recur when excised Responds to steroids	Tends to recur after excision Marginal response to steroid therapy
Timing	Within 8 weeks of injury	3 months after injury to many years
Risk factors	High tension closure Infection Wound dehiscence	Skin type (darkly pigmented skin) Familial predisposition High wound tension
Frequently affected areas	Bony prominences Upper chest Shoulders Upper back Head and neck, especially earlobe, but spares midface	
Symptoms	Pruritus, pain, erythema, and induration	Expansile soft tissue mass
Treatment options*	1. Observation 2. Silicone gel sheets 3. Intralesional steroids or 5-fluorouracil 4. Laser therapy 5. Pressure therapy 6. Surgical excision	1. Intralesional corticosteroid or 5-fluorouracil injections every 3 weeks +/- silicone gel 2. Pressure devices, silicone gel often as an adjunct treatment 3. Laser therapy 4. If no response, consider excision + steroid injections 5. Radiation therapy for severe/refractory cases

*Treatment options are in order of priority

Table 2: Prevention of hypertrophic scarring and keloids.[7,9,10]		
Prevention method	*Effect*	*Example*
Avoidance	Anticipate potential scarring Avoid unnecessary trauma or surgery	Ear piercing, cosmetic removal of benign cutaneous lesions Early treatment of acne and infections
Intraoperative measures	Adjunctive measures to excision can help reduce risk or recurrence	Intralesional corticosteroids or 5-fluorouracil, cryotherapy, radiation therapy
Topical treatment	Keeping wound moist Hastens wound healing, and decreases scar formation	Plain petrolatum, Telfa dressing held in place by tape, DuoDerm, and silicone gel pads
Avoid stretching tension on wound	Limits scar stretching Facilitates wound resting	Protective material like tape, bandages, garments, and silicone gel sheets
Sun protection	Avoids hyperpigmentation	Cover the scar with tape or an adhesive dressing Using broad-spectrum sunscreen with SPF >50

Flowchart 1: The updated international clinical recommendations on scar management algorithm for hypertrophic scars.[8]

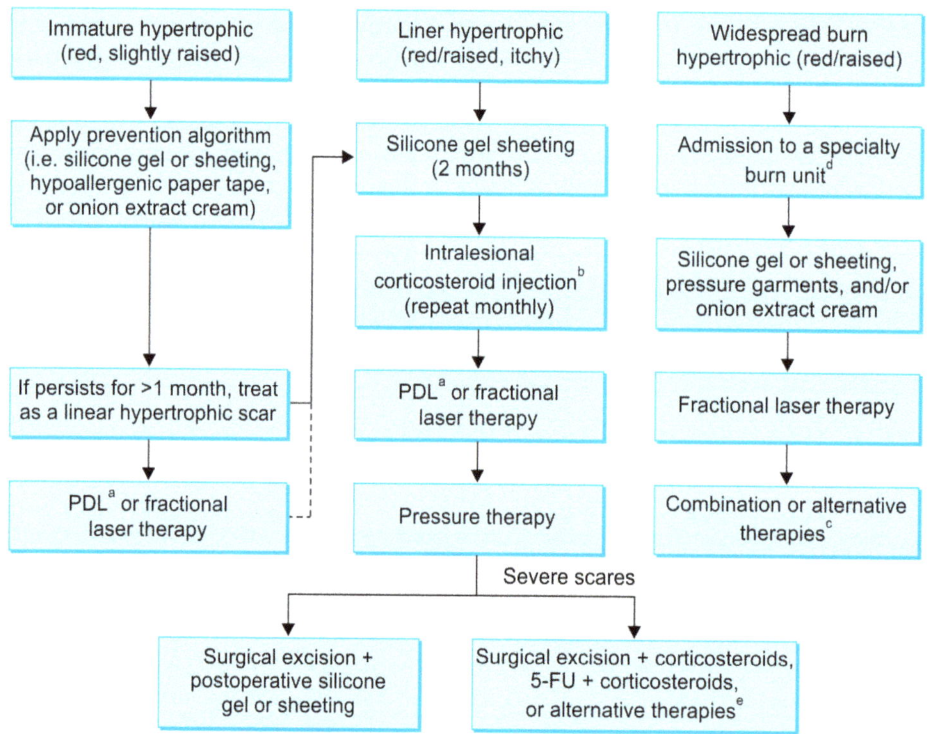

The references in the chart are defined as follows in the article:

(a) Pulse dye laser is preferred initially over ablative fractional laser therapy. (b) Dosing varies based on body site. (c) Intralesional bleomycin or mitomycin C, laser therapy, and cryotherapy. (d) Acute wound care takes precedence over scar prevention or treatment. (e) For burn scars, adjuvant therapies include conservative therapies (e.g., scar massage and physical therapy), surgical scar revisions, or laser treatment

Abbreviations: FU, fluorouracil; PDL, pulsed dye laser.

Source: Curr Opin Otolaryngol Head Neck Surg. 2016 May 7. [Epub ahead of print] Advances in scar management: prevention and management of hypertrophic scars and keloids. Del Toro D1, Dedhia R, Tollefson TT.

- *Steroids*: The local injection of steroids such as triamcinolone acetonide (Kenalog) intradermally or at the dermal-subcutaneous junction can be use as a primary treatment for hypertrophic and keloid scars, or as an adjunct to surgical excision, laser or pressure dressings. Steroids work by decreasing mitosis and inflammatory response, while increasing vasoconstriction, resulting in a flatter, and less pigmented scar by 50–100%.[2] The depth of injection and the amount of product used must be carefully determined as fat atrophy can occur if steroids are injected into the subcutaneous fat or if large amounts are used.

  Although effective, steroid injections require many months before scar flattening occurs and often multiple injections are required to complete the treatment.[11] Patients should be informed that the injections tend to result in a wider scar, and that some permanent depigmentation and skin atrophy can occur. On some occasions, a white residue can also be left in the injected tissues. Also, the injections can result in severe pain, telangiectasias, atrophy, ulceration and rarely necrosis.[2]

- *CO₂ laser*: High-energy pulsed CO_2 lasers are the most frequently used ablative resurfacing lasers.[12] They can be used as a monotherapy to treat keloid and hypertrophic scars, but improved results can be obtained if the technique is combined with injection therapies.[2] The laser generates wavelengths that are absorbed by the water within skin cells, increasing thermal energy and leading to vaporization.[2] The CO_2 laser has a similar effect to dermabrasion and improve pliability, decrease erythema and pruritus and overall, result in a less prominently colored scar.[13] Contrarily to dermabrasion, it offers a bloodless field, which enables the physician to better assess the region to be treated and achieve a flat, smooth surface. Laser treatment can result in pain, persistent erythema, hyper/hypopigmentation, prolonged downtime and increase risk of infections.[2]
- *Excision*: Surgical excision methods are described in detail further in this chapter. Excision may generate good results for hypertrophic scars. They are, however, a last resort for the treatment of keloids because of the high rate of recurrence, even with adjunct therapies such as radiation therapy.[8]
- *Radiation therapy*: The use of radiotherapy is limited to patients with recurrent keloids that are refractory to maximal medical and surgical therapy. Its use for benign conditions is controversial, as there is a potential risk of radiation-induced malignancies such as sarcomas,[14] thus patients should be informed of risks and alternatives. If the patient chooses to follow through with radiation therapy, excision of the scar should be done, followed by immediate photon therapy with 4 Gy, to be repeated on day 2 and day 4 following the procedure.[14] The radiation works by destroying fibroblasts which decreases the previous excessive synthesis of collagen in the wound.[14-16]
- *Others*: Some studies have found benefits of the use of onion extract on scars, but the effects have been shown to be no better than the application of petrolatum emollient, and not as effective as silicone-based products.[8] New injectable agents are still under investigation for scar prevention. These include bleomycin, verapamil and interferon alfa-2a. For the moment, they have limited success and may have significant side effects.

■ DERMABRASION

Indications

Dermabrasion is a form of "skin-sanding" in which the superficial layer of the skin is removed in a controlled way to smooth skin and remove irregularities using a hand-held burr or, more rarely, sterile sandpaper. Undoubtedly, the main indication in scar revision is as a secondary procedure 6–8 weeks after scar revision surgery to smooth raised scars.[17]

Other indications include acne scars, traumatic facial scars (including tattoos), pigmentation disorders, rhinophyma, facial rhytids, cosmetic facial skin resurfacing, or as an adjunct for chemical exfoliation, soft-tissue augmentation and laser procedures[17] in order to enhance results.

The procedure restructures and reorients the collagen fibers parallel to tension lines and epithelial surface, and promotes the migration of epithelial cells from the adnexal appendages to eliminate epidermal defects. It is a time-tested procedure that is less costly than the newer laser treatments, but results in more crusting and downtime.

Contraindications

Dermabrasion is contraindicated for patients who have had treatment with systemic isotretinoin (Accutane) in the previous year because of the potential for hypertrophic scarring.[13] A past history of herpetic infection should elicit the use of antiviral therapy, whereas if active lesions are present, the procedure should be postponed until cleared out. Patients should be screened for bleeding disorders, immunosuppression, transmittable diseases, and previous surgeries to take the necessary precautions.

Method, Surgical Precautions and Types of Burrs

Careful patient selection is crucial in order to generate optimal results from dermabrasion. The procedure should be done within a 4–8 weeks timeframe after injury, during collagen remodeling.[17] As for any procedure, risks and benefits should be explained beforehand, as well as limitations and alternative therapies.

The room should be adequately prepared with optimal lighting and monitoring equipment. Dermabrasion can be done under local regional anesthesia, with IV sedation, or even general anesthesia as needed.[13] Topical refrigerant agents can be used to produce a smooth, firm and anesthetized surface to work on, without distorting skin architecture. A gentian violet stain solution can be used to delineate the areas to be treated and determine depth of the abrasion.[13]

The handheld dermabrader rotates at a speed of 18,000–35,000 revs/minute. There are many interchangeable burrs available, depending on the surface to be treated, including wire brushes, diamond fraises and serrated wheels.[13] The dermabrader should be held at a 90° angle to the wheel rotation and advanced in the direction of wheel rotation.[13] Skin is held taught and the surface is treated gradually, one anatomic unit at a time down to the mid papillary to deep papillary dermis. The surgeon should look for a white coloration to recognize this layer in order to know when to stop dermabrading. The reticular dermis should not be removed as the adnexal structures are essential for subsequent reepithelialization.

Another option for dermabrasion is the use of sterile sandpaper.

Skin Refrigerants and Adjunctive Measures

Skin refrigerants can be applied locally to the skin to be treated in order to obtain a smooth, anesthetized and rigid surface, while diminishing bleeding. Local application of an ice pack or a cryogenic spray containing fluoroethyl or Freon-114 is good option.

Postoperative Care

In the postoperative period, reepithelialization should occur within 5–7 days and erythema is expected to subside within 2–4 months. It is recommended to use a topical antibiotic ointment combined with a semiocclusive dressing until reepithelialization is complete. The ointment will provide a moist environment for the wound and promote reepithelialization, while being unfavorable for bacterial growth.[13] The use of a hydrogel semiocclusive dressing is used to protect the wound and keep the surface clean and moist. If needed, a reinforced tape such as Dermabond can be used to provide support.[13] Silicone sheets can also be added to diminish pruritus and erythema as well as to help eliminate irregularities.[13] A combination of antivirals, antibiotics and steroids is recommended in the postoperative period to prevent complications.[13] The use of topical preparations such as topical vitamin preparations or emollients should be discouraged during the first week after surgery. After this period, their use is left to the discretion of the patient, as there is no evidence supporting or discouraging their use. The use of massages should be encouraged over scar areas once the healing is completed to help realign the collagen fibers, and create a suppler scar by avoiding adhesion to the deeper planes.[13] A recent systematic review compiling the results of ten publications studying the effects of massages on various scars, has concluded that although the evidence in favor of scar massage is weak, it seems to be most effective on surgical scars, such as the ones obtained post-scar revision. It should not be started before 14 days postsurgery, as it could promote hypertrophic scarring.[18]

Complications

The most common complications associated with dermabrasion are pigmentary alterations, erythema, scarring and milia.[13]

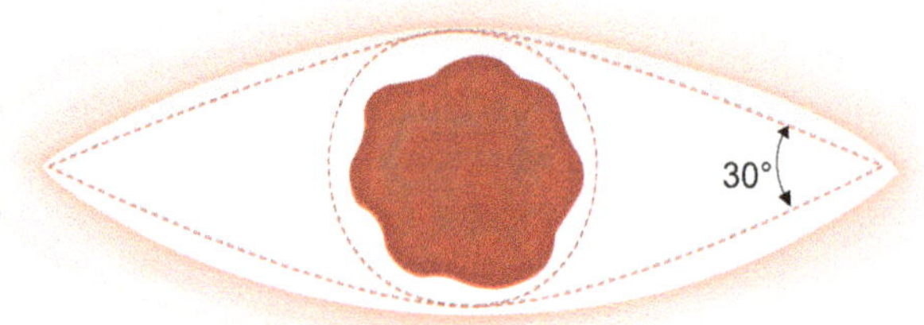

Fig. 4: Fusiform excision.[20]

■ SURGICAL SCAR REVISION METHODS

The decision to proceed with a surgical excision or scar revision should be based on the size, position and orientation of the scar, its relationship to other anatomic units as well as the quality and thickness of the skin around it.[13,19] Once these are assessed, the surgeon can determine the best type of corrective surgery and the ideal scar placement to make it as inconspicuous as possible.

- *Fusiform excision*: Fusiform excision can be used on scars that already benefit from good positioning. The technique involves excising the superficial portion of the scar in a fusiform shape, with extremity angles of 30° or less. It is not necessary to excise the deeper portion of the scar, as it will offer support for the superficial layers and prevent depressions. It might be necessary to undermine the edges of the wound in order to approximate them. Meticulous everting closure in layers should be performed (Fig. 4).[20]

- *Serial excision*: When a scar cannot be surgically removed in a single procedure because of its size, placement or tension, serial excisions can be done in order to gradually advance skin though undermining into the region of the deficit. The number of procedures required will depend on how much scar is to be removed and the elasticity of the surrounding skin.[13]

- *M excision*: The M excision is useful for scars that require excision angles of greater than 30°. It involves separating wide corner angles into two smaller angles by interposing a small triangular flap at the inner corner of the wound. This technique has the advantage of not removing any unnecessary tissue and not lengthening the scar,[13] as well as avoiding a standing cone deformity (Fig. 5).[20]

- *Z-plasty*: Z-plasty is based on the concept of transposition of two triangular skin flaps, which helps diminish distortion created by contractility.[13] In fact, the technique has the particularity of lengthening a contracted scar and can be used to reposition distorted facial landmarks by changing the direction of the scar.[13] The classic procedure uses three equal limbs to create two complementary

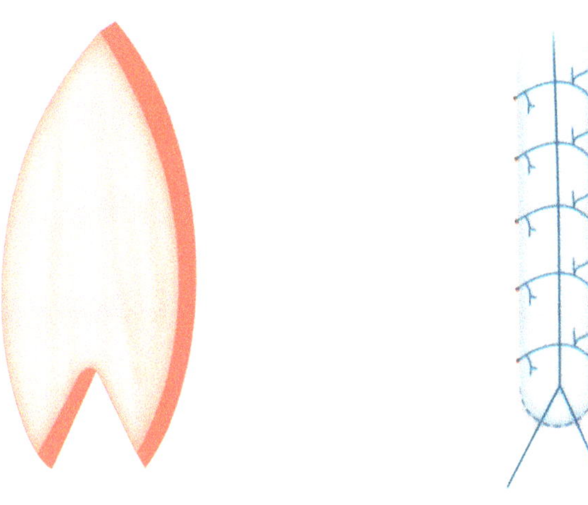

Fig. 5: M-plasty.[20]

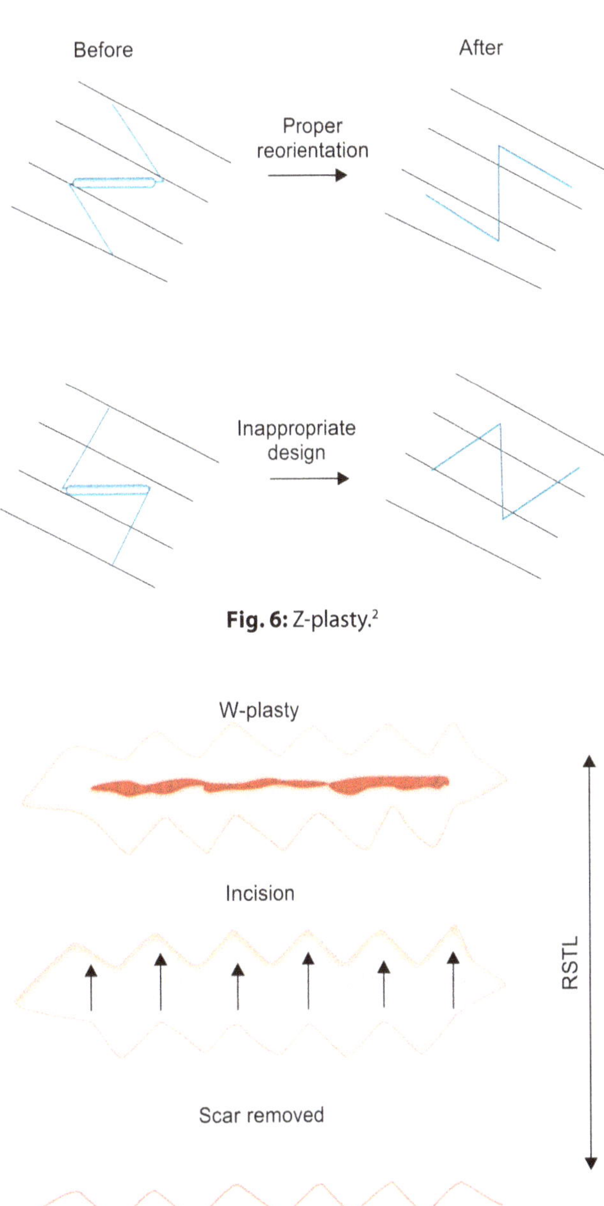

Fig. 6: Z-plasty.[2]

Fig. 7: W-plasty.[2]

RSTL, relaxed skin tension line

triangles. The central limb is positioned on the scar to be corrected. The two other limbs are placed at a 60° angle from either end of the central limb, parallel to each other. The final scar after transposition can be envisioned by tracing a line between the free extremities of the two parallel limbs. Angles of 60°, 45° and 30° can be used, and will respectively lengthen the incision by 75%, 50% and 25%. Angles any less than this can lead to tissue necrosis, whereas angles wider than these can cause deformities and make the transposition difficult.[13] It is not recommended to use Z-plasty to correct a keloid scar, as there is a high rate of recurrence and a potential for further disfigurement (Fig. 6).[2,13]

- *W-plasty*: One of the goals of W-plasty is to irregularize an otherwise straight and obvious scar. Straight scars are more apparent because they reflect light in an even way, making them easy for the eye to follow.[2] W-plasty helps camouflage this by scattering the light, but does not provide optimal concealment because of the predictability of the pattern. The running W-plasty consists of creating multiple small interlocking triangular skin flaps on each side of the wound such that they will interpose once the scar is resected.[13] It is thus an interposition flap instead of a transposition flap, and will not result in lengthening of the scar. W-plasty does require, however, that the surrounding skin possess laxity for closure, as some tissue is resected during the procedure.[13] It is recommended that it combined with a second stage dermabrasion 6–8 weeks postoperatively, in order to smoothen and regularize the scar surface (Fig. 7).[2]

- *Geometric broken lines*: This technique is a more sophisticated way of camouflaging a scar without lengthening it. It should be used on relatively long scars angled 45° or more from RSTLs.[2] It is composed of multiple complementary geometric interposition

flaps on each side of the wound, measuring between 3 mm and 7 mm. Flaps any smaller are difficult to work with, whereas flaps any larger are more noticeable.[13] The shapes used include semicircles, squares, triangles, rhomboids and rectangles, in different orders and sizes.[2] The deep portion of the scar should be preserved to allow for wound effacement. Contrarily to W-plasty, geometric broken lines create an irregularly irregular pattern, which makes the scar less predictable, and thus less noticeable. Dermabrasion should be planned 6–8 weeks after surgery (Fig. 8).[2]

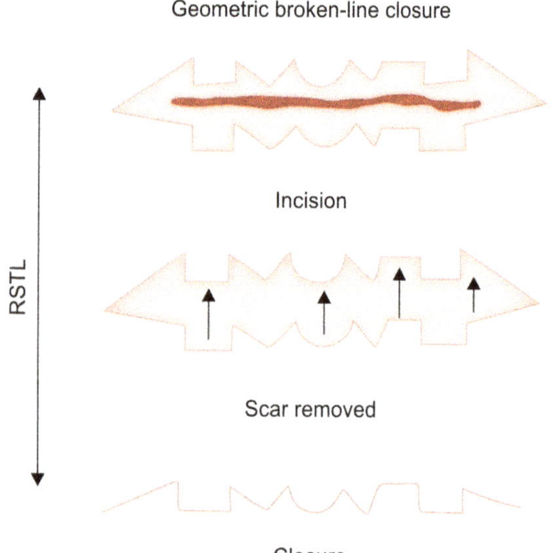

Fig. 8: Geometric broken-line closure.[2]

RSTL, relaxed skin tension line

Table 3: Histological changes in skin expansion.[2]	
Structures	*Histological changes*
Epidermis	• Increase in mitotic activity • Thickness same or slightly increased • Stratified structure preserved
Dermis	• Significant thinning of 30–50% • Thickening of the basal layer • Increased metabolic activity in the fibroblasts and melanocytes • Same number of hair follicles, but density decreases
Subcutaneous tissue	• Adipose tissue thins approximately 50% with loss of adipocytes • Muscle thinning and atrophy • Vascular proliferation • Nerve lengthening with impaired function

OTHER METHODS

- *Nonablative laser resurfacing*: The most commonly used nonablative lasers are the 585-nm pulsed dye laser and the Nd:YAG lasers. The wavelengths generated by these lasers are selectively absorbed by oxyhemoglobin in the microvasculature, while the water in the skin cells is mostly spared. This results in selective tissues ischemia instead of the necrosis seen in ablative laser.[2] The result is diminished scar erythema, pruritus and leveling of the scar. The disadvantages are similar to ablative laser but with less impact.
- *Shave* excision: For narrow, raised or textured lesions with superficial irregularities, such as keloids, shave excision can be performed with a flexible razor blade or with a scalpel.[13] The excision should be done level with normal skin, and caution should be taken to avoid removing the deep dermis. The wound is then left to heal by secondary intention. The technique can be combined with other revision methods.
- *Surgical tattooing/dermatography*: Surgical tattoos can be used to camouflage hypopigmented scars and scars involving areas of alopecia, such as in the eyebrows.[2]

Skin Expansion

Skin expansions are used for scars that cannot be excised in one procedure because of high tension on the wound or anatomic positioning, in lieu of serial excision. The technique requires placing a tissue expander in order to increase available tissue around the scar. Over time, the implant is expanded with saline and the overlying tissues are stretched out, allowing for subsequent scar revision and closure.[2] It is an alternative used less frequently than serial excision because of the inconvenience of multiple appointments, risks of infection and the need for multiple interventions.[2] Table 3 details the histological changes that can be seen in the different layers on the skin as it is subjected to skin expansion.[2]

Fillers

Fillers are usually used to correct atrophic scars. Available fillers include autologous and allogeneic tissue such as fat, xenographic material as well as synthetic material.[2]

Laser Scar Revision

As explained above, ablative and nonablative lasers are an efficient way to treat existing scars or to prevent them, and can be used either as a monotherapy or as an adjunctive treatment.

REFERENCES

1. Mobley SR, Sjogren PP. Soft tissue trauma and scar revision. Facial Plast Surg Clin North Am. 2014;22:639-51.
2. Johnson JT, Rosen CA, Bailey BJ. Bailey's Head and Neck Surgery—Otolaryngology. Philadelphia: Wolters Kluwer Health/Lippincott Williams & Wilkins; 2013.
3. Gold MH. Dermabrasion in dermatology. Am J Clin Dermatol. 2003;4:467-71.
4. Uptodate. Langer's lines of the face. [online] Available from https://www.uptodate.com/contents/image?imageKey=SURG/50913&topicKey=DERM%2F13707&source=preview&search=langer%27s+lines&rank=undefined [Accessed March, 2017].

5. Leventhal D, Furr M, Reiter D. Treatment of keloid and hypertrophic scars: a meta-analysis and review of the literature. Arch Facial Plast Surg. 2006;8:362-8.

6. Pasha R. Otolaryngology, Head & Neck Surgery: Clinical Reference Guide. Australia: Singular; 2001.

7. Uptodate. Keloids and hypertrophic scars. [online]. Available from http://www.uptodate.com/contents/keloids-and-hypertrophic-scars?source=machineLearning&search=keloids&selectedTitle=1%7E73§ionRank=2&anchor=H66627087#H66627087 [Accessed March, 2017].

8. Del Toro D, Dedhia R, Tollefson TT. Advances in scar management: prevention and management of hypertrophic scars and keloids. Curr Opin Otolaryngol Head Neck Surg. 2016;24:322-9.

9. Gold MH, Foster TD, Adair MA, et al. Prevention of hypertrophic scars and keloids by the prophylactic use of topical silicone gel sheets following a surgical procedure in an office setting. Dermatol Surg. 2001;27:641-4.

10. Uptodate. Keloids and hypertrophic scars? [online] Available from https://www.uptodate.com/contents/keloids-and-hypertrophic-scars?source=search_result&search=keloids&selectedTitle=1%7E72#H66627207 [Accessed March, 2017].

11. Sproat JE, Dalcin A, Weitauer N, et al. Hypertrophic sternal scars, silicone gel sheet versus Kenalog injection treatment. Plast Reconstr Surg. 1992;90:988-92.

12. Nehal KS, Levine VJ, Ross B, et al. Comparison of high-energy pulsed carbon dioxide laser resurfacing and dermabrasion in the revision of surgical scars. Dermatol Surg. 1998;24:647-50.

13. Thomas JR, Prendiville S. Update in scar revision. Facial Plast Surg Clin North Am. 2002;10:103-11.

14. Lindsey WH, Davis PT. Facial keloids. A 15-year experience. Arch Otolaryngol Head Neck Surg. 1997;123:397-400.

15. Lu F, Gao J, Ogawa R, et al. Variations in gap junctional intercellular communication and connexin expression in fibroblasts derived from keloid and hypertrophic scars. Plast Reconstr Surg. 2007;119:844-51.

16. Younai S, Venters G, Vu S, et al. Role of growth factors in scar contraction: an in vitro analysis. Ann Plast Surg. 1996;36:495-501.

17. Harmon CB, Zelickson BD, Roenigk RK, et al. Dermabrasive scar revision. Immunohistochemical and ultrastructural evaluation. Dermatol Surg. 1995;21:503-8.

18. Shin TM, Bordeaux JS. The role of massage in scar management: a literature review. Dermatol Surg. 2012;38:414-23.

19. Wolfe D, Davidson TM. Scar revision. Arch Otolaryngol Head Neck Surg. 1991;117:200-4.

20. Medscape. (2016). Basic excisional surgery. [online] Available from http://emedicine.medscape.com/article/1818482-overview [Accessed March, 2017].

Self-assessment Exercise

Q 1. What are the stages of normal skin healing?

Ans. The stages of normal skin healing are as follows:

Inflammation   Proliferation   Remodeling

Q 2. Explain what the relaxed skin tension lines (RSTLs) and Langer's lines are, and how they should be taken into consideration when planning scar positioning.

Ans. The RSTLs are fine lines on the facial skin that are formed by the action of the underlying muscles and as a result, are perpendicular to them. Langer's lines are topological lines formed by the natural orientation of collagen in the dermis. These lines are parallel to underlying muscle fiber. When possible, planned incisions should be placed either parallel to or within a 30–40° angle of RSTLs to give the most pleasing results.

Q 3. Name the different anatomic subunits of the face.

Ans. Facial anatomic subunits include the forehead, eyelids, nose, cheeks, lips and chin.

Q 4. Name 6 surgical scar revision methods and describe what kind of scar they are used on as well as the outline of the technique.

Ans.

- Fusiform excision
- Serial excision
- M excision
- Z-plasty
- W-plasty
- Geometric broken lines

Please refer to the section on surgical scar revision for technique description and indications.

Q 5. Name 2 major differences between keloids and hypertrophic scars and explain the basis of their treatment.

Ans:

- Hypertrophic scars remain in the original injury field and may involute within 18 months. Keloids extend beyond the original injury field and never regress.
- Main treatment options for hypertrophic scars:
  - Observation
    - Silicone gel sheets
    - Intralesional steroids or 5-fluorouracil
    - Laser therapy
    - Pressure therapy
    - Surgical excision
- Main treatment options for keloids:
  - Intralesional corticosteroid or 5-fluorouracil injections every 3 weeks +/- silicone gel
  - Pressure devices, silicone gel often as an adjunct treatment
  - Laser therapy
  - If no response, consider excision + steroid injections
  - Radiation therapy for severe/refractory cases.

Q 6. Name 3 indications and 3 contraindications for dermabrasion.

Ans:

- Dermabrasion is indicated for treating acne scars, traumatic facial scars (including tattoos), pigmentation disorders, rhinophyma, facial rhytids, as well as for cosmetic facial skin resurfacing.

- Dermabrasion is contraindicated for patients who have had treatment with systemic isotretinoin (Accutane) in the previous year because of the potential for hypertrophic scarring. A past history of herpetic infection should elicit the use of antiviral therapy, whereas if active lesions are present, the procedure should be postponed until cleared out. Patients should be screened for bleeding disorders, immunosuppression, transmittable diseases and previous surgeries to take the necessary precautions.

Q 7. Describe how skin expansion affects the epidermis, the dermis and the subcutaneous tissues.

Ans:

Epidermis

- Increase in mitotic activity
- Thickness same or slightly increased
- Stratified structure preserved

Dermis

- Significant thinning of 30–50%
- Thickening of the basal layer
- Increased metabolic activity in the fibroblasts and melanocytes
- Same number of hair follicles, but density decreases

Subcutaneous tissue

- Adipose tissue thins approximately 50% with loss of adipocytes
- Muscle thinning and atrophy
- Vascular proliferation
- Nerve lengthening with impaired function.

Multiple Choice Questions

Q 1. The END POINT of microdermabrasion is which of the following?

A. Erythema
B. Blister formation
C. Frosting
D. Yellow-pale decoloration of skin

Ans: A. Erythema

Q 2. In the 30° Z-plasty technique the length of the scar dimension is INCREASED by which percentage?

A. 10%
B. 25%
C. 30%
D. 35%

Ans: B. 25%

Q 3. Which of the following statements is FALSE about the running W-plasty technique for scar revision?

A. Each limb of the triangles should be 5 mm in length
B. It is used in scars oriented perpendicular to the RSTL (relaxed skin tension lines)

C. The apex of each triangle should be a 60° angle
D. The final triangle at the terminal corners of a running W-plasty should be at a 60° angle

Ans: D. The final triangle at the terminal corners of a running W-plasty should be at a 60 degree angle

Q 4. Which of the following scars is MOST likely to be well camouflaged?

A. 4 cm linear scar depressed and parallel to the RSTL
B. 4 cm linear scar elevated and parallel to the RSTL
C. 4 cm linear scar parallel to the RSTL without depression or elevation
D. 4 cm linear scar perpendicular to the lower eyelid edge

Ans: C. 4 cm linear scar parallel to the RSTL without depression or elevation

Q 5. A 10-year-old boy has a linear vertical forehead scar extending from the hairline to the left eyebrow after facial trauma which occurred 1 year ago. Which is the MOST useful scar revision technique in this case?

A. Multiple Z-plasty
B. Running W-plasty
C. Serial excision
D. Single excision

Ans: B. Running W-plasty

Q 6. After intervention, which of the following scars is the one with the HIGHEST possibility of a POOR cosmetic result?

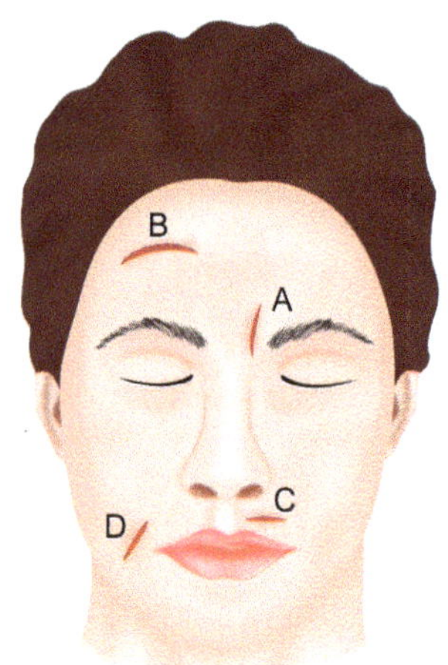

A. A
B. B
C. C
D. D

Ans: C. C

Q 7. Microdermabrasion PRODUCES a controlled removal of the:

A. Papillary dermis
B. Stratum corneum epidermis
C. Superficial reticular dermis
D. Total epidermis

Ans: B. Stratum corneum epidermis

Q 8. Which of the following is the MOST common complication of dermabrasion?

A. Milia

B. Hyperpigmentation

C. Hypopigmentation

D. Skin infection

Ans: A. Milia

Q 9. Dermabrasion is the treatment of CHOICE for which of the following:

A. Postacne scars

B. Traumatic scars

C. Facial wrinkles

D. Actinic keratosis

Ans: A. Postacne scars

Q 10. The use of W-plasty scar revision is CONTRA-INDICATED in which of the following facial areas?

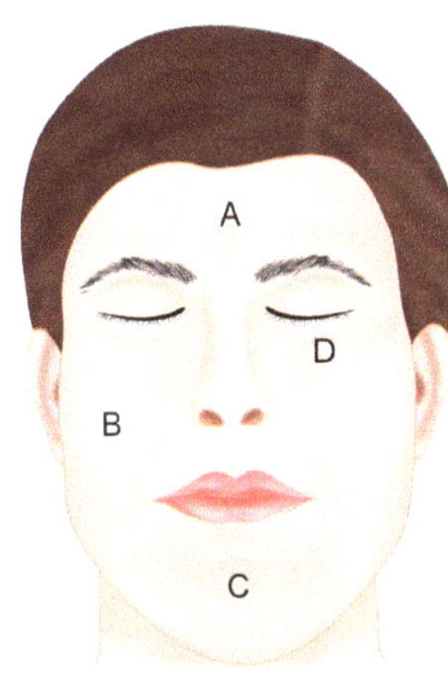

A. A

B. B

C. C

D. D

Ans: D. D

Q 11. Which of the following statements is FALSE regarding Z-plasty?

A. No angles are greater than 90°

B. No angles are less than 30°

C. Arms are no greater than 1 cm on the face

D. Arms have a 2 cm length on the neck

Ans: D. Arms have a 2 cm length on the neck.

Q 12. The angle in a Fusiform Excision as indicated in the drawing SHOULD BE approximately?

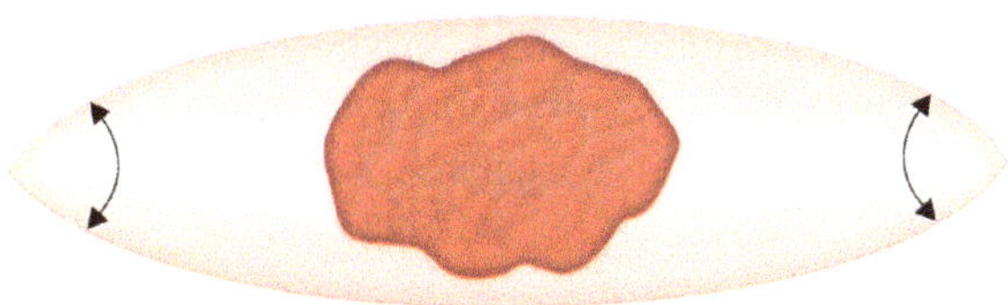

A. 30°

B. 40°

C. 50°

D. 60°

Ans: A. 30°

Q 13. Which of the following is NOT CONSIDERED a "danger zone" in the use of dermabrasion?

A. Maxillary area

B. Zygomatic arch area

C. Malar eminence area

D. Forehead area

Ans: A. Maxillary area

Q 14. Which of the following statements about the running W-plasty technique use in scar revision is FALSE?

A. Each limb of the triangle should be 5 mm in length

B. The apex of the triangle should be a 60° angle

C. The final triangle at the terminal corners of a running W-plasty should be 60° angles

D. Use for scars oriented perpendicular to the RSTL (relaxed skin tension lines)

Ans: C. The final triangle at the terminal corners of a running W-plasty should be 60° angles

Q 15. Which of the following surgical techniques used to treat a long curvilinear scar—not parallel to RSTL—in the cheek is the BEST related to camouflage?

A. Running W-Plasty

B. Multiple M-Plasty

C. Multiple Z-Plasty

D. Geometric broken line closure

Ans: D. Geometric broken line closure

Q 16. Which of the following statements regarding the M-Plasty is FALSE?

A. It is commonly used at the end of the fusiform excision

B. It is commonly used to shorten the final length of the wound

C. The closure of an M-Plasty represents a V-to-Y closure

D. It is commonly used to camouflage a scar

Ans: D. It is commonly used to camouflage a scar

Q 17. Which of the following techniques is the MOST USEFUL in the revision of a circular pin cushion scar deformity?

A. Running W-plasty

B. Geometric broken line closure

C. Multiple Z-plasties

D. Serial excisions

Ans: C. Multiple Z-plasties

**Q 18. A young female actress has requested a scar revision procedure. The scar is on her right cheek and was sustained

3 months ago after a car accident. The scar is 4.5 cm long, linear, slightly elevated and erythematous. The NEXT step in the management for this patient:

A. Dermabrasion
B. W-plasty revision
C. Geometric broken line closure revision
D. No surgery but follow up

Ans: D. No surgery but follow up

Q 19. Which of the following scar revision techniques is the BEST for use on a mature, linear (12 cm), unbroken scar of the left cheek and the lower third of the face?

A. Multiple Z-plasty
B. Running W-plasty
C. Geometric broken-line closure
D. Dermabrasion and laser resurfacing

Ans: C. Geometric broken-line closure

Q 20. Objective preoperative documentation pictures are MOST DIFICULT to obtain for which of the following cosmetic surgeries?

A. Face lift
B. Blepharoplasty
C. Facial scar
D. Otoplasty

Ans: C. Facial scar

Q 21. Which of the following techniques for scar revision IS CORRECTELY described?

A. Simple fusiform excision - ideally the angles should be greater than 60°
B. Serial excision - A period of 12 weeks is required between excisions
C. Geometric broken line closure - It is easier to perform than W-plasty
D. W-plasty - This scar revision will produce wound lengthening

Ans: B. Serial excision - A period of 12 weeks is required between excisions

Q 22. Which of the following statements about MICRODERMABRASION is TRUE?

A. Hypopigmentation is a common complication
B. It can be used safely on the neck
C. Adjunctive use of isotretinoin is not a contraindication
D. It is comparable to a medium-depth peel

Ans: B. It can be used safely on the neck

Q 23. Which of the following statements about facial Z-Plasty is FALSE?

A. The arms are slightly greater than 1 cm
B. It is used to lengthen a scar contraction
C. It is used to rotate the dominant axis of a scar to a more favorable position
D. It is used to avoid a contracture when an incision crosses a concavity

Ans: A. The arms are slightly greater than 1 cm

Q 24. Which of the following statements about Trap-Door deformity is FALSE?

A. It is usually seen after C, U or V-shaped transposition flaps
B. Prevention can be achieved with wide undermining of the surrounding skin
C. Early cases can be treated with intralesional 1 mL triamcinolone acetonide (40 mg/mL) injections
D. Multiple running W-plasty can correct this deformity

Ans: D. Multiple running W-plasty can correct this deformity

Q 25. Which of the following is FALSE about the flap represented in the drawing below?

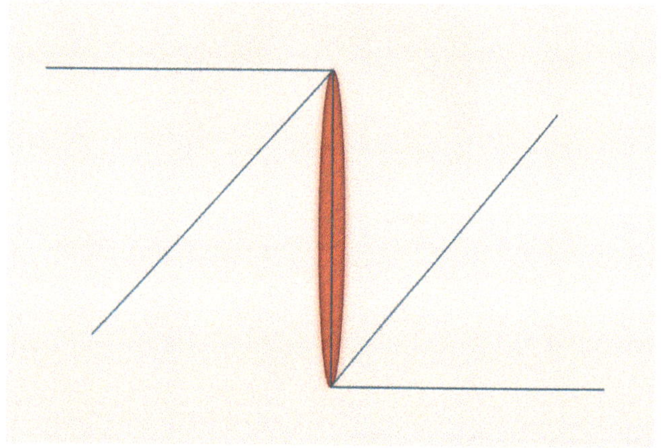

A. It is a serial Z-plasty
B. It is based on a 4-flap 45° Z-plasty
C. The result after completion will be a lengthening created by a 90° Z-plasty
D. It is ideal for the neck surgery

Ans: A. It is a serial Z-plasty

Q 26. Which of the following anatomical areas is LESS LIKELY to develop hypertrophic scarring or keloids?

A. Central third of the face
B. Presternal area
C. Upper back
D. Shoulders

Ans: A. Central third of the face

Q 27. In the execution of serial excisions what is the WAIT TIME between the first and second excision?

A. After the initial scar is healed
B. 1 month
C. 3 months
D. 8 months

Ans: C. 3 months

Q 28. Which of the following facial scars is BETTER NOT revised?

A. 4 cm linear scar within the common border of two aesthetic units
B. 4 cm linear scar perpendicular to the RSTLs
C. 4 cm scar, curved and pin-cushioned
D. 4 cm scar interrupting and crossing an aesthetic unit of the

Ans: A. 4 cm linear scar within the common border of two aesthetic units

Q 29. Which of the following adverse conditions IS ASSOCIATED with wounds closed under a great degree of tension?

A. Decresed tensile strength
B. Hypertrophic scar
C. Infection
D. Keloid

Ans: B. Hypertrophic scar

Q 30. Which of the following is the BEST treatment option for management of this irregular, hypertrophic scar of 8 months duration?

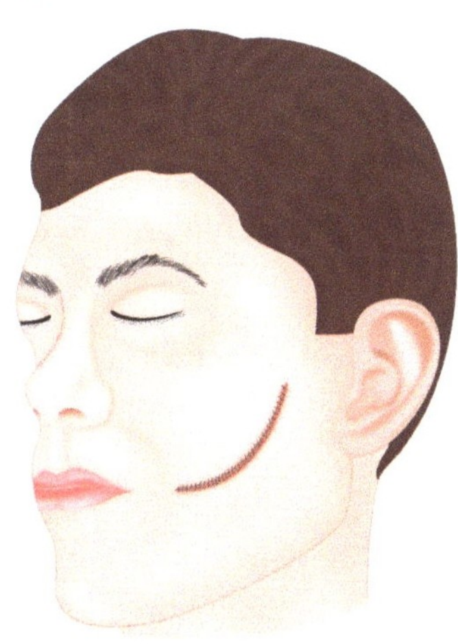

A. Kenalog injections
B. Dermabrasion
C. Laser resurfacing
D. 12 months wait since initial trauma

Ans: D. 12 months wait since initial trauma

Q 31. After scar formation, when is it appropriate to perform Dermabrasion?

A. 2 weeks
B. 4 weeks
C. 8 weeks
D. 10 months

Ans: C. 8 weeks

Q 32. Which of the following scar revision techniques is the one presented in the drawing below?

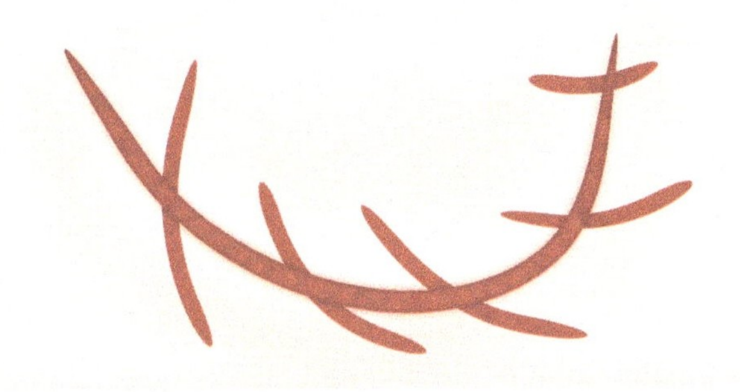

A. Multiple excisions
B. Serial excisions
C. Multiple Z-plasties
D. Running W-plasty

Ans: C. Multiple Z-plasties

Q 33. What will be the theoretical increase in length of the Z-plasty represented in the drawing below?

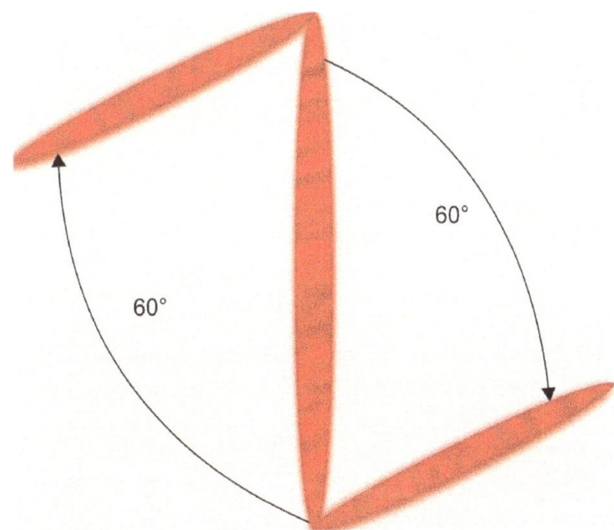

A. 25%
B. 50%
C. 60%
D. 75%

Ans: D. 75%

Q 34. Which of the following scar revision techniques is the ONE used in the drawing?

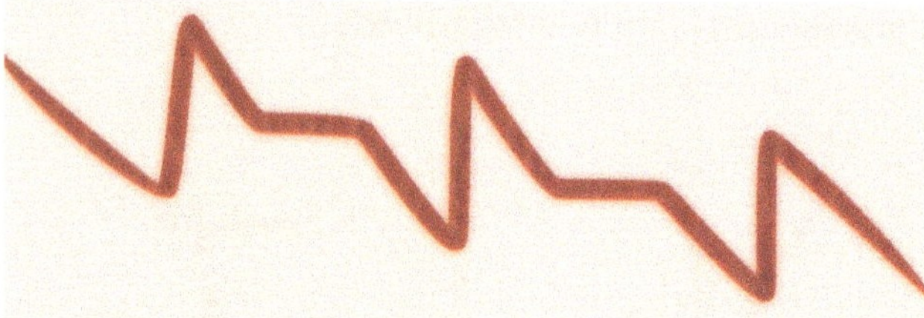

A. Compound Z-plasty
B. Serial Z-plasty
C. Running W-plasty
D. Geometric broken line closure

Ans: B. Serial Z-plasty

Q 35. Which of the following surgical techniques is the one that was used with the final scar result?

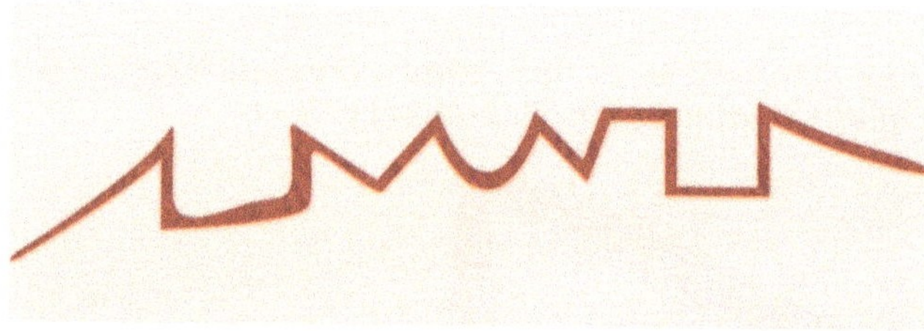

A. Running Z-plasties
B. Running W-plasties
C. Geometric broken-line closure
D. Fusiform excision with scar repositioning

Ans: C. Geometric broken-line closure

Q 36. Which of the following treatment modalities is THE MOST accepted in the treatment and prevention of an hypertrophic scar?

A. Massage therapy
B. Onion extract
C. Vitamin E
D. Silicone gel sheeting

Ans: D. Silicone gel sheeting

Q 37. Which is the MOST common adverse effect of Pulse Dye Laser (PDL)?

A. Transient purpura
B. Edema
C. Hyperpigmentation
D. Hypopigmentation

Ans: A. Transient purpura

Q 38. Which of the following laser is considered "the gold standard" for the treatment of hypertrophic scars and keloids?

A. CO_2 laser
B. Nd:YAG laser
C. Er:YAG laser
D. PDL laser

Ans: D. PDL laser

Q 39. Which of the following topical prevention/treatment for post-surgical scars have NOT been shown to improve scar appearance?

A. Vitamin E
B. Pressure garment
C. Silicone gel sheeting (SGS)
D. Petrolatum ointment

Ans: A. Vitamin E

Q 40. Which of the following statements regarding dermabrasion for facial scars is FALSE?

A. Timing for dermabrasion is usually within the first month of the wound production
B. Penetration into the papillary dermis will produce a diffuse pinpoint bleeding
C. Penetration into the reticular dermis will produce a yellow chamois color appearance
D. Reepithelization usually occurs within 10 days after

Ans: A. Timing for dermabrasion is usually within the first month of the wound production

Q 41. Microdermabrasion is intended to remove which of the following layer of the epidermis?

A. Stratum spinosum of the epidermis
B. Stratum granulosum of the epidermis
C. Stratum lucidum of the epidermis
D. Stratum corneum of the epidermis

Ans: D. Stratum corneum of the epidermis

Q 42. Hyperpigmentation as side effect of dermabrasion will be INCREASED by which of the following?

A. Hydroquinone
B. Kojic acid
C. Tretinoin
D. Estrogens

Ans: D. Estrogens

Q 43. The angle for an M-Plasty, indicated in the drawing, SHOULD BE approximately?

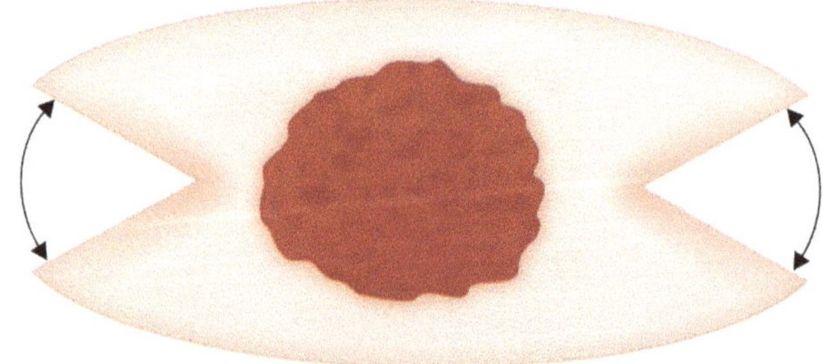

A. 30°   B. 40°

C. 50°   D. 60°

Ans: A. 30°

Q 44. Which of the following statements regarding M-Plasty is TRUE?

A. It is commonly used to lengthen a contracting scar

B. It is commonly used to camouflage an unsightly scar

C. It is commonly used to decrease the volume of healthy skin excised

D. It is commonly used to break a scar into multiple irregular small segments

Ans: C. It is commonly used to decrease the volume of healthy skin excised

Q 45. Which of the following about microdermabrasion is TRUE?

A. It will require mild IV sedation

B. It involves using a closed-loop with aluminum oxide crystals

C. The end point of the technique is signaled by frosting of the skin

D. Treatment sessions must be separated by 6 months

Ans: B. It involves using a closed-loop with aluminum oxide crystals

Q 46. Which of the following photographic parameters is MOST DIFFICULT to adjust in the documentation of a facial scar?

A. Exposure   B. Flash intensity

C. Velocity   D. Depth of field

Ans: A. Exposure

SECTION

4

Nonsurgical Cosmetic Procedures

Section Outlines

Chapter 17

Injectable Botulinum Toxin

Nathalie Gabra

■ INTRODUCTION

Over the last decade, injections of neurotoxins have become the most commonly performed cosmetic procedure. It is an effective, minimally invasive and safe treatment for facial rhytids.

Differences between fillers and neurotoxins:
- *Neurotoxins*: These are used to eliminate or attenuate the dynamic facial wrinkles (produced on animation) by weakening the underlying facial muscles.
- *Fillers*: These are used to attenuate static facial wrinkles or lines that are obvious even at rest.
- Neurotoxins are injected intramuscularly whereas fillers are injected dermally or subdermally.

■ DEFINITION AND PHARMACOLOGY

Main Food and Drug Administration Approved Botulinum Toxin A

- *Onabotulinum toxin A (BoNTA-ONA)*: Sold as Botox (Allergan)
  - Supplied as 50–100 IU vials of powder, dilution with 0.9% NaCl to achieve a concentration of 2–5 U per 0.1 mL, stored in freezer
  - LD50 is 2,800–3,500 U
  - Surrounded by hemagglutinins
  - Refrigerate after reconstitution (up to 24 hours use).
- *Abobotulinum toxin A (BoNTA-ABO)*: Sold as Dysport (Galderma)
  - Supplied as 300–500 IU vials of powder, dilution with 0.9 % NaCl to achieve a concentration of 10 U per 0.1 mL or 10 U per 0.5 mL, stored in freezer
  - Clinically Botox is 2.5–5 (3 is generally accepted) times more potent than Dysport and the dose should be adjusted accordingly
  - Surrounded by hemagglutinins
  - Refrigerate after reconstitution (up to 4 hours use).
- *Incobotulinum toxin A*: Sold as Xeomin (Merz Aesthetics)
  - Supplied as 50–100 IU vials of powder, dilution with 0.9% NaCl to achieve a concentration of 2–5 U per 0.1 mL, *store at room temperature*

- Same potency as Botox
- *Not surrounded by complexing protein*
- Refrigerate after reconstitution (up to 24 hours use).
- *Botulinum toxin B*: Sold as Myobloc (Elan Pharmaceuticals)
  - Food and Drug Administration approved for cervical dystonia
  - Available in 2,500, 5,000 or 10,000 U vials
  - Painful injection, shorter duration of action than type A
  - Higher protein content, more frequent antibody formation
  - Refrigerate after reconstitution (up to 4 hours use).

Mechanism of Action

- *Clostridium botulinum* is a gram-positive anaerobic bacteria that produces 8 different toxins (A, B, C1, C2, D, E, F and G)
- The neurotoxin acts at the pre-synaptic level by temporarily inhibiting the release of acetylcholine (ACh) at the motor end-plates of voluntary muscle
- In fact, the release of ACh is mediated by the assembly of a synaptic fusion complex that allows membrane of the synaptic vesicle that contains ACh to fuse with the neuronal cell membrane
- The toxin enters the neuronal cell membrane by endocytosis and prevents the assembly of this complex and therefore, the release of ACh
- *The effect of botulinum toxin A is reversed by 3–4 months*: First there is growth of new axonal collaterals which create new neuromuscular junctions, then the enzymatic function of the primary (original) nerve is restored and the collaterals regress.

■ HISTORY AND PHYSICAL EXAMINATION

Contraindications to Botulinum Toxin A

- Preexisting neural disorders such as myasthenia gravis, amyotrophic lateral sclerosis, and Eaton-Lambert syndrome
- Sensitivity to any other botulinum toxin product

- Albumin allergy
- Cow's milk protein allergy (in case of Dysport)
- Not recommended to pregnant women or lactating mothers (no safety data).

Common Cosmetic Indications of Botulinum Toxin

- *On-label*:
  - Glabellar rhytids (4 U into each of 5 sites)
  - Crow's feet (4 U into each of 3 sites per side).
- *Off-label*:
  - Forehead wrinkles
  - Bunny lines
  - Smoker's lines/lipstick lines
  - Marionette lines
  - Dimpled chin ("peau d'orange")
  - Gummy smile.

Noncosmetic Indications of Botulinum Toxin

- Overactive bladder or urinary incontinence
- Spasticity
- Cervical dystonia
- Axillary hyperhidrosis
- Blepharospasm
- Strabismus
- Chronic migraine
- Facial contractures, torticollis
- Synkinesis following facial paralysis
- Frey's syndrome, hyperhidrosis
- Sialorrhea
- Muscle tension dysphonia.

■ INJECTION TECHNIQUE

- Informed consent should be obtained after explanation of the procedure, the reason for injection and the potential complications
- Injection site should be documented and pretreatment photography should be obtained
- Mark the patient's face with a pen for all the areas of maximum muscle tension causing the hyperfunctional lines to be treated
- Allow 1–1.5 cm for diffusion of the toxin from each injection point
- Once the marking is complete, the skin could be treated with topical anesthetic to decrease the pain related to the needle entry
- Injection is performed using a 30-G, 31-G or 32-G needle. Apply gentle pressure at the injection site to prevent ecchymosis
- The patient is asked not to rub or massage the injected area for 6 hours to prevent diffusion of the toxin to adjacent muscles and cause unwanted weakness

- If available, an EMG can be used to actively guide the injection in the adequate site and titrate the dose according to the response.

Injection Sites

- *Glabellar rhytids*: It is related to the hyperactivity of the procerus and corrugator muscles. The procerus muscle should be injected at the level of the nasion. Each corrugator muscle should be injected medially and laterally into the belly of the muscle without passing the mid-pupillary and above the superior orbital rim to avoid diffusion into the levator palpebrae, which could cause transient eyelid ptosis. Therefore, the injections should follow a 5-point V pattern with one injection into the procerus muscle and 2 injections in each corrugator muscle. Suggested dosing: 2–5 U of Botox or 6–15 U of Dysport per point (Fig. 1).
- *Transverse forehead rhytids*: The contraction of the frontalis muscle causes elevation of the brow and results in dynamic transverse rhytids. The goal of the treatment is too soften the lines without giving an artificial, unexpressive appearance and avoiding brow ptosis. The patient should be asked to forcefully lift his brow to assess the location of the lines. Injections should be performed in a grid-like fashion across the forehead at 4–5 different sites equally spaced. It is important to stay 1–2 cm above the supraorbital rim to avoid brow or eyelid ptosis. The dose range is between 10 U and 25 U depending on the gender and the "toxin naivety" (Fig. 2).
- *Lateral orbital region "Crow's feet"*: This results from contraction of the lateral orbicularis occuli muscle. It is a very thin muscle and therefore subcutaneous or

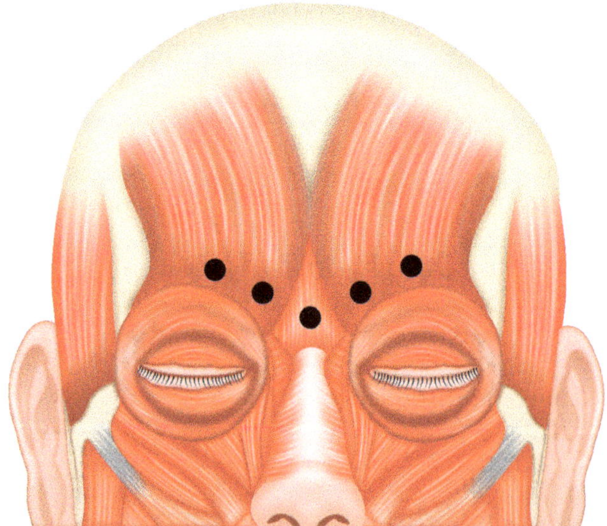

Fig. 1: Injection site and pattern in the corrugator muscles and procerus muscle for the treatment of glabellar rhytids

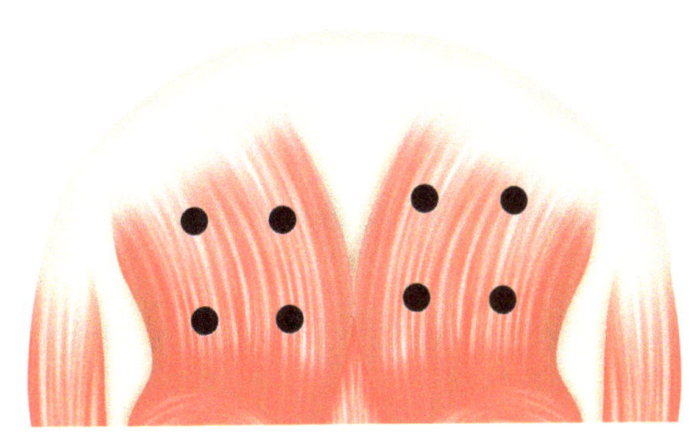

Fig. 2: Injection site and pattern for transverse forehead rhytids

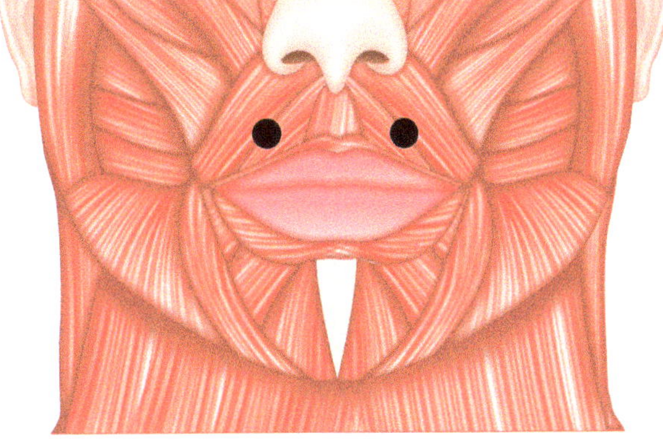

Fig. 4: Injection site and pattern for upper lip rhytids

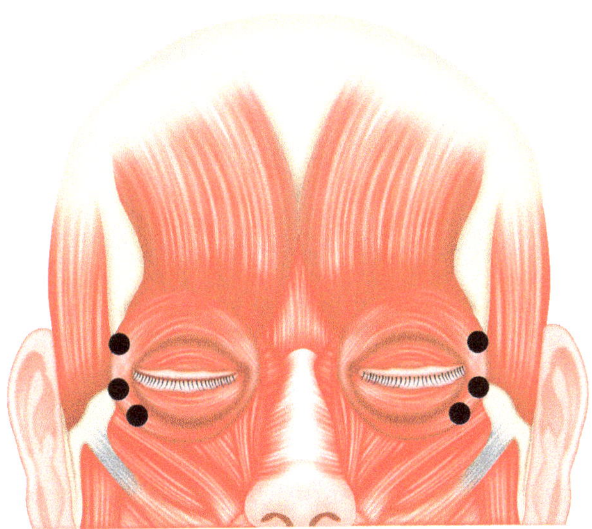

Fig. 3: Injection site and pattern for lateral periobital rhytids "Crow's feet"

intradermal injections are usually sufficient. This site is usually addressed with three injections. The middle injection is placed in line with the lateral canthus, and the remaining two injections are placed 8–10 mm above and below this point (Fig. 3). Total starting dose ranges between 8 U and 16 U of Botox per side for women and 12–16 U of Botox per side for men. It is important to stay at least 1 cm away from the lateral orbital rim to prevent diffusion of the product to the lid retractors and extraocular muscles. Injections should be avoided in patients with upper eyelid ptosis, lagophthalmos or upper facial palsy.

- *Platysmal banding*: The patient should be asked to contract the muscle, and the obvious platysmal bands should be grasped. Each band will require multiple injections about 1–1.5 cm apart from the jawline to the lower neck. Each band should receive about 15 U of Botox or 40 U to 80 U of Dysport. It is important to inject superficially to avoid diffusion to the deeper muscles of the neck, which could cause dysphonia, dysphagia or life-threatening breathing difficulty.
- *Upper lip rhytids*: The orbicularis oris muscle is responsible for dynamic vertical rhytids of the upper lip. Although their appearance is associated with sun exposure and smoking, they are almost universally found with increasing age. The primary function of this muscle is for oral competence and speech. Injections should be performed medial to a vertical line drawn from the lateral nasal ala to the upper lip vermillion. A total of 4 U to 6 U of Botox could be used for this area (Fig. 4).

COMPLICATIONS

- Injection of botulinum toxin A is a relatively safe technique if the appropriate technique, doses and dilutions are adopted. However, given the fact that the effect of the toxin is temporary, so are the complications. Until now, there is no reported death or severe long-term complications from the aesthetic use of botulinum toxin A.
- *Minor local complications include*: Pain, erythema and bruising.
- *Minor systemic side effects include*: Headaches, malaise and fatigue (1%).
- *Upper eyelid ptosis*:
  - Results from the diffusion of the product to the levator palpebrae muscle when injecting the glabella or the periorbital region
  - Usually lasts 2–6 weeks postinjection
  - The use of alpha-adrenergic ophthalmic drops (apraclonidine 0.5%, naphazoline, or phenylephrine 2.5%) can help by stimulating Mueller muscle to

elevate the eyelid. Start two drops BID. Can obtain *2 mm* of elevation.

- *Diplopia*: This results from diffusion to the lateral rectus muscle during injection of Crow's feet.
- *Brow ptosis*: This results from the diffusion of the product while injecting transverse forehead rhytids, can be avoided by remaining 1–1.5 cm above the brow line.
- *Other complications*:
    - Neck weakness (injection of SCM during the treatment of platysmal banding)
    - Oral incompetence or lip weakness
    - Dysphagia or hoarseness.

■ BIBLIOGRAPHY

1. Gart MS, Gutowski KA. Overview of botulinum toxins for aesthetic uses. Clin Plast Surg. 2016;43:459-71.
2. Johnson JT, Rosen CA (Eds). Bailey's Head and Neck Surgery—Otolaryngology, 5th edition. Philadelphia: Wolters Kluwer-Lippincott Williams & Wilkins; 2013.
3. Matarasso A, Deva AK, American Society of Plastic Surgeons DATA Committee. Botulinum toxin. Plast Reconstr Surg. 2002;109:1191-7.
4. Vartanian AJ, Dayan SH. Complications of botulinum toxin A use in facial rejuvenation. Facial Plast Surg Clin North Am. 2003;11(4):483-92.
5. Williams EF, Hove C. Lip construction. In: Paper ID, Holt GR, Larrabee WF (Eds). Facial Plastic and Reconstructive Surgery, 2nd edition. New York: Thieme; 2002.

Multiple Choice Questions

Q 1. Which of the following antibiotics is CONTRAINDI-CATED with the use of Botox?

A. Aminoglycoside
B. Cephalosporin
C. Clindamycin
D. Penicillin

Ans: A. Aminoglycoside

Q 2. Which of the following would benefit the LEAST by using Botulinum Exotoxin A (Botox) injections?

A. Nasolabial folds
B. Horizontal forehead lines
C. Lateral orbital lines ("crow's feet")
D. Glabellar line

Ans: A. Nasolabial folds

Q 3. Which of the following antibiotics is NOT a contraindication for the use of Botulinum Exotoxin A (Botox)?

A. Amikacin
B. Tobramycin
C. Gentamicin
D. Clindamycin

Ans: D. Clindamycin

Q 4. The maximal muscle weakness response after the use of botulinum A toxin injection is:

A. 2 weeks
B. 1 week
C. 36 hours
D. 24 hours

Ans: B. 1 week

Q 5. Which of the following medications is COMPATIBLE with the use of the Botulinum Toxin?

A. Aminoglycosides
B. Penicillamine
C. Calcium channel blockers
D. Statins

Ans: D. Statins

Q 6. Transient lid ptosis can be treated by eye drops causing CONTRACTION of the:

A. Orbicularis oculi muscle
B. Muller muscle
C. Levator palpebrae superioris
D. Levator aponeurosis

Ans: B. Muller muscle

Q 7. Which of the following wrinkles CANNOT adequately treated with Botox?

A. Actinic damage lines
B. Glabellar vertical lines
C. Glabellar horizontal lines
D. Lateral orbital lines (crow's feet)

Ans: A. Actinic damage lines

Q 8. Which of the following statements is the usual dose (per side) of Botox for treatment of crow's feet wrinkles?

A. 5 units
B. 10 units
C. 20 units
D. 35 units

Ans: B. 10 units

Q 9. A patient had botulinum A exotoxin (BTX-A) injected into the forehead. After 3 days there was still no response. Which of the following is TRUE?

A. Reinjection in 3 months
B. Reinjection with a half dose at day 4
C. Reinjection at 2 weeks
D. Reinjection increasing the initial dose at 2 weeks

Ans: C. Reinjection at 2 weeks

Q 10. Which of the following statements about botulinum toxin is TRUE?

A. There are 5 different serotypes of botulinum toxin
B. One unit of botulinum toxin A is defined as the necessary amount to kill approximately 90–100% of a group of 20 g female Swiss-Webster mice
C. Zinc has a critical role in the chemical reaction of botulinum toxin
D. 1 unit of Botox is equivalent to approximately 1 unit of Dysport

Ans: C. Zinc has a critical role in the chemical reaction of botulinum toxin

Q 11. Which of the following serotypes of botulinum toxin is the MOST potent?

A. A

B. B

C. C1

D. D

Ans: A. A

Q 12. Which of the following conditions is NOT A CONTRAINDICATION for the use of botulinum toxin type A?

A. Eaton-Lambert syndrome

B. Myasthenia gravis

C. Psoriasis

D. Multiple sclerosis

Ans: C. Psoriasis

Q 13. HOW MANY units of botulinum neurotoxin A (Botox) are usually needed to achieve a satisfactory reduction in activity of the procerus muscle?

A. 5

B. 15

C. 20

D. 25

Ans: A. 5

Q 14. The "marionette lines" are produced by the hyperactivity of ONE of the following perioral muscles

A. Orbicularis oris

B. Risorius

C. Depressor anguli oris

D. Depressor labii inferioris

Ans: C. Depressor anguli oris

Q 15. Which of the following techniques is the MOST useful in treating glabellar frown lines?

A. Botox injection

B. Chemical peeling

C. CO_2 laser resurfacing

D. Dermabrasion

Ans: A. Botox injection

Q 16. Which of the following is the effect produced by Botulinum Exotoxin A?

A. Inhibits the release of Acetylcholine at the presynaptic level

B. Inhibits the release Acetylcholine at the postsynaptic level

C. Induces the release of Acetylcholine at the presynaptic level

D. Induces the release Acetylcholine at the postsynaptic level

Ans: A. Inhibits the release of Acetylcholine at the presynaptic level

Q 17. What is the human lethal dose of Botulinum toxin A?

A. 500 U

B. 2800 U

C. 5000 U

D. 10000 U

Ans: B. 2800U

Q 18. What is the mechanism of action of Botulinum Toxin A?

A. The neurotoxin acts at the presynaptic level by temporarily inhibiting the release of noradrenaline at the motor end-plates of voluntary muscle

B. The neurotoxin acts at the post-synaptic level by temporarily inhibiting the release of acetylcholine (Ach) at the motor end-plates of voluntary muscle

C. The neurotoxin acts at the postsynaptic level by temporarily inhibiting the release of noreadrenaline at the motor end-plates of voluntary muscle

D. The neurotoxin acts at the presynaptic level by temporarily inhibiting the release of acetylcholine (Ach) at the motor end-plates of voluntary muscle

Ans: D. The neurotoxin acts at the presynaptic level by temporarily inhibiting the release of acetylcholine (Ach) at the motor end-plates of voluntary muscle

Q 19. What is the difference between neurotoxins and fillers for nonsurgical cosmetic procedures?

A. Neurotoxins are used for dynamic facial wrinkles and fillers are used for static facial wrinkles

B. Neurotoxins are used for static facial wrinkles and fillers are used for dynamic facial wrinkles

C. No difference, both are used for static facial wrinkles

D. No difference, both are used for dynamic facial wrinkles

Ans: A. Neurotoxins are used for dynamic facial wrinkles and fillers are used for static facial wrinkles

Q 20. Which one is not a contraindication to the use of Botulinum Toxin A?

A. Myasthenia gravis

B. Eyelid ptosis

C. Albumin allergy

D. Pregnancy

Ans: B. Eyelid ptosis

Q 21. What is the main adverse effect related to the diffusion of the toxin when injecting the glabella and the peri-orbital region?

A. Facial paralysis

B. Hypersensitivity reaction

C. Eyelid ptosis

D. Nasal obstruction

Ans: C. Eyelid ptosis

Q 22. The VERTICAL GLABELLAR frown lines are due to the contraction of which muscle?

A. Corrugator muscle

B. Frontalis muscle

C. Orbicularis oculi muscle

D. Procerus muscle

Ans: A. Corrugator muscle

Q 23. The CREASE noted in the drawing below is PRO-DUCED by:

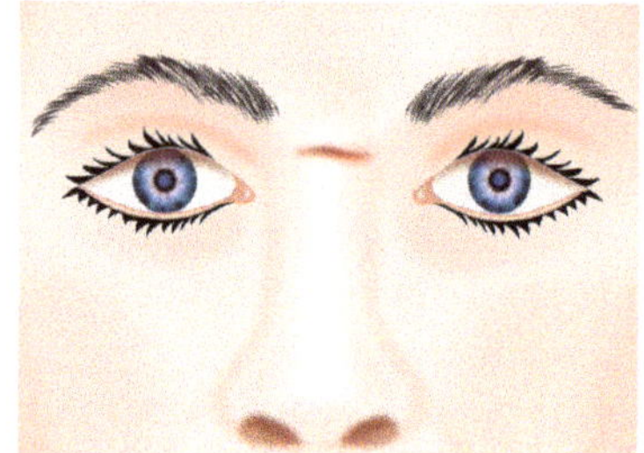

A. Contraction of the frontalis muscle
B. Contraction of the procerus muscle
C. Contraction of the corrugator supercilii muscle
D. Contraction of the orbicularis supercilii muscle

Ans: B. Contraction of the procerus muscle

Q 24. Which of the following muscles arises from the medial end of the orbit (nasal prominence) and runs superiorly and laterally to insert into the deep surface of the skin?

A. Procerus
B. Corrugator supercilii
C. Frontalis
D. Depressor supercilii

Ans: B. Corrugator supercilii

Q 25. What is the percentage of Swiss-Webster mice killed with 1 standard unit of Botulinum toxin A (Botox)?

A. 10%   B. 25%
C. 50%   D. 70%

Ans: C. 50%

Chapter 18

Fillers, Injectables and Implants

Kaitlyn B Zenner, Sapna A Patel, Anisha R Noble, Angelique M Berens

■ INTRODUCTION

The aging face is associated with atrophy, ptosis, and wrinkles which are the result of increased laxity, decreased subcutaneous fat, loss of the dermal papilla, decreased dermal connective tissue (proteoglycans and glycosaminoglycans), and loss of collagen. Periorbital changes include herniation of the periorbital fat, ptosis of the orbicularis muscle, and atrophy of the subcutaneous tissue. The midface descends and experiences volume loss with ptosis and atrophy of infraorbital subcutaneous tissue, malar fat pad, and suborbicularis oculi fat (SOOF). Skeletal atrophy also occurs and exacerbates volume loss.

Fillers, injections, and facial implants can help to restore volume, contour, and symmetry lost as a result of aging, craniofacial deformities, or facial nerve paralysis. These techniques range from in-office procedures to extensive surgical procedures. The ideal injectable or implant should have a predictable duration with minimal migration, be biocompatible, and have low immunogenicity and reactivity. Many materials are available in today's market however each comes with its own risk/benefit profile.

■ ANESTHESIA FOR DERMAL FILLERS

Intradermal injections are more painful than subdermal or supraperiosteal injection and the smallest gauge needle possible should be used. Lidocaine may be infiltrated prior or often comes premixed with the injectable (if not contraindicated by manufacturer recommendations). Nerve blocks can be useful and are most commonly used during lip augmentation. Others may advocate the use of topical anesthesia for more sensitive areas and cold packs are helpful for anesthetic and postprocedural swelling.

■ PROPERTIES OF FILLERS

Lifting ability/elasticity (G') and viscosity are the most important properties of fillers for choosing a filler for a given application. G' helps to ensure stability and allow for lift while viscosity allows for materials to withstand forces once injected (Table 1).

- High G' materials have a higher viscosity making them stiffer which allows for more lift
  - They are better suited for deep fold correction, malar eminence volumizing, and volumizing the temporal hollow

Table 1: Injectable fillers (composition, indications, duration of effect, and contraindicaitons/limitations)

Injectable fillers				
Name	Composition	Indications	Duration	Contraindications/limitations
Collagen				
Cymetra	• Micronized AlloDerm (acellular dermal matrix from human allograft skin)	• Lip augmentation • Nasolabial folds • Burn and scar treatment	• Approximately 3 months but can have cumulative increase with repeat injections	• Not ideal for lip augmentation • Now primarily used for unilateral vocal fold paralysis
Homologous injectable collagen (Dermalogen)	• Injectable acellular collagen from human donor tissue	• Facial wrinkles • Dermal contour defects • Depressed scars	• 3 or 4 injections at 2–4 weeks intervals • 50–75% correction at 3 months • 50% correction at 6 months	• Requires a skin test

Contd...

Contd...

Injectable fillers				
Name	Composition	Indications	Duration	Contraindications/limitations
Hyaluronic acids				
Restylane and Juvederm	• Cross-linked, stabilized heavy (long chain) hyaluronic acid gel	• Glabella • Nasolabial folds • Oral commissures • Depressed acne scars • Lip augmentation	• 50–80% correction after 6 months • Will slowly resorb over time • Higher amount of cross linking (Juvederm Voluma) results in longer duration (18–24 months) of effect	• Tyndall effect: blue tinted hue to skin above injection, most commonly seen in dermal injections. Less likely with Belotero • Delayed edema often occurs
Belotero, Prevelle Silk	• Cross-linked, stabilized light (short chain) hyaluronic acid gel	• Deep wrinkles • Nasolabial folds		
Calcium hydroxyapatite				
Radiesse	• Calcium hydroxyapatite microspheres suspended in an aqueous carboxymethyl-cellulose gel carrier	• Nasolabial folds • Marionette lines • Oral commissures	• 80% maintenance at 12 months	• If injected too superficially will lead to small white nodules on skin surface • Not used in lips because muscle contraction leads to superficial migration and subsequent nodules
Poly-L-lactic acid				
Sculptra	• Poly-L-lactic acid microparticles	• FDA approved for HIV-associated lipoatrophy • Facial wrinkles • Shallow to deep nasolabial folds	• Induces a subclinical inflammatory response resulting in fibroblast and collagen formation • Degraded over 9–24 months	• Granulomas can occur weeks to months after injection • Nodules often occur unless injected below the dermis
Silicone				
Silikon 1,000	• Polymer of dimethylsiloxanes • Augmentation is due to fibroblastic reaction around silicone particles	• Facial wrinkles • Acne scars • Lip augmentation • Facial contour defects • HIV-associated lipoatrophy	• Permanent • Strongly suggest undercorrection • Optimum collagen formation obtained at 12 weeks	• Granulomas can occur weeks to months after injection • Require surgical excision if misplacement occurs
Polymethyl-methacrylate				
Bellafill, Artefill	• Polymethyl-methacrylate microspheres	• Naturally occurring folds and wrinkles of the face • Glabella • Nasolabial folds • Sagging corners of the mouth • Lip augmentation	• Permanent	• Requires skin test • If misplacement occurs only available treatment is wide local excision • Granulomas can occur weeks to months after injection • Smaller particles (<20 µm) more likely to induce inflammation
Autologous biostimulatory agents				
LAVIV	Require a small postauricular punch sample and are then cultured from the patient's own tissue	Scar correction Facial wrinkles Nasolabial folds Glabellar furrows Hypoplastic lips	3–4 injection sessions over 3–6 months 80% correction at 12 months	The cultured fibroblasts should be injected as quickly as possible after shipping (ideally <24 h) to preserve viability
Platelet-rich plasma (PRP)	High concentration plate-lets and growth factors from patient's own blood	Fine lines and wrinkles		Use is off label for these indications, approved for orthopedics

Contd...

Contd...

Injectable fillers				
Name	*Composition*	*Indications*	*Duration*	*Contraindications/limitations*
Autologous fat injections/grafts				
Microlipoinjection	Harvested via liposuction and centrifuged to separate fat and aspirate	Glabella Facial wrinkles Lip augmentation Hemifacial atrophy Nasolabial folds Melolabial folds	30–50% overcorrection because of high rate of resorption	Requires multiple injections and injected fat graft may be replaced by fibrotic tissue
Free fat graft	Harvested from trochanteric and abdominal regions	Larger defects than microlipoinjection.	Higher rate of resorption	Require a second surgical site and scar
Dermal fat graft	Dermal fat remains attached to dermis after de-epithelialization	Large soft tissue defects.	Less resorption than free fat graft	Requires full thickness donor tissue and primary closure

- – The increased viscosity can make injection difficult
- – Used for deep injections (subdermal).
- Low G' materials have a lower viscosity and are more fluid with less lifting ability
  - – They are more effective at filling superficial wrinkles, the lips, the area surrounding the lips, and the skin around the eyes
  - – Used for dermal injections.

■ COMPLICATIONS

Common complications include local discomfort, ecchymosis, and swelling. Depending on what is used, allergic reactions are possible. Injections should be performed by a trained professional due to the possibility of vascular compression or accidental intravascular injection, which may result in complications from blindness, stroke, or skin necrosis. This is typically presents as pain lasting hours after injection and blanched or blue skin in area injected. It is considered a medical emergency; hyaluronic acid based fillers can be reversed with hyaluronidase, and many would advocate utilizing it even if a non-hyaluronic acid filler was utilized. One should also apply nitroglycerin paste, perform warm compress massages, and administer aspirin.

■ FACIAL IMPLANTS

The ideal facial implant is cost-effective, nontoxic, noncarcinogenic, nonantigenic, resistant to infection, chemically inert, easily shaped, will not migrate (or capable of being fixed), autoclavable and capable of maintaining its original form. Resorbable, particles must be more than 40 µm as smaller particles are phagocytosed leading to long-term inflammation. Common implant materials are listed here:

- *Silicone*: Easy to sculpt, encapsulated by tissue, high extrusion rate
- *Alloderm*: Acellular dermal matrix with 65–100% retention depending on mobility of site
- *ePTFE (Gore-Tex)*: Nonresorbable, low risk of infection, and risk of extrusion
- *Polyester fiber (Mersilene)*: Minimal degradation and low risk of infection, tissue ingrowth
- *Acrylics*: Rigid, malleable, and no ingrowth
- *Porous polyethylene (Medpor)*: Low risk of infection and porous to allow for issue ingrowth
- *Metals*: Gold, titanium (osseointegration), and stainless steel (no osseointegration).

Surgical principles differ between solid and semisolid implants. Solid implants require more precise sculpting, larger incision and dissection. Semisolid implants more easily conform to underlying bony structure, require less sculpting, and blend in better with the natural contours of the face.

Midfacial Deformities and Implants for Augmentation

The midface deformities and implants for augmentation are given in Table 2 and Figure 1.

Chin Implants

Chin implants (mentoplasty) is covered in detail in the chin implant chapter.

Table 2: Midface deformities and implants for augmentation

Deformity type	Midface deformity	Augmentation required	Implant predominantly used
I	Primary malar hypoplasia	Projection over malar eminence	"Shell-type" malar implant extends into submalar space for more natural result
II	Submalar deficiency	Anterior projection	Submalar implant (new conform type or generation I submalar implant)
III	Extreme malar-zygomatic prominence	Normal anatomic transition between malar and submalar regions with augmentation of inferior zygoma	Submalar implant (generation II)
IV	Both malar hypoplasia and submalar deficiency	Anterior and lateral projection	"Combined" submalar-shell implant
V	Tear-trough deformity (Infraorbital rim depression/recess)	Site-specific augmentation of infraorbital rim	"Tear-trough" implant

Source: Adapted from Binder WJ. A comprehensive approach for aesthetic contouring of the midface in rhytidectomy. Fac Plast Surg Clin North Am. 1993;1:231–255.

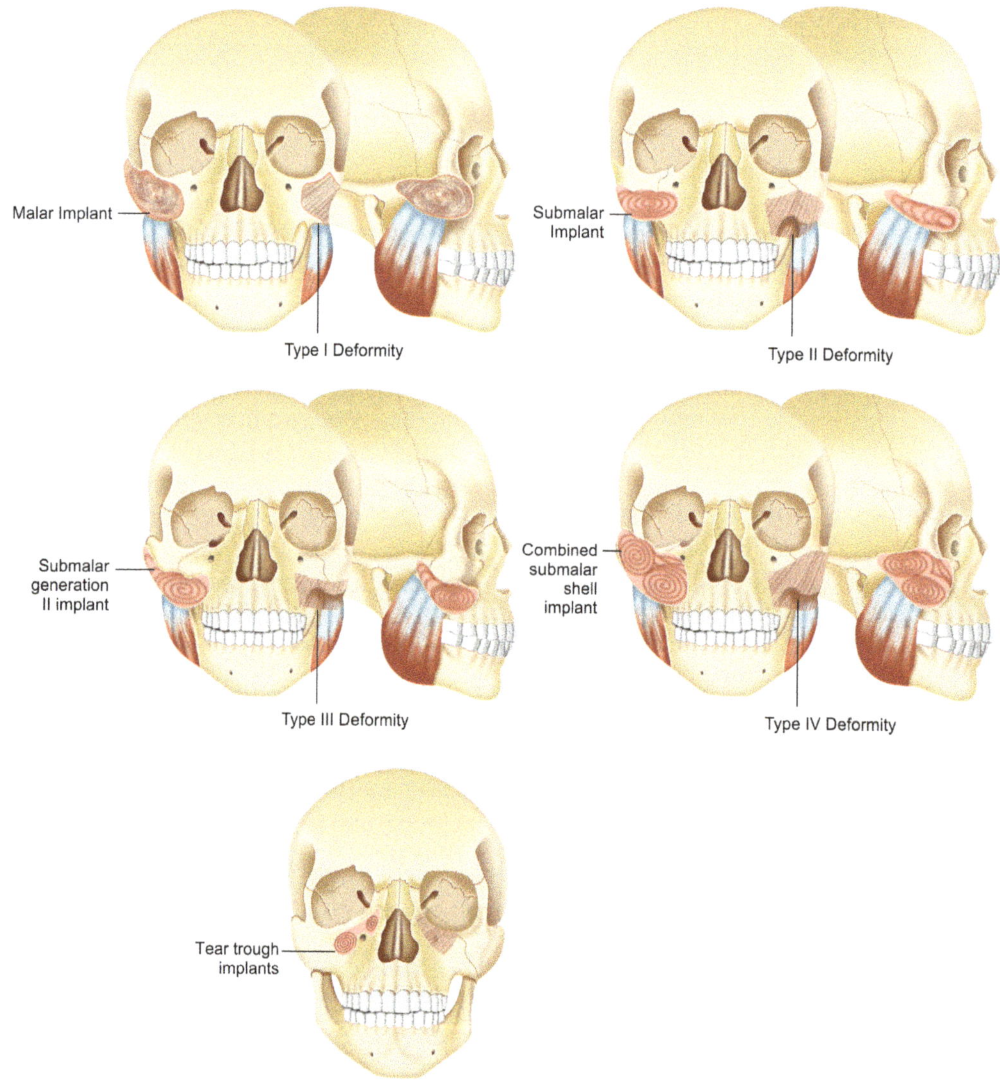

Fig. 1: Midface deformities and implants for augmentation. Each of the midface deformities (Types I–V) can be modified with a corresponding implant type (see Table 2 for more details)

Source: Adapted from Binder WJ. A comprehensive approach for aesthetic contouring of the midface in rhytidectomy. Fac Plast Surg Clin North Am. 1993;1:231–255.

Table 3: Complications of facial implants and interventions to decrease risk	
Complication	*Intervention to decrease risk*
Bleeding/hematoma/ seroma	Full face compression garment Avoid overdissection Control BP during and after the procedure
Infection	Irrigation of surgical site Soaking porous implants in antibiotic solution
Extrusion	Precise technique Adequate soft tissue coverage
Malposition	Larger surface area of implant along bone Adequate dissection of periosteum to create a tunnel/pocket
Displacement or slippage	Appropriate fixation of implant to surrounding tissue
Persistent edema or inflammatory reaction	Appropriate implant fixation decreases excessive movement and continued tissue injury
Neuropraxia	Dissect in the subperiosteal space with malar implants to avoid facial and infraorbital nerves

Complications of Facial Implants

The complications of facial implants are given in Table 3.

Some complications are more common for a particular site or material. Overall, silicone has the highest rate of extrusion and displacement while having the lowest rate of infection. Nasal implants have the highest rate of extrusion, likely from the small amount of soft tissue coverage available at the site. They also have the highest rate of removal for postoperative complications (~10%). Orbital implants have very low rates of complications. The most common complication with malar implants is asymmetry and malposition. They also have the highest rate of infection however this is not increased with an intra-oral incision compare to other approaches (subciliary, transconjunctival, rhytidectomy). The most reliable treatment for infection is removal of implant.

Tissue Expanders (Fig. 2)

- *Indications of soft tissue expanders*:
  - Tissue cannot be closed primarily and tissue from conventional facial flaps is inadequate
  - Adequate tissue is unavailable adjacent to large cutaneous defects of face and neck
  - Primary wound closure not possible and aesthetics require good color, texture, and thickness match.

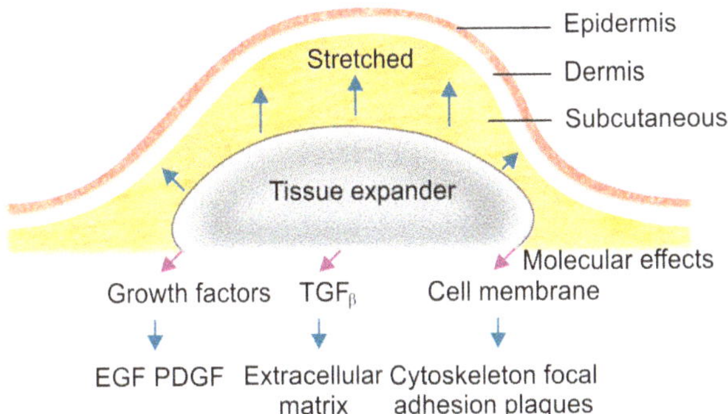

Fig. 2: Biologic response of tissue to tissue expansion. Tissue expanders alter the tissue both physically and chemically. Increased growth factors, transforming growth factor beta (TGFβ), and stress on cell membranes alters the structure of expanded tissues

Abbreviations: EGF, epidermal growth factor; PDGF, platelet-derived growth factor

- *Most common applications*:
  - Extensive burns of the head and neck requiring reconstruction for functional and aesthetic purposes
  - Expansion of postauricular skin prior to external ear reconstruction
  - Expansion of myocutaneous, fascial and free flap tissue
  - Post-traumatic or postoperative alopecia correction
  - Expansion of cheek, neck skin to allow for scar revision, and burn excision.
- *List the physiologic changes in expanded skin*
  Biological creep: Permanent changes in microanatomy and collagen production increases surface area after long period of stretch.
  - Occurs in conventional tissue expanders that are expanded over 4–6 weeks
    » *Epidermis*: Increased mitotic activity of basal cells, enhancing epidermal height; returns to normal within 1–2 years postoperative
    » Dermal thinning with increased fibroblast activity, enhanced collagen synthesis and temporarily enhanced melanin production and skin pigmentation; hair follicles spread out across expanded skin and stiffness, stria, alopecia, diminished sensation
    » *Adipose tissue*: Intolerant of expansion, thins up to 50%; replaced by fibrous tissue
    » Vascular changes: Chronic tissue expansion promotes vascular proliferation.
  Mechanical creep: No change in microanatomy and no net increase in surface area but can recruit adjacent tissue.
  - Occurs in rapid intraoperative tissue expansion; typically with 3 cycles of expansion for 3 minutes.

- *Surgical principles of placement, removal, and serial inflation soft tissue expanders*:
    - Incisions should be placed such that they become incorporated into one margin of the flap
    - Minimize tension on suture lines and reduce likelihood of implant extrusion
    - Balloons should be partially inflated immediately after wound closure to close "dead space" and prevent seroma/hematoma formation
    - Serial inflation starts 1–2 weeks postinitial placement, use frequent small-volume inflations.
- *Technique of expansion (and endpoints) and removal*
    - Using a small gauge needle through the overlying skin into the expander port, insert saline such that brief blanching of overlying skin occurs; repeat this process weekly.
      Injection port types:
        » *Self-contained*: Requires less dissection but has greater risk of rupture
        » *Remote*: Unlikely to rupture but requires more dissection and includes connector tubing between expander and injection port
        » *External valve*: Port is outside of the patient; good for children because eliminates the pain of injection.
    - When appropriate amount of tissue expansion is achieved, expansion is halted; expander is left in place for an additional 2 weeks prior to removal
    - At the time of removal, a final intraoperative expansion can be done for an additional 1–2 cm tissue
    - Following removal of expander and flap advancement takes place.
- *Possible complications and management*
    - Approximately 10% complication rate
    - Most common: Exposure or extrusion of expander
        » *Early*: Expansion aborted
        » *Late*: Expansion completed versus truncated.
    - Infection in head and neck unusual with regards to tissue expanders
    - Ischemia/necrosis of flap rare (likely due to aggressive expansion)
    - Expander failure and deflation are very rare. Usually due to improper inflation or surgical technique.

■ BIBLIOGRAPHY

1. Cuzalina LA, Hlavacek MR. Complications of facial implants. Oral Maxillofacial Surg Clin North Am. 2009;21:91-104.
2. Daines SM, Williams EF. Complications associated with injectable soft-tissue fillers: a 5-year retrospective review. JAMA Facial Plast Surg. 2013;15:226-31.
3. Eppley BL, Dadvand B. Injectable soft-tissue fillers: clinical overview. Plast Reconstr Surg. 2006;118:98e-106e.
4. Flint P, Haughey B, Lund V, et al. Cummings Otolaryngology: Head and Neck Surgery. Philadelphia: Saunders; 2014.
5. Lafaille P, Benedetto A. Fillers: contraindications, side effects and precautions. J Cutan Aesthet Surg. 2010;3:16-9.
6. Papel I, Frodel J, Holt GR, et al. Facial Plastic and Reconstructive Surgery. New York: Thieme Medical Publishers, Inc; 2002.
7. Pasha R, Golub J. Otolaryngology Head and Neck Surgery: Clinical Reference Guide. San Diego, CA: Plural Publishing, Inc; 2014.
8. Rubin J, Yaremchuk M. Complications and toxicities of implantable biomaterials used in facial reconstructive and aesthetic surgery: a comprehensive review of the literature. Plast Reconstr Surg. 1997;100:1336-53.
9. Binder WJ. A comprehensive approach for aesthetic contouring of the midface in rhytidectomy. Fac Plast Surg Clin North Am. 1993;1:231–255.
10. Sclafani AP. What we have learned about soft-tissue augmentation over the past 10 years. JAMA Facial Plast Surg. 2014;16:64-5.
11. Thorn C, Gurtner GC, Chung K, et. al. Grabb and Smith's Plastic Surgery, 7th edition. Philadelphia: Lippincott Williams &Wilkins; 2014.
12. Woodward J, Khan T, Martin J. Facial filler complications. Facial Plast Surg Clin North Am. 2015;23:447-58.

Multiple Choice Questions

Q 1. Which PERCENTAGE is expected to induce skin allergic reaction when using bovine dermal collagen?

A. 1%

B. 3%

C. 5%

D. 10%

Ans: B. 3%

Q 2. Which of the following is THE MOST common complication of tissue expanders?

A. Early infection

B. Late infection

C. Early exposure

D. Late exposure

Ans: D. Late exposure

Q 3. Which of the following metals is THE BEST choice for long-term facial implantation?

A. Stainless steel

B. Vitallium

C. Titanium

D. Chromium

Ans: C. Titanium

Q 4. Which of the following is the recommended wait time prior TO STARTING sequential inflation after insertion of scalp tissue expanders?

A. 2 weeks

B. 3 weeks

C. 4 weeks

D. 6 weeks

Ans: A. 2 weeks

Q 5. Which of the folllowing IMPLANTABLE MATERIALS is an injectable autologous soft tissue material derived from cultured human fibroblasts?

A. Autologen
B. Isolagen
C. Alloderm
D. Dermalogen

Ans: B. Isolagen

Q 6. Which of the following statements is FALSE regarding tissue expanders?

A. The forehead is an ideal location for tissue expansion
B. In the scalp expanders are placed deep to the galea and superficial to the periosteum
C. Nerve tissue tolerates expansion poorly
D. Adipose tissue is intolerant of tissue expansion

Ans: C. Nerve tissue tolerates expansion poorly

Q 7. As a general rule for the selection of a tissue expander its base size SHOULD BE:

A. 1 ½ times the area to be reconstructed
B. 2 times the area to be reconstructed
C. 3 times the area to be reconstructed
D. 4 times the area to be reconstructed

Ans: C. 3 times the area to be reconstructed

Q 8. Which of the following statements regarding calvarial bone grafts is TRUE?

A. The calvarium is an endochondral bone similar to the iliac
B. Calvarial bone grafting is mostly used in nasal dorsal augmentation
C. Calvarial bone grafting is also ideal for struts
D. The calvarial bone graft is taken close to the midline to avoid bleeding

Ans: B. Calvarial bone grafting is mostly used in nasal dorsal augmentation

Q 9. Which of the following statements regarding Zyplast is FALSE?

A. It is a glutaraldehyde cross-linked collagen with a concentration of 35 mg/mL
B. It is less susceptible to collagenase degradation and less immunoresponsive, than Zyderm
C. Overcorrection is necessary
D. It is used mostly for correcting facial rhytids

Ans: C. Overcorrection is necessary

Q 10. Which of the following metallic implants is the BEST tolerated and has the greatest MRI compatibility?

A. Stainless steel
B. Vitalium
C. Titanium
D. Cobalt

Ans: C Titanium

Q 11. Which of the following locations is IDEAL for the use of TISSUE EXPANDERS?

A. Forehead
B. Cheek
C. Neck
D. Temple

Ans: A. Forehead

Q 12. Which of the following synthetic implants has micropores of 30 μm, allows tissue ingrowth, is biocompatible, is soft/pliable, is sculptable, has poor structural support and generally is used for onlay augmentation of the nasal dorsum?

A. Gore-Tex
B. Medpor
C. Mersilene
D. Silastic

Ans: A. Gore-Tex

Q 13. Which of the following substances MOST commonly comprises the prosthetics used in nasal reconstruction?

A. Gelatin-glycerin mixture
B. Poly(methylmethacrylate)
C. Prevulcanized latex
D. Silicone

Ans: D. Silicone

Q 14. Which of the following lip augmentation materials is a PERMANENT injectable filler?

A. Zyplast
B. Artecoll/Artefill
C. Restylene
D. Juvederm

Ans: B. Artecoll/Artefill

Q 15. Which of the following complications is MOST commonly seen in the use of alloplastic mandibular implants?

A. Hematoma
B. Infection
C. Sensory alterations
D. Marginal mandibular branch of the facial nerve injury

Ans: C. Sensory alterations

Q 16. Which of the following is the MOST commonly used chin implant material?

A. Silicone
B. Proplast
C. Gore-Tex
D. Hydroxyapatite

Ans: A. Silicone

Q 17. Which of the following effects is TRUE using soft tissue expanders?

A. Thin epidermis
B. Thin dermis
C. Thick epidermis
D. Decreased skin pigmentation

Ans: B. Thin dermis

Q 18. Which of the following statements regarding collagen is FALSE?

A. There are three types of bovine collagen: Zyderm I, Zyderm II, and Zyplast
B. Zyplast is cross-linked with glutaraldehyde
C. There are three types of human collagen: CosmoDerm I, CosmoDerm II and Cosmoplast
D. Bovine and human collagen will require skin testing prior to the treatment injection

Ans: D. Bovine and human collagen will require skin testing prior to the treatment injection

Q 19. Which of the following statements regarding Hyaluronic acid injectables is FALSE?

A. Hyaluronic acid is one of the components of the extracelullar matrix in the dermis
B. Skin testing is mandatory prior to injection of any form of hyaluronic acid products
C. Restylane is derived from laboratory fermentation of bacterial cultures of equine streptococci
D. Hyaloform is a purified form derived from the rooster combs

Ans: B. Skin testing is mandatory prior to injection of any form of hyaluronic acid products

Q 20. Radiesse is related to which of the following implant materials?

A. Collagen
B. Hyaluronic acid
C. Hydroxyapatite
D. Polyacrylamide

Ans: C. Hydroxyapatite

Q 21. Which of the following statements regarding tissue expanders is TRUE?

A. Tissue expanders are made of silicone
B. The base of the expander should be equal to 1 time the size area to be reconstructed
C. The circular expanders provide the largest gain in surface
D. The tissue expanders are available in two shapes: circular and rectangular

Ans: A. Tissue expanders are made of silicone

Q 22. The PROPER anatomical area—in the scalp—to place the tissue expander is UNDER:

A. The skin
B. The subcutaneous tissue
C. The galea aponeurotica
D. The temporalis muscle

Ans: C. The galea aponeurotica

Q 23. Which of the following statements regarding the physiology of tissue expansion is FALSE?

A. The epidermis has an increased mitotic activity
B. The dermis layer is also increased
C. The muscle tissue demonstrates atrophy
D. The vascular tissue demonstrates proliferation

Ans: B. The dermis layer is also increased

Q 24. What is the MOST common complication noted in tissue expansion?

A. Deflation
B. Migration
C. Infection
D. Exposure

Ans: D. Exposure

Q 25. Which of the following statements regarding tissue expansion used in the head and neck is FALSE?

A. Tissue expanders are made of silicone
B. Tissue expanders have a high rate of infection

C. Tissue expander base size is 2.5 times the area to be reconstructed
D. Tissue expanders work best under the scalp or forehead

Ans: B. Tissue expanders have a high rate of infection

Q 26. Which of the following statements is TRUE regarding SCULPTRA?

A. It is an injectable form dimethylpolysiloxane
B. It is immunologically active
C. Skin testing is necessary prior to treatment
D. It is approved for treatment of facial lipo-atrophy associated with HIV disease

Ans: D. It is approved for treatment of facial lipo-atrophy associated with HIV disease

Q 27. Which of the following shape in tissue expander is the ONE to achieve the MOST GAIN in the tissue surface area?

A. Square
B. Circular
C. Rectangular
D. Crescent

Ans: C. Rectangular

Q 28. Which of the following statements regarding tissue expanders is FALSE?

A. It is indicated in the treatment of male pattern baldness
B. It is indicated in the management of a forehead giant melanocytic nevi
C. It is indicated in the reconstruction of the auricular microtia
D. It is not indicated in previously irradiated areas

Ans: D. It is not indicated in previously irradiated areas

Q 29. Which of the following statements regarding SOFT TISSUE EXPANSION is TRUE?

A. Expanders in the scalp are placed under the periosteum
B. Expanders in the scalp will require a total of 3–4 weeks for complete expansion
C. Expander failure is the most common major complication.
D. Scalp reconstruction after soft tissue expansion is based mainly in advancement flaps

Ans: D. Scalp reconstruction after soft tissue expansion is based mainly in advancement flaps

Q 30. Which of the following statements regarding injectable collagen materials is TRUE?

A. Zyderm I is used in a 25 mg/mL concentration
B. Zyderm II is used in a 50 mg/mL concentration
C. Zyplast is a collagen cross-link with gluteraldehyde
D. Bovine collagen allergic sensitivity is about 5%

Ans: C. Zyplast is a collagen cross-link with gluteraldehyde

Q 31. Which of the following statements regarding the disadvantages of implantable material is FALSE?

A. Cartilage has poor resorption rate predictability
B. Calvarial bone has more resorption than iliac crest

C. Silicone implants have an increased number of extrusions and displacements

D. Acelular dermis is a material useful to cover dorsal nasal irregularities in the thin-skinned patient

Ans: B. Calvarial bone has more resorption than iliac crest

Q 32. Which of the following permanent dermal fillers requires a skin test prior to use?

A. Juvederm

B. Liquid silicone

C. Restylane

D. Bellafill

Ans: D. Bellafill

Q 33. Which of the following IS NOT a property of an ideal implant?

A. Breakdown to particles <40 µm

B. Chemically inert

C. Resistant to infection

D. Cost effective

Ans: A. Breakdown to particles <40 µm

Q 34. Which of the following IS NOT part of the first line management of most facial injection complications?

A. Aspirin

B. Epi pen

C. Nitroglycerin paste

D. Hyaluronidase

Ans: B. Epi pen

Q 35. List the physiologic changes as they occur in expanded skin:

A. Epidermal thinning, dermal thickening, vascular proliferation, adipose atrophy

B. Epidermal thickening, dermal thinning, vascular proliferation, adipose atrophy

C. Epidermal thickening, dermal thinning, reduced vascularity, adipose proliferation

D. Epidermal thinning, dermal thinning, static vascularity, adipose proliferation

Ans: B. Epidermal thickening, dermal thinning, vascular proliferation, adipose atrophy

Q 36. Which of the following tissues IS LESS TOLERANT of EXPANSION?

A. Epidermis

B. Adipose tissue

C. Blood vessels

D. Muscular tissue

Ans: B. Adipose tissue

Q 37. Which of the following statements regarding tissue expansion devices is FALSE?

A. The standard tissue expander is composed of a silastic reservoir, injection port and connecting tubing

B. The rectangular shape device will achieve the least gain in surface area

C. The size of the expander base should be 2.5–3 times the size of the defect to be closed

D. Tissue expander will stimulate proliferation of blood vessels in the expanded area

Ans: B. The rectangular shape device will achieve the least gain in surface area

Chapter 19

Chemical Peels

Angelique M Berens, Michael Duyzend, Sapna A Patel

■ INTRODUCTION

Patients commonly seek facial rejuvenation to reverse the effects of UV radiation, such as premature wrinkling, acne scars, pigment irregularities, actinic keratosis and seborrheic keratosis. Peeling produces a controlled partial thickness chemical burn of the epidermis and papillary dermis, which can improve these conditions. Regeneration of peeled skin from wound margins and follicular and exocrine duct epithelium results in a fresh, orderly, organized epidermis. Extension into the deeper reticular dermis leads to scarring and should thus be avoided. In the dermis, new compact orderly collagen is formed between the epidermis and the underlying damaged dermis, which results in ablation of fine wrinkles and reduction of pigment. Facial skin tends to be thinner, oilier and have a higher density of hair follicles in relation to the rest of the body skin, making it ideal for chemical peels.

■ PATIENT SELECTION CONSIDERATIONS

A full medical history to cover risk factors and thorough head and neck examination with special attention to skin lesions and skin types using the Fitzpatrick scale (Table 1) should be completed. Photoaging should be evaluated using the Glogau scale (Table 2). Evaluate the sebaceous quality of the skin understanding that very sebaceous skin may require additional pre-peel degreasing. The presence of inflammatory skin disorders (e.g. seborrheic dermatitis or psoriasis) can increase the absorption of the peel, and may lead to a deeper peel than intended. Photodocumentation should be obtained.

Counsel patients that chemical peels will improve the texture of the skin but will make no impact on facial architecture. Indications for chemical peels include photodamaged skin, fine rhytids, actinic changes, dyschromias, and acne scars. Contraindications include active herpetic outbreak, scleroderma, and HIV, among others (Box 1). Patients should expect a 2–4 weeks pre-peel regimen followed by an approximately 1 hour office procedure and up to 4 weeks of recovery time, depending on the depth of peel. Preoperative counseling should

Table 1: Fitzpatrick scale.

Skin type	Skin color	Characteristics
I	White; very fair; red or blond hair; blue eyes; freckles	Always burns, never tans
II	White; fair; red or blond hair; blue, hazel or green eyes	Usually burns, tans with difficulty
III	Cream white; fair with any eye or hair color, very common	Sometimes mild burn, gradually tans
IV	Brown; typical Mediterranean caucasian skin	Rarely burns, tans with ease
V	Dark brown; mid-eastern skin types	Very rarely burns, tans very easily
VI	Black	Never burns, tans very easily

include explanation of the preoperative course, procedure, postoperative course, healing time, anticipated results, and potential risks. The specific risk of postinflammatory hyperpigmentation for Fitzpatrick skin types III to V and pre-peel use of 4–8% hydroquinone to reduce the incidence should be discussed.

Use peels with caution in those with a previous history of radiation, as they are at risk of delayed healing and peel breakdown. Regeneration occurs from pilosebaceous units and so the presence of hair follicles is suggestive of sufficient health. Patients with melasma must use hydroquinone, retinoic acid, and sunscreen pre- and post-treatment.

■ PEEL SELECTION CONSIDERATIONS

Peels can be categorized by depth (*superficial, medium, and deep*).

Superficial peels create a youthful look with a target depth of stratum corneum.

- Useful for minor early wrinkles and mild photodamaged skin
- Not useful for dermal pathologies (i.e. wrinkles and furrows)
- Typically takes 1–4 days to heal

Table 2: Glogau scale.

Group I (mild)	Group II (moderate)	Group III (advanced)	Group IV (severe)
Little wrinkling or scarring	Early wrinkling; mild scarring	Persistent wrinkling or moderate acne scarring	Wrinkling: Photoaging, gravitational and dynamic
No keratoses	Sallow color with early actinic keratoses	Discoloration with telangiectasias and actinic keratosis	Actinic keratoses with/without skin cancer or acne scars
28–35 years	35–50 years	50–65 years	60–75 years

Box 1: Contraindications/risk factors (Brody's contraindications).

Relative:
- Darker skin type (Fitzpatrick IV, V, and VI)
- Keloid formation by history
- History of herpes infections
- Cardiac abnormalities
- History of previous facial irradiation
- Marked quantity of villous hair present
- Unrealistic patient expectations
- Physical inability to perform quality postoperative care
- Telangiectasias
- Anticipation of inadequate photoprotection because of, job, vocation, or recreation

Absolute:
- Significant hepatorenal disease
- Human immunodeficiency virus—positive patient
- Significant immunosuppression (hypogammaglobulinemia)
- Emotional instability or mental illness
- Ehlers-Danlos syndrome
- Scleroderma or collagen vascular disease
- Isotretinoin treatment within the previous 6–12 months

Source: Adapted from Brody HJ, Hailey CW. Medium-depth chemical peeling of the skin: a variation of superficial chemosurgery. J Dermatol Surg Oncol. 1989;12:1268-75.

- Creates a level 1 frost
- Repeated superficial peels does not equal medium to deep peels
- *Examples include:*
  - 10–20% *trichloroacetic acid* (TCA)
  - Jessner's combination of two acids and two alcohols, specifically salicylic acid, lactic acid, resorcinol, and ethanol
  - 40–70% glycolic acid (alpha-hydroxy) peels—must rinse off with water after 2–4 minutes or neutralize with sodium bicarbonate. Useful for melasma.

Medium peels target depth of papillary dermis and are useful for epidermal lesions (i.e. actinic keratoses, resurface photoaged skin, dyschromias, repair mild acne scars, and for blending laser resurfacing and deep peels).
- Typically causes level 2 frost
- Can be used in combination (i.e. use superficial peel such as Jessner's or 70% glycolic acid to treat epidermis and then use 35% TCA peel)

- *Examples include:*
  - 30–50% TCA peels
  - Phenol peel: Application time of 60–90 minutes
  - Can do with or without occlusion. Occlude with 0.5 inches of zinc oxide tape to increase depth of penetration to mid-reticular dermis (risky due to possibility of scarring and pigment changes)
  - 70% glycolic acid peel.

Deep peels extend through papillary dermis into reticular dermis leading to new collagen formation. They are used for moderate-to-severe photodamaged skin.
- Conscious sedation or general anesthesia in addition to local blocks typically needed
- *Four stages of healing:*
  - Inflammation—dusky erythema for 12 hours
  - Coagulation—exudates and crusting. Important to use acetic acid soaks multiple times a day to debride and for antibacterial properties
  - Re-epithelialization—starts day 3 to day 10–14; occlusive topical salves promote faster re-epithelialization and less delayed healing
  - Fibroplasia—lasts 3–4 months, neoangiogenesis and collagen formation.
- *Examples include:*
  - Baker Gordon peel—combination of liquid phenol (88%), croton oil (1%), liquid soap (Hibiclens or septisol), and tap water.
    » Croton oil is responsible for the depth of peel, as it is an epidermolytic agent which increases phenol penetration
    » Soap acts as a surfactant to reduce skin tension and increase penetration
    » Get 15–20 seconds of immediate burning which subsides, then pain returns and lasts 6–8 hours
    » Increase absorption by diluting chemicals with water
    » If exposure to eyes, rinse eyes with mineral oil *not* water
    » More than 1% of croton oil results in hypopigmentation and more than 10 days of healing
    » 50% TCA peel is unpredictable due to increased scarring and complications.

- Hetter's solution: Modified Baker-Gordon Peel
  - » Made by varying concentrations of croton oil and phenol for maximal effects with minimal risk.
- *Specific considerations for phenol*:
  - *Toxicity*: Nephrotoxic and cardiotoxic
    - » Phenol is readily absorbed through the skin
    - » 80% excretion through kidney
    - » Can cause diverse arrhythmias as the myocardium is sensitive to phenol.
  - *Precautions*:
    - » Continuous cardiac monitoring during and until 30 minutes after procedure
    - » Oxygen supplementation
    - » Apply phenol to one subunit of the face at a time every 15 minutes to help decrease the systemic phenol load
    - » Gradually apply the peel to decrease phenol absorption
    - » Assure a sufficient fluid load by infusion of intravenous (IV) fluids preoperatively, during the operation, and postoperatively, to avoid circulatory depression due to toxic phenol levels (typically 1 L preoperative and 1 L intraoperative)
    - » Diurese with 20 mg furosemide 10 minutes prior to the application of phenol for increased renal clearance
    - » Administer 75 mg of IV lidocaine hydrochloride prophylactically before phenol administration to decrease occurrence of cardiac arrhythmias
    - » Abort procedure, if there are any signs of EKG abnormalities.

■ PREOPERATIVE PREPARATION

Goals are to have a thin epidermal barrier, enhance uniform active agent penetration, accelerate healing and reduce postoperative side effects. Preoperative routines also assess patients' compliance and tolerance for the postoperative healing phase. Sunscreen (SPF30 or greater) in every pretreatment. Antiviral medications should be used for those undergoing chemical peel in perioral region. Acyclovir 400 mg 1 day before and up to 14 days after peel inhibits viral replication for an intact epidermal cell.

- *Tretinoin 0.05% for 2 weeks*:
  - Binds to nuclear receptors and alters gene expression with fewer MMPs (i.e. collagenases and gelatinases)
  - Linked with increased collagen in dermis, increased hyaluronic acid, compacted stratum corneum, and less UV-B associated collagen breakdown.
  - Accelerates epidermal regeneration.
- Alpha-hydroxy acid 2–3 weeks pretreatment
- *Hydroquinone*:
  - Inhibits tyrosinase → fewer melanin precursors → less new pigment formation
  - Consider, if at high-risk for hyperpigmentation.

- *Topical vitamin C (ascorbic acid)*:
  - Antioxidant
  - Promotes collagen synthesis.
- *Azelaic acid, kojic acid*:
  - Bleaching agent
  - Useful in setting of acne.
- *Others*: Lactic acid, salicylic acid, retinol and glycolic acid.

■ OPERATIVE SET-UP

Preparation

- Degrease (alcohol, acetone, and/or Jessner's solution)
- Antibacterial (if required—chlorhexidine gluconate)
- Topical anesthetics (if required)
  - 20% benzocaine, 6% lidocaine, and 4% tetracaine
  - Local nerve blocks (supraorbital, infraorbital, auriculotemporal, and mental).
- Pain and swelling management
  - Aspirin prior to peels and for first 24 hours
  - Diazepam (5–10 mg PO) for full face peels.
- Keep saline and bicarbonate available to help neutralize TCA or glycolic acid peels; should have mineral oil available for phenol based peels.

Apply peel in the order, forehead to cheeks, nose to chin and eyelids last. Protect sensitive areas of the face (e.g. lips and nasal vestibule) with petrolatum.

There are different levels of frosting based on type of peel used. These are considered the endpoints for the peel (Fig. 1).

- *Level 1*: Erythema with streaky white frost

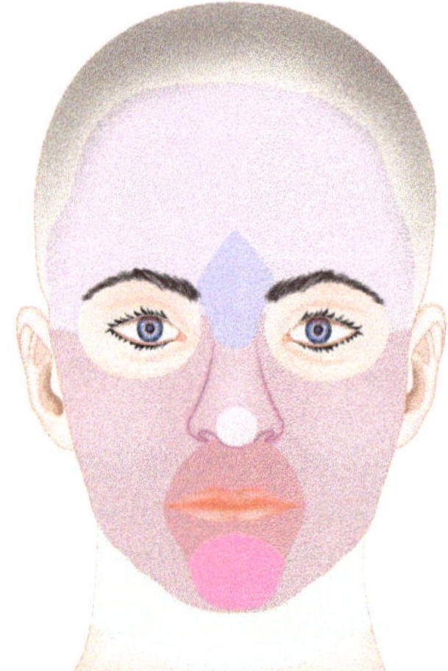

Fig. 1: The schematic shows the difference of skin reactivity to the coaching with trichloroacetic acid (TCA). The darker the area, the higher the number of coats to be applied at the same concentration to achieve the same level of frosting.

Source: Tung RC, Rubin MG. Chemical Peels. Philadelphia: Elsevier/Saunders; 2011.

- *Level 2*: White with erythema seen through
- *Level 3*: Enamel white without erythema; indicative of dermal penetration.

■ POSTOPERATIVE MANAGEMENT

Postoperative management will vary depending on peel depth, but in general acetic acid soak at least six times a day. The area should be kept moist with ointment until re-epithelialization is complete. Advise patients not to pick at the area. Monitor for signs of active herpetic outbreak.

■ COMPLICATIONS

- *Intraoperative*: Incorrect peel medication or solution misplacement
- *Prolonged post-peel erythema (PPPE)*:
  - Usually presents as pain, prolonged erythema, pruritus, burning and/or textural changes in the absence of herpetic vesicles
  - Practitioner should be knowledgeable regarding the expected length of erythema which is dependent on the depth of peel: superficial peels = 15–30 days; medium = 60 days; deep = 90 days
  - *Intrinsic factors* include: Patient sensitivity to peeling agent, preexisting clinical disorder (e.g. rosacea, SLE, eczema, and atopy), pre-existing subclinical disorder (e.g. childhood eczema), contact dermatitis (allergic or irritant) or history of tape allergy
  - *Extrinsic factors* include: Skin pretreatment (retin-A and glycolic acid), peeling technique (aggressive preparation and application technique), and aggressive chemical injury
  - It can result in postinflammatory hyperpigmentation, textural changes, and scarring
  - Location (based on a study of 236 Baker-Gordon peels, Maloney et al.), perioral (55%), periorbital (26%), forehead (4%), full face (19%), and unknown (1%).
- *Outcomes*:
  - In a study of 236 Baker-Gordon peels on 196 patients over a 2-year period, 11% developed PPPE (Maloney et al.)
    None of the major risk factors examined statistically associated with the erythema.
- *Treatment*:
  - Avoidance of possible irritants
  - Emollients
  - Bland topical steroids
  - Acetic acid (0.25%) soaks PRN
- Systemic steroids
- Silicone sheeting
- Pulse dye laser

- *Infection*:
  - Prevent by acetic acid soaks for antibacterial properties and debridement sloughing necrotic tissue
  - Bacterial infections caused by staphylococcus, streptococcus, pseudomonas; signs include delayed healing, purulence, odor, ulceration, etc.
  - Fungal infections should be treated with acetic acid soaks and/or oral/topical antifungals
  - Viral
    » Most commonly due to herpes simplex virus that is reactivated
    » Treat with acyclovir or valacyclovir starting 24 hours before the peel and continue until fully epithelialized; prophylactic dose is different than treatment dose.
- *Pigmentary changes*:
  - At risk for higher Fitzpatrick grades
  - Postinflammatory hyperpigmentation
  - Skin bleaching.
- *Delayed healing*: Treatment is based on cause. This could be due to an infection→ debridement or contact or allergic dermatitis → corticosteroids
- Scarring
- Ectropion
- More peeling in areas of pre-peel inflammation.

■ BIBLIOGRAPHY

1. Botta SA, Straith RE, Goodwin HH. Cardiac arrhythmias in phenol face peeling: a suggested protocol for prevention. Aesthetic Plast Surg. 12:115-7.
2. Brody HJ, Hailey CW. Medium-depth chemical peeling of the skin: a variation of superficial chemosurgery. J Dermatol Surg Oncol. 1986;12:1268-75.
3. Flint PW, Haughey BH, Lund V (Eds). Cummings Otolaryngology: Head and Neck Surgery, 6th edition. Philadelphia, PA: Elsevier, Saunders; 2015.
4. Hetter GP. An examination of the phenol-croton oil peel: part IV. Face Peel results with different concentrations of phenol and croton oil. Plast Reconstr Surg. 2000;105:1061-83.
5. Kligman D, Kligman AM. Salicylic acid peels for the treatment of photoaging. Dermatol Surg. 1998;24:325-8.
6. Maloney BP, Millman B, Monheit G, et al. The etiology of prolonged erythema after chemical peel. Dermatol Surg. 1998;24:337-41.
7. Monheit GD. The Jessner's + TCA peel: a medium-depth chemical peel. J Dermatol Surg Oncol. 1989;15:945-50.
8. Neligan PC, Warren RJ, Van Beek AL (Eds). Plastic Surgery, 3rd edition. London , New York: Elsevier Saunders; 2013.
9. Papel Ira D (Ed). Facial Plastic and Reconstructive Surgery, 3rd edition. New York: Thieme; 2009.
10. Robinson JK (Ed). Surgery of the Skin: Procedural Dermatology, 2nd edition. Edinburgh: Mosby Elsevier; 2010.
11. Tung RC, Rubin MG. Chemical Peels. Philadelphia: Elsevier/Saunders; 2011.

12. Usatine R, Pfenninger J, Stulberg D (Eds). Dermatologic and Cosmetic Procedures in Office Practice. Philadelphia, PA: Elsevier/Saunders: 2012.

13. Weiss JS, Ellis CN, Headington JT, et al. Topical tretinoin improves photoaged skin: a double blind vehicle controlled study. JAMA. 1988;259:527-32.

14. Wong BJ, Arnold MG, Boeckmann JO. Facial Plastic and Reconstructive Surgery Study Guide. New York, NY: Springer; 2016.

Multiple Choice Questions

Q 1. **Which of the following is an absolute CONTRAINDICATION to facial chemical peeling?**

A. Fitzpatrick type IV
B. Fitzpatrick type VI
C. History of herpes infection
D. Recent isotretinoin treatment

Ans: D. Recent isotretinoin treatment

Q 2. **Which of the following chemical peeling agents is the MOST commonly used and the MOST versatile?**

A. Baker-Gordon solution
B. Trichloroacetic acid
C. Glycolic acid
D. Retinoic acid

Ans: B. Trichloroacetic acid

Q 3. **Which of the following components is NOT a component in Jessner's Formula?**

A. Ethanol
B. Glycolic acid
C. Lactic acid
D. Resorcinol

Ans: B. Glycolic acid

Q 4. **Which of the following chemical peeling agents has the HIGHEST risk for scarring?**

A. Trichloroacetic acid 35%
B. Trichloroacetic acid 50%
C. Glycolic acid 70%
D. Pure phenol 88%

Ans: B. Trichloroacetic acid 50%

Q 5. **70% of glycolic acid used as a peeling solution will penetrate to which of the following levels?**

A. Entire epidermis
B. Dermis papillar
C. Upper reticular dermis
D. Midreticular dermis

Ans: A. Entire epidermis

Q 6. **Which of the following statements is FALSE regarding the use of trichloroacetic acid as a chemical peeling agent?**

A Has no systemic toxicity
B Depth of peel is predicted by concentration of solution
C Is unstable and therefore must be mixed fresh before each use
D Neutralization is not needed

Ans: C. Is unstable and therefore must be mixed fresh before each use

Q 7. **Which of the following chemical peels is MOST commonly used for the treatment of fine lower eyelid rhytids during the transcutaneous blepharoplasty skin flap techniques?**

A. 35% trichloroacetic acid
B. 89% phenol
C. Baker-Gordon phenol formula
D. Chemical peeling is not indicated

Ans: D. Chemical peeling is not indicated

Q 8. **Which of the following statements regarding the use of Tretinoin (Retin A) is TRUE?**

A. The liquid preparation is the most commonly used in the treatment of photoaging
B. Dryness of the face is a very uncommon side effect of Tretinoin use
C. Tretinoin therapy is a short-term maintenance therapy, no more than 6 months
D. Desquamation will begin approximately 2 weeks after starting the medication

Ans: D. Desquamation will begin approximately 2 weeks after starting the medication

Q 9. **Which of the following treatments for hyperpigmentation occurring after phenol peeling is INCORRECT?**

A. Hydroquinone cream
B. Hydrocortisone cream
C. Use of Sun-block daily
D. Estrogens

Ans: D. Estrogens

Q 10. **In which type of the PHOTOAGING FITZPATRICK CLASSIFICATION is included a 55-year-old woman who rarely burns, tans profusely and has a brown skin color?**

A. Type II
B. Type III
C. Type IV
D. Type V

Ans: D. Type V

Q 11. **Which of the following chemical peelings is the one MOST LIKELY to produce hypopigmentation changes?**

A. Trichloroacetic acid (TCA) 10%
B. Trichloroacetic acid (TCA) 35%
C. Phenol (Baker-Gordon solution)
D. Glycolic acid 40%

Ans: C. Phenol (Baker-Gordon solution)

Q 12. **Which of the following complications is MOST commonly noted in chemical peeling?**

A. Infection
B. Milia
C. Pigmentary changes
D. Cardiac arrhythmias

Ans: C. Pigmentary changes

Q 13. **Which of the following is of LEAST importance in preoperative evaluation for phenol peeling?**

A. Cardiac status
B. Hepatic status
C. Respiratory status
D. Renal status

Ans: C. Respiratory status

Q 14. Which of the following statements is FALSE regarding chemical peeling in conjunction with rhytidectomy?

A. The combination of chemical peeling and deep-plane rhytidectomy is safe

B. Trichloroacetic acid is the preferred chemical peeling agent for use in combination with rhytidectomy

C. In areas that have not been undermined, chemical peeling can be done in conjunction with rhytidectomy

D. Chemical peeling after rhytidectomy with a long skin flap can be done simultaneously using a superficial peeling agent

Ans: D. Chemical peeling after rhytidectomy with a long skin flap can be done simultaneously using a superficial peeling agent

Q 15. In of the following categories of PHOTOAGING is a 53-year-old woman included who has Glogau Type III periorbital, perioral, forehead and cheek rhytids?

A. Early photoaging with wrinkles in motion

B. Advanced photoaging with wrinkles present at rest

C. Severe photoaging with only wrinkles visible

D. Early photoaging with no wrinkles

Ans: B. Advanced photoaging with wrinkles present at rest

Q 16. Which following is the MOST USEFUL in the treatment of ABSOLUTE hypopigmentation after chemical peeling?

A. Hydroquinone cream

B. Hydrocortisone cream

C. Use of Sunblock daily

D. Camouflage cosmetics

Ans: D. Camouflage cosmetics

Q 17. Which of the following statements regarding the effects of chemical peeling is FALSE?

A. Erythema is not a complication but an expected result lasting for approximately 15 days

B. Prolonged erythema may be treated with topical steroids

C. The areas with a lesser tendency for scarring are the zygomatic arch, the jawline and the chin

D. Hyperpigmentation can be treated with hydroquinone

Ans: C. The areas with a lesser tendency for scarring are the zygomatic arch, the jawline and the chin

Q 18. Mineral oil is BEST used to neutralize chemical peeling with:

A. Trichloroacetic acid (TCA)

B. Baker-Gordon phenol

C. Salicylic acid

D. Jessner's solution

Ans: B. Baker-Gordon phenol

Q 19. From which of the following foods is GLYCOLIC ACID extracted?

A. Sugar cane

B. Sour milk

C. Grapes

D. Lemons

Ans: A. Sugar cane

Q 20. Brown skin that rarely burns and tans more than average is classified as:

A. Fitzpatrick's type II

B. Fitzpatrick's type III

C. Fitzpatrick's type IV

D. Fitzpatrick's type V

Ans: C. Fitzpatrick's type IV

Q 21. The glycolic acid peel is BEST neutralized with:

A. Mineral oil

B. Normal saline

C. Ringer's lactate

D. Diluted sodium bicarbonate

Ans: D. Diluted sodium bicarbonate

Q 22. To which of the following facial subunits is the Baker-Gordon solution is applied FIRST?

A. Forehead

B. Perioral

C. Cheeks

D. Nose

Ans: A. Forehead

Q 23. After phenol chemical face peeling, re-epithelization usually takes:

A. 5 days

B. 10 days

C. 21 days

D. 30 days

Ans: B. 10 days

Q 24. Phenol peeling is NOT recommended in which of the following areas?

A. Neck

B. Forehead

C. Perioral

D. Nose

Ans: A. Neck

Q 25. Which of the following medications is NOT beneficial in the treatment of iatrogenic hyperpigmentation?

A. Tetracycline

B. Hydroquinone

C. Azelaic acid

D. Kojic acid

Ans: A. Tetracycline

Q 26. Which of the following statements is TRUE about hypopigmentation in resurfacing or peeling procedures?

A. Usually resolves with hydroquinone 4% cream

B. Usually seen in the first 2 weeks post-resurfacing or post-peeling

C. It is most likely temporary

D. It is usually permanent

Ans: D. It is usually permanent

Q 27. Which of the following regarding the Baker-Gordon chemical peeling formula is INCORRECT?

A. Phenol 88%, 3 mL

B. Croton oil, 3 drops

C. Septisol, 8 drops

D. Distilled water, 8 mL

Ans: D. Distilled water, 8 mL

Q 28. Which of the following statements about toxicity in chemical face peeling is FALSE?

A. Phenol absorption and toxicity is directly proportional to the concentration of the solution

B. Phenol is cardiotoxic, hepatotoxic and nephrotoxic

C. Phenol absorption and toxicity is directly proportional to the total area of skin treated

D. Phenol toxicity is directly proportional to the concentration of free phenol in the blood and tissues

Ans: A. Phenol absorption and toxicity is directly proportional to the concentration of the solution

Q 29. Which of the following facial areas is MOST COMMONLY scarred after chemical peeling?

A. The forehead

B. The periorbital area

C. The nose

D. The cheek

Ans: C. The nose

Q 30. Which of the following facial esthetic units is done LAST in deep chemical peeling?

A. Cheeks

B. Perioral

C. Nose

D. Periorbital

Ans: D. Periorbital

Q 31. Which of the following Fitzpatrick's Sun-reactive skin type is classified a 40-year-old female patient, who usually burns, and tans with difficulty?

A. I

B. II

C. III

D. IV

Ans: B. II

Q 32. Which of the following complications is THE LEAST in frequency to occur using 35% trichloroacetic acid (TCA) peeling agent?

A. Hypopigmentation

B. Hyperpigmentation

C. Scarring

D. Lines of demarcation between peeled and nonpeeled areas

Ans: C. Scarring

Q 33. The use of retinoid treatments for the face, such as a isotretinoin (accutane), will induce atrophy of the:

A. Keratinocytes cells

B. Sebaceous glands

C. Hair follicles

D. Melanocytes cells

Ans: B. Sebaceous glands

Q 34. Which of the following statements about the use of trichloroacetic acid with concentration for medium depth peeling is TRUE?

A. Patients will require infiltration with local anesthesia and IV sedation

B. The peeling agent will penetrate into the upper reticular dermis

C. The application of the peeling agent will produce severe redness

D. The peeling process for a full-face treatment usually lasts 10 days

Ans: D. The peeling process for a full-face treatment usually lasts 10 days

Q 35. Which of the following components of chemical peeling agents is a SURFACTANT which allows even penetration?

A. Septisol liquid soap

B. Croton oil

C. Lactic acid

D. Resorcinol

Ans: A. Septisol liquid soap

Q 36. What is the mechanism of action of Jessner's Solution?

A. Protein precipitation

B. Keratolysis

C. Keratinocyte discohesion

D. Epidermolysis

Ans: B. Keratolysis

Q 37. Which of the following are NOT used to limit phenol toxicity?

A. IV hydration prior to and during the procedure

B. Limit use of volatile anesthetics

C. Application to each unit and waiting 15 minutes in between

D. Cardiac monitoring during procedure

Ans: B. Limit use of volatile anesthetics

Chapter 20

Skin Resurfacing: Lasers

Kaete A Archer

◾ INTRODUCTION

- There are many causes of facial aging including photoaging and chronologic aging.
- Skin resurfacing is possible with chemical peels, lasers and dermabrasion
  - Dermabrasion less popular due to excessive intraoperative bleeding that can obscure the field resulting in imprecise tissue removal and cosmetic outcomes.
- The general mechanism of resurfacing is to cause dermal collagen reorganization and new collagen deposition by thermal and nonthermal mechanisms
  - Three levels of skin resurfacing:
    » Superficial (epidermis only)
    » Medium (papillary dermis/superficial reticular dermis)
    » Deep (reticular dermis).
  - Difference between ablative and nonablative procedures:
    » Ablative procedures include damage to the surface of the epidermis. Nonablative procedures do not damage the surface of the epidermis.

◾ OVERVIEW OF FACIAL AGING

- *Chronological aging*:
  - Disorganized collagen, thin epidermis, flat dermal-epidermal junction, decreased fibroblasts and collagen
  - Fine rhytids (facial mimetic)
  - Deep rhytids.
- *Photoaging*:
  - Increased or decreased thickness of epidermis, accumulation of elastin fibrils below the dermal-epidermal junction (solar elastosis), increased vascularity, hypercellular dermis.

◾ PREPROCEDURE EVALUATION

- *History*:
  - Main points to address in the preoperative consultation:
    » Important to assess Fitzpatrick phototype and Glogau class of aging
    » Past medical history
    » History of cold sores, herpes simplex viral outbreaks
    » Medication use, history of Accutane use
    » Assess contraindications to laser resurfacing.
  - Contraindications: Contraindications of laser skin resurfacing are described in Table 1.
- *Physical examination*:
  - Ideal patient for resurfacing has a fair complexion (skin phenotype I and II) with lesions amenable to laser treatment and realistic expectations regarding what the surgery can accomplish and what the recovery period will entail.
  - Glogau classification of photoaging (Table 2).
  - Fitzpatrick skin phototype scale (Table 3).

◾ LASERS

- *Method of action*:
  - LASER: Light amplification by stimulated emission of radiation
  - Three most common chromophores and where they are found:
    » Hemoglobin: Dermis
    » Melanin: Epidermis
    » Water: Epidermis and dermis.

Table 1: Contraindications of laser skin resurfacing.

Relative	Absolute
Perpetual UV light exposure	Concurrent isotretinoin use or use within 12–24 months
Collagen vascular or immune disorder	Concurrent bacterial or viral (HSV) infection
Prior lower blepharoplasty (for infraorbital treatment)	Ectropion (for infraorbital treatment)
Keloid or hypertrophic scar tendency	Unrealistic expectations
Koebnerization phenomenon cutaneous diseases	
Prior radiation therapy leading to a loss of adnexal structures	
Extensive fibrosis resulting from prior cosmetic treatments	

(HSV: Herpes simplex virus)

Table 2: Glogau classification of photoaging. Glogau et al. Matarasso.

Type	Photoaging	Age	Makeup
I	Mild pigmentary changes No keratosis Minimal wrinkles	20s–30s	Minimal or no makeup
II	Early senile lentigines visible Keratosis palpable but not visible Parallel smile lines beginning to appear	Late 30s–40s	Usually wears some foundation
III	Obvious dyschromia Telangiectasias Visible keratoses Wrinkles even when not moving	50s +	Wears heavy foundation
IV	Yellow-gray skin color Prior skin malignancies Wrinkled throughout No normal skin	60s–70s	Cannot wear makeup—cracks or cakes

Table 3: Fitzpatrick skin phototype scale

Skin type	Skin color	Tanning response
I	White	Always burns, never tans
II	White	Usually burns, tans with difficulty
III	White	Sometimes mild burn, tan average
IV	Brown	Rarely burns, tans with ease
V	Dark brown	Very rarely burns, tans very easily
VI	Black	No burn, tan very easily

- Laser parameters and which ones can be adjusted by the clinician:
  » Fluence: Adjustable
  » Pulse width: Adjustable
  » Cooling temperature: Adjustable
  » Wavelength: Nonadjustable.
- Main indications:
  » Erbium:YAG (Er:YAG)—Mild photodamage, mild atrophic scars, mild dyspigmentation, refractory melasma, various epidermal and dermal lesions
  » CO_2: Moderate-to-severe photodamage, moderate atrophic scars, diffuse lentigines, mild dermatochalasis, various epidermal and dermal lesions
- *Ablative lasers*:
  - CO_2:
    » Wavelength: 106,00 nm
    » Chromophore: Water
    » Depth: 20–30 µm; reticular dermis
    » Downtime: 7–14 days
    » Indications: Moderate-to-severe photodamage, moderate atrophic scars, diffuse lentigines, mild dermatochalasis, various epidermal and dermal lesions.
  - Fractionated CO_2:
    » Wavelength: 106,000 nm

  » Chromophore: Water
  » Depth: 20–30 µm, reticular dermis
  » Downtime: 7–10 days
  » Indications: Moderate-to-severe photodamage, moderate atrophic scars, diffuse lentigines, mild dermatochalasis, various epidermal and dermal lesions.
- Er: YAG:
  » Wavelength: 2,940 nm
  » Chromophore: Water; Erbium laser light is absorbed 12-18X more efficiently by cutaneous tissue than CO_2 laser light.
  » Depth: 2–5 µm, papillary dermis
  » Downtime: 5–7 days
  » Indications: Mild photodamage, mild atrophic scars, mild dyspigmentation, refractory melisma, various epidermal and dermal lesions.
- *Nonablative lasers* (for each, briefly mention wavelength, chromophore, depth, downtime, main indications, main complications).
  - Fractional resurfacing
  - Neodymium-doped yttrium aluminum garnet (Nd:YAG).
    » Wavelength: 1,064 nm
    » Chromophore: Nonselective heat into dermis with minimal affinity for melanin. Short pulse duration in the nanosecond range is thought to confine injury to the intended target and minimize heat diffusion
    » Depth: Dermis
    » Downtime: None
    » Indications: Irregular skin texture and mild rhytids.

OTHER NONABLATIVE RESURFACING MODALITIES

- *Intense-pulsed light (IPL)*:
  - Define: Intense-pulsed light—IPLs use flashlamps, computer-controlled power supplies, and bandpass filters to generate light pulses of prescribed duration, intensity, and spectral distribution
  - Commercial example: Broadband light, Sciton, Palo Alto, CA
  - Wavelength: Based on light filter used. Common wavelengths are 560 nm filter for reds and 515 nm filter for browns
  - Target: Pigment (browns) and telangiectasia/erythema (reds)
  - Indications: Pigment (browns) and telangiectasia/erythema (reds)
  - Depth: Epidermis and dermis
  - Downtime: None
  - Complications: Thermal damage.
- *Light-emitting diode (LED) phototherapy*:
  - Define: Light-emitting diode (LED) photomodulation is a nonthermal technology used to modulate cellular

activity with light rather than evoke thermal wound healing mechanisms.

- Commercial example: Gentlewaves yellow light 590 nm LED photomodulation unit (Light Bio Science, Virginia Beach, VA, USA)
- Target cellular acting (mitochondria): Downregulation of matrix metalloproteinases (MMPs) upregulation of collagen type I synthesis by fibroblasts increase dermal collagen
- Indications: Rhytids, irregular skin texture, pigmented and vascular signs of photoaging (superficial dyspigmentation in dermis and epidermis), dermal telangiectasia improvement pigmented and vascular signs of:
  » Depth: Epidermis and dermis
  » Downtime: None
  » Complications: No improvement
- *Q-switched lasers*:
  - Define: Nanosecond pulse durations is of three types: (1) ruby, (2) Nd:YAG and (3) alexandrite
  - Commercial example: C6 Q-switched Nd:YAG laser (HOYA Con Bio, Fremont, CA)
  - Wavelength:
    » Ruby 694 μm: Black, blue, green, and purple
    » Nd:YAG 1, 064 nm: Black
    » Nd:YAG 532 nm: Red and orange
    » Alexandrite 755 nm: Blue, green and black.
  - Target: Exogenous tattoo pigment
  - Indications: tattoo removal
    » Best for blue, black: Ruby
    » Best for red brown, brown and orange: Nd:YAG
    » Best for blue and green: Alexandrite
    » Best for purple, and violet: Q-switched 694-nm ruby laser.
  - Depth: Mid-dermis
  - Downtime: Approximately 7 days of crusting, scabbing and wound care
  - *Complications*:
    » Ruby: Highest clearance but increased risk hypopigmentation since 694 nm is absorbed by melanin, textural change and scarring
    » Benstein tattoo Nd:YAG: Best for dark skin because decreased absorption by melanin compared to ruby and alexandrite, and textural changes
    » Alexandrite: Transient hypopigmentation and textural changes
    » Contact dermatitis.
- *Radiofrequency devices*:
  - Define: Resistance of tissue to electrons immediate collagen contraction and long-term collagen remodeling. Resistance of tissue to the movement of electron with KF field converts electrical element to thermal energy (heat).
  - Commercial example: Monopolar radiofrequency (Therma-Cool TC; Thermage, Haywood, CA, USA)

- Target: Water
- Indications: Tighten and contour nonsurgically mild-to-moderate laxity of the skin without significant underlying structural ptosis, improve skin texture and soften fine lines. Best candidates are youthful with minimal facial sagging.
- Depth: 1–2 mm, reticular dermis
- Downtime: None
- Complications: No tightening effect, pain, and thermal damage to overlying skin.

■ SUMMARY TABLES

- *Laser summary*: Laser summary described in Table 3.
- *Summary for condition and procedure*: The condition and procedure of laser described in Table 4.

Table 3: Laser summary.

Laser	Chromophore	Wavelength (nm)
Argon	Oxyhemoglobin	485
KTP	Oxyhemoglobin/melanin	532
PDL	Oxyhemoglobin	585
Ruby	Melanin, black, blue, green, purple violet	694
Alexandrite	Melanin, black, blue, green	755
Nd:YAG	Pigment/oxyhemoglobin Red, red brown, orange, black, blue, oxyhemoglobin	1,064
Ho:YAG	Water	2,100
Er:YAG	Water	2,940
CO_2	Water	10,600

(Nd:YAG: Neodymium-doped yttrium aluminium garnet; Er:YAG: Erbium:YAG; Ho:YAG: Holmium:YAG; PDL: Pulsed dye laser; KTP: Potassium-titanyl-potassium

Table 4: Condition and procedure of laser.

Condition	Most appropriate procedure
Accumulated fat in the lower face, submentum, and neck	Radiofrequency
Actinic damage and other epidermal/dermal lesions	Erbium, CO_2
Mild atrophic scars	Erbium
Moderate atrophic scars	CO_2
Hypertrophic scars and keloids	585nm PDL or CO_2 + 585 nm PDL
Tattoo removal	Q-switched laser (nanosecond pulses)
Mild to moderate dermatochalasis, facial lines, rhytidosis, photodamage (Glogau I-II)	Erbium
Moderate to severe dermatochalasis, facial lines, rhytidosis, photodamage (Glogau III-IV)	CO_2
Melasma and other dyschromias	IPL, Erbium
Rhinophyma	Erbium, CO_2

(PDL: Pulsed dye laser; IPL: Intense-pulsed light)

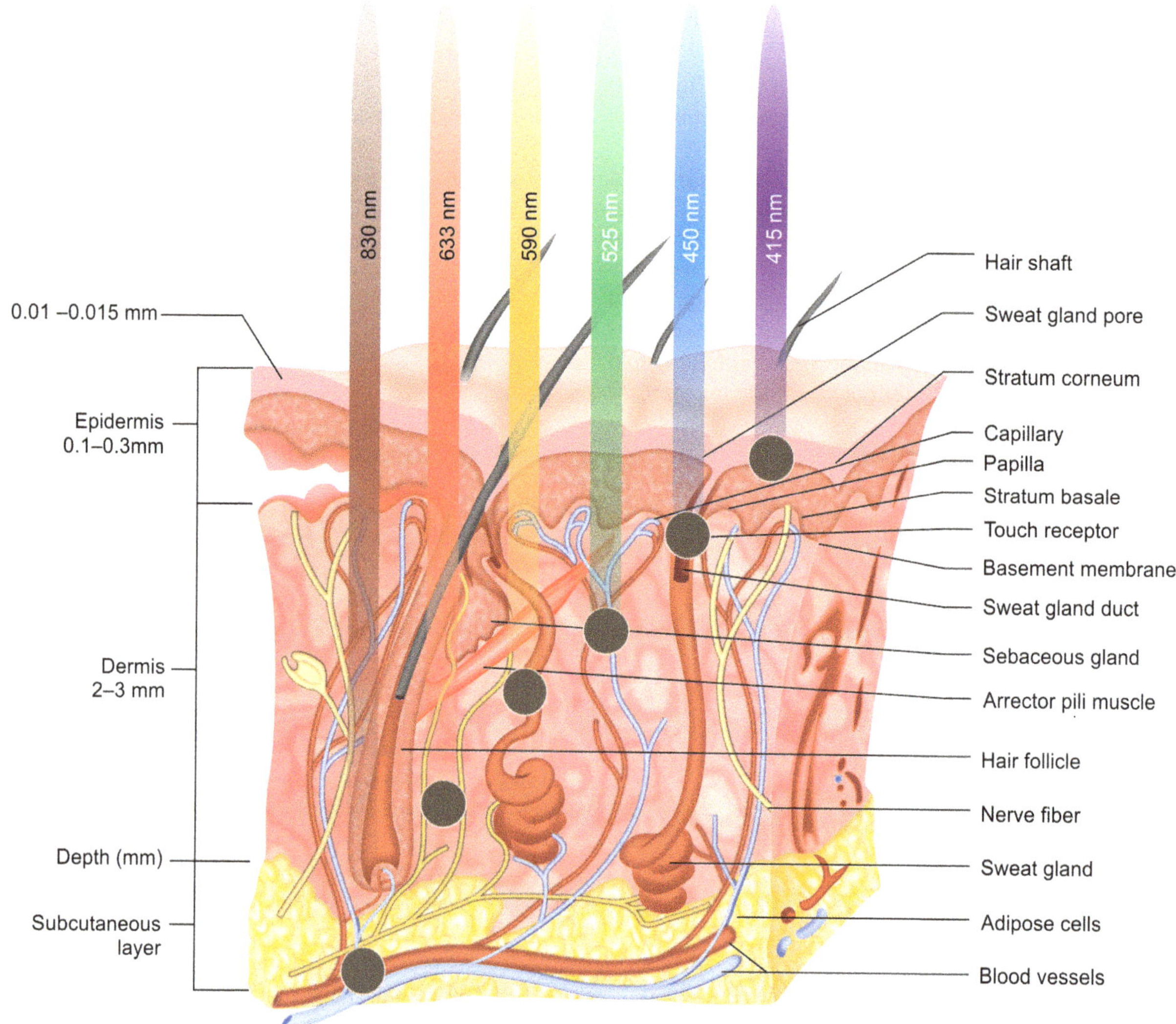

Fig. 1: Interaction of wavelengths with the skin.

POSTPROCEDURE CARE AND COMPLICATIONS

- *Laser skin resurfacing postprocedure care*:
  - Moist wound environment.
- *Laser skin resurfacing complications*:
  - Mild: Prolonged erythema, crusting, edema, allergic/irritant dermatitis, milia, acne exacerbation
  - Moderate: Transient hyperpigmentation, delayed hypopigmentation, localized bacterial/fungal infection, regional herpes simplex viral reaction
  - Severe: Hypertrophic scarring, ectropion, and disseminated infection.

BIBLIOGRAPHY

1. Alster TS, Lupton JR. Treatment of complications of laser skin resurfacing. Arch Facial Plast Surg. 2000;2:279-84.
2. Alster TS. Cutaneous resurfacing with CO_2 and erbium:YAG lasers: preoperative, intraoperative and postoperative considerations. Plast Reconstr Surg. 1999;103:619-32.
3. Alster TS. Laser treatment of hypertrophic scars, keloids and striae. Dermatol Clin. 1997;15:419-29.
4. Atiyeh BS, Dibo SA. Nonsurgical nonablative treatment of aging skin: radiofrequency technologies between aggressive marketing and evidence-based efficacy. Aesthetic Plast Surg. 2009;33:283-94.
5. Bernstein EF. Laser treatment of tattoos. Clin Dermatol. 2006;24:43-55.

6. Bloom BS, Brauer JA, Geronemus RG. Ablative fractional resurfacing in topical drug delivery: an update and outlook. Dermatol Surg. 2013;39:839-48.

7. Bramhall J. Regional anesthesia for aesthetic surgery. Semin Cutan Med Surg. 2002;21:3-26.

8. Duke D, Grevelink JM. Care before and after laser skin resurfacing. A survey and review of the literature. Dermatol Surg. 1998;24:201-6.

9. Fife DJ, Fitzpatrick RE, Zachary CB. Complications of fractional CO_2 laser resurfacing: four cases. Lasers Surg Med. 2009;41:177-84.

10. Gentile RD. (2009). Laser-assisted neck-lift: high-tech contouring and tightening. Facial Plast Surg. 2011;27:331-45.

11. Gilbert DJ. Incorporating photodynamic therapy into a medical and cosmetic dermatology practice. Dermatol Clin. 2007;25:111-8.

12. Goldman MP. CO_2 laser resurfacing of the face and neck. Facial Plast Surg Clin North Am. 2001;9:283-90.

13. Goon PK, Dalal M, Peart FC. The gold standard for decortication of rhinophyma:combined erbium-YAG/CO_2 Laser. Aesthetic Plast Surg. 2004;28:456-60.

14. Grekin RC. Laser resurfacing of the face: is there just one laser? Facial Plast Surg Clin North Am. 2000;8:153-62.

15. Holcomb JD, Turk J, Baek SJ, et al. Laser-assisted facial contouring using a thermally confined 1444-nm Nd-YAG laser: a new paradigm for facial sculpting and rejuvenation. Facial Plast Surg. 2011;27:315-30.

16. Holcomb JD. Laser assisted facelift. Facial Plast Surg. 2014;30:405-12.

17. Holcomb JD. Versatility of erbium YAG laser: from fractional skin rejuvenation to full-field skin resurfacing. Facial Plast Clin North Am. 2011;19:261-73.

18. Massaki AB, Fabi SG, Fitzpatrick R. Repigmentation of hypopigmented scars using an erbium-doped 1.550-nm fractionated laser and topical bimatoprost. Dermatol Surg. 2012;38:995-1001.

19. McMenamin P. Laser face-lifts: a new paradigm in face-lift surgery. Facial Plast Surg. 2011;27:299-307.

20. Nouri K, Rivas MP, Bouzari N, et al. Nonablative lasers. J Cosmet Dermatol. 2006;5:107-14.

21. Rohrich RJ, Gyimesi IM, Clark P, et al. CO_2 laser safety considerations in facial skin resurfacing. Plast Reconstr Surg. 1997;100:1285-90.

22. Ross EV. Laser versus intense pulsed light: competing technologies in dermatology. Lasers Surg Med. 2006;38:261-72.

23. Rostan EF, Fitzpatrick RE, Goldman MP. Laser resurfacing with a long pulse erbium:YAG laser compared to the 950 ms pulsed CO_2 laser. Lasers Surg Med. 2001;29:136-41.

24. Rostan EF. Laser treatment of photodamaged skin. Fac Plast Surg. 2005;21:99-109.

25. Schwartz RJ, Burns AJ, Rohrich RJ, et al. Long-term assessment of CO_2 facial laser resurfacing: aesthetic results and complications. Plast Reconstr Surg. 1999;103:592-601.

26. Weinstein C, Pozner J, Scheflan M. (2001). Combined erbium:YAG laser resurfacing and face lifting. Plast Reconstr Surg. 2001;107:586-92.

27. Weiss RA, McDaniel DH, Geronemus RG, et al. Clinical experience with light-emitting diode (LED) photomodulation. Dermatol Surg. 2007;31:1199-205.

28. Youn JL, Holcomb JD. Ablation efficiency and relative thermal confinement measurements using wavelengths 1,064, 1,320 and 1,444 nm for laser-assisted lipolysis. Lasers Med Sci. 2013;28:519-27.

Multiple Choice Questions

Q 1. Using the CO_2 laser resurfacing technique, the treated area changes from pink to a yellow chamois color. Which LEVEL of tissue penetration has the laser reached?

A. Epidermis   B. Upper reticular dermis
C. Deep reticular dermis   D. Subcutaneous tissue

Ans: B. Upper reticular dermis

Q 2. Which of the following statements regarding CO_2 laser facial resurfacing is TRUE?

A. Neck skin is well-suited for CO_2 laser resurfacing.
B. Deep "ice-pick" acne responds very well to CO_2 laser
C. The initial layer of desiccated white debris has to be left in
D. The reticular dermis level is recognized by its "yellow chamois cloth" appearance

Ans: D. The reticular dermis level is recognized by its "yellow chamois cloth" appearance

Q 3. Which of the following side effects is MOST commonly seen in laser skin resurfacing?

A. Erythema   B. Edema
C. Pruritus   D. Hypopigmentation

Ans: A. Erythema

Q 4. Which of the following represents THE ONSET of a herpes simplex infection after a carbon laser skin resurfacing procedure?

A. Pain   B. Edema
C. Pruritus   D. Vesicles

Ans: A. Pain

Q 5. Which of the following statements comparing the erbium laser to the CO_2 laser in skin resurfacing is FALSE?

A. Erbium laser energy absorption remains very superficial
B. The depth of vaporization after one pass is 25 μm
C. Erbium laser has less postoperative erythema and pigmentation problems
D. Erbium laser is useful in treating deeper wrinkles and severe photodamage

Ans: D. Erbium laser is useful in treating deeper wrinkles and severe photodamage

Q 6. Which of the following infections is the MOST common in the postoperative period after laser skin resurfacing?

A. Herpes simplex virus   B. Staphylococcus aureus
C. Pseudomonas aeruginosa   D. Candida

Ans: A. Herpes simplex virus

Q 7. 48 hours after Er:YAG laser resurfacing a diffuse eruption with small papules developed. Cultures were negative. A potassium hydroxide examination was negative for yeast. A Tzanck smear is positive. The BEST treatment in this particular patient is:

A. Topical corticosteroids
B. Acyclovir PO
C. Topical hydroquinone
D. Ciprofloxacin PO

Ans: B. Acyclovir PO

Q 8. Which of the following facial areas is more prone to delayed healing and scarring after the use of laser resurfacing or chemical peeling techniques?

A. Forehead
B. Neck
C. Temple
D. Cheek

Ans: B. Neck

Q 9. Which of the following lasers achieves the GREATEST depth of penetration?

A. CO_2
B. Er:YAG
C. Nd:YAG
D. Pulsed dye

Ans: C. Nd:YAG

Q 10. Which of the following complications is MOST COMMONLY seen in bipolar radiofrequency resurfacing?

A. Hyperpigmentation
B. Hypopigmentation
C. Herpetic infections
D. Bacterial infections

Ans: A. Hyperpigmentation

Q 11. Which of following statements related to the use of the laser resurfacing is TRUE?

A. Hyperpigmentation does not have an effective treatment
B. Erbium laser resurfacing has more risk of hypopigmentation than CO_2 laser resurfacing
C. True hypopigmentation occurs approximately 10 months after initial treatment
D. Itching and blister formation are the initial presentations of herpetic viral infections

Ans: C. True hypopigmentation occurs approximately 10 months after initial treatment

Q 12. Which of the following will benefit LEAST by laser skin resurfacing?

A. Dynamic rhytids
B. Actinic keratosis
C. Dyschromias
D. Acne

Ans: A. Dynamic rhytids

Q 13. Which of the following lasers is NOT ADEQUATE for the treatment of facial telangiectasias?

A. Long-pulsed alexandrite laser
B. Coper vapor laser
C. Continuous wave yellow dye laser
D. Flashlamp-excited dye (FEDL)

Ans: A. Long-pulsed alexandrite laser.

Q 14. Which of the following anesthesia regimens is adequate in facial Er: YAG laser skin resurfacing?

A. Regional nerve blocks with 0.25% bupivacaine plus 1:200.000 epinephrine
B. Regional nerve blocks with 1% lidocaine plus 1:100.000 epinephrine
C. Regional nerve blocks with 2% lidocaine plus 2:100.000 epinephrine
D. EMLA cream applied 2 hours prior the surgical procedure

Ans: D. EMLA cream applied 2 hours prior the surgical procedure

Q 15. Which of the following statements about bipolar radiofrequency resurfacing is FALSE?

A. Its re-surfacing power is based on a process called coblation
B. The mechanism of resurfacing is basically the same as that used in resurfacing lasers
C. The first pass can separate the epidermal-dermal junction
D. The second pass extends into the papillary dermis

Ans: B. The mechanism of re-surfacing is basically the same as that used in re-surfacing lasers

Q 16. Which of the following is NOT a laser/tissue surface interaction?

A. Absorption
B. Concentration
C. Reflection
D. Scatter

Ans: B. Concentration

Q 17. Which of the following lasers has a visible-wavelength in the electromagnetic spectrum?

A. Argon
B. CO_2
C. Er:YaG
D. Erbium

Ans: A. Argon

Q 18. Which of the following examinations is MOST likely to detect ocular damage after Argon laser?

A. Fluorescein eye drops
B. Direct eye fundus evaluation
C. Corneal and conjunctival under magnification
D. Refraction evaluation

Ans: B. Direct eye fundus evaluation

Q 19. Which of the following lasers is useful to treat facial telangiectasias?

A. Copper vapor
B. CO_2
C. Erbium
D. Ruby

Ans: A. Copper vapor

Q 20. Which of the following statements regarding CO_2 laser resurfacing is FALSE?

A. Topical anesthetic is adequate for a facial CO_2 laser resurfacing

B. Prophylactic antivirals medications for all patients undergoing CO_2 laser resurfacing are mandatory

C. The use of prophylactic antibiotics in CO_2 laser resurfacing in not universally used

D. A typical "yellow chamois" is seen when the laser enters the reticular dermis

Ans: A. Topical anesthetic is adequate for a facial CO_2 laser resurfacing

Q 21. Which of the following laser is considered an ABLATIVE facial laser?

A. Er:YAG laser

B. 532 nm laser

C. 1320 nm Nd:YAG laser

D. Fraxel laser

Ans: A. Er:YAG laser

Q 22. Which of the following lasers is THE BEST or the removal of GREEN tattoo pigments?

A. CO_2

B. Nd:YAG

C. Q-switched ruby

D. Pulse dye laser

Ans: C. Q-switched ruby

Q 23. Which of the following lasers is the one used in the treatment of rhinophyma?

A. Alexandrite

B. CO_2

C. Erbium

D. Ruby

Ans: B. CO_2

Q 24. The FDA has approved radiofrequency in the treatment of which of the following?

A. Telangiectasias

B. Dyschromias

C. Rhytids

D. Hypertrophic scars

Ans: C. Rhytids

Q 25. Which of the following lasers uses a VISIBLE GREEN LIGHT (wavelength 532 nm)?

A. CO_2 laser

B. Nd:YAG laser

C. KTP laser

D. Argon laser

Ans: C. KTP laser

Q 26. What is the ideal relationship between pulse duration and thermal relaxation time?

A. Pulse duration shorter than thermal relaxation time

B. Thermal relaxation time shorter than pulse duration

C. Pulse duration equal to thermal relaxation time

D. Pulse duration twice thermal relaxation time

Ans: A. Pulse duration shorter than thermal relaxation time

Q 27. What is the most abundant chromophore in skin?

A. Hemoglobin

B. Water

C. Melanin

D. None

Ans: B. Water

Q 28. Which Glogau class represents a patient who has obvious dyschromia, telangiectasias, visible keratosis, wrinkles not in motion in her 50s?

A. I

B. II

C. III

D. IV

Ans: C. III

Q 29. Which scar is best for laser resurfacing?

A. Atrophic, shallow

B. Raised

C. Wide

D. Firm

Ans: A. Atrophic, shallow

Q 30. What is an absolute contraindication for cutaneous laser resurfacing?

A. Frequent UV light exposure

B. History of radiation

C. Isotretinoin use in prior 12 months

D. Previous cosmetic facial surgery

Ans: C. Isotretinoin use in prior 12 months

Q 31. Where is tattoo ink located in the skin?

A. Mid dermis

B. Epidermis

C. Superficial dermis

D. Deep dermis

Ans: A. Mid dermis

Q 32. Most common pigment allergy:

A. Red

B. Yellow

C. Blue

D. Green

Ans: A. Red

Q 33. What is the mechanism of action of LED therapy?

A. Thermal damage > collagen remodeling

B. Mitochondrial cytochrome light absorption > increased collagen synthesis

C. Oxygen free radical damage

D. None of the above

Ans: B. Mitochondrial cytochrome light absorption > increased collagen synthesis

Q 34. What is responsibility of laser safety officer?

A. Operating the laser

B. Turning laser to stand by mode

C. Cleaning the laser

D. A and B

Ans: D. A and B

Q 35. What temperature must epidermis reach for tightening to occur?

A. 1–3 deg Celsius

B. 3–5 deg Celsius

C. 5–7 deg Celsius

D. 7–10 deg Celsius

Ans: B. 3–5 deg Celsius

Q 36. Which of the following is the "PRIMARY CHROMO-PHORE" for resurfacing lasers?

A. Water

B. Melanin

C. Melanin

D. Carboxyhemoglobin

Ans: A. Water

Q 37. Which of the following is UNRELATED to laser-tissue interaction?

A. Power density increases proportionally with the diameter (spot size) of the laser system

B. The wavelength is the distance between two successive peaks of the wave

C. The amplitude is the height of the peak and is related to the intensity of the light

D. Frequency, or the period of the light wave, is the amount of the time require for one full wave cycle

Ans: A. Power density increases proportionally with the diameter (spot size) of the laser system

Q 38. Which of the following statements is TRUE about LASER suspension microlaryngoscopy done under general?

A. FIO_2 should not be above of 10%

B. FIO_2 should not be above of 20%

C. FIO_2 should not be above of 30%

D. FIO_2 should not be above of 40%

Ans: D. FIO_2 should not be above of 40%

Q 39. Which of the following techniques is the MOST useful in the treatment of Deep-Pitted Acne Scars located around the oral commissure?

A. CO_2 laser resurfacing

B. Dermabrasion

C. Punch excision with primary closure

D. Chemical peeling

Ans: C. Punch excision with primary closure

Q 40. Which of the following statements about RHINOPHYMA is TRUE?

A. It is more common in female patients

B. It is more common in Asians

C. It represents the fourth stage of evolving rosacea

D. Its major histological findings involve decreased dermal thickening and vascularity

Ans: C. It represents the fourth stage of evolving rosacea

Chapter 21

Hair Restoration

Kirkland N Lozada, Jeffrey Cranford

■ ANATOMY AND PHYSIOLOGY

Follicular unit transplantation (FUT) is based on the concept that hair naturally grows in groupings of 1–4 terminal hair follicles known as a follicular unit. Terminal hair follicles found on the scalp are long, thick, and dark compared to vellus hair follicles, which are short, thin, and cover much of the remainder of the body. The follicular cycle consists of three phases: anagen (growth), catagen (involution), telogen (rest). Each phase has a different duration: anagen, 2–6 years; catagen, 2–3 weeks; and telogen, 3 months. Approximately 90% of scalp hair exists in the anagen phase and up to 100 hairs in telogen phase are shed daily.

■ CAUSES OF ALOPECIA

Scarring Alopecia

Scarring alopecia comprises a spectrum of disorders in which inflammatory mediators affect the upper part of the hair follicle, causing destruction of the stem cell and associated sebaceous gland. Ultimately, scarring and permanent hair loss ensues. During active stages of disease, erythematous, scaly skin may be present at the periphery of lesions and the diagnosis may be confirmed by a punch biopsy. Causes of scarring alopecias include lichen planopilaris, central centrifugal cicatricial alopecia, and systemic processes, such as scleroderma, sarcoidosis, and discoid lupus erythematous. Treatment with hair transplantation must be deferred until there is no evidence of active scalp disease and, even then, caution must be exercised since reactivation of the disease may occur at any time.

Nonscarring Alopecia

Telogen effluvium is characterized by diffuse hair shedding as a result of a synchronized, premature entry of hair follicles into the telogen phase. This is typically prompted by an emotional or physiologic stressor, including fever, childbirth, chronic illness, crash diets, and medication use. Hair loss lags 3 months behind the stressor and generally is fully reversible. *Anagen effluvium* results from the loss of anagen hairs, classically caused by radiation or systemic chemotherapeutics. Rapidly proliferating cells of the hair follicle are affected, resulting in rapid hair loss. Hair typically returns but may differ in texture or color. *Alopecia areata* is an autoimmune disorder that targets hair follicles. Its presentation can vary from sharply demarcated areas of patchy hair loss to diffuse thinning. Characteristic hairs become narrower along the length of the strand, producing an "exclamation point" appearance. Limited success in treatment has been achieved by using topical and intralesional injections of corticosteroids.

Other causes of nonscarring alopecia include thyroid disorders, granulomatous disorders, inflammatory disorders (i.e. seborrheic dermatitis, psoriasis), infectious disorders (i.e. dermatophytes, tinea capitis, and syphilis) and certain drugs [i.e. oral contraceptives, beta blockers, coumadin, selective serotonin reuptake inhibitor (SSRIs), TCAs. *Triangular alopecia* is a rare cause of alopecia, typically presenting in otherwise-healthy children as a triangular-shaped patch of loss that may be complete or be replaced by fine vellum hairs. The compulsive hair pulling of *trichotillomania* results in patchy areas of loss with broken hairs of varying lengths. *Traction alopecia* results from the excessive pulling of hair from hair weaves, braided cornrows, or other means of mechanical stress and can result in permanent hair loss.

Androgenic alopecia (AA) is an androgen-dependent hereditary disorder responsible for the majority of hair loss in men and women. In *male pattern androgenic alopecia* (MPAA) conversion of terminal to vellus hairs occurs as a result of androgen binding to susceptible hair follicles. 5-dihydrotestosterone (DHT) binds to hair follicles with five times the affinity of testosterone and is recognized as being the primary contributor to MPAA. DHT causes hair follicles to miniaturize, decreasing their lifespan and making them finer and shorter. The enzyme responsible for converting free testosterone into DHT is 5α-reductase and is the target of the medication finasteride. Men with MPAA usually have higher levels of 5α-reductase, lower levels

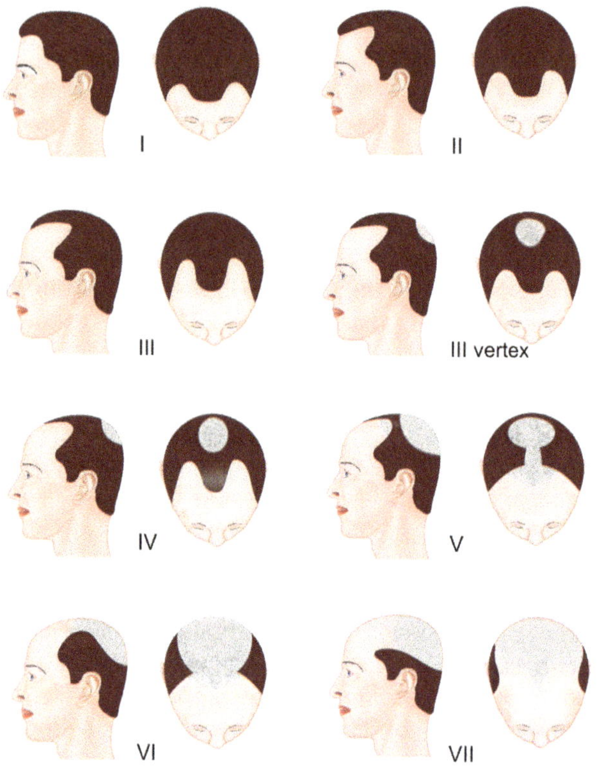

Fig. 1: Norwood classification of male-pattern baldness. Class I: adolescent hairline, rests on upper brow crease. Class II: mature hairline that sits 1.5 cm above the upper brow crease; not considered balding. Class III: deepening of temporal recession; earliest stage of male hair loss. Class III vertex: early hair loss in the vertex. Class IV: further loss in front and vertex but still separated by solid band of hair. Class V: thinning of bridge of hair separating front and vertex. Class VI: complete loss of the connecting bridge of hair. Class VII: extensive loss with remaining hair on sides and rear only.

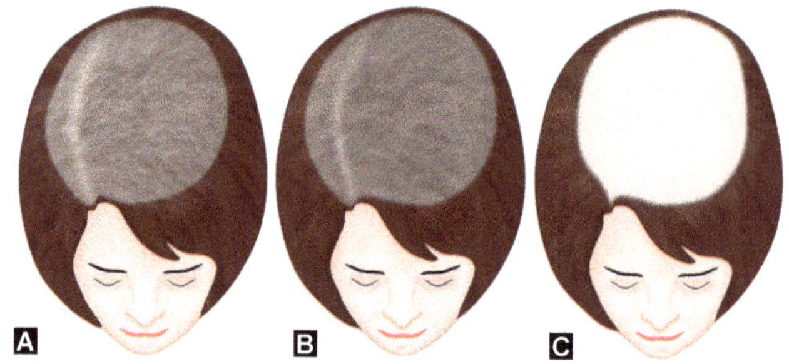

Figs. 2A to C: Ludwig classification for female pattern baldness. (A) Stage I, thinning in the crown but anterior hairline preserved; (B) Stage II, significant widening of the midline part and significant decrease in volume; (C) Stage III, diffuse thinning.

■ PATIENT EVALUATION

A thorough history and physical examination are essential to determine the etiology and treatment of alopecia. In MPAA, a detailed family history gives insight into the future pattern of loss, helping to inform treatment planning. Future hair loss is especially difficult to predict in young patients and results may therefore be met with less satisfaction. Most patients will require multiple surgeries and it is important to assess each patient's motivation and goals. Physical examination should include assessment of hair density and scalp laxity. Additionally, hair color, skin color, and hair texture should be noted, as these factors affect the ultimate appearance of density in implanted regions. In men presenting with alopecia characteristic of MPAA, laboratory testing is not necessary, however, in symptomatic patients a laboratory workup including thyroid function tests and serum iron with ferritin may be performed. Tissue biopsy can be helpful when the etiology is uncertain or to diagnose scarring alopecia, chronic telogen effluvium, and diffuse alopecia areata (AA).

■ TREATMENT

Medical treatment of allopecia consists of the two FDA approved pharmacologic agents for AA: (1) minoxidil and (2) finasteride. *Minoxidil* is a vasodilating calcium channel blocker. Its use for allopecia was discovered when cardiac patients reported increased hair growth while taking minoxidil. Its mechanism of action for hair growth is unknown. Further studies showed about 60% of patients experienced hair growth while taking this drug. It must be used for 4–6 months continuously to show results, which can be marginal and short lived. Discontinuation of the medication results in regression of hair gain over a few months (Saraswat 2007). *Finasteride* inhibits 5α-reductase, which converts testosterone to DHT and is found in the prostate, genitourinary tract, and scalp. Finasteride decreases serum levels of DHT by 70% but clinical results may not be apparent for up to 12 months. Important side

of total testosterone, and higher levels of free (unbound) androgens, including testosterone and DHT Sawaya, 1997. The pattern of clinical hair loss in MPAA is well-defined, occurring first in the frontotemporal region and the vertex. With time, these regions enlarge and coalesce, such that the entire front, top and vertex of the scalp are bald. The distribution of hair loss is commonly described according to the Norwood classification (Fig. 1).

Female pattern androgenic alopecia (FPAA) differs from the classic pattern of MPAA, instead characterized by diffuse central thinning or the "Christmas tree" pattern, where thinning is wider in the frontal scalp. Women typically maintain their anterior hairline and the pathologic role of androgens is less well-understood. FPAA has been classified by Ludwig into three stages: mild, moderate, and severe (Figs. 2A to C). Rarely, women may present with a pattern of loss similar to MPAA and, in such cases, workup for hyperandrogenism must be undertaken.

effects include decreased libido, erectile dysfunction, and ejaculatory dysfunction. The use of both finasteride and minoxidil is beneficial and results in an additive effect because of their different mechanisms of action (Rousso 2014).

When medical management fails to yield adequate results, surgical treatments may be considered. Options include hair transplantation, scalp reduction, scalp flaps, and tissue expanders. *Hair transplantation* re-establishes hair density in non-hair bearing area of the scalp. It can be used to treat many causes of both scarring and non-scarring alopecia. Modern methods of hair transplantation revolve around the harvest of follicular units from the hair bearing scalp and transplanting them into carefully-planned recipient sites to re-create a naturally-appearing hair line. Patients must understand that with AA, hair loss will continue after transplantation and future operations may be necessary (Epstein 2003).

Follicular unit grafting (FUG) consists of harvesting a narrow strip of hearing bearing scalp in the subcutaneous plane with subsequent dissection of follicle units in preparation for grafting. The defect is closed primarily with a trichophytic closure. The harvest area is smaller than other techniques, such as follicular unit extraction.

Follicular unit extraction (FUE) obtains follicle grafts directly from donor scalp using small punches. This avoids excision of scalp tissue and linear scarring. Small donor incisions heal by secondary intention. With this method, a larger donor area is required to obtain the same density of graft hair when compared to FUG.

Microunit grafting consists of the transfer of individual follicular units obtained via FUG/FUE methods. Grafts must be kept in chilled saline and implanted within 6 hours of harvest as any drying of the grafts will negatively impact survival. Planning of the recipient area is perhaps the most important step in hair transplantation. Recipient areas are prepared with small blades or needles, taking care not to damage the underlying blood supply. Ideal spacing of grafts is 1–2 mm apart with increasing distance between grafts when arriving at the hair line (Epstein 2003). It is important to recognize the *direction* of hair growth when planning the recipient site. Areas, such as the eyebrows and eyelashes have unique hair growth patterns that need to be maintained. Eyebrows typically grow in a horizontal/flat direction whereas eyelashes grow perpendicular to the eyelid. Unfavorable cosmetic results will results if hair growth patterns are not respected during grafting.

The anterior *hairline* is typically placed 7.5–9.5 cm above the glabella, with the frontotemporal angle being the most critical part of the overall design. This is the area lateral to vertical lines from the lateral canthus (Rousso 2014). The normal hairline slopes backward as it approaches the frontotemporal recession. Grafting should aim to achieve 50% of the patient's original hair density. Further

transplantation should be avoided as excessive grafting in a small region can inhibit the survival of surrounding follicles. Patients should be counseled that grafted hair will shed after transplantation but will grow back within 3 months.

Scalp reduction surgically removes nonhair bearing scalp regions, leaving resulting defects to be closed primarily. Many different patterns of excision are possible depending on the geometry of scalp needing to be removed. Incisions should be planned along Langer's lines of skin tension. This technique depends on scalp elasticity to close the final defect and patients often require more than one surgery to achieve satisfactory results. Tissue expansion works by mechanical and biological creep in target tissues. It is an adjunct procedure to scalp reduction that can be beneficial. *Stretch back* is a normal phenomenon where skin can stretch around an incision line. This results in areas of nonhear bearing scalp that may need to be grafted to achieve adequate coverage.

Scalp flaps were the standard treatment for alopecia before grafting, but this has fallen out of favor in the modern era of FUT. The *juri* flap is an axial flap based off the posterior branch of the superficial temporal artery which can be rotated to recreate the entire frontal hairline.

■ COMPLICATIONS

Complications include a unesthetically low hairline, large "plug-like" graft size, abnormal hair growth direction, unrealistic coverage (unnatural hairline appearance), *pitting* (depression of skin around grafted hairs), *ridging* (demarcation of native vs transplanted hair), and *slot deformity* (unnatural hair growth patterns after scalp reduction).

■ BIBLIOGRAPHY

1. Epstein SS. Follicular unit hair grafting. Arch Facial Plastic Surg. 2003;5:439-44.
2. Lam SM, Hempstead BR, Williams EF. A philosophy and strategy for surgical hair restoration: a 10-year experience. Dermatol Surg. 2002;28:1035-42.
3. Ludwig E. Classification of the types of androgenetic alopecia (common baldness) occurring in the female sex. Br J Dermatol. 1977;97:247-54.
4. Norwood OT. Male pattern baldness: classification and incidence. South Med J. 1975;68:1359-65.
5. Rousso DE, Kim SW. A review of medical and surgical treatment options for androgenetic alopecia. JAMA Facial Plast Surg. 2014;16:444-50.
6. Saraswat A, Kumar BF. Minoxidil vs finasteride in the treatment of men with androgenetic alopecia. Arch Dermatol. 2003;139;1219-21.
7. Sawaya ME, Price VH. Different levels of 5 alpha-reductase type I and II, aromatase, and androgen receptor in hair follicles of women and men with androgenetic alopecia. J Invest Dermatol. 1997;109:296-300.

Multiple Choice Questions

Q 1. The Telogen effluvium phenomenon will RESOLVE in what time period?

A. 2 weeks
B. 1 month
C. 2 months
D. 3 months

Ans: D. 3 months

Q 2. Which of the following statements regarding hair transplantation is TRUE?

A. Patients with ages between 20 to 25 are better candidates that those with ages between 50 to 55
B. The patient's hair color is the most critical parameter to assess before hair transplantation
C. Micrografts are usually used at the crown
D. Minigrafts are usually used at the vertex

Ans: D. Minigrafts are usually used at the vertex

Q 3. Which of the following statements regarding hair transplantation is TRUE?

A. Minigrafts are used at the most anterior portion of the hairline
B. Minigrafts comprise from 3–8 hair follicles
C. Micrografts are used at the crown and vertex
D. Micrografts have a success rate of approximately 75%

Ans: B. Minigrafts comprise from 3–8 hair follicles

Q 4. Which of the following statements is FALSE regarding the medical treatment of male pattern baldness with finasteride?

A. Finasteride has no affinity for androgen receptors
B. Finasteride works by blocking the peripheral conversion of testosterone to dihydrotestosterone (DHT)
C. The recommended oral dose of finasteride is 5 mg/day
D. Finasteride is a competitive and specific inhibitor of type II 5α-reductase

Ans: C. The recommended oral dose of finasteride is 5 mg/day

Q 5. Which of the following patients is MOST LIKELY to be discouraged from hair transplantation?

A. 20-year-old male
B. 30-year-old male
C. 40-year-old male
D. 50-year-old male

Ans: A. 20-year-old male

Q 6. Which of the following statements is TRUE about the male frontal hairline in hair restoration surgery?

A. The frontal hairline is restored basically with six-hair minigrafts
B. The frontal hairline is better higher than lower
C. The frontal hairline should look almost horizontal from the top and oval from the profile view
D. The frontal hairline should begin 5 cm from the upper aspect of the brow

Ans: B. The frontal hairline is better higher than lower

Q 7. Which of the following statements about the frontal hairline is FALSE?

A. Never place the hairline below the superior border of the upper third of the face
B. The adult male hairline should have a gentle convex curve
C. The distance of the hairline from the midglabellar point should be less than 7 cm
D. Micrografts are mandatory for the frontal hairline

Ans: C. The distance of the hairline from the midglabellar point should be less than 7 cm

Q 8. Which of the following statements about hair replacement surgery is INCORRECT?

A. Standard round grafts are 4 mm punch graft
B. Micrografts contain 1-2 hairs
C. Minigrafts contain 10-12 hairs
D. Micrografts are used in the anterior portion of the hairline

Ans: C. Minigrafts contain 10-12 hairs

Q 9. Which of the following PERCENTAGES APPROXIMATES the survival rate of micrografts in hair replacement surgery?

A. 70%
B. 80%
C. 90%
D. 100%

Ans: D. 100%

Q 10. Which of the following type of male pattern baldness is the one representing a large vertex region of alopecia remaining separated from also a large frontotemporal region of alopecia. The band of hair of separation is narrow and sparse?

A. Type III
B. Type IV
C. Type V
D. Type VI

Ans: C. Type V

Q 11. Which of the following statements regarding the Juri flap is FALSE?

A. It is 25 cm long
B. It is 3 cm wide
C. It will span the entire frontal hairline
D. Dog ear formation is rarely found

Ans: D. Dog ear formation is rarely found

Q 12. Which of the following flaps is the one that BEST describes THE FRECHET'S flap used for management of a crown "slot" defect produced by scalp reduction surgery?

A. It is a long single Z-plasty flap
B. It is an occipital advancement flap
C. It is a bilateral temporo-occipital flap
D. It is a triple hair-bearing transposition flap

Ans: D. It is a triple hair-bearing transposition flap

Q 13. Which of the following statements represent NORMAL HAIR DENSITY in a candidate for hair replacement surgery.?

A. 2 hairs per mm²
B. 4 hairs per mm²
C. 6 hairs per mm²
D. 4 hairs per ½ cm²

Ans: A. 2 hairs per mm2

Q 14. The male pattern baldness represented in the picture below belongs to which of the following classifications?

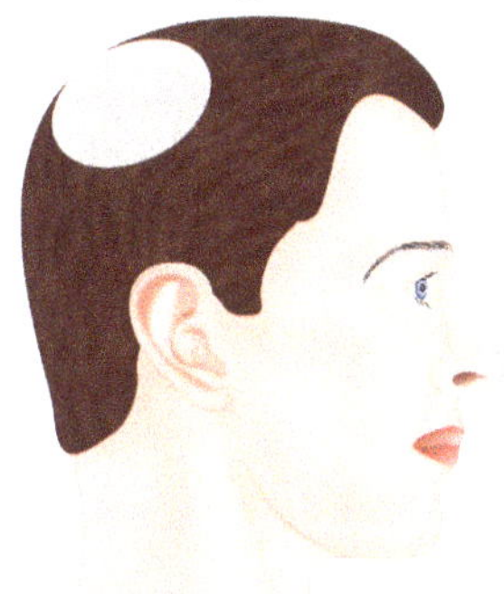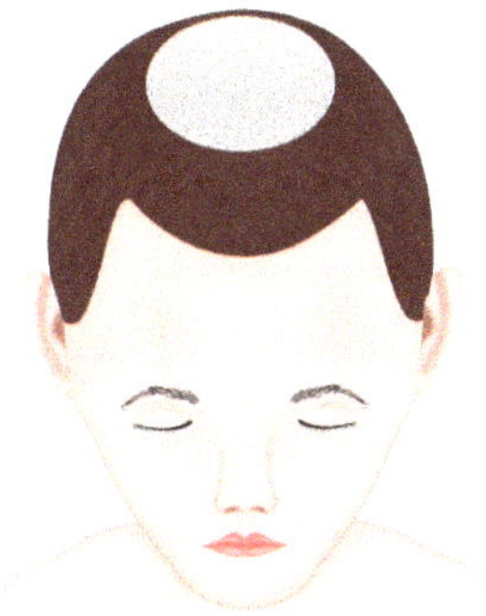

A. Class II

B. Class III

C. Class IV

D. Class V

Ans: C. Class IV

Q 15. Which of the following medications is used for the INITIAL management of female pattern hair loss?

A. Minoxidil

B. Finasteride

C. Nioxin

D. Nizoral

Ans: A. Minoxidil

Q 16. Which of the following medications is NOT approved for management of female pattern hair loss?

A. Minoxidil

B. Finasteride

C. Nioxin

D. Zinc

Ans: B. Finasteride

Q 17. In the normal human scalp, what is the percentage of hair follicules in the TELOGEN PHASE?

A. 1%

B. 5%

C. 10%

D. 20%

Ans: C. 10%

Q 18. Which of the following statements about postoperative care after hair restoration surgery is FALSE?

A. A gentle pressure head dressing is used for 48 hours

B. Head elevation and no bending for 48 hours is mandatory

C. Shampoo and shower are allowed at 48 hours

D. Saline spray and aloevera gel are applied to the grafts at night

Ans: A. A gentle pressure head dressing is used for 48 hours

Q 19. Which of the following statements about hairline design is FALSE?

A. The design should be high

B. The design should include a temporal recession

C. The most anterior point of hairline is placed at 7.0 cm from the midglabellar point

D. The temporal points linking frontal hair with temporal hair should be located at intersection of line drawn from lateral canthus to temporal fringe

Ans: C. The most anterior point of hairline is placed at 7.0 cm from the midglabellar point

Q 20. Which of the following hair colors is the LEAST suited for hair transplantation procedures in patients with light skin and straight hair?

A. Dark brown

B. Red

C. Gray

D. Salt-and-pepper

Ans: A. Dark brown

Q 21. Which of the following arteries supplies the Juri Flap distally and proximally?

A. Anterior branch of the superficial temporal artery and the occipital artery

B. Posterior branch of the superficial temporal artery and occipital artery

C. Anterior and posterior branches of the superficial temporal

D. Anterior branch of the superficial temporal artery and postauricular arteries

Ans: B. Posterior branch of the superficial temporal artery and occipital artery

Q 22. Into which of the following classifications would a patient selected for scalp reduction due to androgenetic alopecia fall?

A. Norwood and Hamilton classification of alopecia class I

B. Norwood and Hamilton classification of alopecia class II

C. Norwood and Hamilton classification of alopecia class VI

D. Norwood and Hamilton classification of alopecia class VII

Ans: C. Norwood and Hamilton classification of alopecia class VI

Q 23. The doll's-hair, or plug-like appearance , in hair restoration is produced most likely by using:

A. Standard 4 mm plug grafts

B. Half/standard 4 mm plug grafts

C. Quarter/standard 4 mm plug grafts

D. Minigrafts

Ans: A. Standard 4 mm plug grafts

Q 24. How many hairs are usually contained in a minigraft used for hair restoration?

A. 1

B. 2

C. 5

D. 10

Ans: C. 5

Q 25. Which of the following type of Hamilton-Norwood alopecia classification is capable to achieve THE BEST and MORE NATURAL result with hair replacement surgery?

A. Type I

B. Type II

C. Type IV

D. Type VI

Ans: C. Type IV

Q 26. Which of the following hair conditions is a CONTRA-INDICATION for a hair replacement surgery?

A. Androgenic alopecia

B. Traumatic alopecia

C. Male pattern alopecia
D. Diffuse female pattern baldness

Ans: D. Diffuse female pattern baldness

Q 27. Which of the following statements regarding hair restoration is FALSE?

A. Hair loss although progressive is always predictable at any age
B. Do not make the hairline too low (higher better than lower)
C. The frontal temporal angle lies on the lateral epicanthal line as hair loss progresses
D. The frontal hairline consists of microirregularity and macroirregularity

Ans: A. Hair loss although progressive is always predictable at any age

Q 28. Which of the following scalp zones is ideal for scalp reduction?

A. Crown
B. Mid-scalp
C. Occipital scalp
D. Temporal scalp

Ans: A. Crown

Q 29. Which of the following alopecia areas is ideal for the use of scalp flaps?

A. Crown
B. Frontal
C. Occipital scalp
D. Temporal scalp

Ans: B. Frontal

Q 30. What is the percentage of hair loss necessary before alopecia becomes noticeable?

A. 20%
B. 30%
C. 50%
D. 60%

Ans: C. 50%

Q 31. Which of the following factors is THE MOST important regarding hair replacement surgery?

A. Hair density
B. Hair thickness
C. Hair color
D. Hair direction

Ans: A. Hair density

Q 32. Which of the following patterns of scalp reduction is the IDEAL for use in hair replacement surgery?

A. S-shape pattern of excision
B. Sagittal midline ellipse pattern of excision
C. U-shaped pattern
D. Pattern tailored to the individual patient

Ans: D. Pattern tailored to the individual patient

Q 33. In which of the following areas will the "halo effect" complication occur after hair replacement surgery?

A. Vertex
B. Occipital
C. Temporal
D. Postauricular

Ans: B. Occipital

Q 34. Which of the following statements about tissue expansion in hair replacement surgery is FALSE?

A. Scalp expansion creates a larger hair-bearing surface area
B. Hair density decreases after scalp reduction
C. Tissue expansion does not affect hair follicle morphology
D. Scalp expansion will be of most benefit in patients with Norwood class VII

Ans: D. Scalp expansion will be of most benefit in patients with Norwood class VII

Q 35. Which of the following structures is the one containing the HAIR MATRIX?

A. The bulb
B. The infundibulum
C. The inner and outer root sheath
D. The isthmus

Ans: A. The bulb

Q 36. Which of the following statements about the hair growth cicle is TRUE?

A. The growth is 90% of hairs in the anagen phase and 10% in the telogen phase
B. The growth is 80% of hairs in the anagen phase and 20% in the telogen phase
C. The growth is 70% of hairs in the anagen phase and 30% in the telogen phase
D. The growth is 60% of hairs in the anagen phase and 40% in the telogen phase

Ans: A. The growth is 90% of hairs in the anagen phase and 10% in the telogen phase

Q 37. Which of the following statements regarding the temporo-parietal-occipital (TPO) flap is FALSE?

A. The TPO flap's blood supply is based on the superficial temporal artery
B. The TPO flap is 25 cm long
C. The TPO flap is 4 cm wide
D. The TPO flap is used for the treatment of frontal male-pattern alopecia

Ans: C. The TPO flap is 4 cm wide

Q 38. Which of the following statements regarding the Juri Flap is TRUE?

A. The Juri flap's blood supply is based on the deep temporal
B. The Juri flap has a 4 cm width
C. The Juri flap is transposed after one delay procedure
D. The Juri flap is undermined in the subperiosteal plane

Ans: B. The Juri flap has a 4 cm width

Q 39. The timing for the SECOND DELAY in the temporo-parietal-occipital (TPO) flap is:

A. 3 days
B. 7 days
C. 2 weeks
D. 3 weeks

Ans: B. 7 days

Q 40.   Which of the following indicates an INCORRECT facial flap/blood supply relationship?

A. Nasolabial flap—Angular artery
B. Median forehead flap—Supratrochlear artery
C. Paramedian forehead flap—Infratrochlear artery
D. Lateral forehead flap—Superficial temporal artery

Ans: C. Paramedian forehead flap-Infratrochlear artery

Q 41.   Which of the following is the ADEQUATE INTERVAL between scalp reductions?

A. 1 month
B. 2 months
C. 3 months
D. 4 months

Ans: C. 3 months

Q 42.   Which of the following statements about scalp reduction is TRUE?

A. It is adequate for Norwood alopecia class I and II
B. It is adequate for Norwood alopecia class V
C. The "Stretch-Back" phenomenon is insignificant
D. It is usually carried out under general anesthesia

Ans: B. It is adequate for Norwood alopecia class V

Chapter 22

Mohs Micrographic Surgery

Sameep Kadakia, Yadranko Ducic

■ INTRODUCTION

Mohs micrographic surgery, initially described by Frederick Mohs in 1930, is a highly accurate method of excising cutaneous malignancies through the use of horizontal sectioning and careful analysis of tumor margins in a three dimensional format.[1,2] Cutaneous malignancies can have unpredictable patterns of multidirectional spread often times not visible to the naked eye. Human skin is a dynamic organ system composed of epidermis, papillary dermis interdigitating with underlying reticular dermis, subcutaneous fat, and adnexa including vessels, nerves, and pilosebaceous units. As tumors can readily access these deeper structures, complete excision is paramount.[3,4] Embryonic fusion planes, fields of mesodermal fusion among the facial processes during the 5th–10th weeks of development, have been thought to offer paths of tumor spread; however, studies remain controversial as fusion planes are typically closed by adulthood.[5-7]

Cutaneous malignancy can be treated by multiple modalities including cryotherapy, radiation, curettage, laser ablation, convention surgical resection, and chemical injection among many others.[8-12] The abovementioned techniques, while employed in certain circumstances, pose the challenge of clearly defining tumor boundaries especially in the setting of microscopic tumor extension. Imaging techniques are limited in determining extension on the microscopic level, which may be readily apparent in macroscopic disease.[4] Another consideration in traditional treatment of cutaneous malignancy lies in the histologic analysis of tumor margins. As tumors are typically sectioned in the vertical plane, with slices obtained several millimeters apart, it is possible to miss tumor extension occurring between slices. The challenge in the treatment of cutaneous malignancy hinges on the balance between complete tumor excision and sparing of uninvolved tissue for functional and aesthetically minded reconstruction.[4]

Mohs micrographic surgery allows for complete excision of skin lesions while sparing uninvolved tissue through a meticulous process of mapping, excision, and repeated histologic analysis.

■ INDICATIONS FOR MOHS MICROGRAPHIC SURGERY

Mohs surgery is commonly offered as initial treatment of any cutaneous malignancy. Locally aggressive or recurrent tumors, tumors occurring in radiated skin, and cutaneous tumors in immunosuppressed patients can all be indications to perform Mohs micrographic surgery.[13-16] Tumors occurring in areas, such as the face, where tissue preservation and esthetics are crucial, arc also best served by Mohs surgery.[4,8,13,17] Some studies suggest a role for Mohs in treating cutaneous malignancies in skin overlying embryonic fusion planes, such as the retroauricular sulcus, philtrum, inner canthus, and nasolabial fold.[18] As mentioned previously, the role of embryonic fusion planes in dictating tumor spread is debated in the literature.

Mohs surgery can be used to address tumors of varying pathology including squamous cell carcinoma (SCC), basal cell carcinoma (BCC), adenoid cystic carcinoma, Merkel cell carcinoma, melanoma, and angiosarcoma among many others.[4] As BCC and SCC are far more common than other pathologies, further discussion on these two subjects is of greater yield. BCC represents the most common skin cancer treated by Mohs surgery. Among the subtypes of BCC, morpheaform, micronodular, and field fire variants should be readily considered for Mohs treatment as aggressive subtypes show greater benefit from Mohs surgery owing to the increased precision of margin analysis.[13] BCC lesions smaller than 3 cm have a Mohs cure rate of 99%, while lesions larger than 3 cm have a cure rate of approximately 93%. Taken together, the overall cure rate of BCC treated with Mohs surgery is greater than 99% according to the literature.[19,20]

Squamous cell carcinoma, the second most common cutaneous malignancy treated with Mohs surgery, has increased likelihood for local metastasis and skip lesions compared to BCC and thus poses a slightly greater challenge in obtaining high cure rates compared to BCC.[19] Despite the increased risk, Mohs micrographic surgery achieves approximately 98% overall 5-year cure rate in patients with

SCC without metastasis. In patients with local metastasis, the success of the procedure decreases to 16%.[19] Tumors less than 2 cm have a reported cure rate of 99% while tumors greater than 2 cm are successfully treated in 82% of patients.[4] SCC has a higher propensity for perineural invasion compared to BCC, especially in lesions greater than 2.5 cm where up to 64% of lesions can have perineural invasion compared to 11% in tumors less than 2.5 cm.[15,21] Although simple excision is typically performed on lesions with carcinoma in situ, lesions with poorly defined borders or suspicious features may be best served by Mohs techniques.[17,22]

The application of Mohs for cutaneous melanoma represents a controversial subject as no prospective trials exist comparing Mohs outcomes with traditional surgical resection. Some studies show cure rates up to 100% for Clark level 2 lesions, with this statistic dropping to 33% for Clark level 4 lesions. Experienced Mohs surgeons have reported an equivalent outcome compared to conventional resection but it is important to note that these are based on select comparative studies.[8,19,23-25]

Mohs surgery offers an accurate form of treating cutaneous malignancy in locations where tissue preservation is crucial for esthetic reconstruction. Compared to radiation therapy or traditional excision, Mohs micrographic surgery is also more cost-efficient.[26] Despite the advantages of Mohs, one must keep in mind that the procedure can be labor intensive and time consuming given the numerous surgical margins that must be analyzed following each subsequent section. A specially trained surgeon and nursing staff must be utilized, a laboratory technician that can prepare horizontal sections, and a trained dermatopathologist. A well-trained team is crucial as the most common cause of cutaneous recurrence following Mohs surgery is technical error.[4]

PROCEDURE: OVERVIEW OF THE FIXED AND FRESH TECHNIQUE

When initially described in the early 1900s, Mohs would routinely perform chemosurgery through the use of zinc chloride as a fixative agent. The use of zinc chloride afforded the advantage of superior hemostasis and high success rates, but was time consuming. This technique of Mohs surgery, later named the fixed technique, was abandoned for the fresh technique which is most commonly employed today.[4] The fixed technique is now only used for specific circumstances; greater than 70% of practitioners use the fresh technique.[27] The fresh technique involves initial tumor outlining followed by infiltration with lidocaine. The raised or soft portion of the tumor can be removed with a curette until the lesion is flush with the skin. Based on the contour of the edges, a Mohs map is created by circumferentially marking the lesion with margins. Tissue is excised at 45° to the skin, subdivided to make thin sections for slide preparation, and then analyzed with frozen section. Each

successive excision is performed based on the margin analysis on each slide. Using this modality, a careful excision is performed with adequate margins while using the Mohs maps and histologic specimen for maintaining a clear record of the procedure. The fresh technique can be completed in a shorter period of time than the fixed technique, typically in less than 1 day, which also facilitates immediately reconstruction. The use of lidocaine decreases the preoperative discomfort associated with zinc chloride fixation. The major disadvantage of the fresh technique is the risk of bleeding and the toxicity from lidocaine use.[4]

The postoperative course following Mohs surgery depends on whether reconstruction is to be performed immediately or in a delayed fashion. If reconstruction is performed at the same time as the initial procedure, then postoperative care consists of incision care through the use of ointments to maintain skin moisture, and possibly wound dressings in the event a portion of the wound is left open to granulate or a skin graft is placed. If reconstruction is to be delayed till a later date, the surgically created defect would require a moist dressing to maintain tissue integrity and prevent infection through direct exposure.

■ RECONSTRUCTIVE OPTIONS

As with any defect, resected tissue should be repaired with similar tissue to restore function and cosmesis. This is especially true in the face where the analysis of subunits is of prime importance. Smooth transitions between facial subunits lend to a perceived sense of harmony and youth.[28] As such, incisions should be hidden in natural skin creases and if a large portion of a subunit is affected, the entire subunits should be reconstructed.[29] The concept of subunit reconstruction has been described extensively for the repair of nasal defects.

The reconstructive surgeon should approach any Mohs defect in keeping with the reconstructive ladder. If lesions can be closed primarily following wide undermining, this would be feasible, if cosmesis is not compromised. If the lesion is not amenable to primary closure, then secondary intention could be considered. Secondary intention in areas such as the skin adjacent to the medial canthus has favorable outcomes; however, secondary intention on a large visible area, such as the cheek may not be the best option and a rotational flap could be employed for closure. Rotational flaps and advancement flaps are commonly used in the closure of Mohs defects, but consideration must be given to the location of the defect and planned donor site as skin thickness and mobility varies in the head and neck. In closing defects with local flaps, often times donor sites may require skin grafting or secondary intention to heal. Lastly, large defects, such as those that may present on the scalp may require the use of free tissue transfer, if other options are not optimal.

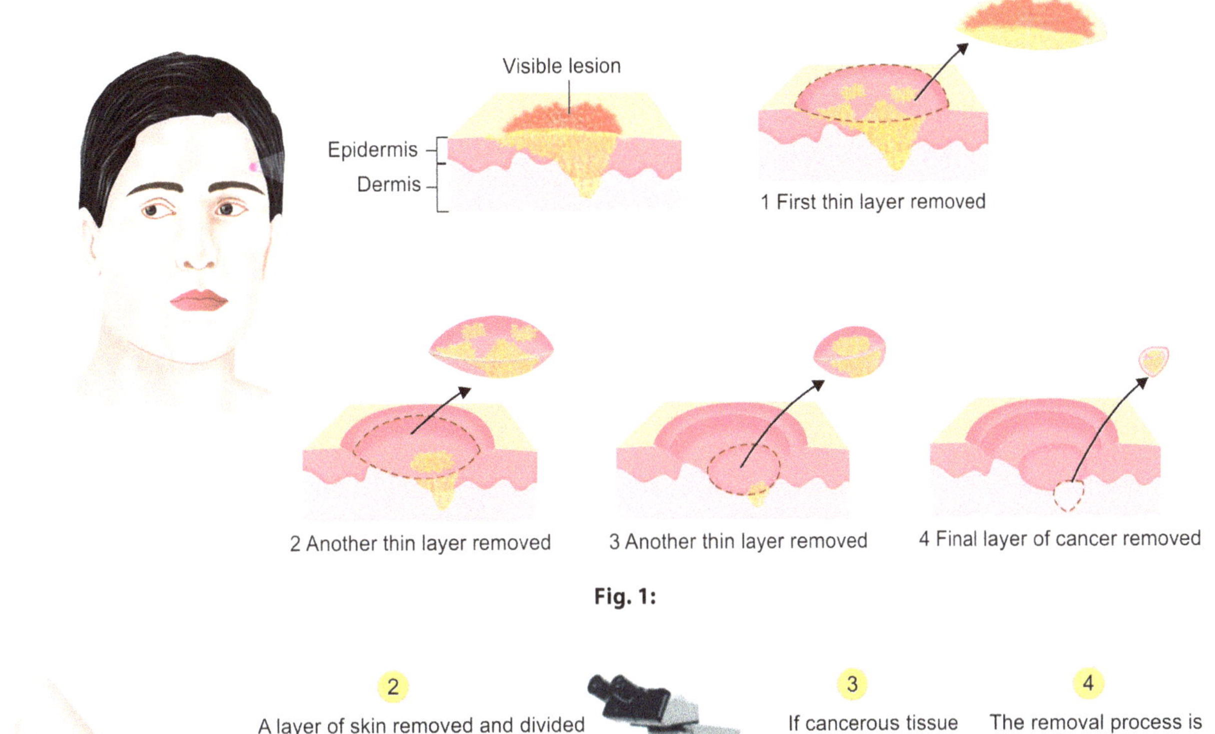

Fig. 1:

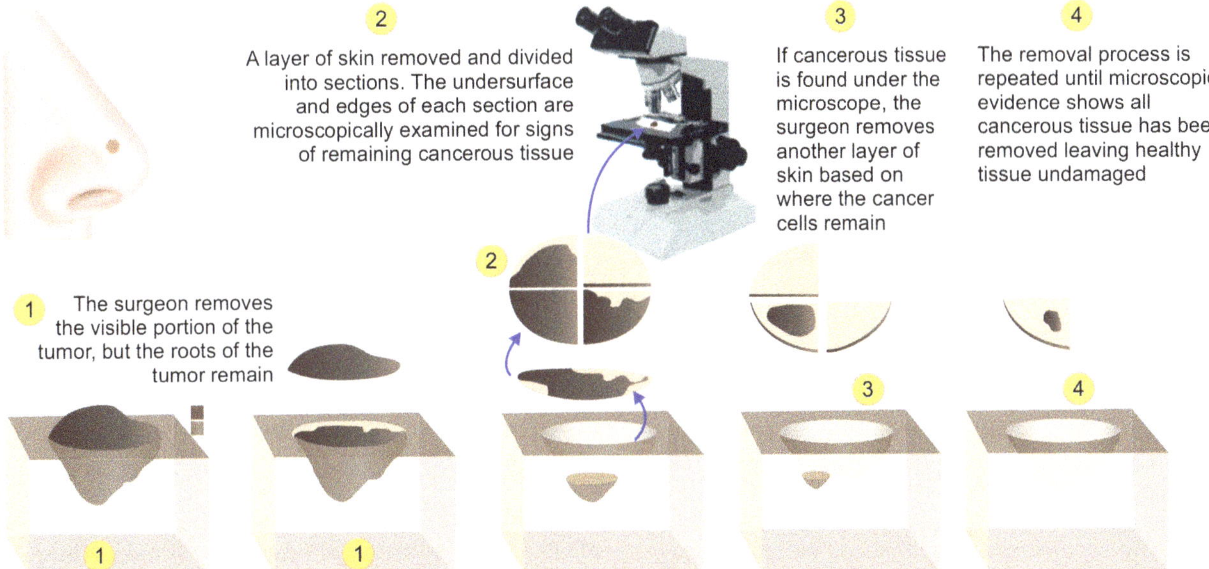

Fig. 2:

■ REFERENCES

1. Mohs FE. Mohs micrographic surgery. A historical perspective. Dermatol Clin. 1989;7(4):609-11.
2. Dinehart SM, Pollack SV. Mohs micrographic surgery for skin cancer. Cancer Treat Rev. 1989;16(4):257-65.
3. Wentzell JM, Robinson JK. Embryologic fusion planes and the spread of cutaneous carcinoma: a review and reassessment. J Dermatol Surg Oncol. 1990;16(11):1000-6.
4. Shriner DL, Mccoy DK, Goldberg DJ, et al. Mohs micrographic surgery. J Am Acad Dermatol. 1998;39(1):79-97.
5. Salasche SJ. Curettage and electrodesiccation in the treatment of midfacial basal cell epithelioma. J Am Acad Dermatol. 1983;8(4):496-503.
6. Lang PG, Duncan IM, Hochman M. Occurrence of subclinical tumor in excised facial subunits. Arch Facial Plast Surg. 2004;6(3):158-61.
7. Granström G, Aldenborg F, Jeppsson PH. Influence of embryonal fusion lines for recurrence of basal cell carcinomas in the head and neck. Otolaryngol Head Neck Surg. 1986;95(1):76-82.
8. Hruza GJ. Mohs micrographic surgery. Otolaryngol Clin North Am. 1990;23(5):845-64.
9. Soura E, Chasapi V, Stratigos AJ. Pharmacologic treatment options for advanced epithelial skin cancer. Expert Opin Pharmacother. 2015;16(10):1479-93.
10. Miller BH, Shavin JS, Cognetta A, et al. Nonsurgical treatment of basal cell carcinomas with intralesional

5-fluorouracil/epinephrine injectable gel. J Am Acad Dermatol. 1997;36(1):72-7.

11. Greenway HT, Cornell RC, Tanner DJ, et al. Treatment of basal cell carcinoma with intralesional interferon. J Am Acad Dermatol. 1986;15(3):437-43.

12. Wheeland RG, Bailin PL, Ratz JL, et al. Carbon dioxide laser vaporization and curettage in the treatment of large or multiple superficial basal cell carcinomas. J Dermatol Surg Oncol. 1987;13(2):119-25.

13. Lang PG, Osguthorpe JD. Indications and limitations of Mohs micrographic surgery. Dermatol Clin. 1989;7(4):627-44.

14. Calhoun KH, Wagner RF. Multidisciplinary treatment of facial skin cancer. Tex Med. 1991;87(12):64-9.

15. Matorin PA, Wagner RF. Mohs micrographic surgery: technical difficulties posed by perineural invasion. Int J Dermatol. 1992;31(2):83-6.

16. Soo K, Carter RC, O'Brian CJ, et al. Prognostic implications of perineural spread in squamous carcinoma of the head and neck. Laryngoscope. 1986;96:1145-8.

17. Albom MJ, Swanson NA. Mohs micrographic surgery for the treatment of cutaneous neoplasms. In: Friedman RJ, Rigel DS, Kopf AW, Harris MN, Baker D (Eds). Cancer of the skin. Philadelphia: WB Saunders; 1991. pp.484-529.

18. Panje WR, Ceilley RI. The influence of embryology of the mid-face on the spread of epithelial malignancies. Laryngoscope. 1979;89(12):1914-20.

19. Mohs FE (Ed). Chemosurgery. Microscopically controlled surgery for skin cancer. Springfield (IL): Charles C Thomas; 1978. pp. 1-29,153-64.

20. Leslie DF, Greenway HT. Mohs micrographic surgery for skin cancer. Australas J Dermatol. 1991;32(3):159-64.

21. Carter RL, Tanner NS, Clifford P, et al. Perineural spread in squamous cell carcinomas of the head and neck: a clinicopathological study. Clin Otolaryngol Allied Sci. 1979;4(4):271-81.

22. Mohs FE, Snow SN, Larson PO. Mohs micrographic surgery for penile tumors. Urol Clin North Am. 1992;19(2):291-304.

23. Kaspar TA, Wagner RF. Mohs micrographic surgery for thin stage I malignant melanoma: rationale for a modern management strategy. Cutis. 1992;50(5):350-1.

24. Brooks NA. Fixed-tissue micrographic surgery in the treatment of cutaneous melanoma. An overlooked cancer treatment strategy. J Dermatol Surg Oncol. 1992;18(11):999-1000.

25. Mohs FE. Chemosurgery for melanoma. Arch Dermatol. 1977;113(3):285-91.

26. Miller PK, Roenigk RK, Brodland DG, et al. Cutaneous micrographic surgery: Mohs procedure. Mayo Clin Proc. 1992;67(10):971-80.

27. Mcgillis ST, Wheeland RG, Sebben JE. Current issues in the performance of Mohs micrographic surgery. J Dermatol Surg Oncol. 1991;17(8):681-4.

28. Tan SL, Brandt MG, Yeung JC, et al. The aesthetic unit principle of facial aging. JAMA Facial Plast Surg. 2015;17(1):33-8.

29. Jergensen ZR, Pezeshk RA, Thornton JF. Rationale and argument for subunit Mohs excision nasal reconstruction. J Cutan Med Surg. 2016;20:343-5.

Multiple Choice Questions

Q 1. Which of the following carcinoma is the MOST common in the eyelid area?

A. Basal cell carcinoma

B. Squamous cell carcinoma

C. Sebaceous carcinoma

D. Adenocarcinoma

Ans: A. Basal cell carcinoma

Q 2. Which of the following region of the eyelid is MOST commonly involved by malignant skin lesions?

A. Upper eyelid B. Lower eyelid

C. Medial canthus D. Lateral canthus

Ans: B. Lower eyelid

Q 3. Which of the following statement is FALSE regarding secondary intention healing in the eyelids after Mohs' surgery?

A. The ideal wound should be superficial

B. The ideal should not expose cartilage

C. The ideal wound should be less than 25% of the entire eyelid surface

D. The ideal candidate should be a young individual rather than an old patient

Ans: D. The ideal candidate should be a young individual rather than an old patient

Q 4. Which of the following statements is TRUE regarding skin seborrheic keratoses?

A. Seborrheic keratoses are due to sun exposure

B. Seborrheic keratoses have a premalignant potential

C. Seborrheic keratoses require a mandatory excision

D. Seborrheic keratoses are superficial lesions

Ans: D. Seborrheic keratoses are superficial lesions

Q 5. Which of the following skin conditions is treated EFFECTIVELY with topical 5-fluorouracil and/or Imiquimod cream?

A. Seborrheic keratoses

B. Dermatosis papulosa nigra

C. Actinic keratosis

D. Basal cell carcinoma

Ans: C. Actinic keratosis

Q 6. In which of the following clinical situations Mohs micrographic surgery is usually NOT necessary?

A. Basal cell carcinoma recurrent of the cheek

B. Basal cell carcinoma nodular type of the cheek

C. Squamous cell carcinoma of cheek greater than 2 cm

D. Basal cell carcinoma morpheaform type of the cheek

Ans: B. Basal cell carcinoma nodular type of the cheek

Q 7. What is the most common symptom of nonmelanoma skin cancer?

A. Asymptomatic

B. Pain

C. Pruritus

D. Bleeding

Ans: A. Asymptomatic

Q 8. Which of the following sites is NOT included in the "mask area" of the face?

A. Eyelids

B. Preauricular

C. Postauricular

D. Forehead

Ans: D. Forehead

Q 9. Which of the following statements regarding the Leser-Trélat sign is FALSE?

A. It is the abrupt appearance of multiple seborrheic keratosis

B. It is also associated with multiple actinic keratosis lesions

C. It is commonly implicated or marker for internal malignancy

D. It is most commonly associated with colon adenocarcinoma

Ans: B. It is also associated with multiple actinic keratosis lesions

Q 10. What major advantage does zinc chloride offer in the fixed technique of Mohs surgery?

A. Improved accuracy

B. Hemostasis

C. Patient comfort

D. Faster procedure time

Ans: B. Hemostasis

Q 11. Which of the following is true regarding embryonic fusion planes?

A. They are unanimously regarded as sites of low resistance to tumor spread

B. Their implication in tumor spread is debated

C. They typically persist into adulthood

D. They represent fusion planes between neuroectodermal cells

Ans: B. Their implication in tumor spread is debated

Q 12. Which of the following is a limitation of Mohs surgery?

A. Increased cost compared to traditional excision

B. Need for highly trained physician, nurse, technician, and pathologist

C. Poor accuracy compared to conventional techniques

D. Patient dissatisfaction

Ans: B. Need for highly trained physician, nurse, technician, and pathologist

Q 13. _True or False:_ Basal cell carcinoma more commonly has skip lesions and local metastasis than squamous cell carcinoma:

A. True

B. False

Ans: B. False

Q 14. _True or False:_ The horizontal sectioning techniques of Mohs offers improved accuracy and margin analysis compared to traditional vertical sectioning.

A. True

B. False

Ans: A. True

Q 15. Which of the following subtypes of basal cell carcinoma (BCC) is the MOST common?

A. Basosquamous carcinoma

B. Morpheaform BCC

C. Nodular BCC

D. Superficial BCC

Ans: C. Nodular BCC

Q 16. Which of the following subtype of melanoma is the MOST common?

A. Nodular melanoma

B. Micronodular melanoma

C. Superficial spreading melanoma

D. Lentigo maligna melanoma

Ans: C. Superficial spreading melanoma

Q 17. Cutaneous malignancy of the external ear is MOST commonly found in the:

A. Antihelix

B. Concha bowl

C. Scapha

D. Tragus

Ans: A. Antihelix

Q 18. What is the PERCENTAGE of basal cell carcinoma skin lesions involving the lower eyelid?

A. 20%

B. 30%

C. 50%

D. 70%

Ans: D. 70%

Q 19. Which of the following statements regarding actinic keratosis is TRUE?

A. Actinic keratosis are common skin lesions with no malignant potential

B. Actinic keratosis result from solar damage and chronic skin trauma

C. Diffuse actinic keratosis can be treated with topical 5-fluorouracil

D. Actinic keratosis can be removed or watched

Ans: C. Diffuse actinic keratosis can be treated with topical 5-fluorouracil

Q 20. Which of the following statements is TRUE in cutaneous malignancies?

A. Squamous cell carcinoma is the most common type of skin cancer

B. Actinic keratosis is the most common precursor of squamous cell carcinoma

C. Nodular basal cell carcinoma has ill-defined borders which cannot be easily detected clinically

D. Cystic basal cell carcinoma has a tendency to spread at embryonic fusion planes

Ans: B. Actinic keratosis is the most common precursor of squamous cell carcinoma

Q 21. Which of the following treatments for actinic keratosis is INCORRECT?

A. Superficial shave excision

B. Cryotherapy

C. 5-fluorouracil

D. Radiation therapy

Ans: D. Radiation therapy

Q 22. Which of the following basal cell carcinoma lesions represented in the drawing below has the LEAST possibility of recurrence?

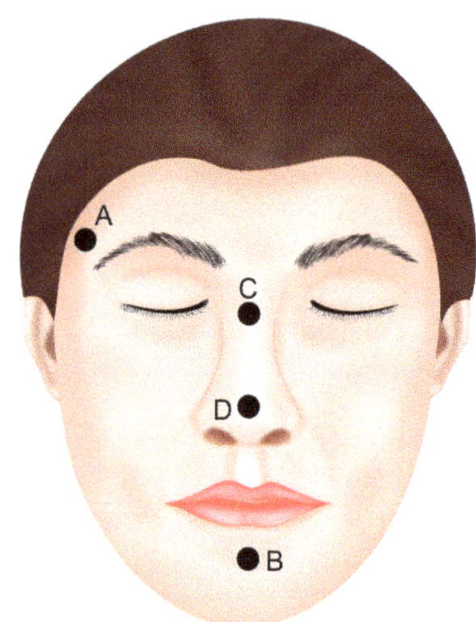

A. A

B. B

C. C

D. D

Ans: B. B

Q 23. A 72-year-old female is referred to you with a biopsy diagnosis of Merkel Cell carcinoma located in the skin for the left temple area. The lesion is firm, raised and ulcerated, measuring 1. 5 cm. What is the BEST treatment option for this particular patient?

A. Wide local excision

B. Wide local excision and prophylactic lymphadenectomy

C. Chemotherapy

D. Radiation therapy

Ans: A. Wide local excision

Q 24. Which of the following pigmented lesions is the MOST invasive with the POOREST prognosis?

A. Lentigo maligna melanoma

B. Superficial spreading melanoma

C. Nodular melanoma

D. Acral lentiginous melanoma

Ans: C. Nodular melanoma

Q 25. A patient has a malignant melanoma in the cheek area with a 3 mm thickness. The current recommended margin for adequate resection is:

A. 1.0 cm

B. 2.0 cm

C. 2.5 cm

D. 3.0 cm

Ans: B. 2.0 cm

Q 26. Which of the following facial areas is NOT considered high-risk for aggressive cutaneous malignancies?

A. Nose

B. Cheek

C. Preauricular

D. Postauricular

Ans: B. Cheek

Q 27. Which of the following facial areas is the MOST common location for recurrence of cutaneous malignancies?

A. Temple

B. Periorbital

C. Nose

D. Scalp

Ans: C. Nose

Q 28. A 72-year-old female is referred to you for a suspected dysplastic nevus of 1 cm with irregular pigmentation and indistinct borders. The BEST biopsy technique in this particular situation is:

A. Incisional biopsy

B. Excisional biopsy

C. Punch biopsy

D. Curettage

Ans: B. Excisional biopsy

Q 29. Which of the following skin lesions is BEST treated with 5-fluorouracil (5-FU)?

A. Superficial basal cell carcinoma

B. Actinic keratosis

C. Seborrheic keratosis

D. Dermatosis papulosa nigra

Ans: B. Actinic keratosis

Q 30. Which of following statement the is FALSE about LENTIGO SENILIS?

A. Lesions are most commonly located on the face and hands

B. Potential malignant degeneration is high

C. Lesions slowly increase in size, the color is uniform and dark brown and the outline is irregular

D. Lesions are best treated by chemical peeling

Ans: B. Potential malignant degeneration is high

Q 31. Which of the following percentages represents the melanomas originating from previous existing moles?

A. 20%

B. 40%

C. 70%

D. 90%

Ans: C. 70%

Q 32. Which of the following statements regarding Pilomatrixoma is TRUE?

A. It is a locally invasive skin neoplasm

B. It is more common in adults than children

C. It is treated with surgical excision

D. It commonly has a high local recurrence rate

Ans: C. It is treated with surgical excision

Q 33. Which of the following areas are THE MOST COMMON SITE for metastasis in patients with facial cutaneous Melanomas treated with adequate margins of wide local excision?

A. Lymph nodes
B. Lung
C. Liver
D. Brain

Ans: A. Lymph nodes

Q 34. Which of the following signs or symptoms raises EARLY SUSPICION OF MELANOMA in an acquired nevus?

A. Pruritus
B. Asymmetry
C. Bleeding
D. Change of color

Ans: A. Pruritus

Q 35. Which of the following statements is TRUE about adequate margins of wide excision in Merkel cell carcinoma?

A. They are undefined
B. They are assisted with frozen sections
C. They are assisted with Mohs surgery
D. An adequate margin is 3 cm.

Ans: A. They are undefined

Q 36. The five year cure rate for primary basal cell carcinoma after Mohs micrographic surgery is reached by which percentage of patients?

A. 85%
B. 90%
C. 95%
D. 99%

Ans: D. 99%

Q 37. For each specimen, what is the percentage of lateral and deep margins that can be checked using the horizontal sectioning technique in Mohs surgery?

A. 90%
B. 95%
C. 99%
D. 100%

Ans: D. 100%

Q 38. Which of the following managements is the IDEAL for treatment of dermatofibrosarcoma protuberans localized in the head and neck area?

A. Currettage followed by electrosurgery
B. Wide surgical excision
C. Mohs surgery
D. Radiation therapy

Ans: B. Wide surgical excision

Q 39. Which of the following statements about Mohs micrographic surgery for basal cell carcinoma is FALSE?

A. Mohs technique is ideal for the treatment of initial basal cell carcinoma
B. Mohs technique is ideal for treatment of recurrent basal cell carcinoma
C. Mohs technique sectioning allows to check 100% of the lateral and deep margins of the each specimen
D. Mohs Technique gives a high five year cure rate of 90%

Ans: D. Mohs technique gives a high five year cure rate of 90%

Q 40. Which of the following treatment options for the management of facial cutaneous basal cell carcinoma is INCORRECT?

A. Cryotherapy
B. Radiotherapy
C. Laser vaporization
D. Topical imiquimod

Ans: C. Laser vaporization

Q 41. Which of the following statements about congenital melanocytic nevi is TRUE?

A. Congenital melanocytic nevi are dark brown, round or oval in shape, and always hairless
B. Congenital melanocytic nevi from 10 to 15 cm are considered large
C. Congenital melanocytic nevi of large size will transform into melanoma in 30% of cases
D. Congenital melanocytic nevi carry a risk of melanoma related to the age of the child

Ans: D. Congenital melanocytic nevi carry a risk of melanoma related to the age of the child

Q 42. Which of the following statements about Merkel cell carcinoma is TRUE?

A. Merkel cell carcinoma is a malignant tumor derived from neuroendocrine cells of neural crest origin
B. Most of the lesions are localized on the trunk
C. They are most commonly seen in the childhood age
D. Wide local excision is the only effective treatment

Ans: A. Merkel cell carcinoma is a malignant tumor derived from neuroendocrine cells of neural crest origin

Q 43. Which of the following characteristics of congenital melanocytic nevi is related to the risk for the development of melanoma?

A. Color
B. Size
C. Shape
D. Hairy

Ans: B. Size

Q 44. What is the minimal size of congenital hairy nevus clinically significant for the development of melanoma?

A. 10 cm
B. 15 cm
C. 20 cm
D. 25 cm

Ans: C. 20 cm

Q 45. Which of the following congenital syndromes is an inherited multisystemic disorder that includes multiple basal cell carcinomas, palmar and plantar pitting, calcification of the dura, jaw cysts and skeletal abnormalities?

A. Xeroderma pigmentosum
B. Epidermoldysplasia verruciformis
C. Nevoid basal cell carcinoma syndrome
D. Muir-Torre syndrome

Ans: C. Nevoid basal cell carcinoma syndrome

Q 46. Which of the following eyelid or periorbital areas is MOST commonly involved by basal cell carcinoma of the skin?

A. Lateral canthal area
C. Medial canthus
B. Lower lid
D. Periorbital area

Ans: B. Lower lid

Q 47. Which of the following is considered a MAJOR criteria in the diagnosis of skin melanoma in the revised Glasgow seven-point checklist?

A. Changes in color
C. Bleeding
B. Crusting
D. Inflammation

Ans: A. Changes in color

Q 48. Which of the following skin nevus is the MOST common in the adult population?

A. Junctional nevus
C. Compound nevus
B. Intradermal nevus
D. Halo nevus

Ans: B. Intradermal nevus

Q 49. A "LARGE" congenital nevus is defined as a lesion of:

A. Greater than 20 cm
C. Between 15 and 10 cm
B. Between 15 and 20 cm
D. Between 5 and 10 cm

Ans: A. Greater than 20 cm

Q 50. Which of the following is the MOST appropriate management for a "LARGE" congenital nevus?

A. Conservative, no surgery
B. Surgery, serial excision in stages
C. Surgery, total excision in one stage
D. CO_2 laser

Ans: B. Surgery, serial excision in stages

Q 51. Which of the following percentages is the approximately chance of developing melanoma in the first two decades of life, in a child with a "LARGE" congenital nevus?

A. 5%
C. 20%
B. 10%
D. 25%

Ans: B. 10%

Q 52. Which of the following is the mainstay in the treatment of the Merkel cell carcinoma?

A. Surgery
C. Chemotherapy
B. Radiation therapy
D. Laser (CO_2)

Ans: A. Surgery

Q 53. Which of the following form of malignant melanoma involves in equal frequency blacks and whites?

A. Superficial spreading melanoma
B. Acral lentiginous melanoma
C. Nodular melanoma
D. Lentigo maligna melanoma

Ans: B. Acral lentiginous melanoma

Q 54. What is the recommended margin of resection for a cutaneous melanoma with a tumor thickness of 3.5 mm?

A. 0.5 cm
C. 1 cm
B. 0.75 cm
D. 2 cm

Ans: D. 2 cm

Q 55. Which of the following nevi are usually the largest?

A. Junctional nevus
C. Compound nevus
B. Intradermal nevus
D. Congenital nevus

Ans: D. Congenital nevus

Q 56. Which of the following nevi are small, less than 1 cm, most common in women than men, dome-shaped blue appearance, and more than 50% of the cases found on the dorsa of the hands and feet?

A. Junctional nevus
C. Intradermal nevus
B. Blue nevus
D. Congenital nevus

Ans: B. Blue nevus

Q 57. Which of the following statements regarding the Halo nevus is FALSE?

A. It is a pigmented melanocytic nevus
B. It is usually malignant in nature
C. It is found in all races
D. It is found equally in boys and girls

Ans: B. It is usually malignant in nature

Q 58. The treatment of CHOICE of dermatofibrosarcoma protuberans of the head and neck is:

A. Surgery
C. Radiation therapy
B. Curettage
D. Chemotherapy

Ans: A. Surgery

Q 59. Which of the following skin neoplasms is associated with the Leser-Trelat sign?

A. Seborrheic keratosis
C. Pilomatricoma
B. Syringoma
D. Sebaceous adenoma

Ans: A. Seborrheic keratosis

Q 60. Which of the following surgical options is the ONE represented in the drawing below?

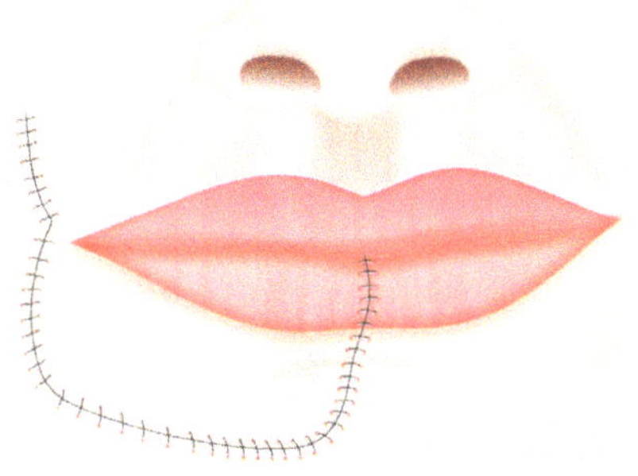

A. Gilles flap
C. Karapandzic flap
B. Estlander flap
D. Abbé flap

Ans: A. Gilles flap

Q 61. Which of the following indicators is the MOST reproducible prognostic factor in malignant melanoma?

A. Clark level
B. Breslow thickness
C. Growth phase
D. Ulceration

Ans: B. Breslow thickness

Q 62. Which of the following statements about Merkel cell carcinoma is TRUE?

A. Local recurrence has very low incidence approximately 2%
B. Wide local lesion is used for recurrence only
C. It is resistant to the chemotherapeutic agents
D. It is a radiosensitive tumor

Ans: D. It is a radiosensitive tumor

Chapter 23

Local Flaps and Grafts

Lina Zahra Benamira

DEFINITIONS

- The repair of facial cutaneous defects can be achieved by numerous options, including: healing by secondary intention, primary closure, local and regional flaps, skin grafts, composite grafts and free tissue transfers.
- Skin *flaps* are a transfer of skin and subcutaneous tissue with direct vascular supply.
- Skin *grafts* consist of epidermis and a partial- to full-thickness of the underlying dermis.
- Unlike flaps, grafts "do not have a blood supply" and initially survive by absorbing transudate from the recipient site.
- Flaps can be classified based on the location of the flap relative to the defect (Table 1).
- Flaps can also be classified based on vascular supply—random versus axial. This chapter will be a specific review of *random cutaneous flaps*, i.e. flaps supplied by musculocutaneous arteries "near the flap base", as opposed to axial flaps which will be covered in another chapter.

CLASSIFICATION

- Another way to describe flaps is based on the method of tissue movement. It can be subdivided in four categories (Figs. 1 to 5):
  1. *Rotation flaps*: Involve use of immediately adjacent tissue "rotated in an arc" around a fix point.
  2. *Advancement flaps*: Involve "linear movement" of tissue directly to the defect.

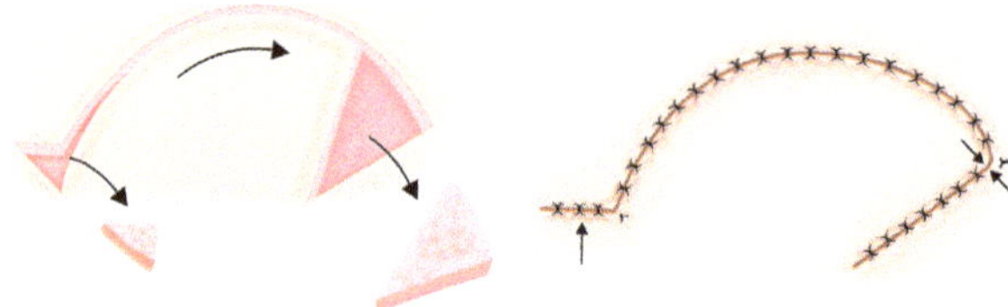

Fig. 1: Rotation flap.

For example: Monopedicled, bipedicled, V-Y or Y-V, Island.
  3. *Transposition flaps*: Involve the transfer of adjacent tissue around a pivot point but in a "linear" fashion.
  For example: Rhomboid, banner-type, and bilobed.
  4. *Interpolation flaps*: Also involve the transfer of adjacent tissue around a pivot point; however, "the base of the flap is not contiguous to the defect", resulting in the formation of a *pedicle*.
  For example: Nasolabial and postauricular.

GRAFTS

- *The process of skin grafts take is subdivided in three stages (Tables 2 and 3):*
  1. *Imbibition*: At 24–48 hours; Formation of a fibrin network between the graft and the wound bed, diffusion of nutrients from the wound bed to the graft through plasma exudates.
  2. *Inosculation*: At 48–72 hours; capillaries from the graft contact capillaries from the wound bed, and neovascularization process is triggered.
  3. *Neovascularization*: The newly formed vascular connections differentiate into afferent and efferent vessels (sometime between 4–7 days).
- *Factors for graft failure include*: Insufficient vascularity of the recipient site, hematoma, seroma, infection, excessive tension, comorbidities (diabetes, smoking, protein and vitamin deficiency) and medication (immunosuppressive agents, steroids, anticoagulants).

Table 1: Flap classification based on location.	
Local	*Tissue adjacent or near to the defect*
Regional	Tissue from outside of the *face, scalp,* or *neck*, where the arterial pedicle is sufficient to reach the facial defect (e.g. pectoralis muscle flap)
Distant	Tissue from a distant location, requiring microvascular anastomosis of vessels

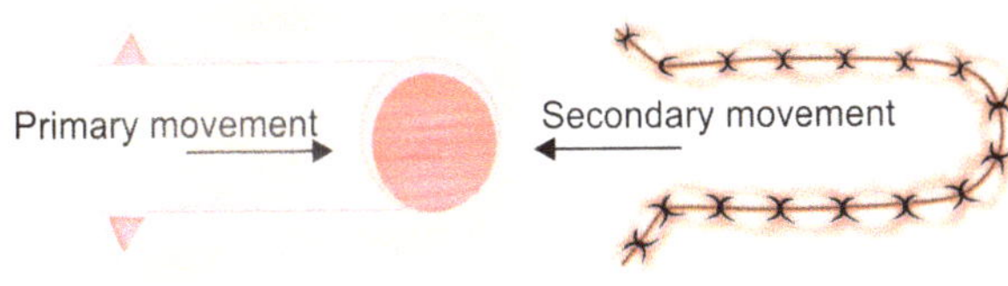

Fig. 2: Unipedicled advancement flap.

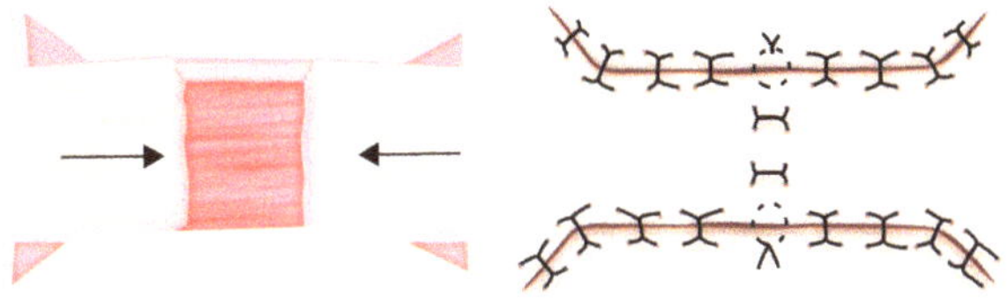

Fig. 3: Bilateral unipedicled advancement flap.

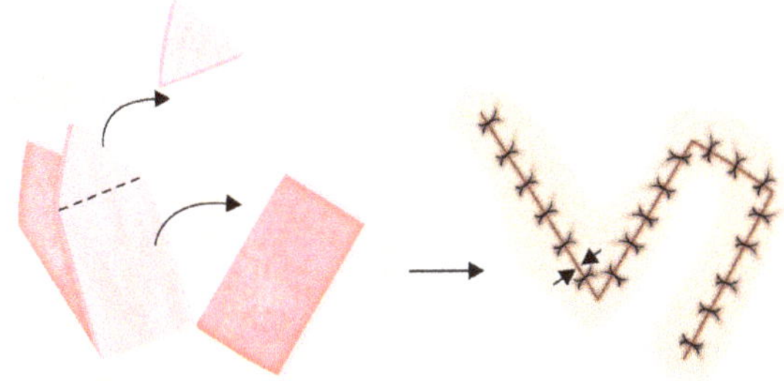

Fig. 4: Transposition flap.

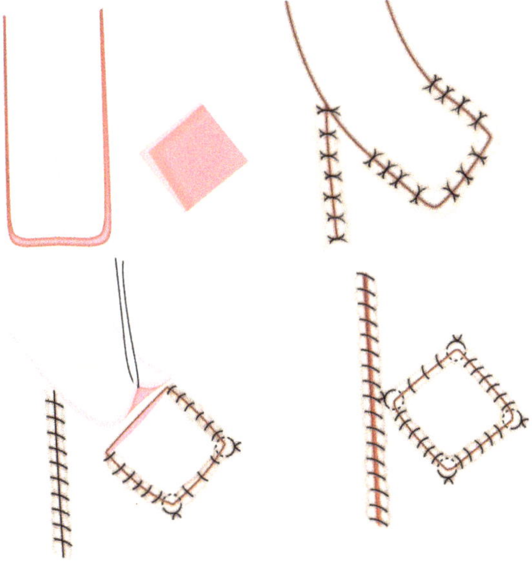

Fig. 5: Interpolation flap.

Table 2: Skin grafts.		
	Split-thickness skin graft	*Full-thickness skin graft*
Advantages	• Better survival • Rapid healing • Less primary contraction	• Minimal secondary contraction • Better texture and pigmentation match with normal skin
Disadvantages	• Poor color and texture match with normal • Propensity to secondarily contract	• Greater primary contraction • Reduced survival rates • Longer healing time

Table 3: Common indications of grafts subtypes.	
FTSG	Superficial defect involving loss of skin with intact muscle and soft tissues
STSG	Large defects of the trunk or extremities away from joints (rarely used to replace facial cutaneous defects)
Dermal grafts	Preventing the contour depression left by the repair of deeper defects
Mucosal grafts	Upper eyelid reconstruction and urethroplasty
Bone grafts	Mandibular and midface reconstruction
Fat grafts	Soft tissue augmentation

RECONSTRUCTION OF SPECIFIC FACIAL SUBSITES

Principles

- Avoid tension on hairline, medial/lateral canthus and oral commissure.
  - *Flap physiology*:
    - » *Stress*: Force applied per cross-sectional area.
    - » *Strain*: Change in length divided by the original tissue length, to which a force is applied.
    - » *Creep*: Strain as a function of time due to constant stress over an extended period of time.
    - » *Stress relaxation*: Decrease in stress when the skin is held in tension at a constant strain for a given time.
  - *Delay phenomenon*: Principle according to which a skin flap should be partially devascularized in a staged procedure prior to its placement in order to increase blood flow at the time of grafting.
  - *Flap prefabrication and prelamination* are complex techniques which are used as an end resort when conventional flaps are not technically or esthetically achievable. *Prefabrication* consists in transferring an intact vascular pedicle under a tissue without an axial vessel and allowing neovascularization to occur over a few weeks before transferring that unit as a free flap to the new recipient site. *Prelamination is* the implantation of tissue in a vascular bed without

manipulating the native blood supply. This technique allows the implanted tissue to become vascularized over time which results in a multilayered composite flap for the reconstruction of multilayer structures (e.g. the nose).

Common Options for Reconstruction of Specific Subsites

- *Forehead*: Primary closure, advancement flaps, rotation flaps (e.g. unilateral and O-to-Z flap), transposition flaps (e.g. rhombic flap), FTSG, STSG (if very large)
- *Eyelids*: Tenzel semicircular rotation flap, tarsoconjunctival bridge, free tarsoconjunctival graft, Mustarde cheek rotation flap
- *Cheeks*: Primary closure, W-plasty, Z-plasty, Rhomberg transposition flap, advancement flap, V-Y advancement flap, FTSG
- *Nose*:
  Multilayer reconstruction for the nose: Staged surgical procedure aiming to replicate the original multilayered anatomy of the nose in complex nasal defects involving the loss of:
  - Mucosal lining
  - Support
  - Skin.
- *Lip*: Primary closure, bilateral advancement flap, adjacent labiomental crease A-to-T flap, nasolabial flap, rotation flap, transposition flap, FTSG
- *Ear*: Chondrocutaneous advancement flap, temporoparietal flap, transposition flaps, thin-tubed flap, banner flap, FTSG
- *Chin*: Primary closure, lateral V-Y advancement flap, laterally based platysmal flap, FTSG
- *Neck*: Bilobed flap and STSG.

■ BIBLIOGRAPHY

1. Ambrozová J, Mesták J, Smutková J. Reconstruction of the lower eyelid after excision of major tumours. Acta Chir Plast. 1993;35:131-45.
2. Chajchir A, Benzaquen I. Fat grafting injection for soft tissue augmentation. Plast Reconstr Surg. 1989;84:921-34.
3. Chiang YC. Combined tissue expansion and prelamination of forearm flap in major ear reconstruction. Plast Reconstr Surg. 2006;117:1292-5.
4. Dhar SC, Taylor GI. The delay phenomenon: the story unfolds. Plast Reconstr Surg. 1999;104:2079-91.
5. Ebrahimi A, Ashayeri M, Rasouli HR. Comparison of local flaps and skin grafts to repair cheek skin defects. J Cutan Aesthet Surg. 2015;8:92-6.
6. Espinoza GM, Prost AM. Upper Eyelid Reconstruction. Facial Plast Surg Clin North Am. 2016;24:173-82.
7. Glogau RG, Haas AF. Skingrafts. Local flaps in facial reconstruction. St-Louis, MO: Mosby; 1995. pp. 247-51.
8. Hinshaw JR, Miller ER. Histology of healing split-thickness, full-thickness autogenous skin grafts and donor sites. Arch Surg. 1965;91:658-70.
9. Johnson J, Rosen C. Bailey's Head and Neck Otolaryngology, 5th edition. 2013.
10. Mathijssen IM, van der Meulen JC. Guidelines for reconstruction of the eyelids and canthal regions. J Plast Reconstr Aesthet Surg. 2010;63:1420-33.
11. Meyers S, Rohrer T, Grande D. Use of dermal grafts in reconstructing deep nasal defects and shaping the ala nasi. Dermatol Surg. 2001;27:300-5.
12. Morey AF, McAninch JW. When and how to use buccal mucosal grafts in adult bulbar urethroplasty. Urology. 1996;48:194-8.
13. Parrett BM, Pribaz JJ. An algorithm for treatment of nasal defects. Clin Plast Surg. 2009;36:407-20.
14. Ratner D. Skin grafting. Semin Cutan Med Surg. 2003;22:295.
15. Siegle RJ. Reconstruction of the forehead. In: Baker SR, Swanson NA (Eds). Local Flaps in Facial Reconstruction. St. Louis, Mo: Mosby; 1995. pp.421-42.
16. Thornton JF, Gosman AA. Skin grafts and skin substitutes and principles of flaps. In: Kenkel JM (Ed). Selected Readings in Plastic Surgery. Dallas: Southwestern, University of Texas; 2004.
17. Tromovitch TA, Stegman SJ, Glogau RG. Forehead. In: Tromovitch TA, Stegmen SJ, Glogau RG (Eds). Flaps and Grafts in Dermatologic Surgery. Chicago, Ill: Yearbook Medical; 1989. pp. 83-92.
18. Yao ST. Vascular implantation into skin flap: experimental study and clinical application: a preliminary report. Plast Reconstr Surg. 1981;68:404-10.

Multiple Choice Questions

Q 1. Which of the following statements is TRUE about a "note flap"?

A. It is a rotation flap
B. It is useful to close a circular defect
C. It is useful to close a fusiform defect
D. It is useful to close a rectangular defect

Ans: B. It is useful to close a circular defect

Q 2. The Z-plasty INVOLVES:

A. An advancement flap
B. An interpolation flap
C. A transposition flap
D. A rotation flap

Ans: C. A transposition flap

Q 3. Which of the following statements about the local flap shown below is TRUE?

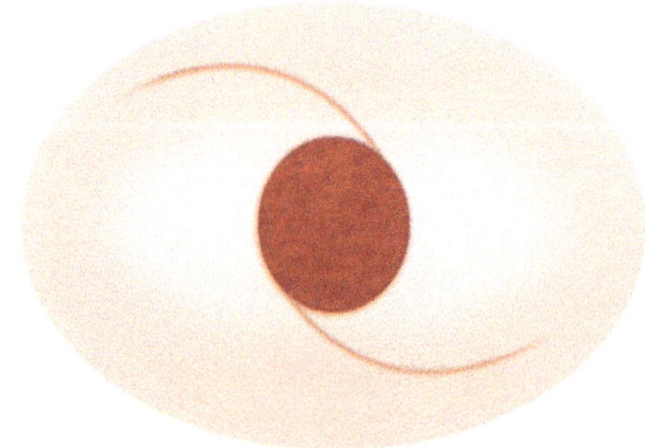

A. It is a bilateral rotation-transposition flap

B. It is also called O-T flap

C. It is useful to close circular defects in the scalp area

D. Using a triple flap instead of two flaps is a disadvantage for closing

Ans: C. It is useful to close circular defects in the scalp area

Q 4. Which of the following statements is FALSE regarding the "O-T" flap?

A. The flap converts a circular defect to a T-shaped scar

B. The disadvantage is that it leaves an unfavorable scar with two perpendicular limbs

C. The advantage is that there is no need for excision of normal tissue

D. The flap has advancement and rotational components

Ans: C. The advantage is that there is no need for excision of normal tissue

Q 5. The IDEAL obtuse angle represented in the rhombic flap (Limberg flap design) shown in the drawing below should be:

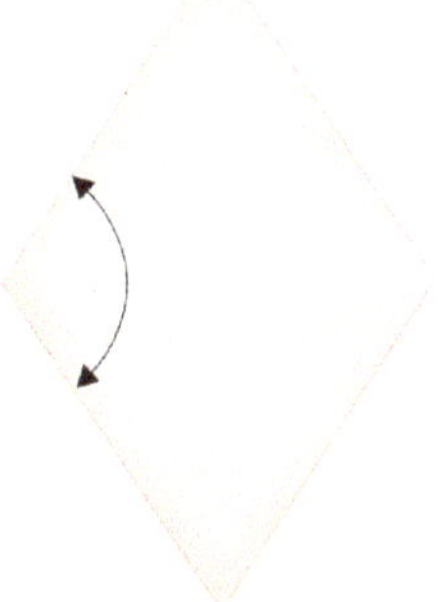

A. 80 degrees

B. 100 degrees

C. 120 degrees

D. 140 degrees

Ans: C. 120 degrees

Q 6. Which of the following lines represents THE VECTOR OF MAXIMAL TENSION in the rhombic flap below?

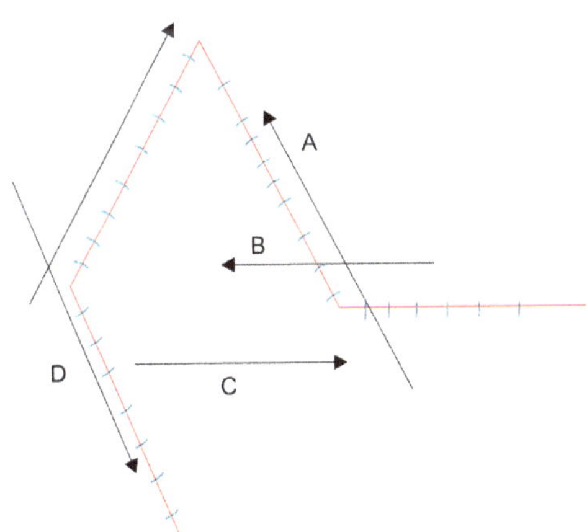

A. A

B. B

C. C

D. D

Ans: A. A

Q 7. The drawing below represents a local flap used to close a facial defect. Which of the following statements BEST describes this reconstructive flap?

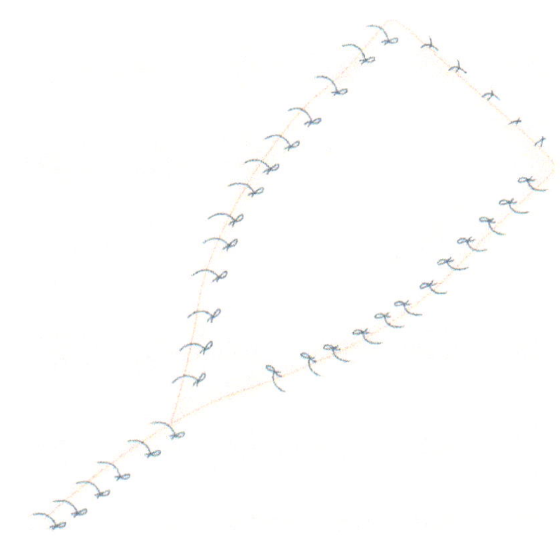

A. Rotation

B. Transposition

C. Advancement

D. Hinge

Ans: C. Advancement

Q 8. The drawing below represents a flap designed to close a defect in the left temple. Which of the following statements is FALSE?

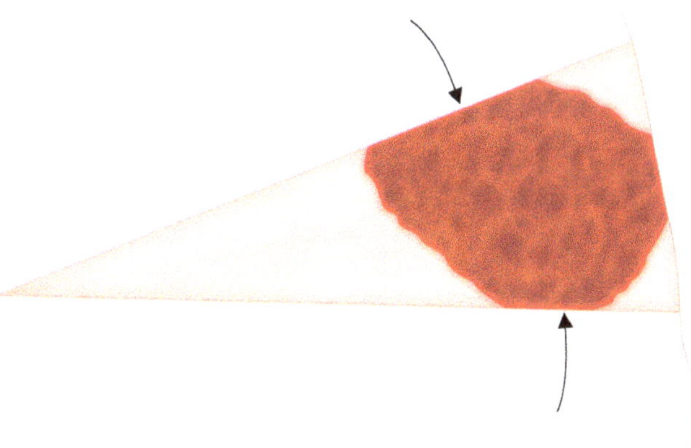

A. It is a O-T flap

B. It has rotation and advancement components

C. It is useful for defects juxtaposed to important aesthetic landmarks

D. The advantage is a very favorable scar running parallel to relaxed skin tension lines (RSTL)

Ans: D. The advantage is a very favorable scar running parallel to relaxed skin tension lines (RSTL)

Q 9. The drawing below represents a rhomboid flap sutured in place. Which of the following areas is the one of MAXIMAL closing tension?

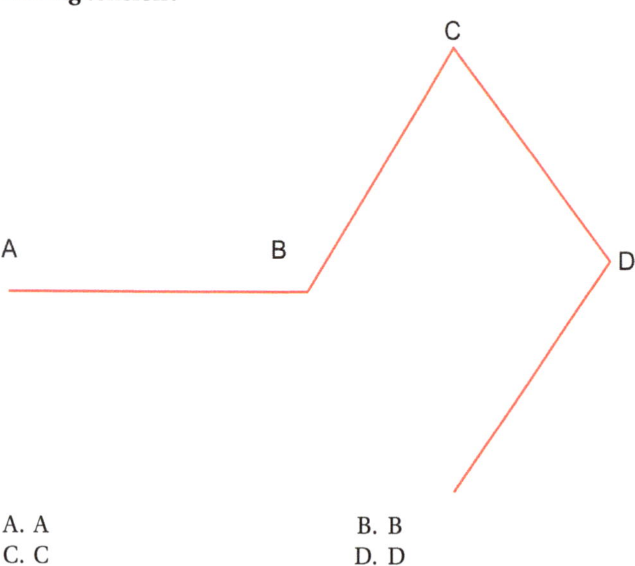

A. A   B. B
C. C   D. D

Ans: B. B

Q 10. Which of the following local flaps is the ONE represented in the drawing below?

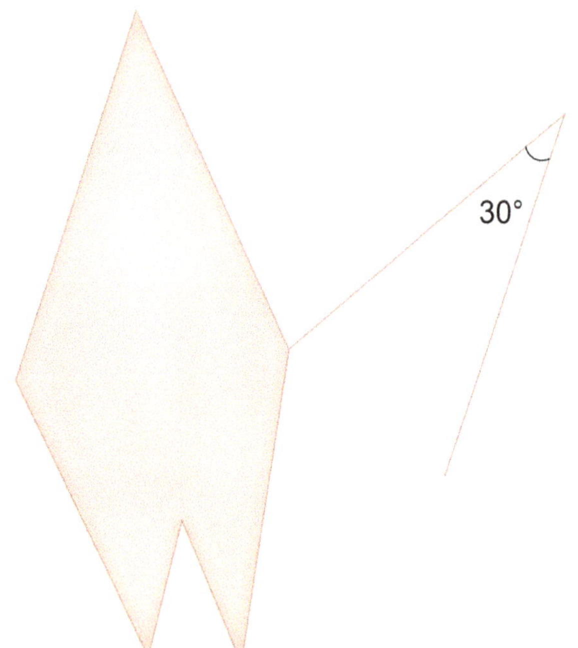

A. Classic rhomboid flap with an M-plasty
B. Limberg flap
C. Webster flap
D. Dufourmentel flap

Ans: C. Webster flap

Q 11. Which of the following local flaps is the one represented in the drawing below?

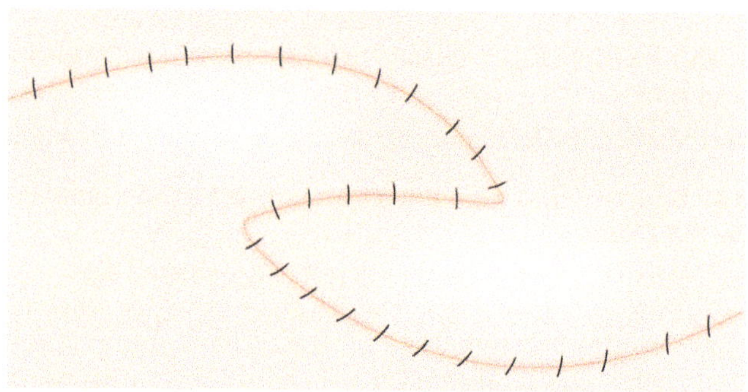

A. Note flap   B. O-T flap
C. O-Z flap   D. V-Y flap

Ans: C. O-Z flap

Q 12. Which of the following is FALSE about local flaps?

A. Provide better donor site match
B. Involve one stage most of the time
C. Based on axial pattern blood supply
D. Allow minimal donor site morbidity

Ans: C. Based on axial pattern blood supply

Q 13. Which of the following statements is TRUE regarding the local flap shown below?

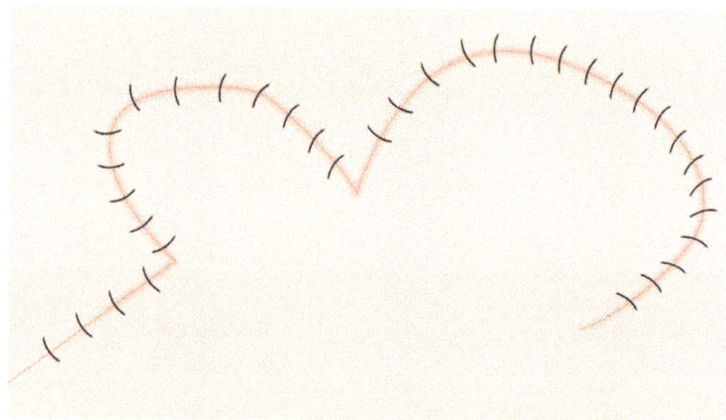

A. The first flap should be ½ the size of the defect
B. The second flap should be slightly smaller than the defect
C. The major disadvantage is a high-risk for pin cushioning
D. This flap distributes tension mainly on the first flap

Ans: C. The major disadvantage is a high risk for pin cushioning

Q 14. Which of the following statements regarding the Zitelli modified bilobe flap is TRUE?

A. Uses narrow angles (60 degrees) between lobes
B. Reduces the pin cushion effect in the nasal skin
C. Best used to repair skin defects of the upper third of the nose
D. Is elevated in the subdermal plane?

Ans: B. Reduces the pin cushion effect in the nasal skin

Q 15. Which of the following statements is TRUE regarding the bilobed flap seen in the drawing below?

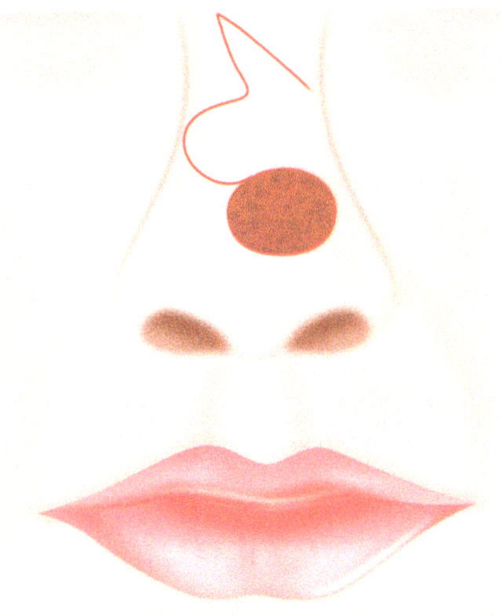

A. It is an advancement/rotation flap
B. It has a total rotation angle of approximately 180 degrees
C. Its major advantage is less pin cushioning compared its counterpart
D. It will leave circular scars that will blend easily with nasal subunits

Ans: C. Its major advantage is less pin cushioning compared its counterpart

Q 16. A nasal subunit deficit will require the removal of the entire subunit, if the percentage of the defect is APPROXIMATELY:

A. 10%–20%
B. 21%–40%
C. 41%–50%
D. 51%–60%

Ans: D. 51%–60%

Q 17. Which of the following statements regarding trap-door deformity is FALSE?

A. It is a bulging elevation of the skin following the use of a transposition flap
B. Early trap-door deformities can be treated with intralesional 1 mL triamcinolone acetonide (40 mg/mL)
C. Long standing trap-door deformities can be treated with multiple Z-plasties
D. Cartilage support replacement during reconstruction will minimize the risk of trap-door formation

Ans: D. Cartilage support replacement during reconstruction will minimize the risk of trap-door formation

Q 18. What PERCENTAGE of shrinkage is expected when using a composite graft of skin and cartilage to correct an alar margin retraction?

A. 1%
B. 5%
C. 10%
D. 20%

Ans: C. 10%

Q 19. Which of the following facial flaps has an AXIAL-PATTERN vascular component?

A. Rhomboid
B. Dufourmentel flap
C. Bilobed flap
D. Nasolabial flap

Ans: D. Nasolabial flap

Q 20. Which of the following techniques is the BEST for reconstruction of a 1.4 cm nose tip defect?

A. Secondary intention
B. Preauricular skin graft
C. Bilobed local flap
D. Nasolabial flap

Ans: C. Bilobed local flap

Q 21. Which of the following statement regarding nasal reconstruction is TRUE?

A. Secondary intention is commonly used to repair small defects of the tip of the nose
B. Large defects involving the tip and ala are best repaired with a nasolabial flap
C. The alar subunit can be repaired with a V-Y flap
D. A small midline defect can be closed primarily leaving a vertical midline scar

Ans: D. A small midline defect can be closed primarily leaving a vertical midline scar

Q 22. Which of the following statements about local flaps is FALSE?

A. Local flaps are accomplished usually in a one stage
B. Local flaps have low donor site morbidity
C. Local flaps have usually an axial pattern blood supply
D. Local flaps do not have enough bulk for deep facial defects

Ans: C. Local flaps have usually an axial pattern blood supply

Q 23. Which of the following is the MOST significant inconvenience of using the costal cartilage for nasal augmentation?

A. Infection
B. Displacement
C. Warping
D. Resorption

Ans: C. Warping

Q 24. Which of the following statements about the reconstruction flap used shown is TRUE?

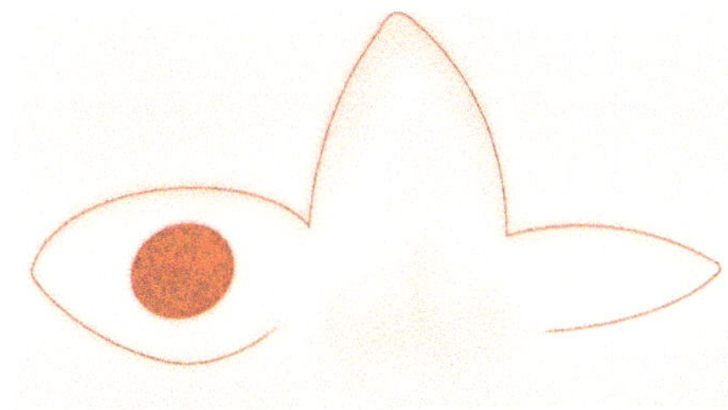

A. Two rotation flaps are used
B. Two advancement flaps are used
C. Two transposition flaps are used
D. One rotation and one transposition flap is used

Ans: C. Two transposition flaps are used

Q 25. Which of the following statements about split-thickness skin grafts (STSGs) is INCORRECT?

A. STSGs contain a portion of the epidermis
B. STSGs have a different texture and lighter color than the neighboring tissue
C. STSGs are cosmetically inferior to full-thickness skin grafts
D. STSGs are less durable than full-thickness skin grafts

Ans: A. STSGs contain a portion of the epidermis

Q 26. What percentage of a full thickness upper eyelid defect can be reconstructed by using THE TENZEL FLAP?

A. 20%   B. 30%
C. 50%   D. 70%

Ans: C. 50%

Q 27. The drawing below depicts the final result after closing a scalp defect. Which of the following flaps is represented?

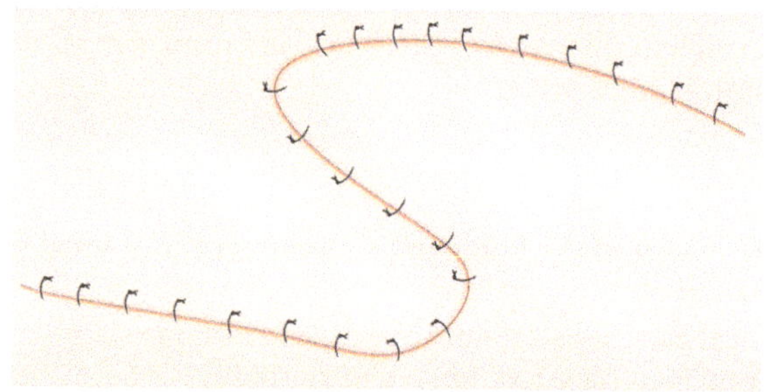

A. Bilateral rotation   B. O-T flap
C. A-T flap   D. Bilobed flap

Ans: A. Bilateral rotation

Q 28. Which of the following defects can be closed with a TRIPLE RHOMBOID flap?

A. A fusiform defect   B. A rectangular defect
C. A circular defect   D. A rhomboid defect

Ans: C. A circular defect

Q 29. Which of the following statements about the reconstruction of the lower eyelid defect depicted in the drawing below is FALSE?

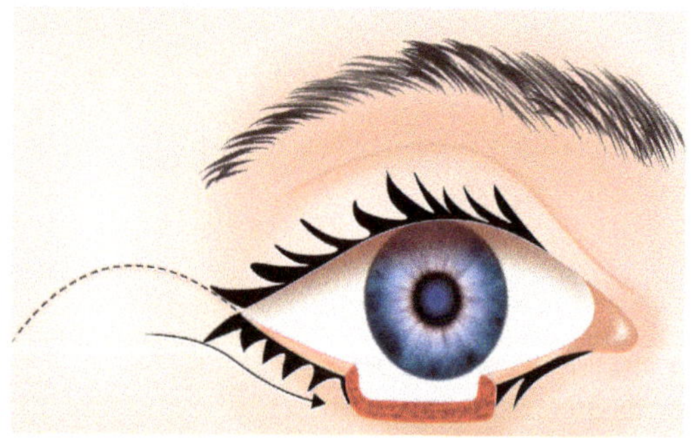

A. The flap is a lateral canthal, semicircular flap
B. The flap is applicable to the lower eyelid only

C. The flap will require canthotomy and cantholysis prior to musculocutaneous elevation
D. The flap is called a Tenzel musculocutaneous flap

Ans: B. The flap is applicable to the lower eyelid only

Q 30. The drawing below represents a transposition flap designed to close a circular defect with a diameter of "d". A tangent is drawn on one side of the circle, parallel to the RSTL. Which of the following measurements represents an adequate proportion between the length "X" and "d"?

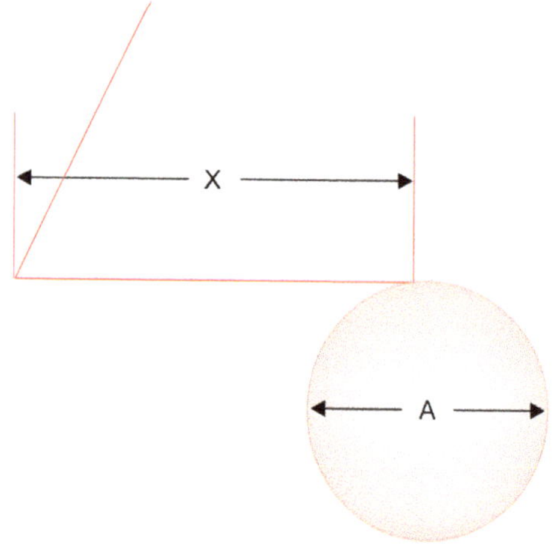

A. X is equal to 1 d   B. X is equal to 1.25 d
C. X is equal to 1.50 d   D. X is equal t o 1.75 d

Ans: C. X is equal to 1.50 d

Q 31. Which of the following statements about the dorsal nasal flap is FALSE?

A. It is a transposition flap
B. It is useful for reconstruction of defects of the distal half of the nasal dorsum
C. The flap is elevated in the submuscular/aponeurotic plane
D. The defect should have a diameter not greater than 2 cm

Ans: A. It is a transposition flap

Q 32. Which of the following flaps is a TRANSPOSITION flap?

A. Paramedian forehead flap   B. Melolabial flap
C. Limberg flap   D. O-T flap

Ans: C. Limberg flap

Q 33. Which of the following is NOT a characteristics of local facial flaps?

A. Similar color and texture
B. Good survival rate
C. Less contracture
D. Good in younger patients

Ans: D. Good in younger patients

Q 34. The drawing below represents a local flap used to closed a circular defect located just below the mid lower eyelid margin. Which of the following statements regarding the flap used is TRUE?

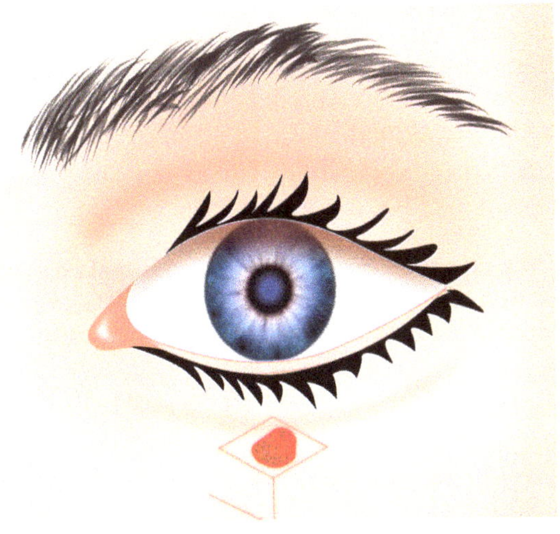

A. It is a Webster flap design
B. It is an improper flap design
C. Most of the scars violate the direction of the RSTLs
D. The vectors of tension are parallel to the eyelid margin

Ans: B. It is an improper flap design

Q 35. Which of the following reconstructive techniques is RARELY used in the repair of nasal defects?

A. Split thickness skin graft
B. Full thickness skin graft
C. Secondary intention healing
D. Bilobed flap

Ans: A. Split thickness skin graft

Q 36. Which of the following is FALSE regarding full thickness skin grafts compared to split thickness skin grafts?

A. Better color
B. Better texture
C. Better survival rate
D. Less contour irregularities

Ans: C. Better survival rate

Q 37. How many possible designs can be constructed with the classic Rhombic flap?

A. 1
C. 3
B. 2
D. 4

Ans: D. 4

Q 38. Which are the amplitude of the angles in the classic Rhombic flap?

A. 30 and 60
C. 60 and 70
B. 60 and 120
D. 45 and 90

Ans: B. 60 and 120

Q 39. Which of the following local facial flap is the ONE represented in the drawing?

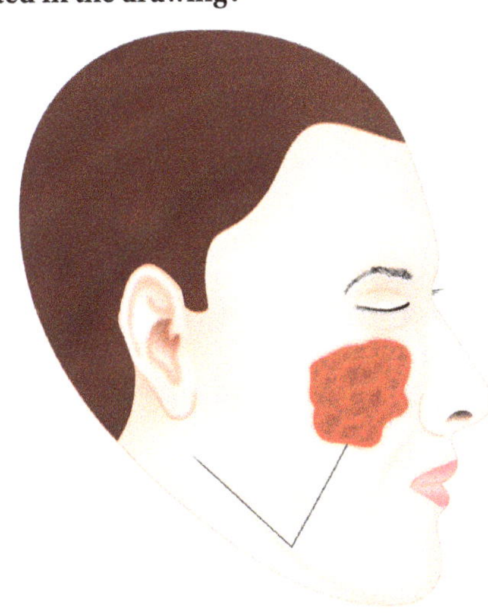

A. Rotation
C. Transposition
B. Interpolation
D. Advancement

Ans: C. Transposition

Q 40. What is the name of the surgical technique used in the repair of the left forehead defect?

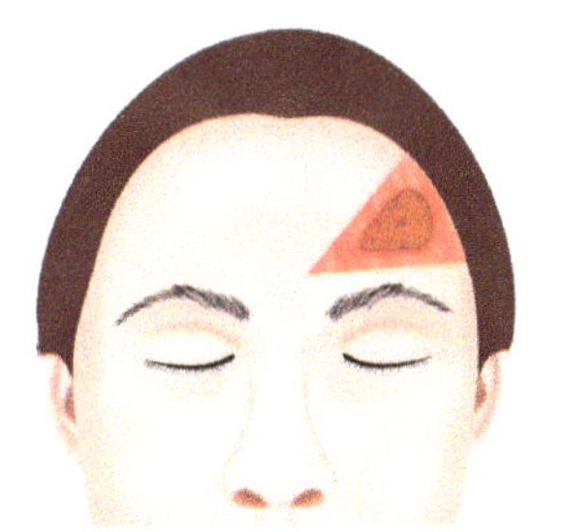
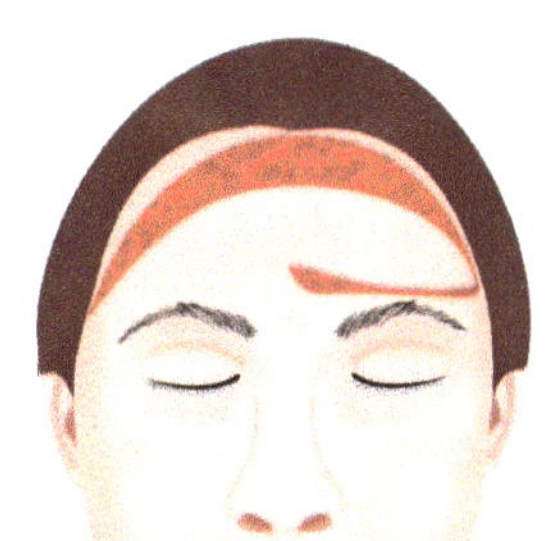
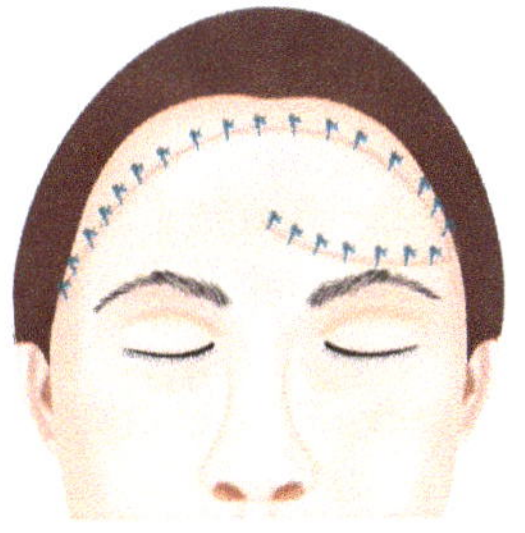

A. Jury flap
C. Orticochea flap
B. Worthen flap
D. Hatchet flap

Ans: B. Worthen flap

Q 41. Which of the following statements is considered a drawback in the use of a single-stage melolabial flap for nasal alar reconstruction?

A. Trap-door deformity
C. Dehiscence
B. Necrosis
D. Stenosis

Ans: A. Trap-door deformity

Q 42. Which of the following organisms is MOST commonly associated with infection produced by medical leeches?

A. *Pseudomonas aeruginosa*   B. *Aeromonas hydrophila*
C. *Bacteroides fragilis*   D. *Staphylococcus aureus*

Ans: B. *Aeromonas hydrophila*

Q 43. Which of the following statements is FALSE about medicinal leech therapy?

A. *Hirudo medicinalis* is the most commonly used leech in compromised flaps
B. *Aeromonas hydrophila* has been found in wound infection when using leeches
C. Monitoring of serum myoglobin is mandatory during leech therapy
D. The use of a third-generation cephalosporin is mandatory for wound infection prophylaxis when using leeches

Ans: C. Monitoring of serum myoglobin is mandatory during leech therapy

Q 44. Which the following surgical managements is the BEST in order to correct a severe right nasal alar retraction?

A. Contralateral cavum concha graft
B. Ipsilateral cavum concha graft
C. Composite cymba concha of the left ear
D. Composite cymba concha of the right ear

Ans: C. Composite cymba concha of the left ear

Q 45. The incidence of infection using alloplastic implants can be REDUCED by soaking the implant with:

A. Gentamicin   B. Erythromycin
C. Methicillin   D. Cefuroxime

Ans: A. Gentamicin

Q 46. Which of the following statements about alloderm is FALSE?

A. Alloderm is fabricated from cadaveric skin
B. Alloderm has an acellular dermis matrix
C. Alloderm carries the complication of migration
D. Alloderm is used as a soft tissue filler and camouflage of grafts

Ans: C. Alloderm carries the complication of migration

Q 47. Which of the following statements regarding cartilage grafts for head and neck augmentation and reconstruction is FALSE?

A. Homologous cartilage grafts resorb more commonly than autografts cartilage
B. Lyophilized cartilage does not need rehydration prior to implantation
C. Nasal autogenous cartilage graft is harvested preserving a dorsal and caudal struts of 10 mm wide
D. Composite helical rim grafting should not be wider than 1.5 cm

Ans: B. Lyophilized cartilage does not need rehydration prior to implantation

Q 48. Which of the following statements about skin graft vascularization is FALSE?

A. Skin grafts initially adhere to the recipient bed by fibrin
B. Skin grafts receive fluid during the first 48 hours by plasmatic imbibition
C. Skin grafts will create after 48 hours connections between preexisting blood vessels and their bed (inosculation)
D. Skin grafts usually attain the normal sensory innervation after healing is complete

Ans: D. Skin grafts usually attain the normal sensory innervation after healing is complete

Q 49. If a skin graft is wrapped in saline soaked gauze and placed in a sterile jar in a refrigerator at 4° C, what is the maximum time that it can be stored before grafting?

A. 72 hours   B. 1 week
C. 2 weeks   D. 3 weeks

An: D. 3 weeks

Q 50. Which of the following statements regarding free composite grafts is FALSE?

A. Inosculation phenomenon occurred within 72 hours
B. Neovascularization phenomenon occurred within 4–5 days
C. Initially the graft will appeared blanched for approximately 24 hours
D. After 24 hours in place the graft becomes cyanotic due to venous congestion

Ans: A. Inosculation phenomenon occurred within 72 hours

Q 51. Which of the following statements about the flap shown below is FALSE?

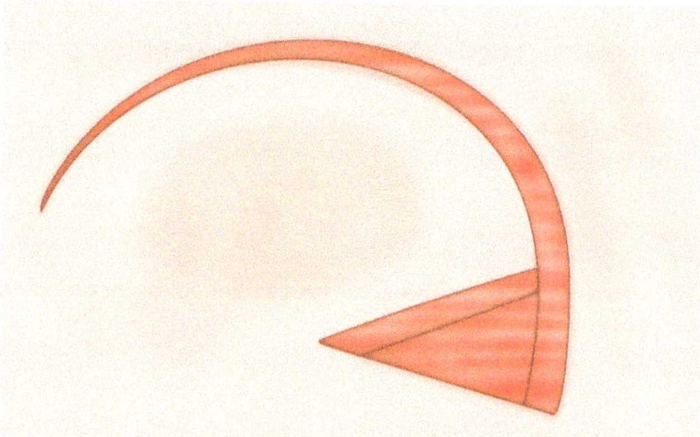

A. The design is a rotation-advancement flap
B. It is useful to close circular cheek defects
C. On the scalp the rotation flap should have 4 times the diameter of the defect
D. Both 90° and 180° arc flaps are used in the design

Ans: C. On the scalp the rotation flap should have 4 times the diameter of the defect

Q 52. Which of the following reconstructive techniques is BEST in order to correct the defect shown in the drawing below?

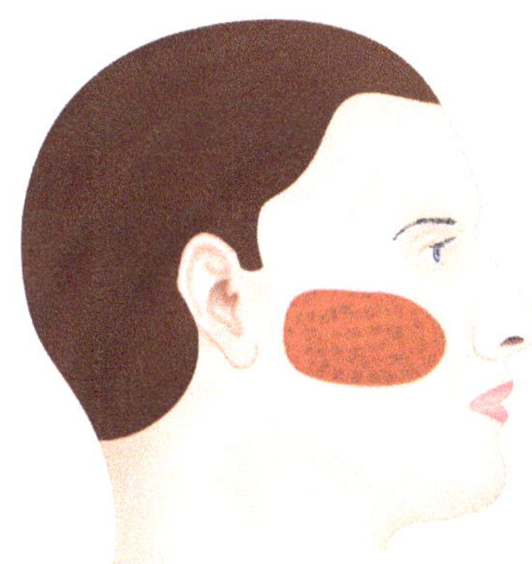

A. Biloped flap

B. Rhomboid flap

C. Bilateral advancement-rotation flap

D. Cheek-neck advancement-rotation flap

Ans: D. Cheek-neck advancement-rotation flap

Q 53. Which of the following facial flaps has a blood supply from the DERMAL AND SUBDERMAL PLEXUS?

A. Nasolabial flap   B. Median forehead flap

C. Dufourmentel flap   D. Lateral forehead flap

Ans: C. Dufourmentel flap

Q 54. Which of the following flaps is the ONE in which the base of the flap is not adjacent to the recipient defect and a second stage is required?

A. Interposition   B. Interpolation

C. Rotation   D. Advancement

Ans: B. Interpolation

Q 55. Which of the following statements is the MOST COMMON COMPLICATION of the cervicofacial rotation-advancement flap?

A. Hematoma   B. Infection

C. Distal ischemic necrosis   D. Facial nerve paralysis

Ans: C. Distal ischemic necrosis

Q 56. Which is the following surgical techniques is BEST for reconstruction of a full-thickness defect involving 40% of the upper lip reaching the oral commissure?

A. Abbé flap   B. Estlander flap

C. Nasolabial flap   D. Rhomboid flap

Ans: B. Estlander flap

Q 57. Which of the following is NOT a topographic subunit of the nose?

A. Nasal dorsum   B. Nasal supratip

C. Nasal tip   D. Soft triangles

Ans: B. Nasal supratip

Q 58. Which of the following areas is NOT appropriate for healing by second intention?

A. Nasal ala

B. Melolabial fold

C. Convex surfaces of the face

D. Posterior auricular sulcus

Ans: C. Convex surfaces of the face

Q 59. Which of the following reconstructive surgical techniques is the BEST for closure of defects encompassing 40% of the lower lip but not involving the oral commissure?

A. The Abbé technique

B. The Estlander technique

C. The Karapandzic technique

D. The Cutler-Beard technique

Ans: A. The Abbé technique

Q 60. Which of the following anatomic sites will heal by the Second-intention with the BEST cosmetic result?

A. Temple   B. Forehead

C. Cheek   D. Chin

Ans: A. Temple

Q 61. Which of the following techniques is the IDEAL for the reconstruction of an upper or lower eyelid defect of up to 50%?

A. Transposition flap

B. Rotational myocutaneous flap from the lateral canthal area, Tenzel flap

C. Two-stage reconstruction, Cutler-Beard technique

D. Two-stage reconstruction, Hughes tarsoconjuntival flap

Ans: B. Rotational myocutaneous flap from the lateral canthal area, Tenzel flap

Q 62. Which of the following surgical techniques have been USED in the reconstruction of the lower lip defect seen in the drawing below?

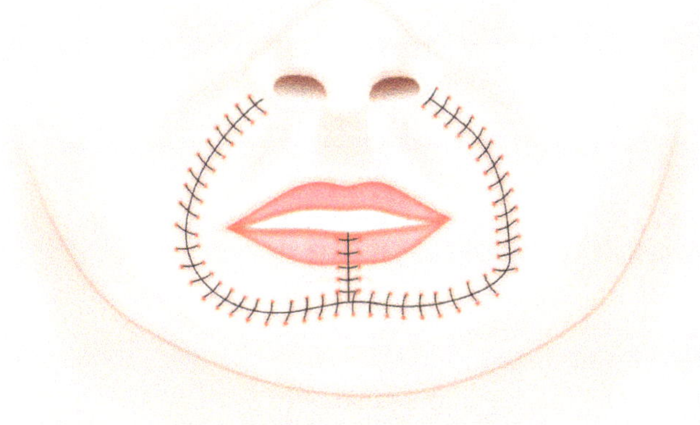

A. Estlander flap   B. Karapandzic flap

C. Bernard-Burrow flap   D. Gillies flap

Ans: B. Karapandzic Flap

Q 63. Which of the following reconstructive techniques is the ONE represented in the drawing below?

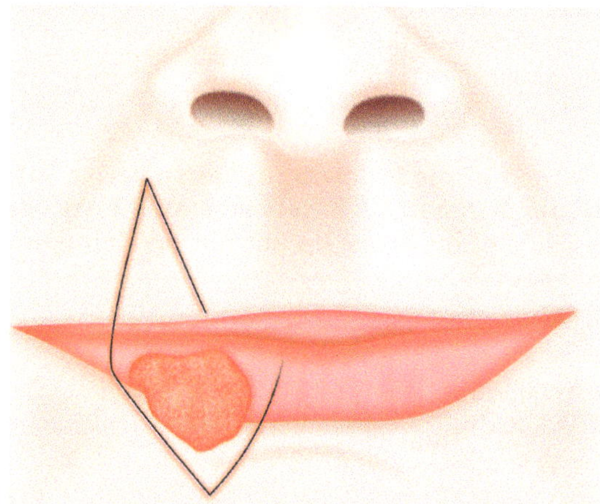

A. Abbé flap
B. Estlander flap
C. Gillies fan flap
D. Bernard-Burrow flap

Ans: A. Abbé flap

Q 64. Which of the following statements regarding nasal reconstruction is TRUE?

A. There are eight aesthetic units in the nose
B. The lobule has thick sebaceous skin
C. The skin of the dorsum is more thick and sebaceous than that of the lobule
D. The structural support of the ala is provided by the lower lateral cartilages

Ans: B. The lobule has thick sebaceous skin

Q 65. Which of the following donor areas for "full-thickness skin graft" is the BEST to cover a superficial defect in the cephalic aspect of the nose?

A. Preauricular
B. Postauricular
C. Supraclavicular
D. Eyelid

Ans: A. Preauricular

Q 66. The number of aesthetic units of the nose is:

A. 6
B. 7
C. 8
D. 9

Ans: D. 9

Q 67. Which of the following statements regarding lip-switch flaps is TRUE?

A. Medial defects are closed with the Estlander flap
B. Commissure defects are closed with the Abbé flap
C. The Abbé flap is a one-stage procedure
D. The Estlander flap usually will require a secondary commissuroplasty

Ans: D. The Estlander flap usually will require a secondary commissuroplasty

Q 68. The reconstructive lip repair represented in the drawing UTILIZES which of the following flaps?

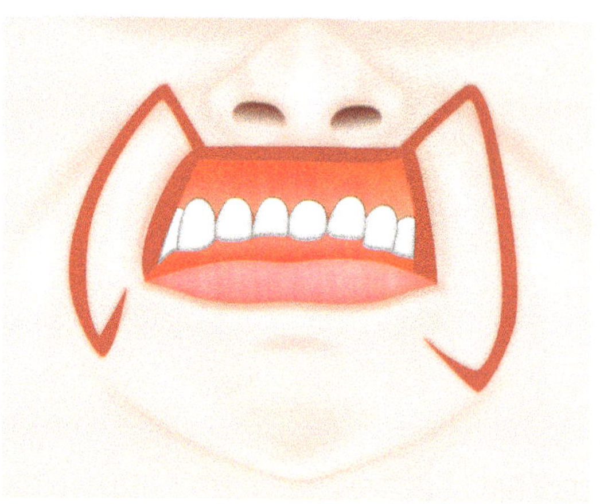

A. Karapandzic flap
B. Abbé flap
C. Estlander flap
D. Gillies flap

Ans: D. Gillies flap

Q 69. Which of the following statements about the Staircase flap used to reconstruct lower lip defects is FALSE?

A. The unilateral staircase flap is useful for lateral lower lip defects of 2 cm or less
B. The bilateral staircase flap is useful for middle and lower lip defects exceeding 2 cm
C. This flap demonstrates wide versatility in closing defects comprising 60% of the lower lip
D. Avoidance of microstomia is one of the advantages of this flap

Ans: D. Avoidance of microstomia is one of the advantages of this flap.

Q 70. Which TECHNIQUE to close a surgical defect of the lower lip is demonstrated in the drawing below?

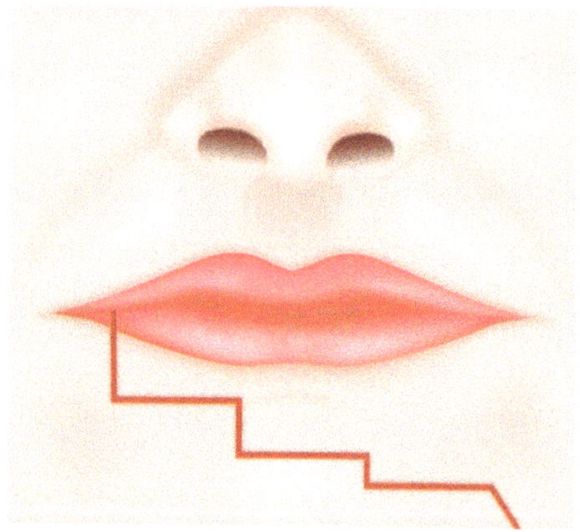

A. Johanson flap
B. Karapandzic flap
C. Parallel Abbé flap
D. Webster flap

Ans: A. Johanson flap

Q 71. Which of the following skin grafts is BEST for covering the anterior floor of the mouth?

A. Split-thickness skin graft (STSG) with 0.005 inches of thickness
B. Split-thickness skin graft with 0.010 inches of thickness
C. Split-thickness skin graft with 0.017 inches of thickness
D. Split-thickness skin graft with 0.025 inches of thickness

Ans: C. Split-thickness skin graft with 0.017 inches of thickness

Q 72. The drawing represents the reconstruction repair of a left upper eyelid defect. Which of the following techniques is REPRESENTED in the picture below?

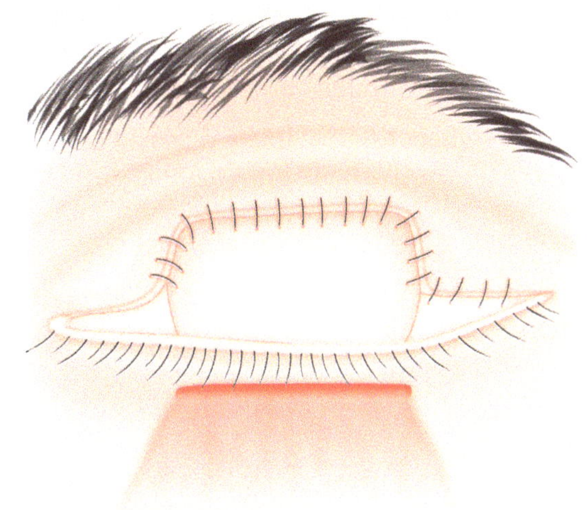

A. Tenzel semicircular flap
B. Mustardé lid repair
C. Cutler-Beard lid repair
D. Hughes flap repair

Ans: C. Cutler-Beard lid repair

Q 73. Which of the following techniques use a semicircular rotational myocutaneous flap from the lateral canthal region to repair a lower or upper eyelid defect of up to 50% of the eyelid margin?

A. Primary closure with lateral canthotomy and inferior cantholysis
B. Tenzel technique
C. Hughes technique
D. Culter-Beard technique

Ans: B. Tenzel technique

Q 74. Which of the following surgical techniques is the BEST for repairing injury to the upper or lower eyelid involving a 25% of tissue loss?

A. Primary closure ± Lateral canthotomy/Lateral cantholysis
B. Semicircular rotation-advancement flap (Tenzel)
C. Pedicled lid switch flap (Mustarde)
D. Bridge flap (Cutler-Beard)

Ans: A. Primary closure ± Lateral Canthotomy/Lateral cantholysis

Q 75. Which of the following reconstruction methods is the LEAST useful for a medium (not possible to use primary closure) midcheek defect ?

A. Secondary intention
B. Rhombic flap
C. Bilobed flap
D. Cheek advancement flap

Ans: A. Secondary intention

Q 76. Which of following statements about Scalp Reconstruction is FALSE?

A. Skin grafting provides a suboptimal cosmetic result
B. Skin grafts will take in pericranium or drilled calvarial bone
C. Local flaps must be designed larger and longer than those in other areas
D. The local flaps used are rotation in design only due to the lack of elasticity

Ans: D. The local flaps used are rotation in design only due to the lack of elasticity

Q 77. Which of the following statements regarding the Arc of Rotation in the scalp is TRUE?

A. The arc of rotation in the scalp should be 3 times the wound diameter
B. The arc of rotation in the scalp should be 4 times the wound diameter
C. The arc of rotation in the scalp should be 5 times the wound diameter
D. The arc of rotation in the scalp should be 6 times the wound diameter

Ans: D. The arc of rotation in the scalp should be 6 times the wound diameter

Q 78. Which of the following statements about the local flap designed below is FALSE?

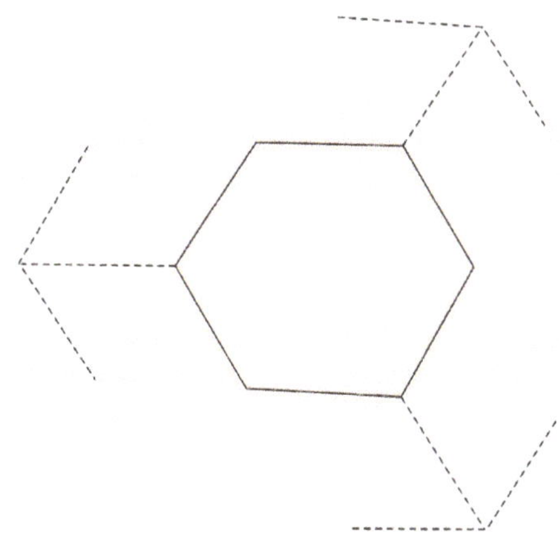

A. It is based on the principles of the Limberg flap
B. It will allow designs in 2 different ways
C. It will closed large circular defects
D. Its main disadvantage is "trap-door" contracture

Ans: D. Its main disadvantage is "trap-door" contracture

Q 79. In a Periocular Surgical Zone II Full-thickness Eyelid Excision, what is the maximal eyelid defect that can be closed primarily with the assistance of canthotomy and cantholysis?

A. Defect less than 30% of eyelid width
B. Defect less than 40% of eyelid width
C. Defect less than 50% of eyelid width
D. Defect less than 60% of eyelid width

Ans: C. Defect less than 50% of eyelid width

Q 80. Which of the eyelid and periocular surgical zones is the one indicate by the letter "X"?

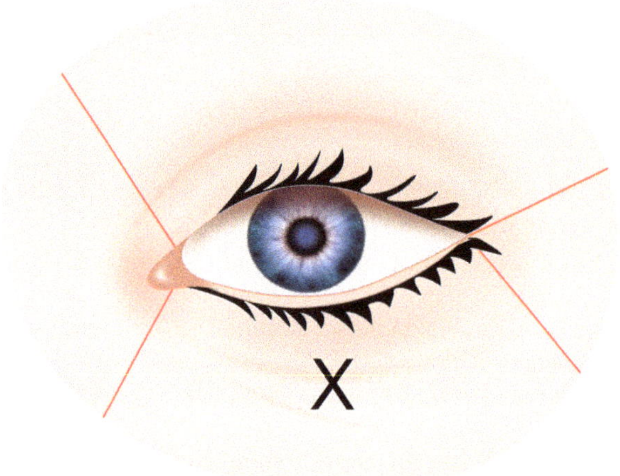

A. Zone I
B. Zone II
C. Zone III
D. Zone IV

Ans: B. Zone II

Q 81. Your must close an 8 cm X 8 cm circular defect on the malar surface of the face of a 47-year-old man, using the "Round Block" "Purse-String" Suture. Multiple large numbers of concentric redundant skin folds are formed with such closure associated with a considerable distortion of nearby structures. Which of the following managements is the best to use in this particular situation?

A. Full thickness skin graft to decrease skin tension
B. Conservative management for 1 month
C. Chemical peeling after healing is completed
D. Botulinum toxin injection during the healing process

Ans: B. Conservative management for 1 month

Q 82. Which of the following reconstruction techniques is THE BEST for closing 9 cm X 12 cm defect of the scalp with bone exposure?

A. Bilateral rotation advancement flap
B. Skin grafting after drilling down to the diploic layer of the bone
C. Pectoralis myocutaneous flap
D. Orticochea "Banana Peel" flap

Ans: D. Orticochea "Banana Peel" flap

Q 83. Which of the following reconstruction lip techniques is UNLIKELY to produce microstomia?

A. Abbé flap
B. Estlander flap
C. Karapandzic flap
D. Gillies flap

Ans: D. Gillies flap

Q 84. Which of the following statements regarding The orticochea ("Banana Peel") flap for scalp defects is FALSE?

A. The technique will require the mobilization of the entire scalp
B. The technique is based in two large and wide scalp flaps
C. The technique will serve well for scalp defects up to 30% of the total scalp area
D. The technique is based on axial flaps

Ans: B. The technique is based in two large and wide scalp flaps

Q 85. When is there near complete return of sensory and motor function after placement of the Abbé Cross Lip Flap?

A. 6 months
B. 8 months
C. 10 months
D. 12 months

Ans: D. 12 months

Q 86. Which of the following flaps is the ONE represented in the drawing below?

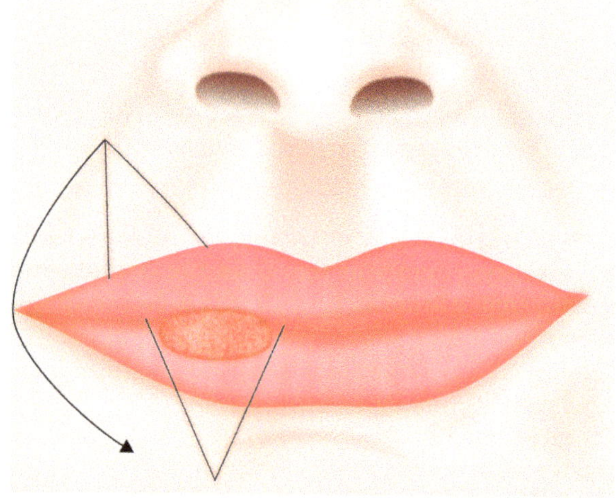

A. McGregor
B. Gillies
C. Abbé
D. Estlander

Ans: C. Abbé

Q 87. Which of the following lip reconstruction techniques is MOST likely responsible for producing a rounded commissure?

A. Bilateral cross-lip flap
B. Estlander flap
C. Bernard-Burrow-Webster flap
D. Gillies flap

Ans: B. Estlander flap

Q 88. Which of the following is FALSE regarding the Hughes procedure for lower eyelid reconstruction?

A. It is one-stage technique of eyelid reconstruction
B. It is used in near total full-thickness lower eyelid defect
C. The tarsoconjuntival flap is combined with a full-thickness skin graft
D. The tarsoconjuntival flap can be combined also with a myocutaneous flap from the lower eyelid

Ans: A. It is one-stage technique of eyelid reconstruction

Q 89. What is the BEST reconstruction option to repair one third full-thickness surgical defect of the lower lip?

A. Primary repair
B. Abbé flap
C. Estlander flap
D. Gillies flap

Ans: A. Primary repair

Q 90. Which of the following statements regarding the "STAIRCASE" method presented below used for lip reconstruction is FALSE?

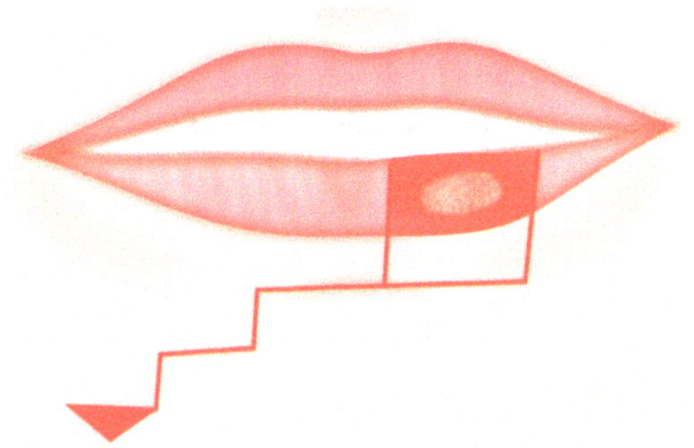

A. It is used for defects greater than two-third of the lower lip
B. The major advantage is the excellent cosmesis and well camouflage skin incision design
C. Each horizontal "step" used in the reconstruction measures half the defect
D. The orbicularis muscle fibers are not altered and the lip innervation is preserved

Ans: B. The major advantage is the excellent cosmesis and well camouflage skin incision design

Q 91. Which of the following anatomic sites will heal by the Second intention with the WORST cosmetic result?

A. Temple
B. Concave surface of the eye
C. Antihelix
D. Chin

Ans: D. Chin

Q 92. Which of the following surgical techniques is the BEST for reconstruction of a full-thickness defect comprising 50% of the upper lip and NOT INVOLVING the oral commissure?

A. Abbé flap
B. Estlander flap
C. Rhomboid flap
D. Nasolabial flap

Ans: A. Abbé flap

Q 93. Which of the following full-thickness eyelid defects is IDEAL for use of the lateral canthotomy with cantholysis technique?

A. 30%
B. 55%
C. 60%
D. 75%

Ans: A. 30%

Q 94. Which of the following facial defect shapes is BEST corrected using a Rotation Flap?

A. Circular
B. Square
C. Rectangular
D. Triangular

Ans: D. Triangular

Q 95. The proper design of an Scalp rotation flap will require:

A. An arc 3 times the diameter of the defect
B. An arc 4 times the diameter of the defect
C. An arc 5 times the diameter of the defect
D. An arc 6 times the diameter of the defect

Ans: D. An arc 6 times the diameter of the defect

Chapter 24

Regional Tissue Transfer for Head and Neck Reconstruction

Catherine Dufour-Fournier

▉ INTRODUCTION

Coverage of defects is always a challenge for surgeons. Many options are available depending on the location and extent of the defect. Grafts consist of a tissue transfer without any vascular supply, relying on neovascularization to survive. Local flaps are flaps with a fixed pedicle, but with often a random vascularization and situated next to the defect. Microvascular free flaps consist of free tissue transfer from a location far from the defect taken with its blood supply, consisting of one or more arteries and veins that are anastomosed to local veins and arteries at the recipient site.

This chapter will cover the subject of axial regional flaps, which are flaps based on a vascular pedicle and used in an axial pattern. They can have one or more main arterial vascular supply that is enough to feed the region used for the flap, called an angiosome.

▉ SELECTED FLAPS

Paramedian Forehead

The paramedian forehead flap is mainly used for nasal defect reconstruction. It can also be used for upper lip or cheek defects. It is based on the supratrochlear artery, a terminal branch of the ophthalmic artery. Its main contraindications include previous radiation, surgery or trauma to the area where the vascular pedicle is located. The main advantages are versatility, ease of harvest, and color match. The main disadvantage of this flap is the need for a multistep procedure in order to eventually divide the pedicle and possible further cosmetic revisions.

Deltopectoral

The deltopectoral flap is less used nowadays due to the wide variety of regional and free flaps available. Its main indications are for pharyngoesophageal reconstruction, but it can also be used for reconstruction of skin defects up the cheek area. The arteries are perforators of the internal mammary. Specific contraindications are previous coronary bypass surgery, mastectomy, pacemaker or pectoralis major flap. Advantages are its ease of harvest and a good color match. Disadvantages are the need for a two-step procedure, the necessity of a skin graft to the donor site and the unreliability of the distal tip of the flap.

Temporoparietal

The temporoparietal flap is a versatile flap for reconstruction of the upper part of the head and neck region. It can be used for auricular reconstruction, orbitomaxillary defects or even skull base reconstruction. The contraindications are trauma, radiation or surgery in the area of the vascular pedicle. The flap is easy to harvest and is very reliable. It could cause alopecia in some cases.

Temporalis

The temporalis flap was initially used to repair various defects of the head and neck region such as oral or oropharyngeal defects. It is now mainly used for reanimation of the midface region in facial paralysis rehabilitation. Its major contraindications are radiation, surgery or trauma to the region of the vascular pedicle. The main advantages of this flap are its ease of harvest and the avoidance of a two-step procedure. The main disadvantage is that when the flap is used for facial reanimation, a skin incision in the nasolabial fold, causing a visible scar, is necessary.

Pectoralis Major

The pectoralis major flap has been the go-to flap for oncological reconstruction of the head and neck for decades and is still widely used as a primary reconstruction option in parts of the world. It is based on the pectoral branch of the thoracoacromial artery, with a minimal contribution from internal mammary artery perforators and the lateral thoracic artery. In Europe and North America, it is now mostly used for vessel coverage in previously irradiated patients or for salvage surgery. It has no major contraindication and can even be used if the donor site and artery has been irradiated in the past. The pectoralis major flap has a wide variety of advantages, including its ease of harvest, its versatility and reliability, its rich vascularity and its ability to cover large areas. On the other hand, this flap can be bulky and its

Table 1: Summary of regional tissue transfer for head and neck reconstruction					
Flap	*Main artery*	*Indications*	*Contraindications*	*Advantages*	*Disadvantages*
Paramedian forehead	Supratrochlear	Main: Nasal defect Other: Upper lip Cheek	Radiation/Surgery/ Trauma to the area of the vascular pedicle	Easy to harvest Versatility Color match	Multistep procedure
Deltopectoral	Internal mammary	Pharyngoesophageal reconstruction Skin defects up to the cheek	Previous coronary bypass surgery Prior mastectomy, pacemaker or pectoralis major flap	Easy to harvest Color match	Two-stages Can require skin graft Unreliable distal tip
Temporoparietal	Superficial temporal	Auricular reconstruction Orbitomaxillary defects Skull base reconstruction	Radiation/Surgery/ Trauma to the area of the vascular pedicle	Ease of harvest Reliability	Alopecia
Temporalis	Anterior and posterior deep temporal	Main: Facial paralysis rehabilitation (midface) Other: Oral, oropharyngeal, nasopharyngeal defects	Radiation/Surgery/ Trauma to the area of the vascular pedicle	Ease of harvest Avoidance of a two-stage flap	External scar
Pectoralis major	Pectoral branch of thoracoacromial	Vessel coverage in previously irradiated patients Salvage surgery	No major contraindications	Ease of harvest Reliable Versatile Rich vascularity Covers a lot of territory	Bulky Limited reach above zygoma Breast area deformation
Latissimus dorsi	Thoracodorsal artery	Defects of most sites of the head and neck	Previous axillary dissection	Ease of harvest Reliable Versatile Can reach above zygoma up to vertex	Requires patient repositioning Can be bulky Difficulty in tunneling flap in the axilla

Trapezius
  Superior island
  Lateral island
  Lower island
	Paraspinal perforators Transverse cervical Dorsal scapular	Superior: Posterolateral neck defects Lateral: Lateral and anterior neck defects Lower: Posterior neck and scalp defects	Radiation/Surgery/ Trauma to the area of the vascular pedicle	Ease of harvest Color match	Requires patient repositioning Two-stages Can require skin graft Shoulder mobility

SCM	Superior: Occipital Inferior: Transverse cervical	Mucosal and cutaneous defects Contour restoration	Previous neck dissection	Ease of harvest Color match	Contour deformity Limited use with neck dissection Limited size skin paddle Unreliable skin paddle
FAMM	Facial or angular	Inferiorly based: Floor of mouth, tongue, retromolar trigone defect Superiorly based: Palate defects	Previous neck dissection Previous neck irradiation Oral cavity diffuse dysplasia	Ease of harvest Reconstruct mucosal defects with mucosa	Two-stages Vulnerable pedicle

(SCM: Sternocleidomastoid; FAMM: Facial artery musculomucosal).

harvest can cause visible deformities of the chest area. It also has a limited reach above the zygoma.

Summary of regional tissue transfer for head and neck reconstruction is given in Table 1.

Latissimus Dorsi

The latissimus dorsi flap is based on the thoracodorsal artery. This flap is a versatile flap used for most defects of the head and neck region. The only specific contraindication for this flap is a previous axillary dissection. The flap is easy to harvest, reliable, versatile and can reach above the vertex for reconstruction purposes. The insetting of the flap is its main disadvantage, because of its bulk and the difficulty to tunnel it through the axilla. The harvesting and the insetting of the flap are also done in different patient positions on the table, requiring to reposition the patient during surgery.

Trapezius

The trapezius flap can be divided in three individual flaps, all coming from the same area but with a different axial vascularization and utilization. The superior island flap is based on the paraspinal perforators and is used for posterolateral neck defects. The lateral island flap is based on the transverse cervical artery and is used for lateral and anterior neck defects. The lower island flap is based on the dorsal scapular artery and is used for posterior neck and scalps defects. The only contraindication to the use of theses flaps is trauma, surgery or radiation in the area of the vascular pedicle. All three types of trapezius flaps are easy to harvest and give a good color match. However, harvesting the flaps requires prone positioning, and the procedure could be a two-stage procedure. Moreover, it could require a skin graft and the shoulder mobility can be affected.

Sternocleidomastoid

The sternocleidomastoid (SCM) flap is used for different mucosal and cutaneous defects, but is particularly useful for contour restoration after surgeries like parotidectomy. It can be based on two arteries depending of which part of the muscle and skin is harvested. The superior part is based on the occipital artery and the inferior part on the transverse cervical artery. However, it is not possible to use this flap in the context of a previous neck dissection, making it a lot harder to use in an oncological context. The flap is relatively easy to harvest and gives a good color match, but the available skin paddle is very small and poorly reliable. Removing part of the SCM on one side for the flap gives rise to contour deformity that can be unsightly.

Facial Artery Musculomucosal

The facial artery musculomucosal (FAMM) flap is primarily used for the repair of mucosal defects of the oral cavity. This flap can be pedicled superiorly or inferiorly on the facial/angular artery. When inferiorly based, its main indications are tongue, floor of the mouth and retromolar trigone defects. When superiorly based it is mainly used for palatal repairs. It is not recommended to use it when there if diffuse dysplasia of the oral cavity and a history of neck dissection or irradiation. This flap is the only one that covers mucosal defects with mucosa. It is relatively easy to harvest. A disadvantage is that it can be a two-step procedure and that the vascular pedicle is vulnerable, particularly if it is inserted between the upper and lower teeth.

■ CONCLUSION

There are many options available for the reconstructive surgeon in the head and neck. When evaluating a patient preoperatively, one needs to always address the problem to come keeping all options in mind. Regional axial flaps are, for the most part, easy to harvest with generally reliable and good results. Most defects can be covered using one of the many regional flap options. In the actual era of free flaps and microvascular reconstruction, the place of regional axial flap has greatly diminished, but it is important not to forget their existence and usefulness in a vast array of situations.

■ BIBLIOGRAPHY

1. Al Felasi MA, Bissada E, Ayad T. Reconstruction of an inferior orbital rim and cheek defect with a pedicled osteomyocutaneous submental flap. Head Neck. 2016;38:E64-7.
2. Ayad T, Xie L. Facial artery musculomucosal flap in head and neck reconstruction: a systematic review. Head Neck. 2015;37:1375-86.
3. Blondeel PN, Van Landuyt KH, Monstrey SJ, et al. The Gent consensus on perforator flap terminology: preliminary definitions. Plast Reconstr Surg. 2003;112:1378-83.
4. Braasch DC, Lam D, Oh ES. Maxillofacial reconstruction with nasolabial and facial artery musculomucosal flaps. Oral Maxillofac Surg Clin North Am. 2014;26:327-33.
5. Fernandes R. Local and Regional Flaps in Head & Neck Reconstruction: A Practical Approach. Ames, Iowa: John Wiley & Sons Inc.; 2014.
6. Gullane PJ, Arena S. Palatal island flap for reconstruction of oral defects. Arch Otolaryngol. 1977;103:598-9.
7. Helling ER, Okoro S, Kim G 2nd, et al. Endoscope-assisted temporoparietal fascia harvest for auricular reconstruction. Plast Reconstr Surg. 2008;121:1598-605.
8. Janis JE (Ed). Essentials of Plastic Surgery, 2nd edition. St. Louis, Missouri Boca Raton: Quality Medical Publishing, CRC Press/Taylor & Francis Group; 2014.
9. Levin LS. The reconstructive ladder. An orthoplastic approach. Orthop Clin North Am. 1993;24:393-409.
10. McGregor IA, Morgan G. Axial and random pattern flaps. Br J Plast Surg. 1973;26:202-13
11. Mathes SJ, Nahai F. Classification of the vascular anatomy of muscles: experimental and clinical correlation. Plast Reconstr Surg. 1981;67:177-87.
12. Millard DR Jr. Wide and/or short cleft palate. Plast Reconstr Surg Transplant Bull. 1962;29:40-57.

13. Moubayed SP, Labbe D, Rahal A. Lengthening temporalis myoplasty for facial paralysis reanimation: an objective analysis of each surgical step. JAMA Facial Plast Surg. 2015;17:179-82.
14. Moubayed SP, Rahal A, Ayad T. The submental island flap for soft-tissue head and neck reconstruction: step-by-step video description and long-term results. Plast Reconstr Surg. 2014;133:684-6.
15. Nicoli F, Orfaniotis G, Gesakis K, et al. Supraclavicular osteocutaneous free flap: clinical application and surgical details for the reconstruction of composite defects of the nose. Microsurgery. 2015;35:328-32.
16. Parhiscar A, Har-El G, Turk JB, et al. Temporoparietal osteofascial flap for head and neck reconstruction. J Oral Maxillofac Surg. 2002;60:619-22.
17. Pribaz J, Stephens W, Crespo L, et al. A new intraoral flap: facial artery musculomucosal (FAMM) flap. Plast Reconstr Surg. 1992;90:421-9.
18. Rigby MH, Hayden RE. Regional flaps: a move to simpler reconstructive options in the head and neck. Curr Opin Otolaryngol Head Neck Surg. 2014;22:401-6.
19. Sataloff RT. Sataloff's Comprehensive Textbook of Otolaryngology: Head and Neck Surgery. New Delhi: Jaypee Brothers Medical Publishers; 2015.
20. Smart RJ, Yeoh MS, Kim DD. Paramedian forehead flap. Oral Maxillofac Surg Clin North Am. 2014;26:401-10.
21. Urken ML. Atlas of Regional and Free Flaps for Head and Neck Reconstruction: Flap Harvest and Insetting, 2nd edition. Philadelphia: Wolters Kluwer Health/Lippincott Williams & Wilkins; 2012.

Self-assessment Exercise

Q 1. What are the rungs of the reconstructive ladder?

Ans:
- Secondary intention
- Primary intention
- Delayed primary closure
- Skin grafting
- Tissue expansion
- Local tissue transfer
- Free tissue transfer

Q 2. Describe the Mathes and Nahai classification of musculovascular pedicles.

Ans:
- Type I – Single pedicle
- Type II – Single dominant pedicle in mid belly of muscle, several minor distally (platysma, SCM, trapezius)
- Type III – Two dominant pedicles (orbicularis oris, rectus abdominis)
- Type IV – Multiple similar size pedicles along the belly
- Type V – Single dominant pedicle and multiple secondary segmental pedicles (pectoralis major, latissimus dorsi)

Q 3. Name five classification schemes for flaps.

Ans:
- Vascularity
- Composition
- Method of transfer
- Geometric shape
- Method of local transfer (local flaps)

Q 4. What are the four main types of local flaps?

Ans:
- Advancement – Monopedicled, Bipedicled, V-Y, or Hinged
- Rotation
- Transposition (Rhomboid, Dufourmental, Bilobed)
- Interpolation– Linear, can be classified as pivotal, but base located some distance away from defect (Paramedian Forehead, Nasolabial, Postauricular)

Q 5. Name the blood supply of the following regional skin flaps (paramedian forehead, temporoparietal, nasolabial, SCM, trapezius, deltopectoral, pectoralis major).

Ans:
Paramedian forehead – Supratrochlear and supraorbital arteries
Temporoparietal – Superficial temporal artery and vein
Nasolabial – Angular artery of the facial
SCM –
- Upper third: Occipital (dominant); secondary branches from posterior auricular
- Middle third: Superior thyroid
- Lower third: Suprascapular (most common), transverse cervical or thyrocervical trunk direct branch

Trapezius –
- Lateral island flap: Transverse cervical (dominant)
- Superior island flap: Occipital and paraspinous perforators
- Inferior (lower) island flap: Descending branch of transverse cervical and dorsal scapular

Deltopectoral – 1st-4th perforators from internal mammary artery
Pectoralis major – Thoracoacromial artery, lateral thoracic (supplies inferior 1/5th), and internal mammary artery perforators

Q 6. Name the four contraindications to a palatal island flap.

Ans:
- Defect larger than remaining palate
- Absence of internal maxillary artery
- Prior palatal surgery
- Prior radiation therapy

Q 7. Name three regional flaps that are also commonly used as microvascular free flaps.

Ans:
- Temporoparietal fascial flap
- Submental island flap
- Latissimus dorsi flap

Q 8. Name ten bone-containing regional flaps.

Ans:

- Temporoparietal osteofascial flap
- Submental island osteomyocutaneous
- Supraclavicular osteocutaneous flap
- Deltopectoral acromion flap
- Temporalis-calvarial flap
- Trapezius osteomyocutaneous
- SCM osteomyocutaneous
- Pectoralis major and sternum
- Pectoralis major and rib
- Latissimus dorsi and rib

Q 9. What planes are found above and below the temporoparietal fascial flap?

Ans:

- Deep to the flap is the superficial layer of the deep temporal fascia
- Superficial to the flap is the skin and subcutaneous tissue

Q 10. Name six advantages of the pectoralis major flap.

Ans:

- Rich vascularity
- Large skin territory
- Ability to close skin primarily
- Long arc of rotation
- Good bulk
- Ease of harvest

Multiple Choice Questions

Q 1. Which of the following statements about the paramedian forehead flap is FALSE?

A. It is an axial flap
B. It is mostly supplied by the infratrochlear vessels
C. It is useful for reconstruction of any or all nasal subunits
D. The single-vessel paramedian forehead flap has a pedicle of approximately 1.5 cm wide at its origin

Ans: B. It is mostly supplied by the infratrochlear vessels

Q 2. Which of the following regarding the diagnosis of flap venous congestion is FALSE?

A. A pinprick demonstrates dark venous blood
B. The flap has an edematous appearance
C. The flap has a purplish blue color
D. The flap's color blanches with pressure but does not refill

Ans: D. The flap's color blanches with pressure but does not refill

Q 3. Which is the following statements regarding the Trapezius Myocutaneous Flap is TRUE?

A. The lateral trapezius island myocutaneous flap is the most reliable of the three trapezius flaps
B. The superior trapezius myocutaneous flap is the least reliable of the three trapezius flaps

C. The superior trapezius myocutaneous flap is not compromised by neck dissection
D. The lateral trapezius island is based on the paraspinous perforator arteries

Ans: C. The superior trapezius myocutaneous flap is not compromised by neck dissection

Q 4. Which of the following Pedicle Flaps has the LARGEST AREA of tissue transfer and the GREATEST REACH of any:

A. Pectoralis major flap
B. Latissimus dorsi flap
C. Temporalis muscle flap
D. Trapezius flap

Ans: B. Latissimus dorsi flap

Q 5. Which statement regarding the Latissimus Dorsi Musculocutaneous Flap is FALSE?

A. It has an axial blood supply from the thoracodorsal artery
B. The thoracodorsal nerve innervates the latissimus dorsi
C. The skin paddle width can reach more than 10 cm
D. Primary closure is always possible even in large skin paddle defects

Ans: D. Primary closure is always possible even in large skin paddle defects

Q 6. Which of following statements regarding facial flap survival is FALSE?

A. Delaying the flap involves incising the borders and leaving it "in situ" for 2 weeks
B. Hyperbaric oxygen has a proven beneficial effect on facial flaps with arterial ischemia
C. Most common vascular problems in facial flaps are due to congestion
D. Medicinal leeches are beneficial when arterial ischemia is present

Ans: D. Medicinal leeches are beneficial when arterial ischemia is present

Q 7. Which of following aesthetic nasal subunits is BEST resurfaced using a melolabial interpolation flap?

A. Lobule
B. Ala
C. Dorsum
D. Sidewall

Ans: B. Ala

Q 8. When is the PROPER time to divide the paramedian forehead flap?

A. 7 days
B. 14 days
C. 21 days
D. 30 days

Ans: C. 21 days

Q 9. The BAKAMJIAN FLAP has its blood supply from:

A. The transverse cervical artery
B. The perforating branches of the internal mammary artery
C. The thoracodorsal artery
D. The thoracoacromial artery

Ans: B. The perforating branches of the internal mammary artery

Q 10. Execution of the Juri Flap is accomplished in HOW MANY STAGES?

A. 1   B. 2
C. 3   D. 4

Ans: D. 4

Q 11. Which of the following statements regarding the superior trapezius flap is TRUE?

A. It is the least reliable of the three trapezius flaps
B. Its blood supply is the transverse and dorsal scapular arteries
C. Its blood supply is compromised by a previous neck dissection
D. It is a reliable flap for coverage of exposed major neck vessels after radiation therapy

Ans: D. It is a reliable flap for coverage of exposed major neck vessels after radiation therapy

Q 12. Which of the following statements related to the classification of the midforehead flap is TRUE?

A. It is a rotation flap   B. It is a transposition flap
C. It is an interpolation flap   D. It is a hinged flap

Ans: C. It is an interpolation flap

Q 13. Which of the following represents THE PERCENTAGE of a muscle atrophy occurring after muscular flap transfer?

A. 10%   B. 20%
C. 30%   D. 40%

Ans: D. 40%

Q 14. Which of the following arteries is the one indicated by the black arrow in the drawing below?

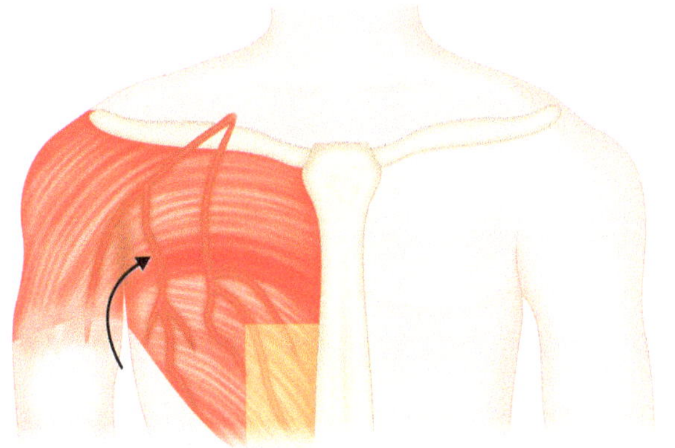

A. Thoracoacromial artery   B. Lateral thoracic artery
C. Transverse cervical artery   D. Dorsal scapular artery

Ans: B. Lateral thoracic artery

Q 15. Which of the following statements regarding the flap below is FALSE?

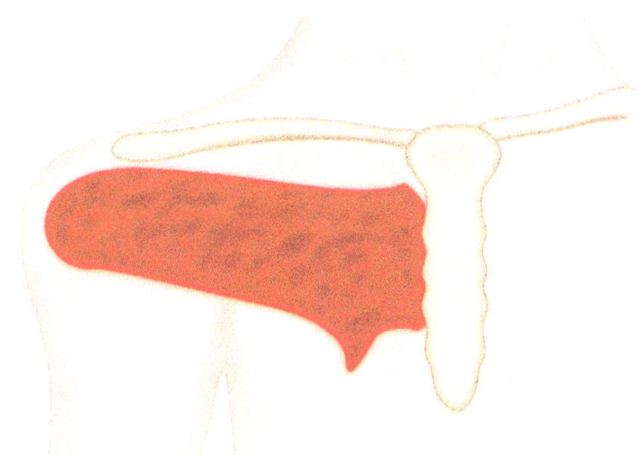

A. It is based on the branches from the internal mammary arterial system
B. It perfused predominately by the first internal mammary artery
C. 2/3 of medial aspect an Axial flap, and the distal third is a Random flap
D. The deltoid and pectoralis fascias are included in the flap

Ans: B. It perfused predominately by the first internal mammary artery

Q 16. Which of the following reconstructive flaps is THE BEST CHOICE after wound breakdown with exposed major neck vessels post radical neck dissection and radiation therapy?

A. Deltopectoral flap   B. Lateral trapezius flap
C. Lower trapezius flap   D. Superior trapezius flap

Ans: D. Superior trapezius flap

Q 17. Which of the following events is MOST commonly associated with the Superior Trapezius Flap?

A. Necrosis   B. Dehiscence
C. Venous congestion   D. Limited arc of rotation

Ans: D. Limited arc of rotation

Q 18. Which of the following represents an INCORRECT relationship between flap and blood supply?

A. Rectus myocutaneous free flap - deep superior epigastric vessels
B. Forehead flap/Supraorbital and supratrochlear arteries
C. Latissimus dorsi flap/Thoracodorsal artery
D. Deltopectoral flap/Internal mammary arteries

Ans: A. Rectus Myocutaneous free flap - deep superior epigastric vessels

Q 19. Which of the following statements about the anterior scalping flap of Converse is INCORRECT?

A. It is an option for reconstruction of subtotal or total nasal tissue losses

B. Most of the incision is hidden behind the hairline
C. The working portion of the flap is raised from the medial portion of the forehead
D. The defect in the forehead is filled with a full thickness skin graft (FTSG) from the postauricular area

Ans: C The working portion of the flap is raised from the medial portion of the forehead

Q 20. Which of the following reconstructive techniques will give the BEST cosmetic result in the repair of a defect of the entire lobule of the nose?

A. Full thickness skin graft
B. Bilobed flap of the dorsum
C. Nasolabial flap
D. Paramedian forehead flap

Ans: D. Paramedian forehead flap

Q 21. Which of the following arteries is the one represented in the drawing below?

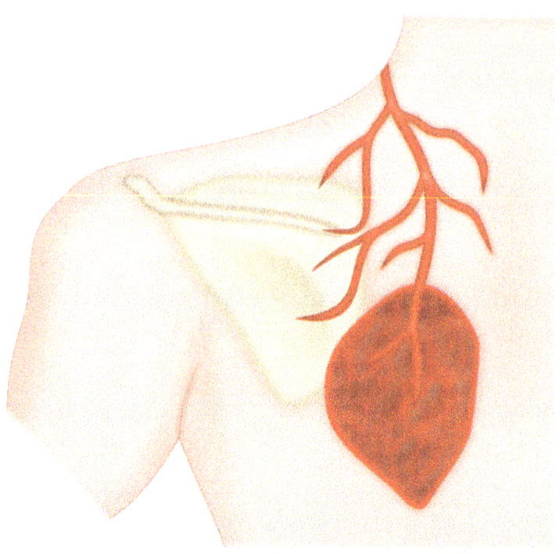

A. Occipital artery
B. Paravertebral perforators arteries
C. Transverse cervical artery
D. Dorsal scapular artery

Ans: C. Transverse cervical artery

Q 22. The paramedian forehead flap has its BLOOD SUPPLY from:

A. The supraorbital artery
B. The supratrochlear artery
C. The angular artery
D. The anterior branch of the superficial temporal artery

Ans: B. The supratrochlear artery

Q 23. A patient has a partial thickness defect of approximately 12 mm in the right nasal ala after using Mohs' microsurgery for a squamous cell carcinoma. Which of the following reconstructive techniques is the BEST in this particular case?

A. Full thickness skin grafting
B. Full thickness skin grafting after granulation tissue is formed in the surgical bed
C. Nasolabial flap
D. Bilobed flap

Ans: C. Nasolabial flap

Q 24. Which of the following reconstructive techniques is the BEST for a surface nasal defect involving the columella and lobule?

A. Paramedian forehead flap
B. Bilobed flap of the dorsum
C. Rhomboid flap of the dorsum
D. Full thickness skin graft

Ans: A. Paramedian forehead flap

Chapter 25

Free Tissue Transfer in Head and Neck Reconstruction

Brittany Barber, Khalid Ansari, Daniel O'Connell, Hadi Seikaly

■ INTRODUCTION

The latter half of the twentieth century brought a remarkable evolution in reconstruction of defects of the head and neck with the era of microvascular reconstruction. We have seen impressive advances and refinements in techniques, donor sites, and monitoring, leading to widespread use of free tissue transfer in head and neck reconstruction.[1] This chapter reviews free tissue transfer options, intraoperative considerations, and postoperative management of patients undergoing major head and neck cancer reconstruction.

■ MUSCLE AND MYOCUTANEOUS FLAPS

Rectus Abdominis

The rectus flap can be harvested as a muscle, myofascial, myosubcutaneous, or myocutaneous flap, as well as a rotational flap.[2]

Advantages of the rectus flap include the convenient two-team approach, an inconspicuous donor site, a large volume of soft tissue, and a long pedicle. Applications of the rectus flap include large soft tissue replacement such as in total glossectomy, skull base reconstruction, and extensive scalp reconstructions. The arcuate line is used as a landmark for the deep inferior epigastric (DIE). Below the arcuate line, the posterior rectus sheath is absent, meaning that the anterior rectus sheath may not be harvested below this line and must be reapproximated to avoid herniation.

Anatomy

- *Artery*: Deep inferior epigastric and deep superior epigastric (DSE) arteries.
- *Vein*: Deep inferior epigastric and deep superior epigastric veins.
- *Nerve*: Intercostal nerves; no reliable neurotization.

Latissimus Dorsi

The latissimus dorsi free flap was initially utilized for its large quantity of soft tissue in skull base reconstruction. Later descriptions of an innervated flap allowed for its utility in total glossectomy and large scalp defects (with skin grafting).[3,4] The latissimus flap can be elevated with the subscapular system of flaps, allowing for additional soft tissue bulk with a bony component. It is also more recently used for single-stage facial reanimation.

Anatomy

- *Artery*: Thoracodorsal artery (primary, enters the latissimus muscle 8–10 cm below midaxilla level) and intercostal perforating vessels (secondary).
- *Vein*: Thoracodorsal vein.
- *Nerve*: Thoracodorsal nerve (branch of posterior cord of brachial plexus).[5,6]

Gracilis

The gracilis flap was initially popularized for facial reanimation.[7] Its thin muscle can be reinnervated to restore synchronous mimetic movement when the proximal aspect of the facial nerve is not available, using a two-stage procedure with a cross-face sural nerve graft. The skin paddle is supplied by musculocutaneous perforators in the proximal third, with unpredictable vascularity. Therefore, the gracilis is usually used as a muscle-only flap.

Anatomy

- *Artery*: Terminal branch of the adductor artery.
- *Vein*: Venae comitantes.
- *Nerve*: Anterior branch of the obturator nerve.[8]

■ FASCIAL AND FASCIOCUTANEOUS FLAPS

Radial Forearm

The radial forearm free flap (RFFF) is considered the workhorse flap in head and neck reconstruction for its versatility, reliable anatomy, long pedicle, and accessible donor site.[9] Applications for the RFFF include small (<200 cm^2) defects of the oral cavity, oropharynx, hypopharynx, total pharyngoesophagus, palate, skin and scalp, and skull base.

An incomplete superficial palmar arch and/or lack of communication between deep and superficial palmar arch; combination of both puts blood supply to thumb and forefinger at risk. Therefore, the flap requires a negative preoperative Allen's test.

10 to 12 cm of radius with less than or equal to 40% circumference can be harvested for osseous reconstruction.

It can be transferred with palmaris longus or brachioradialis muscle for total lip reconstruction or facial reanimation.[10]

Anatomy

- *Artery*: Radial artery (20 cm long; 2–2.5 mm in diameter, courses in lateral intermuscular septum and separates flexor carpi radialis and brachioradialis muscles).
- *Vein*: Venae comitantes and/or cephalic vein (drainage can be maintained independently with superficial or deep system).
- *Nerve*: Lateral antebrachial cutaneous (terminal branch of the musculocutaneous nerve), medial and posterior antebrachial cutaneous can be harvested with very large flaps.

Lateral Arm

The lateral arm flap (LAF): It has similar applications to that of the RFFF, including the oral cavity, oropharynx, hypopharynx, and other sites.[11] However, its distinguishing feature is the variation in skin thickness available within the flap, providing thicker skin for tongue base reconstruction alongside thinner skin used for pharyngeal wall reconstruction.[12] It can be harvested as a fascial, fasciocutaneous, or composite flap, with a portion of triceps muscle and/or a 1 × 10 cm section of humerus bone.[13] It has however fallen out of favor due to a short (8–10 cm) and small sized pedicle (artery 1.25–1.75 mm).[14]

It can be harvested as an osteocutaneous flap (1 × 10 cm bony segment). Less than 6 cm or one-third of the arm circumference can allow for primary closure.

Anatomy[15-17]

- *Artery*: Posterior radial collateral artery (PRCA) (travels in the intermuscular septum between the brachioradialis and triceps).
- *Vein*: Venae comitantes and/or cephalic vein.
- *Nerve*: Posterior cutaneous nerve of the arm (must also identify and preserve the radial nerve and posterior collateral cutaneous nerve of the forearm).

Temporoparietal Fascia Flap

The temporoparietal fascia flap (TPFF) can be used as a free or pedicled flap.[18,19] It can be transferred with hair-bearing scalp, split thickness calvarial bone grafts, or auricular cartilage.[20] Applications of the TPFF include reconstruction of the oral cavity, hair-bearing lip, skull base, auricle, and scalp.

Anatomy

- *Artery*: Superficial temporal artery; parietal branch (the frontal temporal artery can be safely dissected 3–4 cm anteriorly before encountering temporal branch of facial nerve).
- *Vein*: Superficial temporal vein.
- *Nerve*: None.

Anterolateral Thigh

The anterolateral (ALT) thigh flap: It can be harvested as a septocutaneous or musculocutaneous flap, and can include tendons or muscles to enhance its reconstructive potential.[21] The ALT can allow for a larger skin paddle for moderate-to-high volume defects, and can be used if the RFFF is unavailable. Applications of the ALT include oral cavity, oropharynx, larynx, pharyngeal, and skull base defects.[22,23] Perforators of the artery exist on a line drawn from the anterior superior iliac spine (ASIS) to the lateral edge of the patella, between the midpoint and upper-to-middle thirds of the line.

Anatomy

- *Artery*: Descending branch of the lateral circumflex femoral artery.
- *Vein*: Venae comitantes.
- *Nerve*: Lateral femoral cutaneous; runs axially.

■ COMPOSITE FLAPS

Scapula

The scapular free flap (SFF) has become a versatile composite flap in head and neck reconstruction.[24,25] Its long vascular pedicle, thin and hairless skin, curved bony contour, and multidimensional in setting potential make it an excellent composite option for complex multi-surfaced defects. The SFF is primarily used for oromandibular reconstruction, but possesses inadequate bone stock alone for osseointegrated dental implantation. The scapular tip flap, based on the angular branch of the thoracodorsal artery, may be used for its thicker bone segment.[26]

Harvesting both the circumflex scapular and thoracodorsal systems (including latissimus dorsi flap) at the level of the subscapular vessels = "mega" flap.

Anatomy

- *Artery*: Circumflex scapular artery (CSA, two cutaneous branches: (1) horizontal—scapular flap; (2) vertical—parascapular flap) or angular branch of thoracodorsal artery (for scapular tip flap).

- *Vein*: Circumflex scapular vein (CSV) or thoracodorsal vein (parallels arterial system) *CSA/CSV traverses the triangular space defined by the teres major, teres minor, and the long head of the triceps muscle.*
- *Nerve*: No reliable neurotization.

Iliac Crest

The iliac crest (IC) osteocutaneous free flap was adapted to include the internal oblique muscle to provide a thicker soft tissue substrate for reconstruction.[27,28] Urken et al. have used this flap extensively for oromandibular reconstruction for its long (up to 16 cm), curved bony segment, long pedicle, mobile muscle tissue, and potential for osseointegration.[29] The main disadvantages are risk of hernia, gait distortion, sensory changes, and limited skin paddle mobility.

Anatomy

- *Artery*: Deep circumflex iliac artery (DCIA).
- *Vein*: Deep circumflex iliac vein.
- *Nerve*: Lateral cutaneous branch of twelfth thoracic nerve.

Fibular Osteocutaneous

The free fibular flap (FFF) is considered the workhorse of oromandibular reconstruction.[30] Other applications include midface and palatal reconstruction. It boasts a long and reliable pedicle, a contoured bone segment, and a thin skin paddle. The FFF can also be a sensate flap if transferred with the lateral sural cutaneous nerve.

Skin perforators can course through the posterior intermuscular septum as septocutaneous or musculocutaneous perforators through the flexor hallucis longus and soleus. Lateral intramuscular septum (IMS) is estimated by a line connecting the lateral epicondyle inferiorly with the fibular head superiorly. The distal one-third of the line allows for the highest quantity of skin perforators. Inadequate blood supply to skin occurs in 8.5–15%.[30,31]

Anatomy

- *Artery*: Peroneal artery (branch of posterior tibial artery).
- *Vein*: Venae comitantes.
- *Nerve*: Lateral sural cutaneous nerve (branch of the common peroneal nerve).

■ VISCERAL FLAPS

Free Jejunal Flap

Primary applications pertain to circumferential hypopharyngeal and cervical esophagus defects.[32,33]

Anatomy

- *Artery*: Segmental jejunal arteries of the superior mesenteric artery.
- *Vein*: Analogous jejunal veins.
- *Nerve*: Intrinsic nervous supply resumes with revascularization.

Free Omentum

The omentum is a double-layered curtain of peritoneum that hangs over the greater curvature of the stomach and transverse colon. Although infrequently used, it has utility in coverage of osteomyelitic or osteoradionecrotic bone, facial contouring, large scalp defects, and coverage of exposed vessels.[34]

Anatomy

- *Artery*: Right (and left) gastroepiploic arteries.
- *Vein*: Right (and left) gastroepiploic veins.

Summary of neurovascular supply to various free flap options along with advantages and disadvantages of their use is given in Table 1.

■ TOPICS IN MANAGEMENT

Perioperative Considerations

Existing data has correlated higher volumes of perioperative crystalloid administration (>130 mL/kg/day or >7 liters intraoperatively) with medical and flap complications.[35,36] The ideal range of crystalloid infusion in the 24-hour postoperative period has been stated as 3.5–6.0 mL/kg/hour.[37]

Anticoagulation

- *Intraoperative*: Intraoperative medications administered during microvascular anastomosis often include 4% xylocaine or papaverine for topical vasodilation, heparin solution (100 U/cm^3) for luminal irrigation, and/or streptokinase or urokinase for lysis of intraluminal thrombus. A previous study by Chen et al. demonstrated no effect on the incidence of complications, including microvascular thrombosis, with intraoperative administration of systemic heparin.[38]
- *Postoperative*: Options for anticoagulation include daily aspirin, low molecular weight heparin, dextran, or a combination thereof. Controversy exists regarding the necessity, or lack thereof, of postoperative anticoagulation in microvascular free tissue transfer. A study by Ashjian et al. demonstrated no significant difference in complications (bleeding or thromboembolism) with either aspirin or low molecular weight heparin prophylaxis following oncologic free tissue transfer. However, when compared to aspirin, administration of

Table 1: Summary of neurovascular supply to various free flap options along with advantages and disadvantages of their use

Flap	Artery	Vein	Nerve	Advantages	Disadvantages
Muscle and myocutaneous flaps					
Rectus	Deep inferior epigastric and deep superior epigastric	Deep inferior epigastric and deep superior epigastric	Intercostal nerves	Large quantity soft tissue bulk, discrete donor site, long vascular pedicle	Limited tissue mobility, abdominal wall hernia, and wound dehiscence
Gracilis	Terminal branch of the adductor artery	Venae comitantes	Anterior branch of the obturator nerve	Thin, pliable muscle for facial reanimation, discrete donor site, muscle bulk modifiable	Vascular supply to overlying skin variable
Fascial and fasciocutaneous flaps					
Radial forearm	Radial	Venae comitantes; cephalic vein	Lateral (or medial) antebrachial cutaneous	Thin, pliable, versatile, reliable anatomy, long pedicle, large skin paddle	Limited bulk, skin graft required for donor site, anatomic variations possible
Lateral arm	PRCA	Venae comitantes; cephalic vein	Posterior cutaneous nerve of the arm	Variable thickness, nonessential donor artery	Donor site appearance, elbow pain, hair growth at recipient site[41]
Temporoparietal fascia	STA	STV	None	Several composite options, thin and pliable soft tissue, hair-bearing	Alopecia over donor site, risk to temporal branch of facial nerve, small pedicle
Anterolateral thigh	Descending branch of LCFA	Venae comitantes	Lateral femoral cutaneous	Large quantity of tissue, primary closure	Anatomic variability, history of vasculopathy with bypass graft is contraindication
Composite flaps					
Scapula	CSA or thoracodorsal artery	CSV or thoracodorsal vein	No reliable neurotization	Diversity of reconstruction on single pedicle, abundant skin and soft tissue, three-dimensional maneuverability	Requires intricate positioning, two-team approach difficult, thin bone stock
Latissimus dorsi	Thoracodorsal artery	Thoracodorsal vein	Thoracodorsal nerve	Multitude of reconstruction options, two potential skin paddles, discrete donor site	Difficult positioning, occasional unreliable vascular supply to skin paddle
Iliac crest	Deep circumflex artery	Deep circumflex vein	Lateral cutaneous branch of twelfth thoracic nerve	Large and curved bone segment, tall and thick bone stock, skin and muscle options, discrete donor site	Risk of hernia, gait distortion, sensory changes, limited skin paddle mobility
Fibula	Peroneal artery	Venae comitantes	Lateral sural cutaneous nerve	Thick bone stock for DI, reliable and sensate skin paddle, two-team approach	Weakness of toe flexion, potential ankle instability, skin graft required

Contd...

Contd...

Flap	Artery	Vein	Nerve	Advantages	Disadvantages
Visceral flaps					
Jejunal	Segmental jejunal arteries of the SMA	Segmental jejunal veins of the SMA	Intrinsic	Potential for shorter time to oral alimentation, low incidence of fistula[42]	Requires laparotomy, postoperative dysphagia caused by peristalsis, stricture formation, poor vocalization with tracheoesophageal puncture[43]
Free omentum	Right (and left) gastroepiloic arteries	Right (and left) gastroepiloic veins	None	Thin, pliable tissue, lower fistula rates and strictures in laryngopharyngectomy defects[44]	Laparotomy morbidity including gastric leak, gastric outlet obstruction, contraindicated in peptic ulcer disease

(PRCA: Posterior radial collateral artery; STA: Superficial temporal artery; STV: Superficial temporal vein; LCFA: Lateral circumflex femoral artery; CSA: Circumflex scapular artery; CSV: Circumflex scapular vein; SMA: Superior mesenteric artery).

dextran was found to be associated with an increased incidence of systemic complications.[38]

Monitoring

- Frequent postoperative evaluation remains the gold standard for assessing flap viability.[39] Specific characteristics to assess include color, capillary refill, turgor, surface temperature, presence of bleeding, skin graft adherence, and auditory assessment of blood flow.
- Adjunctive measures for assessment may include pulse oximetry, Doppler ultrasonography, external cutaneous paddles for buried flaps, laser Doppler flowmeter devices, and implantable anastomotic Dopplers.[40]

▌ REFERENCES

1. Paper I. Facial Plastic and Reconstructive Surgery, 2nd edition. New York: Thieme Medical Publishers; 2002.
2. Taylor GI, Corlett RJ, Boyd JB. The versatile deep inferior epigastric (inferior rectus abdominis) flap. Br J Plast Surg. 1984;37:330-50.
3. Baudet J, Guimberteau J, Nascimento E. Successful clinical transfer of two free thoraco dorsal axillary flaps. Plast Reconstr Surg. 1976;58:680-8.
4. Tansini I. Spora it mio processo di amputazione della mamella per cancre. Riforma Medica. 1896;12:3-5.
5. Schultes G, Karcher H, Gaggl A. Sensate myocutaneous latissimus dorsi flap. J Reconstr Microsurg. 1998;14:541-3.
6. Russell RC, Pribaz J, Zook E, et al. Functional evaluation of the latissimus donor site. Plast Reconstr Surg. 1978;78:336-44.
7. Harii K, Ohmori K, Torii S. Free gracilis muscle transplantation of the oral cavity following partial and total glossectomy. Arch Otolaryngol Head Neck Surg. 1994;120:589-601.
8. Strauch B, Yu H. Atlas of microvascular surgery: anatomy and operations. Laryngoscope. 2001;111:1192-6.
9. Soutar DS, Scheker LR, Tanner SB, et al. The radial forearm flap: a versatile method for intraoral reconstruction. Br J Plast Surg. 1993;36:1-8.
10. Daya M. Simultaneous total upper and lower lip reconstruction with a free radial forearm-palmaris longus tendon and brachioradialis chimeric flap. J Plast Reconstr Aesthet Surg. 2010;63:e75-6.
11. Song R, Song Y, Yu Y, et al. The upper arm free flap. Clin Plast Surg. 1982;9:27-35.
12. Civantos FJ, Burkey BB, Lu F, et al. Lateral arm microvascular flap in head and neck reconstruction. Arch Otolaryngol Head Neck Surg. 1997;123:830-6.
13. Clymer MA, Burkey BB. Other flaps for head and neck use: temporoparietal fascial free flap, lateral arm free flap, omental free flap. Facial Plast Surg. 1996;12:81-9.
14. Gordon J, Small JO. The addition of muscle to the lateral arm and radial forearm flaps for wound coverage. Plast Reconstr Surg. 1992;89:563-6.
15. Katsaros J, Tan E, Zoltie N, et al. Further experience with the lateral arm free flap. Plast Reconstr Surg. 1991;87:902-10.
16. Moffett T, Madison S, Derr J, et al An extended approach for the vascular pedicle of the lateral arm free flap. Plast Reconstr Surg. 1992;89:259-67.
17. Rivet D, Buffet M, Martin D, et al. The lateral arm flap: an anatomic study. J Reconstr Microsurg. 1987;3:121-32.
18. Brown WJ. Extraordinary case of horse bite: the external ear completely bitten off and successfully replaced. Lancet. 1898;1:1533-34.
19. Monks GH. The restoration of a lower eyelid by a new method. N Engl J Med. 1898;139:385-7.
20. Cheney ML. Temporoparietal fascia. In: Urken ML, Cheney ML, Sullivan MJ, Biller HF (Eds). Atlas of Regional and Free Flaps for Head and Neck Reconstruction. New York: Raven Press, 1995.
21. Song YG, Chen GZ, Song YL. The free thigh flap: a new free flap concept based on the septocutaneous artery. Br J Plast Surg. 1984;37:149-59.
22. Lueg EA. The anterolateral thigh flap: radial forearm's "big brother" for extensive soft tissue head and neck defects. Arch Otolaryngol Head Neck Surg. 2004;130:813-8.
23. Wong CH, Wci FC. Anterolateral thigh flap. Head Neck. 2010;32:529-40.
24. Saijo M. The vascular territories of the dorsal trunk: a reappraisal for potential flap donor sites. Br J Plast Surg. 1978;31:200-4.
25. Gilbert A, Teot L. The free scapular flap. Plast Reconstr Surg. 1982;69:601.
26. Wagner A, Bayles SW. The angular branch: maximizing the scapular pedicle in head and neck reconstruction. Arch Otolaryngol Head Neck Surg. 2008;134:1214-7.

27. Taylor GI, Townsend P, Corlett R. Superiority of the deep circumflex iliac vessels as the supply for free groin flaps: experimental work. Plast Reconstr Surg. 1979;64:595-604.

28. Ramasastry SS, Tucker JB, Swartz WM, et al. The internal oblique muscle flap: an anatomic and clinical study. Plast Reconstr Surg. 1984;73:721-30.

29. Urken ML, Vickery C, Weinberg H, et al. The internal oblique-iliac crest osseomyocutaneous microvascular free flap in head and neck reconstruction. J Reconstr Microsurg. 1989;5:203-14.

30. Taylor GI, Miller GD, Ham FJ. The free vascularized bone graft. A clinical extension of microvascular techniques. Plast Reconstr Surg. 1975;55:533-44.

31. Wei FC, Seah CS, Tsai YC, et al. Fibula osteoseptocutaneous flap for reconstruction of composite mandibular defects. Plast Reconstr Surg. 1994;93:294-304.

32. Carrel A. The surgery of blood vessels. John Hopkins Hosp Bull. 1907;19:18-28.

33. Seidenberg B, Rosenak SS, Hurwitt ES, et al. Immediate reconstruction of the cervical esophagus by a revascularized isolated jejunal segment. Ann Surg. 1959;142:162-71.

34. Baudet J. Reconstruction of the pharyngeal wall by free transfer of the greater omentum and stomach. Int J Microsurg. 1979;1:53.

35. Clark JR, McCluskey SA, Hall F, et al. Predictors of morbidity following free flap reconstruction for cancer of the head and neck. Head Neck. 2007;29:1090-101.

36. Haughey BH, Wilson E, Kluwe L, et al. Free flap reconstruction of the head and neck: analysis of 241 cases. Otolaryngol Head Neck Surg. 2001;125:10-7.

37. Zhong T, Neinstein R, Massey C, et al. Intravenous fluid infusion rate in microsurgical breast reconstruction: important lessons learned from 354 free flaps. Plast Reconstr Surg. 2011;128:1153-60.

38. Chen CM, Ashjian P, Disa JJ, et al. Is the use of intraoperative heparin safe? Plast Reconstr Surg. 2008;121:49e-53e.

39. Chubb D, Rozen WM, Whitaker IS, et al. The efficacy of clinical assessment in the postoperative monitoring of free flaps: a review of 1140 consecutive cases. Plast Reconstr Surg. 2010;125:1157-66.

40. Abdel-Galil K, Mitchell D. Postoperative monitoring of microsurgical free tissue transfers for head and neck reconstruction: a systematic review of current techniques—part I. Noninvasive techniques. Br J Oral Maxillofac Surg. 2009;47:351-5.

41. Graham B, Adkins P, Scheker LR. Complications and morbidity of the donor and recipient sites in 123 lateral arm flaps. J Hand Surg Br. 1992;17:189-92.

42. Alford EL. Free jejunal transfer. Facial Plast Surg. 1996;12:69-73.

43. Reece GP, Bengtson BP, Schusterman MA. Reconstruction of the pharynx and cervical pharynx and cervical esophagus using jejunal transfer. Clin Plast Surg. 1994;21:125-36.

44. Clymer MA, Burkey BB. Other flaps for head and neck use: temporoparietal fascial free flap, lateral arm free flap, omental free flap. Facial Plast Surg. 1996;12:81-9.

Multiple Choice Questions

Q 1. The thoracodorsal artery is the primary source of BLOOD SUPPLY for the:

A. Pectoralis major flap

B. Trapezius flap

C. Latissimus dorsi flap

D. Deltopectoral flap

Ans: C. Latissimus dorsi flap

Q 2. In microvascular anastomosis, which of the following medications SHOULD NOT BE USED postoperatively in order to lessen the likelihood of vessel thrombosis?

A. Ibuprofen

B. Heparin

C. Dextran

D. Prednisone

Ans: A. Ibuprofen

Q 3. Which of the following statements regarding intraoperative management of microvascular flaps is TRUE?

A. End-to-side anastomosis is not useful in microvascular anastomosis

B. Interrupted stitches with 5-0 nylon are used for anastomosis

C. The use of anastomotic devices in free-tissue transfer is contraindicated

D. If the lumen size of the vessels mismatch the surgeon can use the fish-mouth and unequal bites techniques for closing

Ans: D. If the lumen size of the vessels mismatch the surgeon can use the fish-mouth and unequal bites techniques for closing

Q 4. The vast majority of microvascular surgeons prefer WHICH OF THE FOLLOWING TECHNIQUES in order to monitor flap status postoperatively?

A. Clinical assessment

B. Doppler ultrasonography

C. Doppler flowmetry

D. Photoplethysmography

Ans: A. Clinical assessment

Q 5. Which of the following statements is TRUE regarding the Radial Forearm Free Flap?

A. The Esmarch bandage and tourniquet control of the upper extremity are unnecessary in its harvesting

B. The Allen test is not required in younger patients

C. The risk of pathologic fracture after harvesting radial bone is insignificant

D. The medial and lateral antebrachial nerves are fundamental in obtaining a sensate flap

Ans: D. The medial and lateral antebrachial nerves are fundamental in obtaining a sensate flap

Q 6. Which of the following statements is TRUE regarding the Lateral Arm Free Flap?

A. Primary closure of the donor site is extremely difficult to accomplish

B. The lateral arm flap has only one venous drainage system the deep venous system

C. The variability of the lateral arm skin thicknesses is one of this flap's advantages

D. The lateral arm flap is based on the anterior radial collateral

Ans: C. The variability of the lateral arm skin thicknesses is one of this flap's advantages

Q 7. Which of following statements is TRUE regarding the Rectus Myocutaneous Free Flap?

A. It is based on the deep inferior epigastric vessels

B. Closure of the defect requires a full skin thickness graft

C. The most common complication is necrosis of the donor site

D. The main disadvantage is a short vascular pedicle available for anastomosis

Ans: A. It is based on the deep inferior epigastric vessels

Q 8. Which of the following statements is FALSE regarding the Latissimus Dorsi Free Flap?

A. The primary pedicle is the thoracodorsal artery and vein

B. Harvesting of the flap will require a lateral decubitus position

C. The location of the latissimus flap will allow a two-team approach

D. Its pedicle is long and has large vessel diameters

Ans: C. The location of the latissimus flap will allow a two-team approach

Q 9. Which of the following statements regarding the Fibula Osteocutaneous Free Flap is TRUE?

A. The maximal size of bone segment available with this flap is approximately 15 cm

B. The fibula free flap is based on the anterior tibial artery

C. The skin paddle is supplied by the septocutaneous perforators from the peroneal artery

D. The closure of the leg donor site can always be accomplished primarily

Ans: C. The skin paddle is supplied by the septocutaneous perforators from the peroneal artery

Q 10. Which of the following techniques of monitoring is the MOST commonly used in the Jejunum Free Flap?

A. Visual monitoring of exteriorized segment of jejunum

B. Hydrogen clearance analysis

C. Photoplethysmography

D. Analysis of venous blood close to the transferred segment

Ans: A. Visual monitoring of exteriorized segment of jejunum

Q 11. Which of the following vascularized donor sites provides the BEST free flap for total mandible reconstruction?

A. Rib

B. Scapula

C. Fibula

D. Iliac crest

Ans: C. Fibula

Q 12. Which of the following statements regarding the Fibula Osteocutaneous Free Flap is FALSE?

A. The fibula free flap will require preserving 3 cm of bone both proximally and distally

B. The peroneal artery provides the primary blood supply for the overlying skin of the lateral aspect of the calf and the fibula

C. 25 cm of fibular bone can be harvested without marked

D. The fibula free flap is the ideal for reconstruction of subtotal and total defects of the mandible

Ans: A. The fibula free flap will require preserving 3 cm of bone both proximally and distally

Q 13. Which of the following statements regarding the Jejunal Free Flap is TRUE?

A. It is rarely used in circumferential defects of the cervical esophagus

B. It is harvested only by laparoscopic approach

C. The second loop of jejunum is usually used

D. Isoperistalytic orientation of the jejunum is not mandatory

Ans: C. The second loop of jejunum is usually used

Q 14. Which of the following statements is FALSE regarding oromandibular reconstruction with free-tissue transfer?

A. The fibula free flap is the workhorse flap for oromandibular reconstruction defects

B. The fibula free flap will allow for osseointegrated implants

C. Through and through defects of the oral cavity are best reconstructed with use of the fibula free flap

D. The Fibula Free Flap has reconstructive capacity in cases up to and including near-total mandibulectomy

Ans: C. Through and through defects of the oral cavity are best reconstructed with use of the fibula free flap

Q 15. Which of the following statements is TRUE regarding flap failure after microvascular flap anastomosis?

A. Thrombosis of the artery is more common than the thrombosis of the vein

B. The failure of arterial anastomosis occurres within the first 24 hours

C. The failure of venous anastomosis occurres within the first 12 hours

D. Bleeding will cause flap failure and therefore, aspirin is contraindicated in the postoperative period

Ans: B. The failure of arterial anastomosis occurres within the first 24 hours

Q 16. Which of the following is NOT USEFUL in the postoperative prevention of vessel thrombosis in free-tissue transfer of microvascular flaps?

A. Aspirin

B. Statins

C. Prednisone

D. Heparin

Ans: B. Statins

Q 17. Which of the following measurements represents the MAXIMUM BONE SEGMENT AVAILABLE in a FIBULAR OSTEOCUTANEOUS FREE FLAP?

A. 20 cm

C. 30 cm

B. 25 cm

D. 35 cm

Ans: B. 25 cm

Q 18. Which of the following statements about the FIBULAR OSTEOCUTANEOUS FLAP is FALSE?

A. The peroneal artery and vein provide the primary blood supply to this flap

B. The sensory input to the flap is provided by the direct innervation of the common peroneal nerve

C. Flap elevation is usually done with a thigh tourniquet inflated to 350 mm Hg

D. A segment of 8 cm of fibula is preserved proximally and distally

Ans: B. The sensory input to the flap is provided by the direct innervation of the common peroneal nerve.

Q 19. Which of the following MEASUREMENTS refers to the distal radius bone segment that can safely be harvested in a composite reconstruction using a Radial Forearm Free Flap?

A 10 cm

C 20 cm

B 15 cm

D 25 cm

Ans: A. 10 cm

Q 20. Which of the following statement represents the principal vascular supply in the iliac crest composite flap for oromandibular reconstruction?

A. The superficial circumflex iliac artery (SCIA)

B. The deep circumflex iliac artery (DCIA)

C. The superior deep branch of the gluteal artery

D. The ascending branch of the lateral circumflex femoral artery

Ans: B. The deep circumflex iliac artery (DCIA)

Q 21. Which of the following represents the highest percentage of pathologic fracture reported after harvest of radial bone foream free flap?

A. 20%

C. 40%

B. 30%

D. 50%

Ans: C. 40%

Q 22. The Radial Foream Flap has the HIGHEST INCIDENCE of which of the following complications?

A. Partial loss of donor-site skin

B. Partial loss of donor-site skin with exposure of tendons

C. Donor-site cold intolerance

D. Lack of superficial radial nerve sensation in the donor-site

Ans: D. Lack of superficial Radial Nerve sensation in the donor -site

Q 23. Which of the following flap monitors IS THE BEST TOOL for reliable detection of early problems in flap perfusion?

A. Laser-Doppler flowmetry

B. Pulse oximetry

C. Photoplethysmography

D. Dupplex Doppler ultrasonography

Ans: A. Laser-Doppler flowmetry

Q 24. What is the LEAST amount of bone required to be left in place when harvesting the Osteocutaneous Free Flap represented in the drawing below?

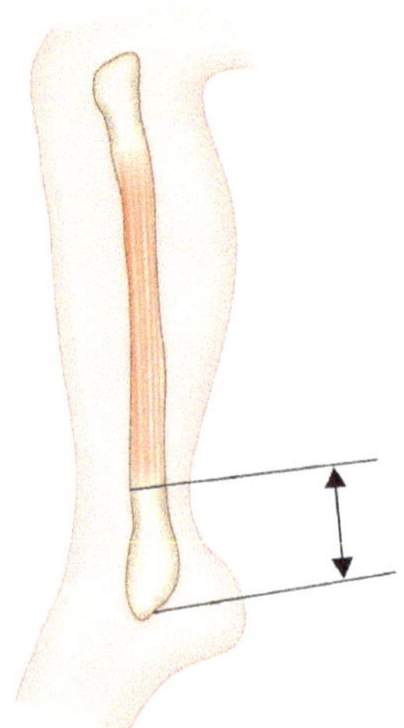

A. 4 cm

C. 12 cm

B. 8 cm

D. 14 cm

Ans: B. 8 cm

Q 25. Which of the following statements about Osteocutaneous Flaps is TRUE?

A. Fibular flaps allow a maximal 20 cm bone length

B. Fibular flaps require that a 10 cm segment of fibular bone be left superiorly and inferiorly

C. Scapular flaps allow a maximal 10 cm bone length availability

D. Iliac crest flaps allow a maximal 10 cm bone length availability

Ans: C. Scapular flaps allow a maximal 10 cm bone length availability

Q 26. Which of the following statements about Microvascular Reconstruction is FALSE?

A. Vessels in the vascular pedicle are skeletonized, freeing the artery from the vein

B. Vessels are transected and irrigated intermittently with dilute heparinized saline solution

C. Vessels should be handled by the intima

D. End-to-End Technique is the most commonly used in arterial anastomosis

Ans: C. Vessels should be handled by the intima

Q 27. Which of the following statements about the Radial Forearm Free Flap is FALSE?

A. It is a fascial flap

B. It is a fasciocutaneous flap

C. It also can be harvested without a bone

D. It does not carry sensory innervation

Ans: D. It does not carry sensory innervation

Q 28. Which of the following statements regarding the radial forearm free flap is TRUE?

A. It is a thick, non-pliable flap

B. It is based in the posterior radial collateral artery

C. The medial and lateral antebrachial nerves can be incorporated into the flap

D. The donor site can be closed primarely

Ans: C. The medial and lateral antebrachial nerves can be incorporated into the flap

Q 29. Which of following statements about the Rectus Myocutaneous Free Flap is TRUE?

A. The rectus abdominal muscle has a dual blood supply from the deep inferior and superior epigastric arteries

B. The deep inferior and superior epigastric arteries are branches of the internal iliac artery

C. The rectus myocutaneous free flap is based in the superior epigastric artery and vein

D. The rectus myocutaneous free flap should be designed below the arcuate line

Ans: A. The rectus abdominal muscle has a dual blood supply from the deep inferior and superior epigastric arteries

Q 30. Which of the following statements about Microvascular Reconstruction is TRUE?

A. The vessels should be handled by the intima

B. The most common arterial anastomosis is End-to-Side

C. Microvascular anastomosis involves the use of 9-0, interrupted or continuous stitches, with slow absorbing

D. The disadvantage of the continuous suture technique is narrowing at the anastomosis of the vessel lumen

Ans: D. The disadvantage of the continuous suture technique is narrowing at the anastomosis of the vessel lumen

Q 31. Which of the following statements about the Fibular Osteomyocutaneous Free Flap is FALSE?

A. The arterial supply is based on the peroneal artery

B. The skin paddle is supplied by septocutaneous perforators from the intermuscular septum

C. The sensory input to the flap is based on the lateral sural cutaneous nerve

D. This flap offers the longest length of available revascularizedbone (30 cm)

Ans: D. This flap offers the longest length of available revascularized bone (30 cm)

Q 32. Which of the following flaps is the most USEFUL in Anterior Skull Base Reconstruction?

A. Rectus myocutaneous

B. Radial forearm

C. Lateral arm

D. Lateral thigh

Ans: A. Rectus myocutaneous

Q 33. Which of the following statements about Jejunum Free Flap is FALSE?

A. It is an adequate option for hypopharyngeal reconstruction

B. The second loop of the jejunum is usually used

C. The flap should be oriented in an isoperistaltic fashion

D. Externalizing a small segment of jejunum outside the neck is not necessary

Ans: D. Externalizing a small segment of jejunum outside the neck is not necessary

Q 34. Which of the following percentage about the overall Jejunal Free Flap success rate is TRUE?

A. 90%

B. 80%

C. 70%

D. 60%

Ans: A. 90%

Q 35. Which of the following statements regarding the Radial Forearm Free Flap is TRUE?

A. It will require mandatory harvesting of bone segment

B. The lateral antebrachial nerve is used to obtain a sensate

C. Allen's test is rarely used for preoperative assessment

D. Primary closure of the donor site is usually accomplished

Ans: B. The lateral antebrachial nerve is used to obtain a sensate flap

Q 36. Which of the following free tissue transfer flaps used for Head and Neck Reconstruction is considered IDEAL for total mandibular reconstruction?

A. Fibula osteocutaneous free flap

B. Scapular osteocutaneous free flap

C. Iliac crest osteocutaneous flap

D. Radius osteocutaneous free flap

Ans: A. Fibula osteocutaneous free flap

Q 37. Which of the following statements about the Radial Forearm Flap is FALSE?

A. It is a fascial flap

B. It is a fasciocutaneous flap

C. It can be harvested with or without bone

D. It is based on the radial and ulnar arteries

Ans: D. It is based on the radial and ulnar arteries

Q 38. Which one of the following anatomical structures is NOT related to the Triangular Space in the design of the Scapula Free Flap?

A. Long head of the triceps
B. Teres minor muscle
C. Teres major muscle
D. Serratus anterior muscle

Ans: D. Serratus anterior muscle

Q 39. Which of the following statements about Jejunal Free Flap is TRUE?

A. It is an unreliable flap when used for 360° circumferential pharyngoesophageal defects
B. The maximum length of jejunum harvested is 15 cm
C. The second arcade of jejunum is the best for pharyngeal reconstruction
D. Isoperistaltic orientation of the jejunum is unnecessary

Ans: C. The second arcade of jejunum is the best for pharyngeal reconstruction

Q 40. Which of the following mm Hg is recommended in order to INFLATE the thigh tourniquet used in the harvesting of a Free Fibula flap?

A. 150 mm Hg
B. 250 mm Hg
C. 350 mm Hg
D. 500 mm Hg

Ans: C. 350 mm Hg

Q 41. Which of the following statements is FALSE regarding the radial forearm free flap?

A. It is thin and pliable flap
B. Versatile
C. Forearm defect can be close primarily
D. Osteocutaneous flap with 10 cm of radius is possible

Ans: C. Forearm defect can be close primarily

Q 42. What is the MAIN ADVANTAGE of the free Lateral Arm Flap versus the free Radial Foream Flap?

A. Thin and pliable skin
B. Primary closure of the donor defect is possible
C. It has more bone available
D. Allen test results is the most important consideration of avoid hand ischemia

Ans: B. Primary closure of the donor defect is possible

Q 43. Which of the following is FALSE regarding the Lateral Arm Free Flap?

A. It is based on the posterior radial collateral artery
B. The radial artery is also a main part of vascular pedicle
C. It has dual venous drainage
D. The cutaneous paddle is approximately to one third of the circumference of the arm

Ans: B. The radial artery is also a main part of vascular pedicle

Q 44. Which of the following is a MORBIDITY MOST commonly related to the Superficial Temporal Parietal Fascia Flap?

A. Skin necrosis
B. Infection
C. Alopecia
D. Bleeding

Ans: C. Alopecia

Q 45. Which of the following microvascular flaps is MOST COMMONLY used in facial reanimation?

A. Lateral arm
B. Superficial temporal parietal fascia
C. Gracilis
D. Radial forearm

Ans: C. Gracilis

Q 46. Which of the following statements regarding the fibular osteocutaneous flap is TRUE?

A. The longest possible segment of fibular bone for harvesting is 20 cm
B. The fibular bone can be contoured to reconstruct only small to medium mandibular defects
C. An 8-cm segment of fibular is necessary above and below for ankle and knee stability
D. Posterior split in the immediate postoperative period is usually not necessary

Ans: C. An 8-cm segment of fibular is necessary above and below for ankle and knee stability

Q 47. Which of the following statements regarding the Radial forearm flap is FALSE?

A. It can be harvested as fascial, fasciocutaneous or osteocutaneous flap
B. It has a very small vessel diameter with limited pedicle
C. It is adequate for reconstruction of total lower lip reconstruction
D. It can be harvested with the inclusion of the lateral antebrachial cutaneous nerve

Ans: B. It has a very small vessel diameter with limited pedicle

Q 48. Which of the following Free Tissue Transfer is the BEST to cover the dead space produced after total maxillectomy with orbital exenteration?

A. Radial forearm
B. Latissimus dorsi
C. Rectus abdominis
D. Transverse rectus abdominis

Ans: C. Rectus abdominis

Q 49. Which of the following DOMINANT pedicles related to these Free Tissue Transfer Flaps is FALSE?

A. Radial forearm flap—Radial artery
B. Lateral arm flap—Posterior radial collateral artery

C. Scapular flap—Circumflex artery
D. Latissimus dorsi flap—Intercostal arteries

Ans: D. Latissimus dorsi flap—Intercostal arteries

Q 50. How many mm Hg is the tourniquet inflated in preparation for harvesting the Radial Forearm Free Flap?

A. 100 mm Hg
B. 150 mm Hg
C. 250 mm Hg
D. 350 mm Hg

Ans: C. 250 mm Hg

Q 51. What AMOUNT OF BLOOD can a medical leech remove during its active feeding period?

A. 1.5 mL
B. 2.5 mL
C. 3.5 mL
D. 4.5 mL

Ans: B. 2.5 mL

Q 52. Which of the following wait periods is APPROPRIATE prior to reconstruction of complex cutaneous facial defects after oncologic resection?

A. 6 months
B. 8 months
C. 10 months
D. 12 months

Ans: D. 12 months

Q 53. Which of the following tissue adhesives is commonly used primarily for VASCULAR ANASTOMOSIS?

A. Tisseel
B. BioGlue
C. Bytyl-cyanocrylate
D. 2-Octyl cyanoacrylate

Ans: B. BioGlue

Chapter 26

Facial Paralysis and Reanimation

Arvind K Badhey, Samuel N Helman

■ INTRODUCTION

The facial nerve [cranial nerve (CN) VII], is an important and complicated structure due to its multiple functions. The most clinically obvious being the control of the facial musculature, including muscles, which activate speech, expression, emotion, and mastication. These functions alone demonstrate the value of the facial nerve to social interaction—vastly widening the implications of nerve injury.[1]

Paralysis of the facial nerve can involve any of the substructures and segments. The etiology of injury can originate anywhere along the course of the nerve from within the brainstem to the most peripheral terminal branches. While the idiopathic causes of facial nerve paralysis known as Bell's palsy is the most common cause, etiologies can broaden to viral syndromes, bacterial infections, trauma, neoplasms and iatrogenic injury (Box 1).[2]

■ RELEVANT ANATOMY

Facial Nerve Fibers

Special visceral efferent/motor fibers (SVE): Nerves originate from the facial motor nucleus and go on to innervate muscles of facial expression, stapedius, posterior belly of digastric, and stylohyoid muscle.

General somatic afferent/sensory fibers (GSA): Nerve fibers travel with the nervus intermedius, splitting to become the posterior auricular branch—sensation of the posterior ear.

Box 1: Causes of facial nerve paralysis

- *Congenital:* Birth trauma, Mobius syndrome, myotonic dystrophy, CHARGE syndrome, vascular malformation
- *Infectious: Herpes zoster:* Ramsay Hunt syndrome, Otitis media, Lyme disease
- *Toxins and trauma:* Temporal bone fractures, iatrogenic surgical injuries, diphtheria toxin vaccination, ethylene glycol poisoning
- *Tumor:* Cholesteatoma, acoustic neuroma, facial neuroma, parotid neoplasms, metastases
- *Endocrine:* Diabetes, hypothyroidism, porphyria, myasthenia gravis
- *Neurological:* Pontine infarction, traumatic external carotid artery aneurysm
- *Systemic:* Hypertension, pseudotumor cerebri

General visceral efferent/motor fibers (GVE): Fibers originate from the superior salivary nucleus, and goes on to exit the skull base either with the chorda tympani or vidian nerve, fibers synapse at either the pterygopalatine ganglion or the submandibular ganglion, eventually innervating the submandibular, sublingual, nasal, or lacrimal gland.

Special visceral afferent/sensory: Special sensory fibers leave the solitary nucleus travel, with cell bodies within the geniculate ganglion, with the chorda tympani and eventually the lingual nerve to receive taste sensation from the anterior two-thirds of the tongue.[3]

Course of the Facial Nerve

The path of the facial nerve can be divided into segments: Intracranial, meatal (13–15 mm, brainstem to internal auditory canal), labyrinthine (3–4 mm, internal auditory canal to geniculate ganglion), tympanic (8–11 mm, geniculate ganglion to pyramidal eminence), mastoid (10–14 mm, pyramidal eminence to stylomastoid foramen), and extratemporal (15–20 mm, stylomastoid foramen to terminal branches).[4,5]

Major Branches

The facial nerve gives off 10 major branches:

1. The *greater (superficial) petrosal nerve* with fibers synapsing at pterygopalatine ganglion and innervating the lacrimal gland.
2. The *nerve to stapedius*.
3. The *chorda tympani* composed of special sensory fibers for taste and parasympathetic innervation of the submandibular and sublingual gland.
4. The *posterior auricular nerve*.
5. The *nerve to posterior Belly of digastric*.
   The nerves which innervate the muscles of facial expression all extend from the *pes anserinus*, a branching point within the parotid gland, dividing temporozygomatic and cervicofacial portions.
6. The *temporal* branch innervates forehead muscles (the frontalis, corrugator, and upper orbicularis oculi) and typically has isolated terminal branches with no cross-connections with other branches.

7. The *zygomatic* innervates the lower orbicularis oculi with multiple anastomoses with buccal branches.
8. The *buccal* branch innervates the zygomaticus muscles and superior labial muscles (levator anguli oris, buccinator, and orbicularis oris) with cross-anastomoses with zygomatic branches.
9. The *marginal mandibular*, supplies innervation to the depressor muscles of the mouth and lips, and exists also as a terminal branch.
10. Finally, the *cervical* which innervates the platysma.

Surgical Landmarks for Main Trunk

Exiting through the stylomastoid foramen, the facial main trunk can be difficult distinguish without reliable surgical landmarks. From the "tragal pointer", the facial nerve can be found 1 cm anterior, inferior, and deep. The nerve is also 6–8 mm deep from the most inferior portion of the *tympanomastoid suture line*. The nerve itself lies in the same plane as *posterior belly of the digastric*. If the case is complicated or the above methods are not suitable, two additional options are (1) *retrograde dissection* of a distal branch, or (2) identification of the vertical segment of the nerve via an *intramastoid approach*.

Extratemporal Branches

Similar to the main trunk, specific branches of the extratemporal facial nerve can only be identified by utilizing precise surface and dissection landmarks. The frontotemporal branch after branching from the pes anserinus can be found along *Pitanguy's line*, a line drawn from 0.5 cm inferior to the tragus to 1.5 cm above the lateral brow. The zygomaticobuccal branch can be found midway along *Zuker's line*, a line from the root of the helix to the lateral commissure of the mouth. The marginal mandibular branch can be found typically 1 cm inferior from the lower border of the body of the mandible.

Microscopic Anatomy

Nerve anatomy can be broken into three portions of endoneurium, perineurium, and epineurium. Where each bundles either; individual axons and the endoneural tube, endoneural tubules, or nerve sheaths and vasculature respectively. When approaching nerve injury, the Sunderland criteria (Table 1) is a useful system to classify the prognosis and management of a particular injury.[6,7]

■ WORK UP OF FACIAL NERVE PARALYSIS

It is critical to evaluate wide differential and obtain through history and physical examination to rule in or out specific diagnosis. Within a history a clinician should focus on onset, duration, and progression. Specific assessment of previous infections, trauma, surgeries, or toxin exposure helps further categorizes etiology. Attentions should be paid to associated symptoms of pain, otalgia, vision changes, and hearing loss can succinctly narrow the differential. Finally, facial nerve paralysis is associated with five functional deficits that be assessed; lagophthalmos and ectropion, nasal obstruction, oral incompetence, mastication and articulation difficulties.

A complete and thorough head and neck examination should be conducted, with attention paid to facial symmetry, paresis versus paralysis, eye closure, and tear production. Utilizing the House-Brackmann scale (Table 2), allows clinician's to easily describe their findings on a numerical basis.

Imaging and Testing

Imaging for facial paralysis in indicated under certain circumstances as defined by the American Academy of Otolaryngology (AAO) guidelines; second paralysis on the same side, paralysis of isolated branches, paralysis associated with other cranial nerve involvement, or no sign of recovery after 3 months. The MRI is the primary test of choice with focus on visualization of the IAC. If MRI is contraindicated, a CT can be used with further evaluation of bony anatomy.

Other ancillary tests such as a baseline audiogram can be important for temporal injuries or if intratemporal access is expected. A wealth of neurostimulatory examinations exists to aid in the facial paralysis workup. They include

Table 1: Sunderland's criteria				
	Sunderland class	*Seddon*	*Description*	*Recovery*
Mild	I	Neurapraxia	Conduction block, nerve in continuity	<3 months
	II	Axonotmesis	Noncontinuity, nerve intact, axonal sprouting/Wallerian degeneration	1 mm per day
	III		Excessive scarring of endoneurium that hinders axon regeneration	<1 mm per day, slowed by scar formation, based on extent of involved fascicles
	IV		Nerve still in-continuity, scar blocks regeneration	Required surgical intervention to reestablish transduction by removing scar and reanastomosing nerve
Most severe	V	Neurotmesis	Rupture of nerve, no continuous fiber	Requires surgical intervention

the most common, Electroneurography (ENoG), which utilizes an evoked electromyography (EMG) within the post-acute timer period 24–72 hours after onset, but should not be performed after 14 days. ENoG demonstrating a more than 90% degeneration poses a poor prognosis for recovery. After 14 days EMG, it can be used to measure the existence of functional motor units. EMG is typically indicated if an injury lasts more than 12 months, to identify which facial muscles are functional and thus amenable to reinnervation procedures. Other rarely used tests include, nerve excitability test (NET), maximal stimulation test (MST), topognostic tests (Schirmer, stapedial reflex, salivary flow test, taste testing, and salivary pH), which all are fairly low-yield.[5,8] Depending on the etiology a blood workup of treponemal studies (VDRL/FTA-Abs, and Lyme titers), complete blood count (CBC), and an angiotensin-converting-enzyme (ACE) level can be useful.

■ MANAGEMENT

Acute Phase

Eye care in all cases:[9-11]
- Eye drops
- Ointment
- Lacrisert, contacts or occlusive bubble
- Taping
- Patch
- Tarsorrhaphy
- Lateral canthoplasty
- Gold or platinum weight insertion
- Palpebral spring
- Wedge resection of lower lid (irreversible)
- Lateral tarsal stripping (irreversible).

Treat the underlying cause when possible:[5]
- *Bell's palsy*: Corticosteroids, antiviral therapy, decompression when indicated
- *Herpes zoster*: Corticosteroids and antiviral therapy
- *Melkersson-Rosenthal*: Corticosteroids
- *Lyme*: Antibiotics
- *Otologic disease*: Treat middle ear disease
- *Penetrating injury*: Explore and primary repair (ideally within 72 hours) if lateral to a vertical line perpendicular to lateral canthus
- *Iatrogenic injury*: Primary repair if possible
- *Temporal bone trauma*: Only explore and primary neurorrhaphy if disruption is clearly seen on imaging and surgical access is possible.

■ LONG-TERM REHABILITATION

Considerations

- *Timing*:
  - Muscles atrophy after 18 months

- Electromyography should be performed if facial paralysis of 12 months duration to identify if muscles can be reinnervated and have not atrophied
  - Bell's palsy should not be rehabilitated before 12 months due to potential for recovery.
- *Presence of partial movement*:
  - Muscles may have been preserved longer than 18 months
  - Optimizes results of XII-VII graft.
- Status of the proximal and distal VII
- Status of the main three donor nerves (XII, nerve to masseter, contralateral VII)
- Patient age and health status
- Prior radiation (decreases grafting success rate)
- *Patient smile pattern*:
  - The "zygomaticus smile", driven by the actions of the zygomaticus major and when present minor, and buccinator muscles is present in the majority (67%) of individuals, followed by the "canine" smile (30% of individuals) resulting from action of zygomaticus and levator labii superioris muscles, and the rare (2%) "full-denture" smile which is the result of simultaneous action of lip elevators and depressor musculature.
- *Goals of surgery*:
  - *Functional*: Eye protection and oral competence
  - *Cosmetic*: Symmetry and volitional facial expression.
- *Ranking of best procedures in terms of outcome (good review question)*:
  - *Best*: Procedures that restore neural input
  - *Second*: Restoring nonfunctioning muscle by functioning muscle with another neural input
  - *Third*: Static techniques.

Optimal techniques for reinnervation from most favorable to least favorable:[12]
- Observation (if nerves are intact) for 12 months as spontaneous recovery may occur
- Primary repair
- Cable grafting with sural nerve, medial antebranchial cutaneous nerve, or greater auricular nerve (GAN) "nerve substitution".
  - Hypoglossal nerve, nerve to masseter.
- Cross-face grafting:
  - May be augmented with the "babysitter procedure" (cite Terzis et al.).
- *Order of priority for reinnervation*:
  - Midface branches (buccal and zygomatic)
  - Marginal mandibular
  - Frontal
  - Cervical.
- Neural input may recover up to 3 years after injury.[13-16]

Specific facial nerve rehabilitation techniques when reinnervation is not possible are divided into specific techniques for each facial third.
- *Upper third*: Brow, upper, and lower eyelids.[17]
  - The brow is optimally managed with direct brow lift

Table 2: House-Brackmann grading system.

Grade	Description	Function	Resting appearance	Dynamic appearance
1	Normal	Normal	Normal	Normal
2	Mild dysfunction	Weakness with effort, mild synkinesis	Normal	Mild oral and forehead asymmetry; complete eye closure with minimal effort
3	Moderate dysfunction	Obvious asymmetry with movement, noticeable synkinesis or contracture	Normal	Mild oral asymmetry, complete eye closure with effort, slight forehead movement
4	Moderately severe dysfunction	Obvious asymmetry, disfiguring asymmetry	Normal	Asymmetrical mouth, incomplete eye closure, no forehead movement
5	Severe dysfunction	Barely perceptible movement	Asymmetric	Slight oral/nasal movement with effort, incomplete eye closure
6	Total paralysis	None	Asymmetric	No movement

- The upper eyelid is optimally managed with eyelid implants
- The lower eyelid is optimally managed with lateral tarsal stripping
- Botox for synkinesis, hypertonia, Bogorad's syndrome.

- *Midface*: Nose, nasolabial folds, oral commissure.
  - External nasal valve cartilage can be managed with a fascia lata sling, securing sesamoid cartilages of the nare laterally to temporalis fascia. Suture suspension techniques can be placed medial (to define a flattened fold) or lateral (to flatten a prominent fold) to the nasolabial fold
  - Midface techniques also focus on correcting the patient's smile in accordance with their "smile type". There are a number of static and dynamic approaches to achieve proper emotive smile.
    - » Static slings (autogenous, allogenic-alloderm, synthetic-ePTFE/Goretex)[18]
    - » Dynamic:
      - Regional muscle transfer (one stage)
        - ◊ Orthodromic temporalis transfer
        - ◊ Traditional temporalis transfer
        - ◊ Masseteric transfer
      - Free muscle transfer (requires two stages with cross-face nerve grafting at least 6 months prior, second stage is performed when a positive Tinel's sign is present).[19,20]
        - ◊ Gracilis (most often used)
        - ◊ Latissimus dorsi
        - ◊ Pectoralis minor.

- *Lower face*: Lower lip, chin, and neck.[21]
  - Lower lip vector aberrancies
  - Chemodenervation of the contralateral lip by botulinum toxin
  - Transecting the fibers of the contralateral depressor labii inferioris
  - Digastric or platysma muscle transfer to dynamically reanimate the lower lip
  - Mentalis dimpling can be treated with botulinum toxin and aberrant activity of the platysma can be treated with botulinum or platysmectomy.[22]

OUTCOME MEASURES

Patient-reported Outcome Measures

Facial Clinimetric Evaluation Scale (FaCE) and Facial Disability Index (FDI), however there has yet to be a specific assessment tool specifically for quality of life outcomes.[23]

Clinician Reported Outcome Measures

Sunnybrook Measures

Facial Grading System based on: Resting symmetry, voluntary excursion, and degree of synkinesis. All areas of the face and standard expressions are used to create composite scale from 0 to 100. Provides range of assessments requiring more in-depth physical examination.[24]

Quantitative Assessments

- FaCE, and FDI.[25]
- House-Brackmann grading system (Table 2).

REFERENCES

1. Medscape. (2015). Facial nerve anatomy. [online]. Available from http://emedicine.medscape.com/article/835286-overview [Accessed March, 2017].
2. Flint P, Haughey B, Niparko J, et al. Cummings Otolaryngology: Head and Neck Surgery. London: Elsevier Health Sciences; 2010.
3. Anatomy-Medicine.com. (2016). The facial nerve. [online] Available from http://anatomy-medicine.com/nervous-system/113-the-facial-nerve.html [Accessed March, 2017].
4. Kochhar A, Larian B, Azizzadeh B. Facial nerve and parotid gland anatomy. Otolaryngol Clin. 2016;49:273-84.
5. Pasha R, Golub JS. Otolaryngology Head and Neck Surgery: Clinical Reference Guide, 4th edition. North America: Plural Publishing; 2014.

6. Drnathbrachialplexus.com. (2016). Nerve injury. [online] Available from http://www.drnathbrachialplexus.com/brachial_plexus/images/Nerve_injury_table_1_1.jpg [Accessed March, 2017].

7. Cleveland Clinic. (2006). Classification of peripheral nerve trauma. [online] Available from http://clinicalgate.com/trauma-of-the-nervous-system-peripheral-nerve-trauma/ [Accessed March, 2017].

8. Iowa Head and Neck Protocols Wiki. (2014). Acute facial paralysis evaluation. [online] Available from https://iowaheadneckprotocols.oto.uiowa.edu/display/protocols/Acute+Facial+Paralysis+Evaluation [Accessed March, 2017].

9. Engström M, Berg T, Stjernquist-Desatnik A, et al. Prednisolone and valaciclovir in Bell's palsy: a randomised, double-blind, placebo-controlled, multicentre trial. Lancet Neurol. 2008;7:993-1000.

10. Salinas RA, Alvarez G, Daly F, et al. Corticosteroids for Bell's palsy (idiopathic facial paralysis). Cochrane Database Syst Rev. 2010:CD001942.

11. Lee V, Currie Z, Collin J. Ophthalmic management of facial nerve palsy. Eye. 2004;18:1225-34.

12. Moradzadeh A, Borschel G, Luciano JP, et al. The impact of motor and sensory nerve architecture on nerve regeneration. Exp Neurol. 2008;212:370-6.

13. Spira M. Anastomosis of masseteric nerve to lower division of facial nerve for correct of lower facial paralysis. Preliminary report. Plast Reconstr Surg. 1978;61:330-4.

14. Hontanilla B, Marré D. Comparison of hemihypoglossal nerve versus masseteric nerve transpositions in the rehabilitation of short-term facial paralysis using the Facial Clima evaluating system. Plast Reconstr Surg. 2012;130:662e-72e.

15. Biglioli F, Colombo V, Rabbiosi D, et al. Masseteric-facial nerve neurorrhaphy: results of a case series. J Neurosurg. 2016;1-7.

16. May M, Sobol SM, Mester SJ. Hypoglossal-facial nerve interpositional-jump graft for facial reanimation without tongue atrophy. Otolaryngol Head Neck Surg. 1991;104:818-25.

17. Chi JJ. Management of the eye in facial paralysis. Facial Plast Surg Clin North Am. 2016;24:21-8.

18. Chen G, Yang X, Wang W, et al. Mini-temporalis transposition: a less invasive procedure of smile restoration for long-standing incomplete facial paralysis. J Craniofac Surg. 2015;26:518-21.

19. Azizzadeh B, Pettijohn KJ. The gracilis free flap. Facial Plast Surg Clin. 2016;24:47-60.

20. Sharma P, Zuker RM, Borschel GH. Gracilis free muscle transfer in the treatment of pediatric facial paralysis. Facial Plast Surg. 2016;32:199-208.

21. Hayashi A, Yoshizawa H, Natori Y, et al. Assessment of T-shape double fascia graft for lower lip deformity from facial paralysis: a questionnaire survey. J Plast Reconstr Aesthet Surg. 2016;69:427-35.

22. Papel ID, Capone RB. Botulinum toxin A for mentalis muscle dysfunction. Arch Facial Plast Surg. 2001;3:268-9.

23. Ho AL, Scott AM, Klassen AF, et al. Measuring quality of life and patient satisfaction in facial paralysis patients: a systematic review of patient-reported outcome measures. Plast Reconstr Surg. 2012;130:91-9.

24. Ross B, Fradet G, Nedzelski JM. Development of a sensitive clinical facial grading system. Otolaryngol Head Neck Surg. 1996;114:380-6.

25. Kahn J, Gliklich R, Boyev K, et al. Validation of a patient-graded instrument for facial nerve paralysis: the FaCE scale. Laryngoscope. 2001;111:387-98.

Multiple Choice Questions

Q 1. Which of the following statements regarding the palpebral spring is TRUE?

A. It is a passive animation method used in the management of lagophthalmos due to facial paralysis
B. The lower end should be wrapped in a sheet of Gelfim
C. Both gravity and pressure are factors that help to restore eyelid function
D. The distance between the spring arms should be 1.5 times the palpebral aperture

Ans: D. The distance between the spring arms should be 1.5 times the palpebral aperture

Q 2. A patient has an idiopathic left facial paralysis. Which of the following indicates a POOR prognosis?

A. Sudden onset
B. Disturbance of taste
C. No acoustic stapedial reflux
D. Loss of Bell's phenomenon

Ans: D. Loss of Bell's phenomenon

Q 3. Which of the following statements regarding Gracilis Muscle free tissue transfer is TRUE in microvascular dynamic facial reanimation?

A. The nerve supply is from the posterior branch of the obturator nerve
B. The blood supply is from branches of the superficial femoral artery
C. It is the most commonly used muscle in the two-stage technique
D. The time between the two stages of reanimation is 6 months

Ans: C. It is the most commonly used muscle in the two-stage technique

Q 4. Which of the following statements about gold weight implantation used in the upper eyelid for facial paralysis is FALSE?

A. Gold weight implantation is a lid loading and gravity-dependent procedure
B. Gold weight implantation can be performed under local anesthesia
C. Gold weight implantation usually leaves a visible bump on the upper eyelid when it is closed
D. Gold weight implantation is placed in a pocket with the sides of the two fenestrations facing caudally

Ans: D. Gold weight implantation is placed in a pocket with the sides of the two fenestrations facing caudally

Q 5. Which of the following statements regarding temporalis muscle for facial reanimation is TRUE?

A. Successful in restoring a smile in 60% of the patients
B. Successful in improving mouth functioning in 70% of the patients
C. The midportion of the temporalis muscle is used
D. At tunneling the temporalis muscle is sutured to the corner of the mouth without overcorrection

Ans: C. The midportion of the temporalis muscle is used

Q 6. Which of the following muscles used in Facial Reanimation is innervated by the Thoracodorsal Nerve and supplied by the thoracodorsal artery?

A. Pectoralis major
B. Pectoralis minor
C. Latissimus dorsi
D. Serratus anterior

Ans: C. Latissimus dorsi

Q 7. Which of the following muscles is MOST COMMONLY used in Facial Reanimation?

A. Gracilis
B. Serratus anterior
C. Pectoralis minor
D. Extensor digitorum brevis

Ans: A. Gracilis

Q 8. After Facial Nerve birth trauma what is the percentage of complete return of Facial Nerve Function?

A. 30%
B. 50%
C. 70%
D. 90%

Ans: D. 90%

Q 9. Which of the following transposition-grafting is MOST COMMOMLY used in facial nerve paralysis rehabilitation?

A. Hypoglossal-Facial
B. Spinal accessory-Facial
C. Glossopharyngeal -Facial
D. Ansa hypoglossi-Facial

Ans: A. Hypoglossal-Facial

Q 10. Prefabricated gold eyelid implants are MOST COMMONLY USED in which size?

A. 0.5 g
B. 1.0 g
C. 1.5 g
D. 2.0 g

Ans: B. 1.0 g

Q 11. Which of the following nomenclatures referencing the terminal ramifications of the facial nerve is INCORRECT?

A. Temporal
B. Ocular
C. Buccal
D. Mandibular

Ans: B. Ocular

Q 12. The SURAL NERVE is located in which of the following areas?

A. Medial to the saphenous vein and posterior to the lateral malleolus of the ankle
B. Medial to the saphenous vein and posterior to the medial malleolus of the ankle
C. Lateral to the saphenous vein and posterior to the lateral malleolus of the ankle
D. Lateral to the saphenous vein and anterior to the lateral malleolus of the ankle

Ans: C. Lateral to the saphenous vein and posterior to the lateral malleolus of the ankle

Q 13. Which of the following degrees of nerve injury is related to disruption of endoneurium leaving the perineurium intact?

A. First-degree injury
B. Second-degree injury
C. Third-degree injury
D. Fourth-degree injury

Ans: C. Third-degree injury

Chapter 27

Craniomaxillofacial Trauma

Paul Covello

■ INITIAL EVALUATION OF THE TRAUMA PATIENT

Essentials of Advanced Trauma Life Support

The evaluation and management of acute trauma is complex and dynamic. A systematic approach ensures efficient and effective identification, stratification, and intervention of life-threatening conditions. A brief summary of advanced trauma life support (ATLS) protocols is provided below.

Primary Survey and Resuscitation (Table 1)

Adjuncts to Primary Survey

- *Monitors*: Arterial blood gas, ventilator rate, end-tidal CO_2, and electrocardiography
- *Catheters*: Urinary and gastric
- *Radiographs [portable anteroposterior (AP)]*: Chest, abdomen, pelvis, and cervical spine
- Focused assessment sonography for trauma (FAST) or diagnostic peritoneal lavage (DPL).

Secondary Survey and Management (Table 2)

Adjuncts to Secondary Survey

- Performed to confirm suspected injuries only after life-threatening conditions have been identified and stabilized.
- *Imaging*: Computed tomography scan (head, chest, abdomen, and/or spine), contrast studies, angiography, and extremities.
- Endoscopy and ultrasonography.

■ REEVALUATION

- Document all changes in the patient's condition and their response to resuscitative efforts.
- Judicious use of analgesics.
- Continued monitoring.

Transfer

- *Communicate*: Events, interventions, rationale for transfer, and needs during transfer.

Table 1: Components of the ATLS primary survey (ABCDE).	
Airway and cervical spine protection	*Assess:* Patency and obstruction *Manage:* Jaw-thrust → clear foreign bodies → oropharyngeal airway → definitive airway (intubation vs surgical cricothyroidotomy) → transtracheal jet ventilation *Maintain:* Cervical spine in neutral position with manual immobilization *Reinstate:* Immobilization with cervical spine device
Breathing: Ventilation and oxygenation	*Assess:* Chest/neck exposure, depth and rate of respirations, tracheal deviation, chest movements, use of accessory muscles, percussion, auscultation *Manage:* Administer oxygen, ventilate, alleviate tension pneumothorax, seal open pneumothorax, capnography, and pulse oximetry
Circulation with hemorrhage control	*Assess:* Hemorrhage, pulse, skin color, and blood pressure *Manage:* Insert two large-caliber intravenous (IV) catheters, obtain blood work [complete blood count (CBC), chemistries, pregnancy, type and cross-match], warmed fluid resuscitation and blood replacement
Disability: Neurological examination	Glasgow coma scale (8 or less = 50% risk of mortality or vegetative state) *Eye opening:* Spontaneous (4), speech (3), pain (2), and none (1) *Motor Response:* Obeys (6), localizes (5), withdraws (4), flexion (3), extension (2), and none (1) *Verbal response:* Oriented (5), confused (4), inappropriate (3), incomprehensible (2), and none (1) Pupils (size and reaction) Lateralizing signs and spinal cord injury
Exposure and environmental control	Completely undress the patient, but prevent hypothermia

Table 2: Detailed information of secondary survey and management.

System	Establishes/identifies	Assess	Finding	Confirm by
Level of consciousness	Severity of head injury	Glasgow Coma Scale score	<8: Severe 9–12: Moderate 13–15: Minor	CT scan Repeat without paralyzing agents
Pupils	Type of head injury Presence of eye injury	Size Shape Reactivity	Mass effect Diffuse axonal injury Ophthalmic injury	CT scan
Head	Scalp injury Skull injury	Inspect for lacerations and skull fractures Palpable defects	Scalp laceration Depressed skull fracture Basilar skull fracture	CT scan
Maxillofacial	Soft-tissue injury Bone injury Nerve injury Teeth/mouth injury	Visual deformity Malocclusion Palpation for crepitus	Facial fracture Soft-tissue injury	Facial-bone X-ray CT scan
Neck	Laryngeal injury Cervical spine injury Vascular injury Esophageal injury Neurologic deficit	Inspection Palpation Auscultation	Laryngeal deformity Subcutaneous emphysema Hematoma Bruit Platysmal penetration Pain or tenderness of cervical spine	Cervical spine X-ray film Angiography Esophagoscopy Laryngoscopy
Thorax	Thoracic wall injury Subcutaneous emphysema Pneumothorax/hemothorax Bronchial injury Pulmonary contusion Thoracic aortic disruption	Inspection Palpation Auscultation	Bruising, deformity, paradoxic motion Chest wall tenderness Crepitus Diminished breath sounds Muffled heart tones Mediastinal crepitus Severe back pain	Chest X-ray CT scan Angiography Bronchoscopy Tube thoracostomy Pericardiocentesis Transesophageal ultrasonography
Abdomen/flank	Abdominal wall injury Intraperitoneal injury Retroperitoneal injury	Inspection Palpation Auscultation Determine path of penetration	Abdominal wall pain or tenderness Peritoneal irritation Visceral injury Retroperitoneal organ injury	DPL/ultrasonography CT scan Laparotomy Contrast GI studies Angiography
Pelvis	Genitourinary (GU) tract injuries Pelvic fractures	Palpate symphysis pubis for widening Palpate bony pelvis for tenderness Determine pelvic stability (only once) Inspect perineum Rectal/vaginal examination	Genitourinary tract injury (hematuria) Pelvic fracture Rectal, vaginal, and perineal injury	Pelvic X-ray film GU contrast studies, including urethrogram, cystogram, intravenous pyelography Contrast-enhanced CT scan
Spinal cord	Cranial injury Cord injury Peripheral nerve injury	Motor response Pain response	Unilateral cranial mass defect Quadriplegia Paraplegia Nerve root injury	Plain spine X-rays CT scan MRI
Vertebral column	Column injury Vertebral instability Nerve injury	Verbal response to pain, lateralizing signs Palpate for tenderness Deformity	Fracture versus dislocation	Plain X-ray CT scan MRI
Extremities	Soft-tissue injury Bone deformities Joint abnormalities Neurovascular defects	Inspection Palpation	Swelling, bruising, pallor Malalignment Pain, tenderness, and crepitation Absence/diminished pulses Tense muscular compartments Neurologic deficits	Specific X-rays Doppler examination Compartment pressure Angiography

CT, computed tomography; DPL, diagnostic peritoneal lavage; GI, gastrointestinal; MRI, magnetic resonance imaging.

EVALUATION OF THE MAXILLOFACIAL COMPLEX

Once the patient has been stabilized, a more detailed evaluation of the maxillofacial complex must be performed for proper identification of soft tissue injuries, fractures, and dental trauma. Key anatomical areas and pertinent finds are described in Table 3.

EMERGENCIES REQUIRING IMMEDIATE ATTENTION

Compromised Airway

Definition (ASA): The clinical situation in which a conventionally trained anesthesiologist experiences difficulty with facemask ventilation of the upper airway, difficulty with tracheal intubation, or both (Flowchart 1).

Airway Assessment (LEMON)

- *Look:* External characteristics
- *Evaluate (3-3-2 Rule):*
  - Three fingers: Distance between maxillary and mandibular incisors
  - Three fingers: Distance between chin and hyoid

- Two fingers: Distance between floor of mouth and thyroid notch.
- *Mallampati:*
  - I: Soft palate, uvula, fauces, pillars
  - II: Soft palate, uvula, fauces
  - III: Soft palate, base of uvula
  - IV: Hard palate only.
- *Obstruction:* Trauma (maxillofacial, laryngeal, and tracheal), bleeding, vomiting, epiglottitis, oropharyngeal or neck abscess/hematoma.
- *Neck mobility:* Cervical stabilization.

Traumatic Injuries

Common injuries requiring immediate identification and intervention are described in Table 4.

IMAGING OF THE MAXILLOFACIAL SKELETON

Computed Tomography Scan

For the evaluation of facial bone trauma in the adult patient, non-contrast CT is preferred because it offers rapid acquisition, high resolution imaging of bone, adequate visualization of soft tissue structures, multiple planes (axial, coronal, and sagittal), and the ability for three-dimensional rendering.

Table 3: Anatomical area and its pertinent findings (Cunningham).

Anatomical area	Pertinent findings (Cunningham)
Scalp and soft tissues	Abrasions, contusions, lacerations, tissue avulsion, and bleeding
Forehead	*Soft tissue:* Ecchymosis, and edema *Osseous structures:* Step deformity and depression
Naso-orbital-ethmoid complex	*Periorbital soft tissue:* Ecchymosis, edema, epiphora, telecanthus (intercanthal distance is normally 50% of interpupillary distance), rounded medial canthus, shorted palpebral fissure *Conjunctiva:* Injection, subconjunctival hemorrhage, and chemosis *Medial canthus:* Rounded medial canthus, shortened palpebral fissure *Osseous structures:* Crepitus, mobility, step deformity, depression of nasal bridge *Bowstring test:* Movement of medial canthal tendon with lateral traction of the lateral canthal tendon *Cerebrospinal fluid (CSF) leak*
Nose	*Perinasal soft tissue:* Ecchymosis, and edema *Osseous structures:* Crepitus, mobility, step deformity, depression or deviation *Nasal Septum:* Perforation, deviation, and hematoma *CSF leak*
Orbit	*Periorbital soft tissue:* Telecanthus and epiphora *Eyelid:* Ptosis and lagophthalmos *Conjunctiva:* Injection, subconjunctival hemorrhage, and chemosis *Globe position:* Dystopia, hypoglobus, proptosis, enophathlmos *Anterior chamber:* Hypema, corneal abrasion or laceration *Posterior chamber:* Vitreous bleeding and retinal detachment *Visual:* Reduced visual acuity, diplopia (monocular vs binocular) *Pupils:* Anisocoria, relative afferent pupillary defect (RAPD)-Marcus pupil (asymmetric response to light), irregular shape, fixed and dilated *Extraocular movement:* Gaze restriction (Entrapment ± Oculocardiac reflex) *Intraocular pressure (normal = 12–22 mm Hg)* Increased (retrobulbar hematoma) and decreased (globe rupture)
Malar area	*Soft tissue:* Ecchymosis and edema *Conjunctiva:* Injection, subconjunctival hemorrhage (flame sign), and chemosis *Osseous structures:* Crepitus, mobility, step deformity, depression, asymmetry

Contd...

Contd...

Anatomical area	Pertinent findings (Cunningham)
Ear	*Periorbital soft tissue:* Ecchymosis (battle sign) and edema *Ear canal:* Laceration, perforation, blood, CSF, and tympanic membrane
Maxilla	*Soft tissues:* Lacerations, ecchymosis, edema, and avulsion *Osseous structures:* Mobility, palatal expansion, and step deformity
Mandible	*Soft tissues:* Lacerations, ecchymosis, edema, and avulsion *Osseous structures:* Mobility, and step deformity *Temporomandibular joint:* Crepitus, deviation, step deformity, and trimus
Dentoalveolar	*Soft tissues:* Lacerations, ecchymosis, edema, and avulsion *Teeth:* Fractured, mobile, avulsed, embedded into soft tissue *Alveolus:* Step deformity and mobility *Occlusion:* Instability, altered contacts (open or premature), and crossbite
Neck	*Zones:* I: Clavicles to cricoid cartilage II: Cricoid cartilage to angle of mandible (warrants exploration) III: Angle of mandible to skull base *Vascular compromise:* Expanding hematoma, hemorrhage, airway compromise, diminished or absent pulses, differential peripheral blood pressure (right vs left), and clavicular fracture *Aerodigestive compromise:* Dysphagia, hoarseness, air bubbling from wound, crepitus, dyspnea, and subcutaneous emphysema
Cranial nerves	*Ocular/orbital injuries:* Optic (II), oculomotor (III), trochlear (IV), abducens (VI) *Maxillofacial injuries:* Trigeminal (V) and facial (VII) *Neck injuries:* Glossopharyngeal (IX), Vagus (X), spinal accessory (XI), and hypoglossal (XII)

Flowchart 1: ATLS algorithm for airway management

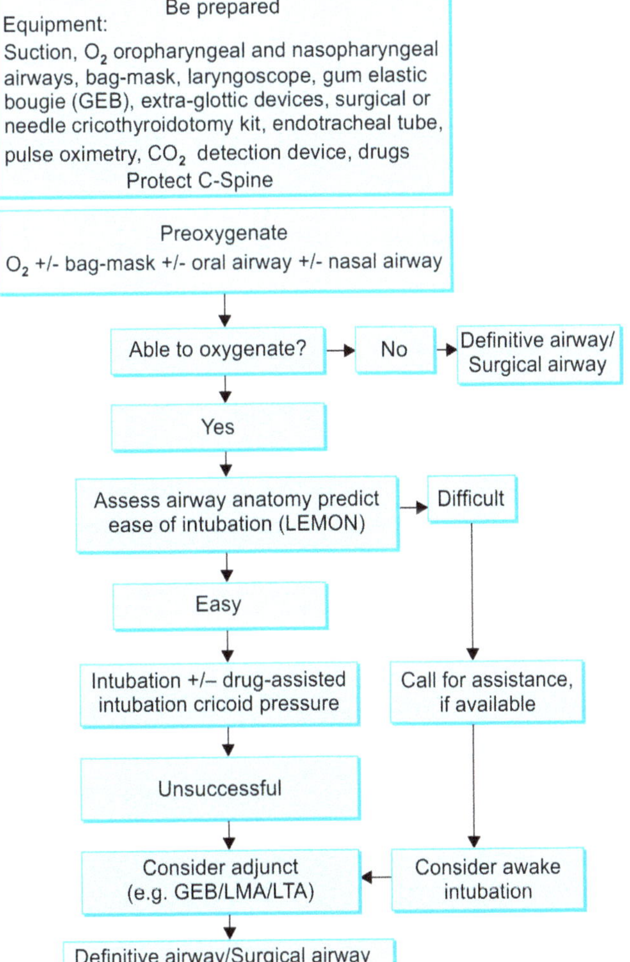

Table 4: Traumatic injuries and its identification.

Injury	Identification
Intracranial hemorrhage	• Altered mental status, focal neurological changes → CT scan • Central midfacial injuries are more commonly associated with CNS trauma
CSF leak	• Rhinorrhea, otorrhea → β2 transferrin or β-trace protein
Globe rupture	• Full-thickness scleral or corneal wound, shallow anterior chamber, decreased intraocular pressure (relative to opposite eye). • May also present with bullous 360° subconjunctival hemorrhage, limited extraocular motility, peaked pupil, or lens material in anterior chamber
Entrapment	• Gaze limitation, diplopia, possible oculocardiac reflex (bradycardia, nausea, and syncope)
Retrobulbar hematoma	• 3 or more of the following: severe pain, decreased vision, proptosis with resistance to retropulsion, chemosis, limited extraocular motility, diplopia, diffuse subconjunctival hemorrhage, increased intraocular pressure (relative to opposite eye), and afferent pupillary defect
Superior orbital fissure syndrome	• Pupillary dilation (CN III), ophthalmoplegia (CN III, IV, VI), ptosis and loss of superior palpebral fold (CN III), hypesthesia of the supraorbital and supratrochlear nerves with loss of the corneal reflex (CN V), and proptosis from engorgement of the ophthalmic vein and lymphatics
Orbital apex syndrome	• Similar to superior orbital fissure syndrome with loss of visual acuity (CN II)
Septal hematoma	• Tender bulging of the nasal mucosa overlying the septum, possible obstruction of airflow

Abbreviations: CT, computed tomography; CNS, central nervous system; CSF, cerebrospinal fluid.

Sources: Lima V, Burt B, Leibovitch I, et al. Orbital compartment syndrome: the ophthalmic surgical emergency. Surv Ophthalmol. 2009;54(4):441-9. Matsuba HM, Thawley SE. Nasal septal abscess: unusual causes, complications, treatment, and sequelae. Ann Plast Surg. 1986;16(2):161-6. Pappachan B, Alexander M. Correlating facial fractures and cranial injuries. J Oral Maxillofac Surg. 2006;64(7):1023-9. Romaniuk VM. Ocular trauma and other catastrophes. Emerg Med Clin North Am. 2013;31(2):399-411. Zachariades N, Vairaktaris E, Papavassiliou D, et al. The superior orbital fissure syndrome. J Maxillofac Surg. 1985;13(3):125-8. Zachariades N, Vairaktaris E, Papavassiliou D, et al. Orbital apex syndrome. Int J Oral Maxillofac Surg. 1987;16(3):352-4.

Table 5: Projection and assessment of computed tomography scan.

Projection	Assessment
Posterior-anterior	Midface fractures, mandible fractures
Lateral cephalic	Airway, retropharyngeal soft tissue, anterior and posterior maxillary antral walls, alveolar ridge, midface fractures, and nasal fractures
Caldwell's lateral oblique	Midface, paranasal sinuses, orbits, zygomatic buttresses, nasal fossa, and mandible
Waters' view	Midface, orbital rims, zygomatic arches, anterior facial structures
Submentovertex	Zygomatic arches and midface fractures
Towne's view	Condyles, inferior orbital floor, inferior orbital rim, maxillary sinuses

Table 6: Injury and management of soft tissue.

Injury	Management
Abrasion	Gently cleansed with mild soap solution and irrigated with normal saline
Contusion	Observation, but may need to evacuate large hematomas
Laceration	Debridement, irrigation with normal saline, layered closure
Avulsion	Skin grafting, local flaps, or free-tissue transfer
Animal and human bites	• Liberal amounts of irrigation and primary closure • Small puncture wounds (i.e. cat bites) are associated with a twofold risk of infection • Antibiotic coverage should include *Pasteurella multocida*

Plain Films

For isolated injuries, two-dimensional plain film radiography offers adequate visualization of specific structures, cost efficiency, and a decreased dose of radiation. Commonly used projections for the evaluation of maxillofacial structures are described in Table 5.

■ SOFT TISSUE INJURY MANAGEMENT

Classification of Injuries

Nearly all facial trauma involves some variation of soft tissue injury. Commonly used terminology is defined in Table 6.

Timing of Soft Tissue Repair

Golden Period (Hammer and Prein, 1995)

Repair of simple wounds involving body areas other than the head are less likely to heal after a period of 19 hours. If kept clean, simple wounds involving the head (including face and scalp) are unaffected by the interval between injury and repair.

Phased Management of the Severe Facial Trauma Patient (Futran, Farwell, Smith, Johnson, and Funk, 2005)

• *Phase I*: Initial encounter
  – Advanced trauma life support trauma management and stabilization

- Identification and management of life-threatening injuries
- Establishment of occlusal relationships
- Debridement of foreign material and nonviable tissue
- Stenting of soft tissue envelop with bone grafts and reconstruction plates for segmental defects.
- *Phase II*: Definitive reconstruction
  - Free tissue transfer for reconstruction of maxillomandibular defects and soft tissue coverage
  - Free bone graft reconstruction of upper face, nasal profile, and periorbital area
  - Nasolacrimal repair.
- *Phase III*: Aesthetic and prosthetic refinement
  - Major flap debulking and contouring
  - Dental rehabilitation with tissue-borne, implant-retained, or implant-borne prosthesis
  - Final oral commissuroplasty
  - Facial prosthetic rehabilitation
  - Cosmetic tattooing
  - Adjunctive cosmetic measures.

Basic Principles in Repairing Specific Soft Tissue Injuries

Scalp (Welch and Boyne, 1991)

- Layers include skin, dense connective tissue, galea aponeurotica, loose areolar tissue, and pericranium (SCALP).
- The arterial adventitia blends intimately with the dense connective tissue layer, which serves a scaffold preventing contraction of cut vessels.
- Two layered closure (galea aponeurotica and skin) limits bleeding and re-establishes a protective barrier.
- The use of drains and a pressure dressing for 48 hours minimizes soft tissue edema.
- Scalp veins that connect with a dural sinus via an emissary vein must be recognized to minimize subgaleal hemorrhage and decrease infection.
- Avulsive injuries may be repaired with a split thickness skin graft if the pericranium is intact.
- Advancement flaps or tissue expansion may be necessary for secondary reconstruction.
- Care should be taken to avoid damage to hair follicles during scar revision by making incisions parallel to healthy hair follicles.

Eyelid and Nasolacrimal Apparatus (Beadles and Lessner, 1994; Smit and Mourits, 1999)

- *Important landmark*: Gray line (muscle of Riolan).
- The anterior, middle, and posterior lamella should be repaired to ensure proper function.

- The tarsus is reapproximated to maintain appropriate lid support.
- Muscle attachments of the levator aponeurosis and Muller's muscle should be identified and reattached to the tarsal plate to prevent ptosis.
- Defects up to 25% of the eyelid length can be closed primarily without resultant entropion.
- Skin grafts, if indicated, can be harvested from the opposite eyelid.
- Lacerations to the medial third of the eyelid should be inspected for damage to the canaliculus.
- Monocanalicular injuries do not require repair, as a single functioning canaliculus provides sufficient lacrimal drainage to prevent epiphora.
- Ends of a lacerated duct are reapproximated over a stent (Crawford tube), which is left in place for 8–12 weeks.
- Secondary dacryocystorhinostomy is indicated in patients with persistent epiphora.

Ear (Punjabi, Haug, and Jordan, 1997)

- Hematomas involving the auricle should be incised and drained, preventing fibrosis and the development of a "cauliflower ear" deformity.
- Following repair, a pressure dressing is required to avoid reformation of hematoma.
- Suturing cartilage should be avoided, if possible, because it may lead to devitalization of cartilage and provide a nidus for infection.
- Avulsive injuries 1 cm or less can be reattached and allowed to revascularize.
- Larger avulsive injuries can be managed with the "pocket principle", in which the detached ear is dermabraded, reattached to the stump, buried beneath a posterior auricular skin flap, revascularlized, uncovered 2–3 weeks later, and allowed to re-epithelialize.

Lip

- *Landmark*: A single suture should be placed to reapproximate the vermillon border.
- Avulsive injuries up to one-fourth of the length of the lip can be closed primarily.
- Advancement, rotational, and cross-lip flaps are used to reconstruct large avulsive injuries.

Parotid Gland (Lewkowicz, Hasson, and Nahlieli, 2002)

- Laceration of the parotid capsule is inspected, cleaned, and sutured.

- Evaluation of trauma to the parotid duct should include cannulation and injection of methylene blue or saline.
- If no extravasation is noted, maintain catheter in place for 1 week and repair facial wound.
- If extravasation is noted and direct anastomosis is successful, stent for 2 weeks.
- If extravasation is noted and direct anastomosis is unsuccessful, the proximal end is ligated.
- Following initial management, external pressure dressing should be applied for 48 hours to prevent sialocele.

Facial Nerve (Coker, 1991)

- Lacerations distal to a vertical line extending from the lateral canthus to mental foramen do not require direct anastomoses due to significant peripheral innervation.

■ FACIAL FRACTURES

Frontal Sinus

Classification (Manolidis and Hollier, 2007) (Fig. 1)

- *Type I*: Linear, minimally displaced fractures of the outer wall
- *Type II*: Comminuted or depressed anterior table fractures (± nasofrontal duct involvement)
- *Type III*: Comminuted fractures of anterior and posterior sinus walls
- *Type IV*: Comminuted fractures of anterior and posterior sinus walls (+ dural injury)
- *Type V*: Comminuted fractures of anterior and posterior sinus walls (+ dural injury and tissue/bone loss).

Management (Bell, Dierks, Brar, Potter, and Potter, 2007)(Flowchart 2)

- *Goals*: Provide an esthetic outcome, restore function, and prevent complications.
- *Procedures*: Repair of anterior table, obliteration, and cranialization.

Nasal Bones (Flowchart 3)

Classification (Rohrich and Adams, 2000)

- *Type I*: Simple unilateral
- *Type II*: Simple bilateral
- *Type III*: Comminuted
    - IIIa: Unilateral
    - IIIb: Bilateral
    - IIIc: Frontal
- Type IV: Complex (Nasal Bone and Septal Disruption)
    - IVa: Septal hematoma
    - IVb: Open nasal laceration
- *Type V*: Naso-orbital-ethmoid

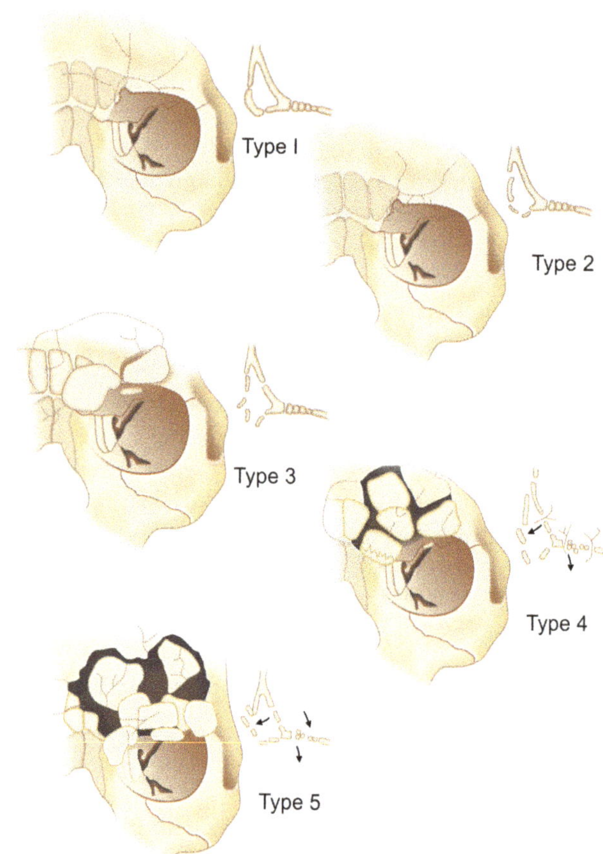

Fig. 1: Manolidis and Hollier classification of frontal sinus fractures.

Naso-Orbital-Ethmoid (Fig. 2)

Classification (Markowitz et al. 1991)

- *Type I*: Single central fragment with attachment of medial canthal tendon intact
- *Type II*: Comminuted central fragment with attachment of medial canthal tendon intact
- *Type III*: Comminuted central fragment with violation of medial canthal tendon
- *Modifiers*: Unilateral, bilateral, open, closed.

Management (Ellis, 1993)

- *Exposure*:
    - Superior: Coronal incision, gull-wing incision, open sky approach, existing lacerations
    - Medial: Lynch incision (curved incision over lateral nasal bone, anterior to MCL)
    - Inferior: Lower eyelid (subciliary, subtarsal, infraorbital), transconjunctival, or transbuccal

Flowchart 2: Algorithm for the management of frontal sinus fractures

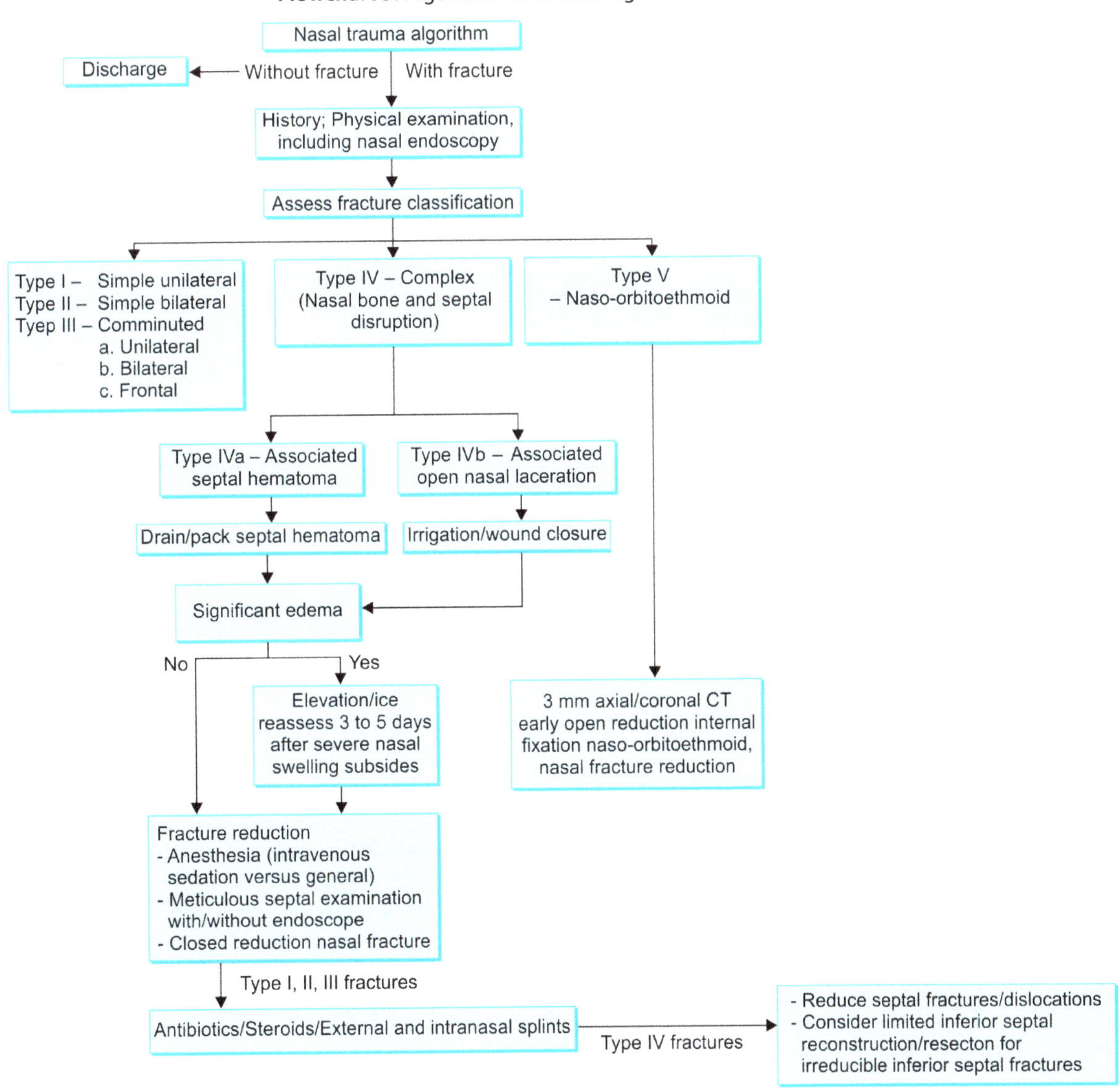

Abbreviation: NOE, naso-orbital-ethmoidal.

Flowchart 3: Algorithm for the management of nasal trauma

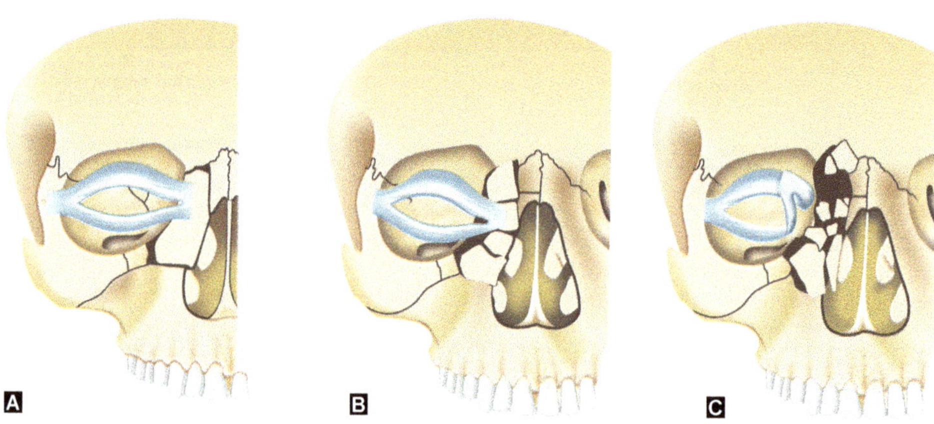

Fig. 2: Markowitz classification of naso-orbital-ethmoid fractures; (A) Type I – single central fragment with intact medial canthal tendon, (B) Type II – comminuted central fragment with intact medial canthal tendon; (C) Type III – comminuted central fragment with violation of the medial canthal tendon.

- – Preferred combination: Coronal incision with lower eyelid incision.
- *Identification of medial canthal tendon*:
  - – Failure to identify tendon or perform medial canthopexy may result in telecanthus.
- *Reduction/reconstruction of medial orbital rims (Fig. 3)*
  - – Most important step in preserving intercanthal distance
  - – Fixation: Transnasal wires (horizontal mattress) with or without bone plates.
  Reconstruction of medial orbital wall:
  - – Failure to repair may result in enophthalmos, diplopia, infraorbital nerve anesthesia, epiphora, and restricted ocular motility
  - – Material: Autogenous (rib, calvaria), titanium mesh, polytetrafluoroethylene (PTFE).
- *Transnasal canthopexy*:
  - – The MCT should be secured posteriorly and superiorly to its native insertion.
- *Nasolacrimal apparatus repair*:
  - – If a sac or duct laceration exists, attempt stenting
  - – Delayed assessment and secondary dacryocystorhinostomy if obstruction exists.
- *Nasal reconstruction*:
  - – Four key principles (Potter, Muzaffar, Ellis, Rohrich, and Hackney, 2006):
    1. Rigid fixation of the nasal pyramid and restoration of nasal height and length
    2. Restoration of tip projection
    3. Septal reduction and reconstruction
    4. Lateral nasal wall augmentation.
- *Soft tissue readaptation*:
  - – Thermoplastic or Denver splints are placed to help redrape the soft tissues into the naso-orbital valley.

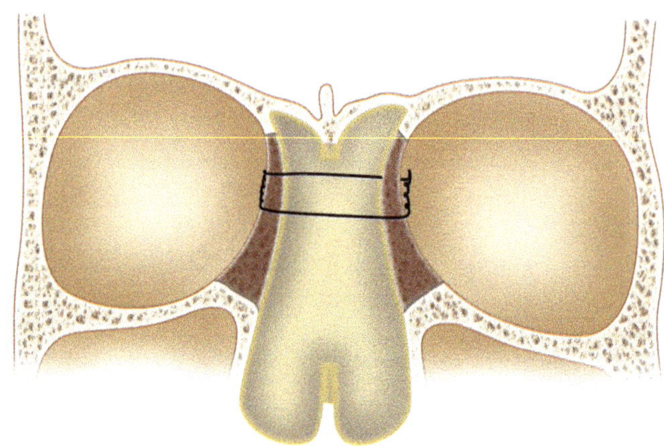

Fig. 3: Fixation of the medial orbital rims with the transnasal wire technique.

Zygoma

Classification

- *Direction of displacement on a Waters' view radiograph (Knight and North, 1961)*:
  - – Group I: No significant displacement
  - – Group II: Isolated zygomatic arch fractures
  - – Group III: Unrotated body fractures
  - – Group IV: Medially rotated body fractures
  - – Group V: Laterally rotated body fractures
  - – Group VI: Complex fractures (additional fracture lines across the main fragment).
- *Pattern of segmentation and displacement on CT imaging (Manson, Markowitz, Mirvis, Dunham, and Yaremchuk, 1990)*:
  - – Low-energy: Little or no displacement with incomplete fracture at one or more articulations

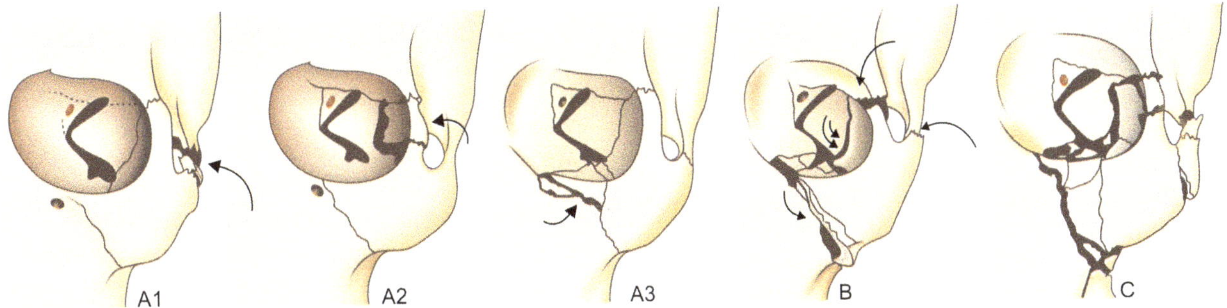

Fig. 4: Zingg classification of zygoma fractures; (A) Type A1 – isolated zygomatic arch; (B) Type A2 – isolated lateral orbital rim; (C) Type A3 – isolated infraorbital rim; (d) Type B – mono-fragment zygomatic fracture; (e) Type C – multi-fragment zygomatic fracture.

- – Middle-energy: Mild to moderate displacement with complete fracture at all articulations, varying degrees of comminution
- – High-energy: Comminution of the greater wing of the sphenoid in the lateral orbit and lateral displacement with posterior segmentation of the zygomatic arch
- *Fragmentation (Zingg et al. 1992) (Fig. 4):*
  - – Type A1: Isolated zygomatic arch
  - – Type A2: Isolated lateral orbital rim
  - – Type A3: Isolated infraorbital rim
  - – Type B: Mono-fragment zygomatic (tetrapod) fractures
  - – Type C: Multi-fragment zygomatic fractures.

Management

- *Isolated zygomatic arch*:
  - – No treatment indicated for nondisplaced or minimally displaced fractures
  - – Reduction without fixation via indirect approach: Gilles (temporal) or Keen (transoral)
  - – Reconstruction of midface width and AP projection in severely displaced or comminuted fractures may require a coronal incision for direct exposure.
- *Zygomatic complex fractures (Ellis and Kittidumkerng, 1996) (Flowchart 4).*

Flowchart 4: Algorithm for the management of zygomatic complex fractures

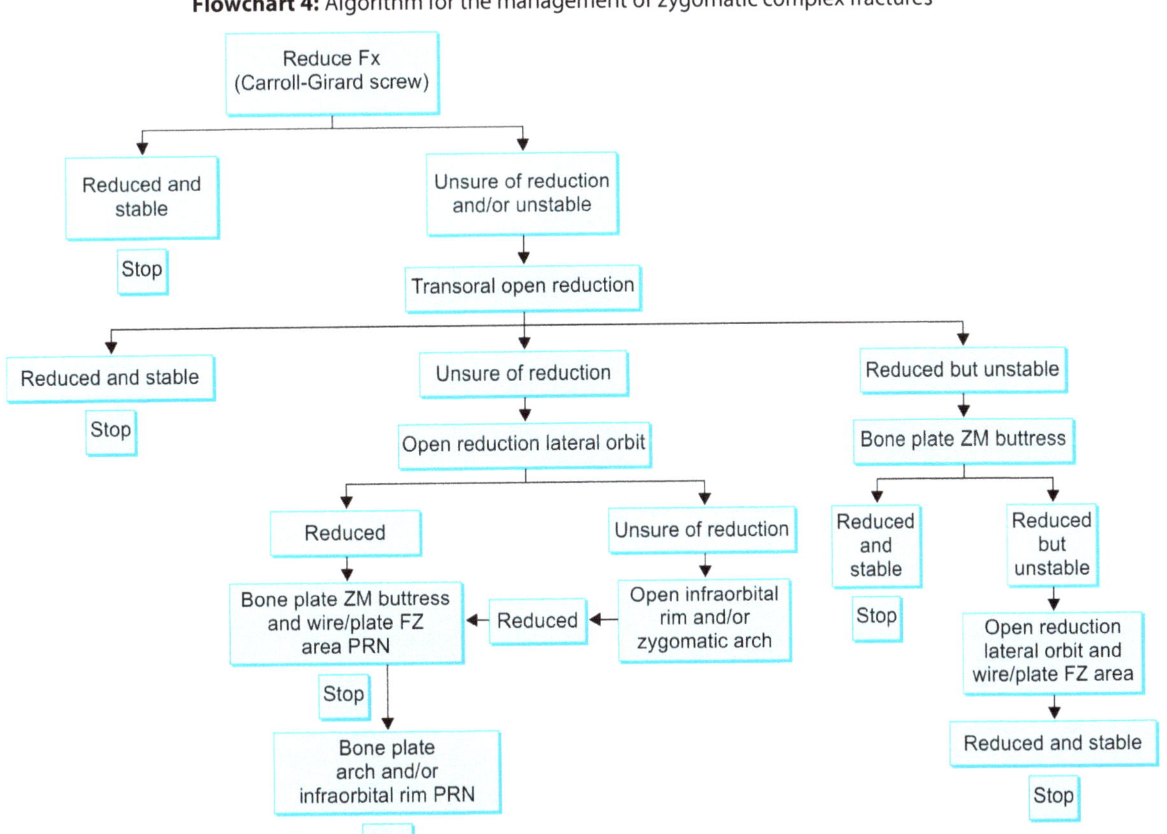

Internal Orbit

Classification

It is described by size and location of defect.
- *Fracture patterns (Hammer, 1995)*:
  - Linear: No defect, periosteal attachments intact
  - Blow-out: Defect less than 2 cm in diameter, limited to one wall
  - Complex: Larger than 2 cm in diameter, two or more walls affected.

Management

Functional and cosmetic considerations (Ochs et al. 2009).
- *Timing (Burnstine, 2002) (Flowchart 5)*:
  - Immediate: Diplopia with CT evidence of entrapped muscle and non-resolving oculo-cardiac reflex; "white-eyed blow-out fracture" in young patients, early enophthalmos/hypoglobus with facial asymmetry.
  - Within 2 weeks: Symptomatic diplopia with positive forced duction and CT evidence of entrapment with minimal clinical improvement; large floor fracture with latent enophthalmos/hypo-ophthalmos, and progressive infraorbital hypesthesia.
  - Observation: Minimal diplopia with good ocular motility and no significant enophthalmos/hypo-ophthalmos.

Maxilla

Classification

- *LeFort (McRae and Frodel, 2000)(Fig. 5)*:
  - LeFort I: Low horizontal fracture pattern that disrupts the tooth-bearing segment of the maxilla, extending transversely above the tooth roots through the maxillary sinus, nasal septum, pyramidal process of the palatine bone, and pterygoid process of the sphenoid.
  - LeFort II: Central, pyramidal fracture, extending from the maxillary tuberosity through the infraorbital rim, and through the nasofrontal suture.
  - LeFort III: Craniofacial dysjunction, extending transversely through the zygomaticofrontal suture, lateral, posterior, and medial orbital walls, and nasofrontal suture.
- *Palatal fractures (Hendrickson et al. 1998) (Fig. 6)*:
  - Type I (alveolar): Fracture of tooth-bearing segments; anterior or posterolateral

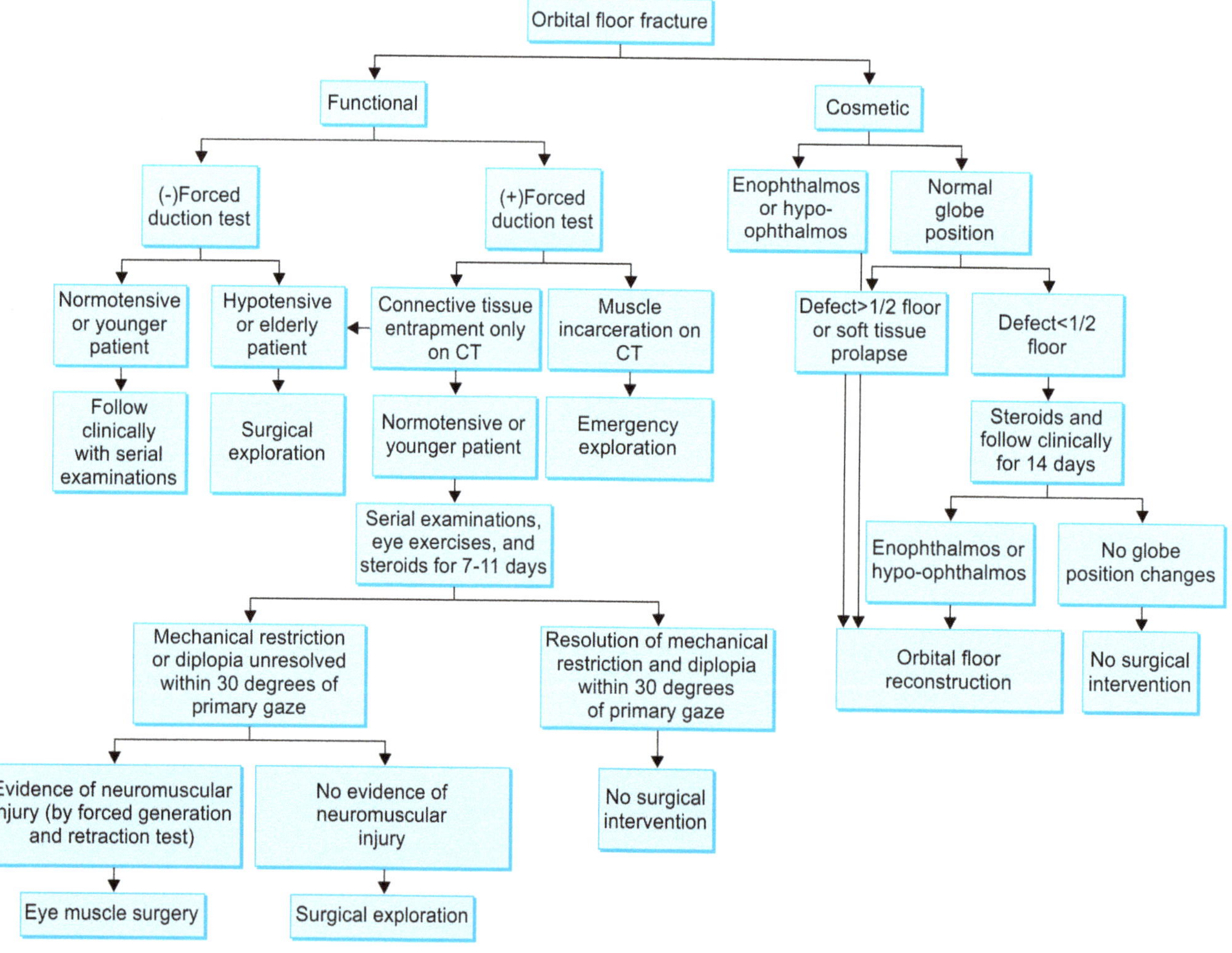

Flowchart 5: Functional and cosmetic considerations for the management of orbital floor fractures

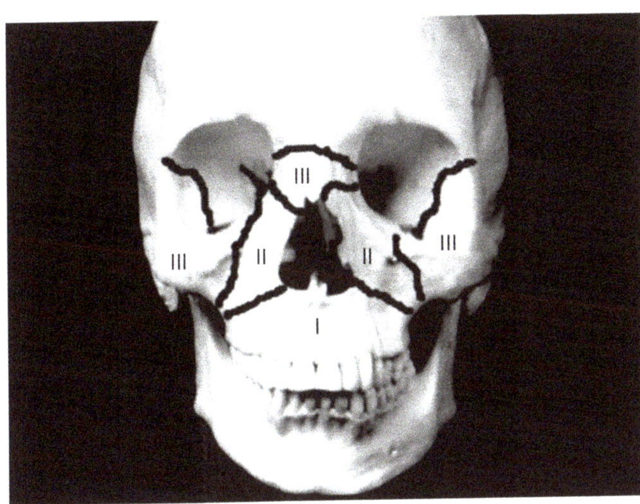

Fig. 5: LeFort classification of maxillary fractures.

- Type II (sagittal): Midline split of the palate
- Type III (para-sagittal): Lateral to the midline
- Type IV (complex): Oblique, transverse, or comminuted fractures of the palate and/or alveolus
- Type V (transverse palatal): Division of the palate and maxilla in a coronal plane.

Management (Kelly et al. 1990)

- *Goal*: Re-establish pre-morbid occlusion and normal facial width, height, and projection.
- *Sequence*: Placement of maxillomandibular arch bars, exposure of fractures, disimpaction and reduction of fracture segments, establish occlusion and maxillomandibular fixation, plate fixation of buttresses, plate fixation of fracture segments, and soft tissue repair.

Mandible (Figs. 7 to 9 and Flowchart 6)

Classification

- *Location*: Dentoalveolar, symphysis, parasymphysis, body, angle, ramus, condyle, and coronoid.
- *Subclassification of condylar fractures*:
  - Fracture level: Condylar head (intracapsular), condylar neck, and subcondylar

- Dislocation at fracture: Medial override, lateral override, no override, and fissure
  - Condylar head relation to articular fossa: No displacement, slight displacement, moderate displacement, and dislocation.
- *Fracture pattern*:
  - Greenstick: Incomplete fracture, involving only one cortex
  - Simple (closed): No communication with external environment
  - Compound (open): Communication with external environment through skin or mucosa
  - Complex (complicated): Simple or compound fracture associated with significant soft tissue injury
  - Comminuted: Multiple, communicating fracture segments
  - Multiple: Two or more fractures within the same bone that do not communicate
  - Pathologic: Fracture secondary to preexisting disease
  - Atrophic: Fracture secondary to mechanical weakening of edentulous mandible (less than 20 mm in height)
  - Indirect: Fracture occurring at a site distant from the area of impact
  - Impacted (telescoped): Fracture with overriding segments.
- *Biomechanics*:
  - Favorable (stable): Fracture line and the vector of muscle pull keep the fracture buttressed and appropriately reduced
  - Unfavorable (unstable): The fracture line and vector of muscle pull cause displacement.

Management and Fixation Techniques

Goals of therapy: Establish a reproducible and stable occlusion, restore form and function (mastication, opening, excursive movements), avoid internal derangement of the temporomandibular joint, and avoid growth disturbances.

- *Maxillomandibular fixation*:
  - Techniques: Arch bars, intermaxillary fixation (IMF) screws, interdental wiring techniques (e.g. Ivy loops, Essig's wiring, Gilmer's wiring, Risdon's wiring), skeletal suspension wires.

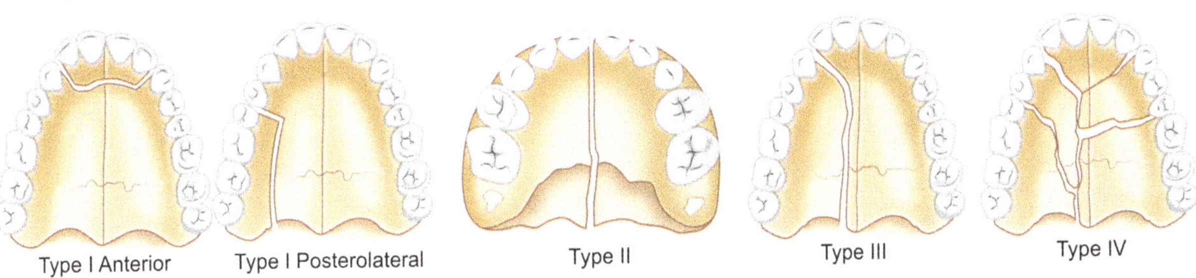

Fig. 6: Hendrickson classification of palatal fractures.

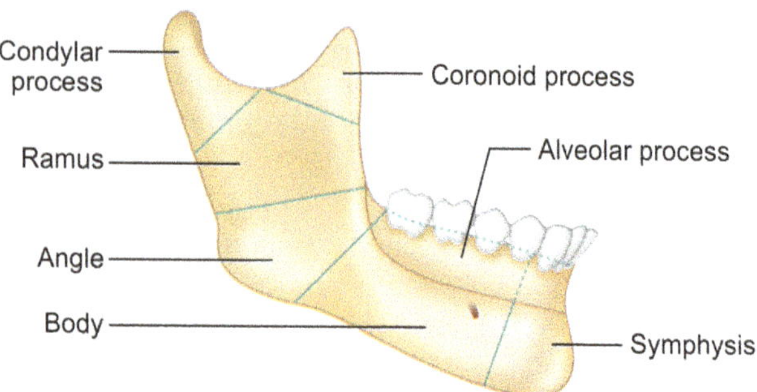

Fig. 7: Classification of mandibular fractures by location.

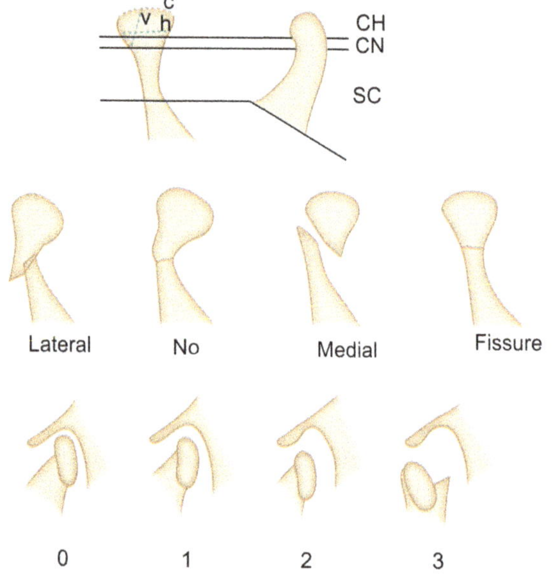

Fig. 8: Subclassification of mandibular condyle fractures; (A) Fracture level: CH = condylar head; CN = condylar neck; SC = subcondyle; (B) Dislocation: Lateral override, no override, medial override, fissure; (C) Displacement: No displacement (0), slight displacement (1), moderate displacement (2), dislocation (3).

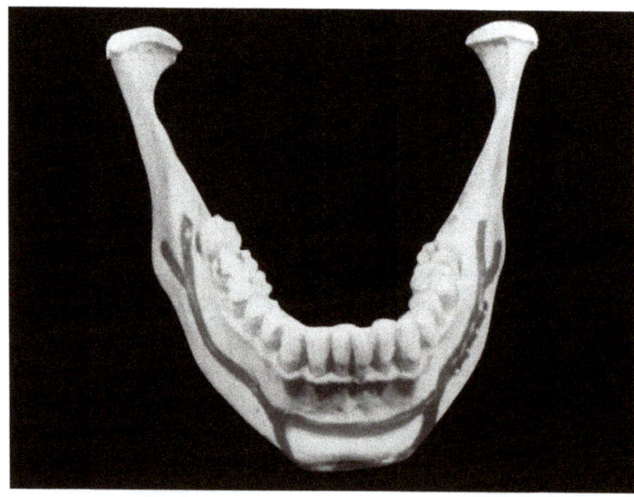

Fig. 9: Champy's ideal lines of mandibular osteosynthesis.

- *Load-sharing*: Stability at the fracture site is created by the frictional resistance between bone ends and the fixation hardware.
  - Examples: Lag screw and compression plating
  - Contraindications: Comminuted or defect fractures.
- *Load-bearing:* The fixation plate bears the forces of function at the fracture sites, accomplished with a locking reconstruction plate.
  - Uses: Atrophic edentulous fractures, comminuted or defect fractures, and complex mandibular fractures.
- *Ideal lines of osteosynthesis (Champy, Lodde, Schmitt, Jaeger, and Muster, 1978):*
  - Horizontal ramus: Masticatory forces create tension along the alveolar border and compression along the lower border
  - Anterior mandible: Masticatory forces create torsion
  - Monocortical miniature fixation plates along the ideal lines of osteosynthesis provide sufficient resistance to masticatory forces for adequate load-sharing fixation.
- *Indications for open reduction and internal fixation of condylar fractures (Zide and Kent, 1983):*
  - Absolute: Severe medial or lateral displacement, inability to reproduce stable occlusion, foreign body invasion
  - Relative: Medical contraindications (e.g. seizures, psychiatrics, alcoholism, intellectual disability), bilateral fractures in edentulous patients, bilateral fractures with concurrent comminuted midface fractures, bilateral fractures with preexisting gnathologic issues (i.e. retrognathia or prognathia).

For noncondylar mandibular fractures, the algorithm shown in Flowchart 6 may be followed.

Dentoalveolar (Figs. 10 and 11)

Classification

- *Ellis and Davey*:
  - I: Enamel only
  - II: Enamel and dentin
  - III: Pulpal involvement
  - IV: Root.
- *Andreasen*:
  - Crown infraction
  - Crown fracture confined to enamel and dentin (uncomplicated)
  - Crown fracture directly involving pulp (complicated)
  - Uncomplicated root fracture
  - Complicated crown-root fracture
  - Horizontal root fracture.

Management (Leathers and Gowans, 2013)

- *Alveolar process fracture*:
  - Occur predominantly in the incisor and premolar regions

Flowchart 6: Algorithm for the management of noncondylar mandibular fractures

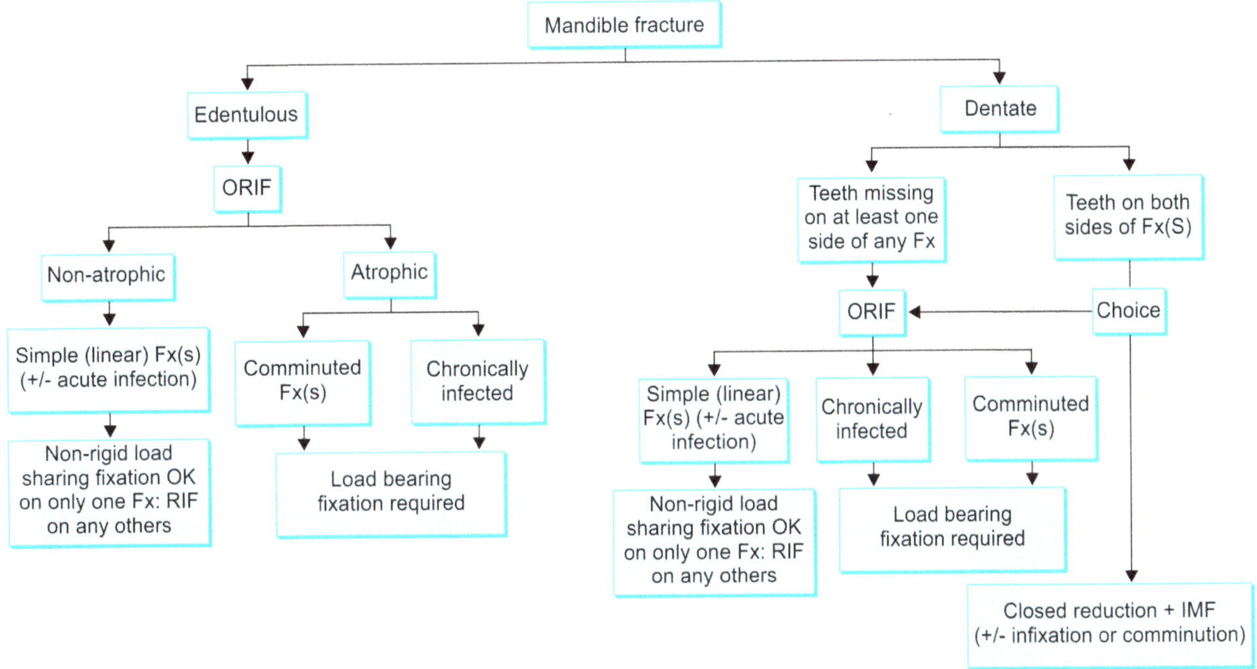

ORIF, Open reduction and internal fixation.

Source: Adapted from Ellis E 3rd. An algorithm for the treatment of noncondylar mandibular fractures. J Oral Maxillofac Surg. 2014;72:939-49.

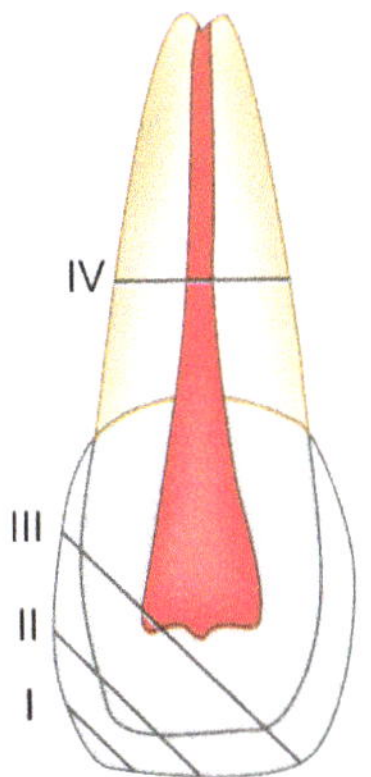

Fig. 10: Ellis and Davey classification of dental fractures; Type I: Enamel only; Type II: Enamel and dentin; Type III: Pulpal involvement; Type IV: Root.

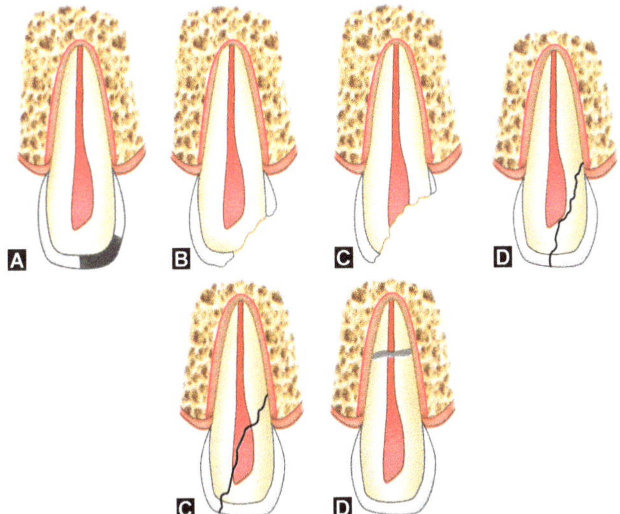

Fig. 11: Andreasen classification of dental fractures; (A) Crown infraction; (B) Crown fracture confined to enamel and dentin (uncomplicated); (C) Crown fracture directly involving pulp (complicated); (D) Uncomplicated root fracture; (E) Complicated crown-root fracture; (F) Horizontal root fracture

- Reduction and then stabilization with rigid splint, Erich arch bar, or Essig wiring technique.
- *Tooth avulsion (Fig. 12):*
  - The tooth should be held by the crown only in order to preserve the periodontal ligament
  - Tooth storage: Solutions that mimic the pH and osmolality of physiologic conditions (Hank solution and Viaspan), cow's milk, or the patient's saliva
  - Timing of re-implantation: Within 2 hours (the periodontal ligament becomes irreversibly necrotic after 2 hours)

- Stabilization: Acid-etch/resin splint (semi-rigid) is method of choice for a period of 7–10 days
- Following stabilization, tooth vitality and prognosis are repeatedly assessed to ascertain the need for endodontic therapy or tooth removal

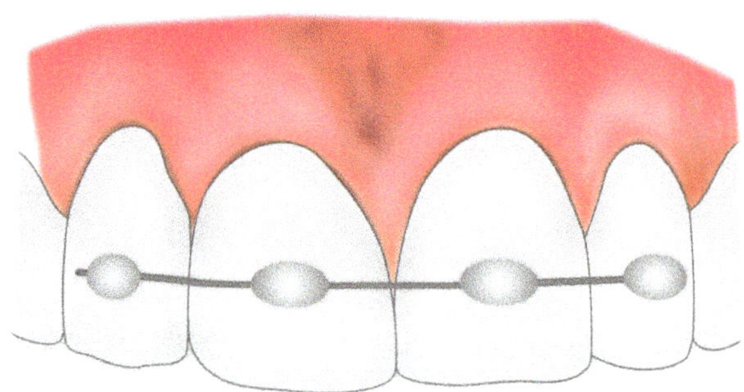

Fig. 12: Tooth avulsion.

- Dental radiographs of teeth and supporting structures should be taken at baseline, 6 weeks, 6 months, 12 months, and annually for 5 years.
- *Delayed sequelae*:
  - Internal or external root resorption, pulpal necrosis, dental ankylosis, alveolar fracture malunion, and soft tissue dehiscence.

MANAGEMENT OF COMPLEX PANFACIAL FRACTURES (KELLY ET AL. 1990)

Historical Perspective

Prior to rigid fixation, war injuries with tissue loss were managed in an "inside-out" and "bottom-up" approach, in which reconstruction began with the mandible and proceeded in a caudal to cranial direction.

Goal

Re-establish pre-morbid occlusion and normal facial width, height, and projection (Fig. 13).

Sequencing

- *Option 1—re-establish the maxillomandibular unit as the first major step (bottom-up)*:
  - Archbars and maxillomandibular fixation are used to re-establish the unit
  - Sagittal split of the palate requires either an intact mandibular arch, reconstruction of the mandibular arch first, or the fabrication of splints to aid in the re-establishment of proper width
  - Once the maxillomandibular unit is established, reduction and fixation proceeds in a caudal direction, starting at the level of the calvarium.
- *Option 2—starting with the reduction and fixation at the level of the calvarium and working in a caudal direction (top-down)*:
  - Cranial unit: Frontal bone fracture fragments are removed, frontal sinus is obliterated or cranialized, sinus and cranial base bone grafting is completed, anterior sinus wall is reconstructed and stabilized

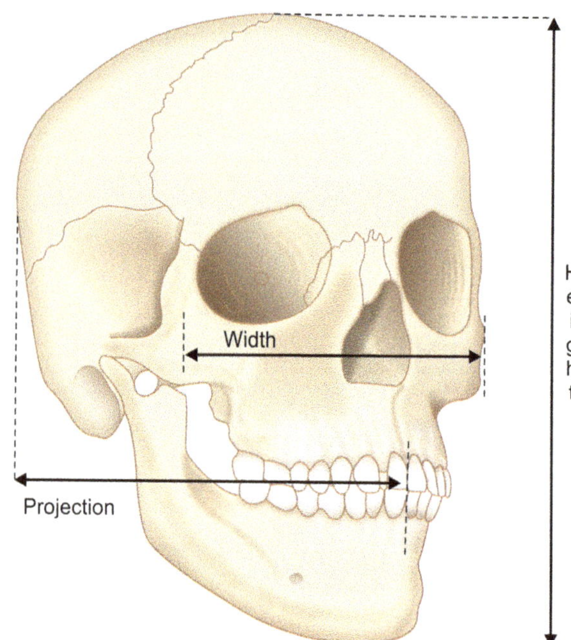

Fig. 13: Pre-morbid occlusion.

to the supraorbital rim (forming the frontal bar), remaining frontal bone fragments are assembled, orbital roof reconstruction is then performed
- Upper midfacial unit: Naso-orbital-ethmoidal fractures are reconstructed and linked to the frontal bar with rigid fixation, the zygomatic arch and zygoma are reduced and fixated, the inferior orbital rim is fixated, the zygomaticofrontal suture is fixated, and the orbital floor is reconstructed
- Lower facial unit: Mandibular symphyseal, body, ramus, and then condylar fractures are reduced and stabilized
- Linking upper and lower facial units: The four anterior maxillary buttresses (bilateral piriform and zygomaticomaxillary) are reduced and fixated, bone defects are grafted if necessary.

PEDIATRIC FACIAL TRAUMA

Anatomical Considerations

- The cranium-to-face ratio is 8:1 at birth, 4:1 by age 5, and 2.5:1 as an adult.
- Skeletal maturity of the facial skeleton occurs at 14–16 years of age in females and 16–18 years of age in males.
- The greater cancellous-to-cortical ratio of bone renders the pediatric maxillofacial complex more malleable.
- Osteogenesis and bone remodeling occur at a more rapid rate than that of an adult.
- Succedaneous (adult) teeth began to replace the deciduous dentition by the age of 6.

Fracture Patterns

- Greenstick fractures are more common due to the cancellous-to-cortical ratio of bone, especially at growth centers.
- During infancy, cranial injuries are far more common than nasal, midfacial, and mandibular fractures due to the relatively larger proportion of the cranium to the facial skeleton.
- Children have more soft tissue covering the maxillofacial skeleton, which results in fewer fractures but the potential for severe soft tissue injuries.

Fixation

- *Wires*:
  - Skeletal wiring (e.g. piriform aperture, circum-zygomatic, and circummandibular) may be required to supplement circumdental wiring to maintain adequate maxillomandibular fixation during the period of mixed dentition.
- *Titanium plates*:
  - Care must be taken to avoid developing tooth buds of the maxilla and mandible
  - Growth may lead to plate migration, precluding their use in frontal fractures
  - If indicated, titanium plates and screws are removed 6 months to 1 year after initial repair.
- *Resorbable plates*:
  - Made of various polymer of polylactic and polyglycolic acids
  - Advantage: Eliminates the need for reoperation to remove implants
  - Disadvantage: Structural weakness compared to titanium.

■ BIBLIOGRAPHY

1. American College of Surgeons. Advanced Trauma Life Support®. Student Course Manual, 9th edition. Chicago, IL: American College of Surgeons; 2012.
2. AO Surgery Reference at www2.aofoundation.org
3. Aziz SR, Ziccardi VB. Management of pediatric facial fracture. In: Fonseca R, Barber HD, Powers M, Frost DE (Eds). Oral and Maxillofacial Trauma, 4th edition. St Louis, Missouri: Saunders, Elsevier, 2013.
4. Beadles KA, Lessner AM. Management of traumatic eyelid lacerations. Semin Ophthalmol. 1994;9(3):145-51.
5. Bell RB, Dierks EJ, Brar P, et al. A protocol for the management of frontal sinus fractures emphasizing sinus preservation. J Oral Maxillofac Surg. 2007;65(5):825-39.
6. Burnstine MA. Clinical recommendations for repair of isolated orbital floor fractures: an evidence-based analysis. Ophthalmology. 2002;109(7):1207-10.
7. Champy M, Lodde JP, Schmitt R, et al. Mandibular osteosynthesis by miniature screwed plates via a buccal approach. J Maxillofac Surg. 1978;6(1):14-21.
8. Coker NJ. Management of traumatic injuries to the facial nerve. Otolaryngol Clin North Am. 1991;24(1):215-27.
9. Cunningham LL. Early assessment and treatment planning of the maxillofacial trauma patient. In: Fonseca R, Barber HD, Powers M, Frost DE (Eds). Oral and Maxillofacial Trauma, 4th edition. St. Louis, Missouri: Saunders, Elsevier, 2013.
10. Ellis E 3rd, Kittidumkerng W. Analysis of treatment for isolated zygomaticomaxillary complex fractures. J Oral Maxillofac Surg. 1996;54(4):386-400.
11. Ellis E 3rd. Sequencing treatment for naso-orbito-ethmoid fractures. J Oral Maxillofac Surg. 1993;51(5):543-58.
12. Futran ND, Farwell DG, Smith RB, et al. Definitive management of severe facial trauma utilizing free tissue transfer. Otolaryngol Head Neck Surg. 2005;132(1):75-85.
13. Hammer B, Prein J. Correction of post-traumatic orbital deformities: operative techniques and review of 26 patients. J Craniomaxillofac Surg. 1995;23(2):81-90.
14. Hammer B. Orbital Fractures: Diagnosis, Operative Treatment, Secondary Corrections. Seattle Toronto Bern Göttingen: Hogrefe and Huber Publishers, 1995.
15. Hendrickson M, Clark N, Manson PN, et al. Palatal fractures: classification, patterns, and treatment with rigid internal fixation. Plast Reconstr Surg. 1998;101(2):319-32.
16. Kellman RM, Tatum SA. Pediatric craniomaxillofacial trauma. Facial Plast Surg Clin North Am. 2014;22(4):559-72.
17. Kelly KJ, Manson PN, Vander Kolk CA, et al. Sequencing LeFort fracture treatment (Organization of treatment for a panfacial fracture). J Craniofac Surg. 1990;1(4):168-78.
18. Knight JS, North JF. The classification of malar fractures: an analysis of displacement as a guide to treatment. Br J Plast Surg. 1961;13:325-39.
19. Leathers RD, Gowans RE. Office-based management of dental alveolar trauma. Atlas Oral Maxillofac Surg Clin North Am. 2013;21(2):185-197.
20. Lewkowicz AA, Hasson O, Nahlieli O. Traumatic injuries to the parotid gland and duct. J Oral Maxillofac Surg. 2002;60(6):676-80.
21. Lima V, Burt B, Leibovitch I, et al. Orbital compartment syndrome: the ophthalmic surgical emergency. Surv Ophthalmol. 2009;54(4):441-9.
22. Manolidis S, Hollier LH Jr. Management of frontal sinus fractures. Plast Reconstr Surg. 2007;120(7 Suppl 2):32s-48s.
23. Manson PN, Markowitz B, Mirvis S, et al. Toward CT-based facial fracture treatment. Plast Reconstr Surg. 1990;85(2):202-12.
24. Markowitz BL, Manson PN, Sargent L, et al. Management of the medial canthal tendon in nasoethmoid orbital fractures: the importance of the central fragment in classification and treatment. Plast Reconstr Surg. 1991;87(5):843-53.
25. Matsuba HM, Thawley SE. Nasal septal abscess: unusual causes, complications, treatment, and sequelae. Ann Plast Surg. 1986;16(2):161-6.
26. McRae M, Frodel J. Midface fractures. Facial Plast Surg. 2000;16(2):107-13.
27. Ochs MW, Johns FR, Marciani RD. Orbital trauma. In: Fonseca R, Marciani R, Turvey T. Oral and Maxillofacial Surgery, 2nd edition. St. Louis, Missouri: Saunders, Elsevier, 2009.
28. Pappachan B, Alexander M. Correlating facial fractures and cranial injuries. J Oral Maxillofac Surg. 2006;64(7):1023-9.

29. Potter JK, Muzaffar AR, Ellis E, et al. Aesthetic management of the nasal component of naso-orbital ethmoid fractures. Plast Reconstr Surg. 2006;117(1):10e-18e.
30. Punjabi AP, Haug RH, Jordan RB. Management of injuries to the auricle. J Oral Maxillofac Surg. 1997;55(7):732-9.
31. Rohrich RJ, Adams WP Jr. Nasal fracture management: minimizing secondary nasal deformities. Plast Reconstr Surg. 2000;106(2):266-73.
32. Romaniuk VM. Ocular trauma and other catastrophes. Emerg Med Clin North Am. 2013;31(2):399-411.
33. Smit TJ, Mourits MP. Monocanalicular lesions: to reconstruct or not. Ophthalmology. 1999;106(7):1310-2.
34. Welch TB, Boyne PJ. The management of traumatic scalp injuries: report of cases. J Oral Maxillofac Surg. 1991;49(9):1007-14.
35. Zachariades N, Vairaktaris E, Papavassiliou D, et al. Orbital apex syndrome. Int J Oral Maxillofac Surg. 1987;16(3):352-4.
36. Zachariades N, Vairaktaris E, Papavassiliou D, et al. The superior orbital fissure syndrome. J Maxillofac Surg. 1985;13(3):125-8.
37. Zide MF, Kent JN. Indications for open reduction of mandibular condyle fractures. J Oral Maxillofac Surg. 1983;41(2):89-98.
38. Zingg M, Laedrach K, Chen J, et al. Classification and treatment of zygomatic fractures: a review of 1,025 cases. J Oral Maxillofac Surg. 1992;50(8):778-90.

Multiple Choice Questions

Q 1. Which of the following is INCORRECT in the management of a severe human bite?

A. Intravenous bolus of a second-generation cephalosporin
B. Debridement of the wound
C. Tetanus prophylaxis
D. Primary closure

Ans: D. Primary closure

Q 2. Which of the following incisions is NOT USED in the approach and repair of a Le Fort I, Le Fort II or Le Fort III fracture?

A. Sublabial incision (gingivolabial)
B. Zygomatic arch incision (Gillies approach)
C. Bicoronal incision
D. Subciliary incision

Ans: B. Zygomatic arch incision (Gillies approach)

Q 3. Which of the following surgical approaches is the ONE used in the treatment of an isolated zygomatic arch fracture with no comminution?

A. Intraoral approach
B. Lateral brow approach
C. Hemicoronal approach
D. Gillies approach

Ans: D. Gillies approach

Q 4. Which of the following fractures of the mandible is BEST visualized with a radiographic Towne's view?

A. Condyle
B. Body
C. Angle
D. Coronoid process

Ans: A. Condyle

Q 5. Which of the following statements is TRUE regarding mandible plating techniques?

A. Wiring fractured bony fragments together will produce "primary" bone healing
B. Dynamic compression plates (DCP) will not require a tension band across the upper alveolar border of the mandible
C. Eccentric dynamic compression plates (EDCP) will require a miniplate along the upper alveolar border of the mandible
D. A tension band can be a miniplate or an arch bar to be used in conjunction with dynamic compression plates

Ans: D. A tension band can be a miniplate or an arch bar to be used in conjunction with dynamic compression plates

Q 6. Which of the following statements regarding compression plating in mandible fractures is FALSE?

A. Compression plates are placed along the basal border of the mandible
B. Strong compression plates alone applied with large screws will overcome the distracting forces with high success rates
C. Tension bands are used with compression plate techniques
D. A miniplate above the inferior alveolar nerve and arch bars attached to the teeth are forms of tension bands

Ans: B. Strong compression plates alone applied with large screws will overcome the distracting forces with high success rates

Q 7. Which of the following surgical approaches is BEST for the management of a Le Fort III fracture?

A. Facial degloving
B. Bicoronal incision flap
C. Bilateral sublabial and subciliary incisions
D. Bilateral lateral rhinotomy and frontozygomatic incision

Ans: B. Bicoronal incision flap

Q 8. Which of the following mandible plating techniques is the one MOST USEFUL in the management of an atrophic mandible fracture?

A. Dynamic compression plates
B. Eccentric dynamic compression plates
C. Mandible reconstruction plates (MRP)
D. Multiple monocortical miniplates

Ans: C. Mandible reconstruction plates (MRP)

Q 9. The four-hole plating system shown below was used to repair a mandible symphysis fracture. Which type of plating is the ONE shown below?

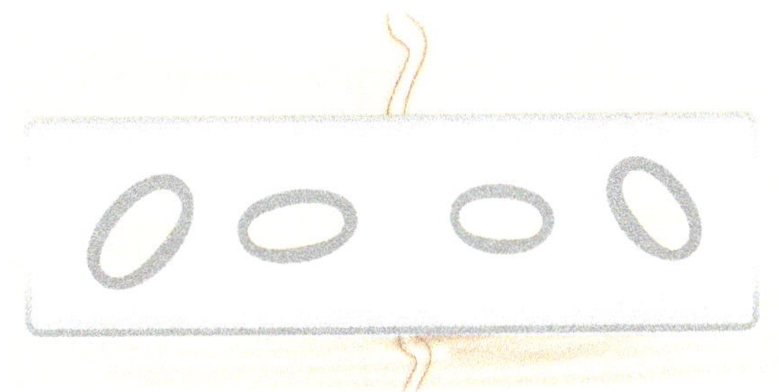

A. Dynamic compression plate system
B. Eccentric dynamic compression plate system
C. Reconstruction plate
D. Titanium hollow screw reconstruction plate (THORP)

Ans: B. Eccentric dynamic compression plate system

Q 10. Which of the following mandible fractures has the HIGHEST incidence of infection?

A. Angle
B. Symphysis/Parasymphisis
C. Body
D. Ramus

Ans: A. Angle

Q 11. The MOST common complication after the reduction of a zygomatic fracture is:

A. Diplopia
B. Enophthalmus
C. Ectropion or inferior scleral show
D. Malar depression

Ans: D. Malar depression

Q 12. Which of the following mandible fractures is usually managed by CLOSED REDUCTION in a dentate, adult patient?

A. Symphysis
B. Body
C. Angle
D. Condyle

Ans: D. Condyle

Q 13. Which of the following is a SOURCE of major bleeding when harvesting a calvarial bone graft?

A. Sigmoid sinus
B. Sagittal sinus
C. Inferior petrosal sinus
D. Superior petrosal sinus

Ans: B. Sagittal sinus

Q 14. The arrow indicates a third molar tooth in an adult mandible. According to the UNIVERSAL NUMBER SYSTEM this tooth is number:

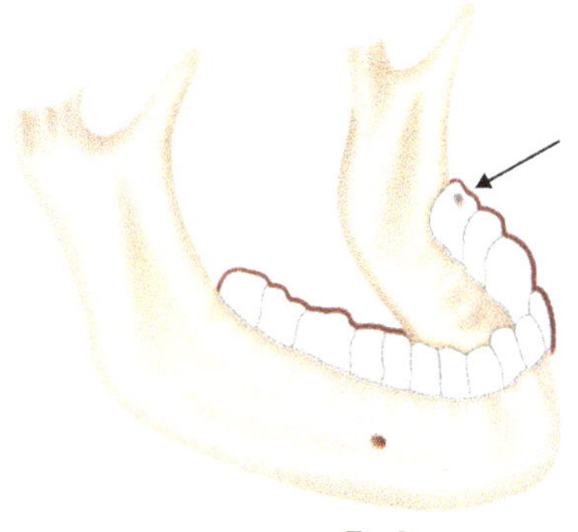

A. 1
B. 9
C. 16
D. 17

Ans: D. 17

Q 15. A mandibular symphysis fracture is usually associated with:

A. Coronoid fracture
B. Condyle fracture
C. Ramus fracture
D. Angle

Ans: B. Condyle fracture

Q 16. Which of the following statements IS FALSE regarding Tension Band Principles applied to a mandibular fracture (dentulous area)?

A. A tension band must overcome the distracting forces at the alveolar border
B. An arch bar can be used as a tension band
C. Bicortical fixation plates are ideal as a tension band
D. A miniplate can be used as a tension band in any mandibular fracture

Ans: C. Bicortical fixation plates are ideal as a tension band

Q 17. What is the time limit that will allow the surgeon to utilize the nerve stimulator intraoperatively to assist in the identification of distal branches of a severed facial nerve?

A. 24 hours
B. 36 hours
C. 48 hours
D. 72 hours

Ans: D. 72 hours

Q 18. Which of the following mandibular fracture managements is the one MOST USEFUL in the reparation of comminuted mandibular body fracture with traumatic bone loss?

A. Multiple miniplates
B. Dynamic compression plates
C. Eccentric dynamic compression plates
D. Mandibular reconstruction plates

Ans: D. Mandibular reconstruction plates

Q 19. The MOST common cause of a "twisted" nose is?

A. Trauma
B. Iatrogenic
C. Congenital
D. Cocaine use

Ans: A. Trauma

Q 20. Which of the following managements is the BEST for isolated fractures of the coronoid process of the mandible?

A. Analgesics and follow-up
B. Maxillomandibular fixation (MMF)
C. Miniplates
D. Microplates

Ans: A. Analgesics and follow-up

Q 21. Which of the following rigid fixation technique used for open reduction of mandibular fractures has lateral holes angled in a superior/medial direction to provide compression at the superior area of the mandibule (Tension side)?

A. Dynamic compression plates
B. Eccentric dynamic compression plate
C. Reconstruction plate (RP)
D. Mandibular external fixator

Ans: B. Eccentric dynamic compression plate (EDCP)

Q 22. In which of the following anatomical areas is silk the RECOMMENDED material for wound closure?

A. Margin of the helix
B. Margin of the eyelid
C. Margin of the brow
D. Margin of the tragus

Ans: B. Margin of the eyelid

Q 23. Which of the following statements regarding mandibular fractures is TRUE?

A. Mandibular fractures that are directed inferiorly and anteriorly are classified as horizontally unfavorable
B. Almost all condylar fractures are managed by open
C. When a symphysis fracture is identified, a subcondylar fracture should be rule out
D. Almost all symphysis-parasymphysis mandibular fractures are managed by closed reduction

Ans: C. When a symphysis fracture is identified, a subcondylar fracture should be rule out

Q 24. The drawing below REPRESENTS a:

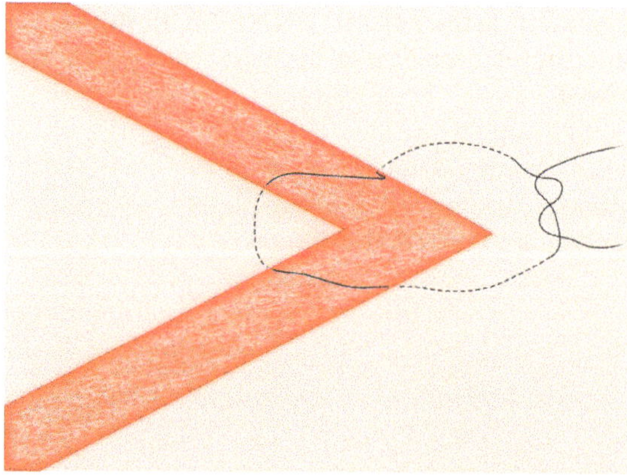

A. Vertical mattress closure
B. Horizontal mattress closure
C. Subcutaneous interrupted closure
D. Horizontal half-buried mattress closure

Ans: D. Horizontal half-buried mattress closure

Q 25. Which of the following facial plating systems CORRECTLY related to the indication?

A. Miniplates—Le Fort fractures
B. Microplates—Zygomatic buttress fractures
C. Dynamic compression plates—highly comminuted mandibular fractures
D. Eccentric dynamic compression plates—glabellar region fractures

Ans: A. Miniplates—Le Fort fractures

Q 26. Which of the following indications is INCORRECT for Three-Dimensional Plating?

A. Comminuted calvarial fractures
B. Orbital defects
C. Blow-out factures
D. Angle of the mandible fractures

Ans: D. Angle of the mandible fractures

Q 27. Which of the following treatments is CORRECT for frostbite of the auricle?

A. Rapid rewarming with moist cotton pledgets at a warm-water temperature of 40° C for 20 minutes
B. Rubbing first with snow then rapid rewarming with moist cotton pledgets at a warm-water temperature of 40°C for 20 minutes
C. Slow rewarming with moist cotton pledgets, first at a warm-water temperature of 35° C for 20 minutes, then at 40°C for 10 minutes
D. Slow rewarming with moist cotton pledgets at a warm-water temperature of 35° C for 30 minutes

Ans: A. Rapid rewarming with moist cotton pledgets at a warm-water temperature of 40°C for 20 minutes

Q 28. A 20-year-old patient has a penetrating injury, stab wound to the right side of his neck. (See drawing below.) The patient arrived at the ER, stable, alert and oriented. He has a huge hematoma in the lower aspect of his neck. The peripheral pulse in his right arm is weak. Which of the following is the MOST APPROPRIATE management for this particular patient?

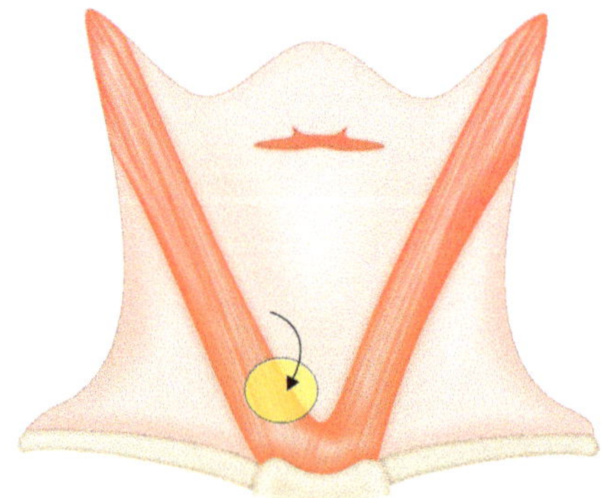

A. Zone I neck injury, immediate neck exploration
B. Zone I neck injury, angiography prior to neck exploration
C. Zone III neck injury, immediate neck exploration
D. Zone III neck injury, angiography prior to neck exploration

Ans: B. Zone I neck injury, angiography prior to neck exploration

Q 29. The mandible fracture represented below is DEFINED as:

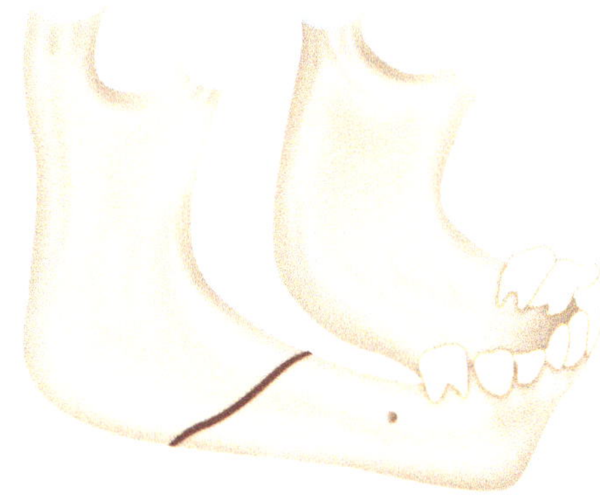

A. Type II, favorable
B. Type II, unfavorable
C. Type III, favorable
D. Type III, unfavorable

Ans: B. Type II, unfavorable

Q 30. Which of the following locations is that region overlying the zygomatic arch ("danger zone") where injury to the temporal branch of the facial nerve is MOST likely?

A. It is between 1.5 cm anterior to the helical root and 1 cm posterior to the anterior end of the arch
B. It is between 1 cm anterior to the helical root and 1.5 cm posterior to the anterior end of the arch
C. It is between 1.8 cm anterior to the helical root and 2 cm posterior to the anterior end of the arch
D. It is between 2.5 cm anterior to the helical root and 2.5 cm posterior to the anterior end of the arch

Ans: C. It is between 1.8 cm anterior to the helical root and 2 cm posterior to the anterior end of the arch

Q 31. Which of the following teeth are NOT RECOMMENDED to be used with maxillo-mandibular fixation (MMF) for a long-term basis?

A. Incisors
B. Canines
C. Premolars
D. First molars

Ans: A. Incisors

Q 32. Which of the following is the most COMMON etiology for loss of eyebrow hair?

A. Trauma
B. Body piercing
C. Trichotillomania
D. Endocrinopathies

Ans: A. Trauma

Q 33. Which of the following statements regarding the management of mandibular pediatric fractures is INCORRECT?

A. Most mandibular fractures can be managed with intermaxillary fixation
B. Intermaxillary fixation is usually maintained for 8 weeks
C. Ivy loops are adequate for intermaxillary fixation between the upper and lower jaw
D. Reduction and fixation should be done early usually within the first 72 hours

Ans: B. Intermaxillary fixation is usually maintained for 8 weeks

Q 34. Which of the following statements about frontal sinus fractures is TRUE?

A. Isolated anterior table fractures are the most common variety
B. Associated facial fractures occur approximately 65% of the time
C. Treatment of facial fractures is standardized
D. Complications usually occur 6 months after fracture

Ans: B. Associated facial fractures occur approximately 65% of the time

Q 35. Which of the following statements about penetrating neck wounds is FALSE?

A. All neck injuries Zones I, II and III, that penetrate the platysma should be explored
B. Symptomatic patients with penetrating neck injury to the Zone III requires angiography prior to neck exploration
C. Asymptomatic patients with penetrating neck injury to the Zone I, requires mandatory angiography prior to neck exploration
D. Penetrating neck injury to the Zone I and III, in both asymptomatic or symptomatic patients requires routine angiography

Ans: A. All neck injuries Zones I II and III, that penetrate the platysma should be explored

Q 36. Which of the following statements about Le Fort fractures is FALSE?

A. Le Fort II fracture is the most common Le Fort fracture pattern
B. Serious concomitant intracranial injury is common
C. Serious concomitant ophthalmologic injury is also common
D. MRI with contrast is the examination of choice for evaluation of these fractures

Ans: D. MRI with contrast is the examination of choice for evaluation of these fractures

Q 37. Which of the following statements about penetrating neck trauma is FALSE?

A. Zone I compromises the root of the neck inferior to the inferior border of the cricoid cartilage
B. Zone II is the zone of the neck between the angle of the mandible and the inferior border of the cricoid cartilage

C. Zone III is the zone compromising the neck superior to the angle of the mandible up to the skull

D. Zone II is the least common site of entry

Ans: D. Zone II is the least common site of entry

Q 38. Which of the following anatomical areas of the mandible is MOST COMMONLY ASSOCIATED with the HIGHEST incidence of infection?

A. Symphysis-Parasymphysis   B. Angle
C. Body   D. Condyle

Ans: B. Angle

Q 39. Which of the following facial areas has FIRST PRIORITY for reconstruction after burns to the face?

A. Eyelids   B. Ears
C. Cheeks   D. Nose

Ans: A. Eyelids

Q 40. Which of the following facial areas has LEAST PRIORITY for reconstruction after burns to the face?

A. Eyelids   B. Ears
C. Cheeks   D. Nose

Ans: B. Ears

Q 41. Which of the following statements regarding electrical injury in children is FALSE?

A. Electrical injury occurs most commonly under 4 years of age
B. Partial-thickness lateral commissure burns are usual
C. Intense edema is followed by sloughing of necrotic tissue and bleeding
D. Commissure splinting can be useful for 6–12 months

Ans: B. Partial-thickness lateral commissure burns are usual

Q 42. Which of the following is the IV FLUID OF CHOICE in Adult Burn Replacement Therapy?

A. Lactated Ringer's solution   B. Normal saline solution
C. Half normal saline solution   D. 5% dextrose in water

Ans: A. Lactated Ringer's solution

Q 43. An unrecognized laceration to the Levator Aponeurosis of the upper eyelid will result in:

A. Lagophthalmos   B. Ectropion
C. Entropion   D. Ptosis

Ans: D. Ptosis

Q 44. A 15-year-old boy suffered blunt neck trauma due to a bicycle handle bar injury. The physical examination and work up revealed massive endolaryngeal edema with airway obstruction, mucosal lacerations with exposed cartilage and an immobile left vocal cord. In which of the following classifications of laryngotracheal injury, according to the Schaefer and Fuhrman, is the injury mentioned above included?

A   I   B   II
C   III   D   IV

Ans: C. III

Q 45. Which of the following reconstruction techniques represents the one used for the Ear Avulsion (with near total loss) shown below?

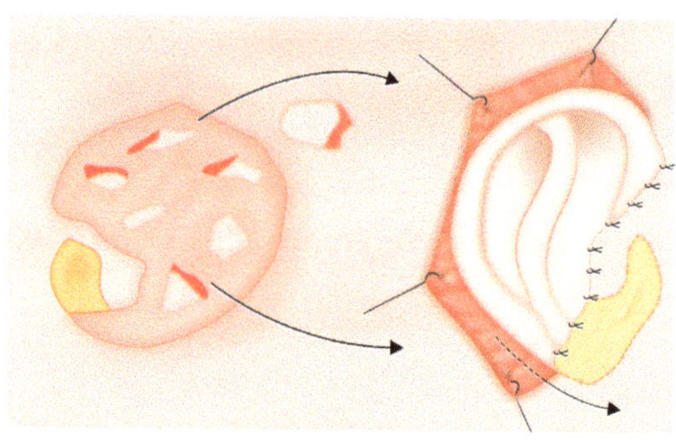

A. The Baudet
B. The Dieffenbach
C. The Tunnel technique of Converse
D. The Davis

Ans: A. The Baudet

Q 46. Which is the appropriate maximal timing to close primarily facial wounds?

A. 24 hours   B. 36 hours
C. 48 hours   D. 72 hours

Ans: B. 36 hours

Q 47. Which of the following statements regarding the extent of the estimated burned surface area is FALSE?

A. Each arm constitutes 9% of the total body surface area
B. Each leg constitutes 18% of the total body surface area
C. The head and neck 18% of the total body surface area
D. The anterior portion of the trunk constitutes 18% of the total body surface area

Ans: C. The head and neck 18% of the total body surface area

Q 48. Which of the following statements about the topical antibacterial agent Sulfamylon (Mafenide) is FALSE?

A. It will penetrate the eschar
B. No hypersensitivity is known
C. It is painful at application
D. It produces metabolic acidosis with a compensatory respiratory alkalosis

Ans: B. No hypersensitivity is known

Q 49. Which of the following facial plating systems is the ONE represented in the drawing below?

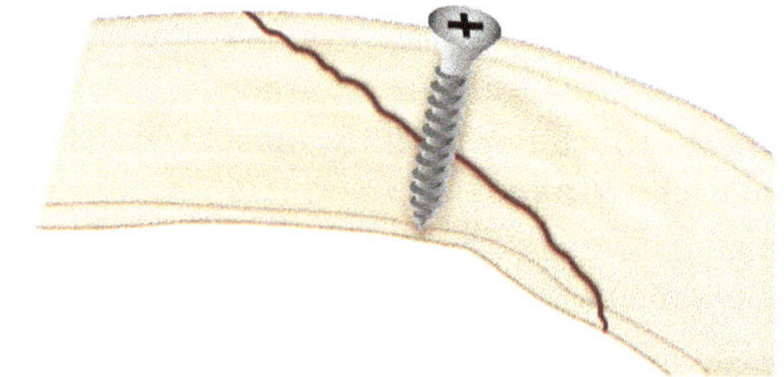

A. Dynamic compression plate system

B. Eccentric dynamic compression plate system
C. Mandibular reconstructive system
D. Lag screw system

Ans: D. Lag screw system

Q 50. Which of the following recommendations is the KEY to the PROPER management of human and animal penetrating wounds?

A. Copious irrigation
B. Debridement
C. Amoxicilin-clavulanate IV
D. Delayed primary closure

Ans: A. Copious irrigation

Q 51. Which of the following statements about oral commisure electrical burns is FALSE?

A. The timing of management is controversial
B. Immediate excision and repair will produce excision of normal tissue
C. Delayed excision and repair carries the risk of labial artery bleeding
D. 90% of cases will require late flaps for commissure reconstruction

Ans: D. 90% of cases will require late flaps for commissure reconstruction

Q 52. Which of the following statements about oral commisure electrical burns is FALSE?

A. 2 weeks after the burn it is necessary to distinguish between vital and nonvital tissue
B. Usually the amount of tissue destruction is less than expected at the initial evaluation
C. The reconstruction stage can start 2-weeks postinjury
D. The acrylic obturator with commisure splint is useful in preventing contracture

Ans: B. Usually the amount of tissue destruction is less than expected at the initial evaluation

Q 53. Which of the following statement regarding frontal sinus fracture is FALSE?

A. Extreme force is required to fracture the anterior table of the frontal sinus
B. Associated serious injuries are common in 2/3 of the patients
C. Combined fractures involving anterior table, posterior table and nasofrontal recess occur in 2/3 of patients
D. Follow-up is limited to 1 year

Ans: D. Follow-up is limited to 1 year

Q 54. Which of the following represents THE BEST course of action after a deep puncture knife wound to Zone III of the neck with swelling and hematoma at the level of puncture entry? The patient is an hemodynamically stable 22 years old male.

A. Direct laryngoscopy and Barium swallow
B. Chest and lateral neck X-rays
C. Angiography
D. CT of neck and base of skull

Ans: C. Angiography

Q 55. Which of the following statements regarding maxillofacial fractures is FALSE?

A. Le Fort I level fracture is more frequently encountered than the Le Fort II
B. Le Fort II level fracture is more frequently encounter than the Le Fort III
C. Le Fort III is the least frequently encounter of the Le Fort
D. All Le Fort can involved the pterygoid plates

Ans: A. Le Fort I level fracture is more frequently encountered than the Le Fort II

Q 56. Which of the following management is the BEST for obstruction distal to the common canaliculus of the lacrimal drainage system?

A. Endoscopic dacryocystorhinostomy
B. Conjunctivorhinostomy
C. Canalicular dilatation
D. Canalicular stenting

Ans: A. Endoscopic dacryocystorhinostomy

Q 57. Which of the following dissection techniques regarding the hemicoronal and coronal flaps in the lateral region of the dissection should NOT be executed?

A. Dissection is done superficial to the superficial layer of the deep temporal fascia
B. Dissection with identification of the superficial temporal fat and its covering fascia
C. Dissection in a subfascial plane over and lateral to the superficial fat pad
D. Dissection below to the deep layer of the deep temporal fascia

Ans: D. Dissection below to the deep layer of the deep temporal fascia

Q 58. What percentage of sensitivity, when used in combination, the barium swallow and the esophagoscopy have for the identification of esophageal perforation after a gunshot to the neck?

A. 60%
B. 70%
C. 80%
D. 90%

Ans: D. 90%

Q 59. Which of the following creams used in burn injuries is painful, penetrates the eschar, cover pseudomonas and may induce hyperchloremic acidosis?

A. Silver nitrate
B. Silver sulfadiazine (Silvadene)
C. Mafenide acetate (Sylfamylon)
D. Bacitracin ointment

Ans: C. Mafenide Acetate (Sylfamylon)

Q 60. Which of the following represents ADEQUATE management of a displaced fracture of the body of the Mandible in a 7-year-old patient?

A. Soft diet, analgesics and antibiotics
B. Closed reduction with fixation using orthodontic splints

C. Open reduction with ivy loop fixation
D. Open reduction with maxillomandibular fixation

Ans: B. Closed reduction with fixation using orthodontic splints

Q 61. Which of the following is NOT RECOMMENDED in facial wound suturing techniques?

A. Skin hooks are very useful in handling soft tissue
B. Gentle inversion of the wound edges
C. The principle of "halving" is frequently used
D. Approximation of the tissue without strangulation

Ans: B. Gentle inversion of the wound edges

Q 62. In which of the following locations sutures can remain the LONGEST PERIOD of time?

A. Scalp
C. Pinna

B. Face
D. Neck

Ans: A. Scalp

Q 63. What is the NORMAL intercanthal distance represented in the drawing?

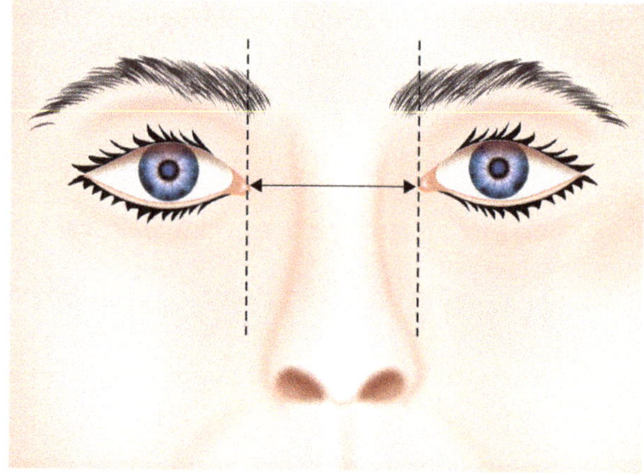

A. 25 mm
C. 40 mm

B. 35 mm
D. 55 mm

Ans: B. 35 mm

Q 64. Which of the following statement regarding the mandibular plating system presented below is FALSE? (See drawing below)

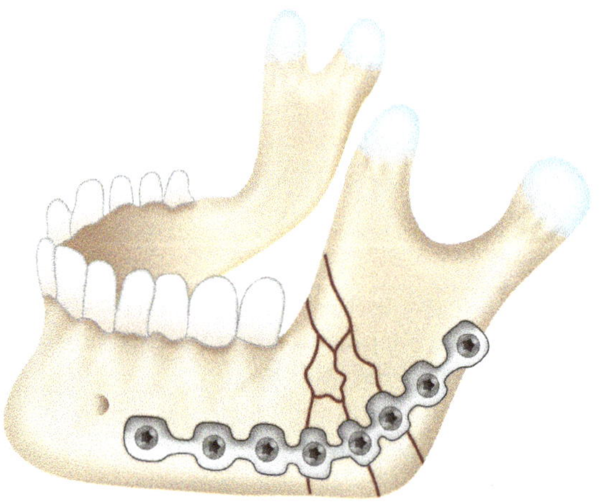

A. This plate is an eccentric dynamic compression plate system
B. This plate will require bicortical fixation
C. This plate is indicated in mandibular fractures related to shotgun wounds
D. This plate is used also in atrophic mandibles

Ans: A. This plate is an eccentric dynamic compression plate system

Q 65. Which of the following statements regarding Eccentric Dynamic Compression Plates is FALSE?

A. Eccentric dynamic compression plates need additional hardware to insure compression at the alveolus
B. Eccentric dynamic compression plates have outside screws holes with incline ramps set obliquely at 45–90° to the long axis of the plate
C. The outer set of screw holes glides superiorly to produce compression at the level of the alveolus
D. The inner set of screw holes glides toward the fracture, providing compression at the inferior mandibular border

Ans: A. Eccentric dynamic compression plates need additional hardware to insure compression at the alveolus

Q 66. Frontal sinus fractures are ASSOCIATED with serious injuries in:

A. 10%
C. 50%

B. 25%
D. 75%

Ans: D. 75%

Q 67. The BEST test to identify Cerebrospinal fluid (CSF) in a salty nasal and postnasal drainage is:

A. Halo test
C. Glucose test

B. Beta-2 transferrin
D. Protein test

Ans: B. Beta-2 transferrin

Q 68. Which of the following anatomical areas is the "danger zone" of the temporal branch for the facial nerve as it passes over the zygomatic arch?

A. The region between 0.5 cm anterior to the helical root and 0.5 cm posterior to the anterior end of the zygomatic arch
B. The region between 1.5 cm anterior to the helical root and 1 cm posterior to the anterior end of the zygomatic arch
C. The region between 1.5 cm anterior to the helical root and 1.5 cm posterior to the anterior end of the zygomatic arch
D. The region between 1.8 cm anterior to the helical root and 2 cm posterior to the anterior end of the zygomatic arch

Ans: D. The region between 1.8 cm anterior to the helical root and 2 cm posterior to the anterior end of the zygomatic arch

Q 69. Which of the following statements regarding frontal sinus anatomy is TRUE?

A. By the age of 10, the frontal sinus is fully developed
B. The sensory innervation is provided by the ophthalmic branch of the trigeminal nerve
C. The ostium lies posterior to the anterior ethmoid cells
D. The posterior table of the frontal sinus is usually thicker than the anterior table

Ans: B. The sensory innervation is provided by the ophthalmic branch of the trigeminal nerve.

Q 70. Which of the following is the average INTERCANTHAL DISTANCE?

A. 25 mm

B. 35 mm

C. 40 mm

D. 45 mm

Ans: B. 35 mm

Q 71. Which of the following is the average INTERPUPILLARY distance?

A. 40 mm

B. 50 mm

C. 70 mm

D. 80 mm

Ans: C. 70 mm

Q 72. The drawing below represents the medial orbital wall in particular the frontoethmoidal suture. What is the measurement of the area indicated by the arrow marked with X ?

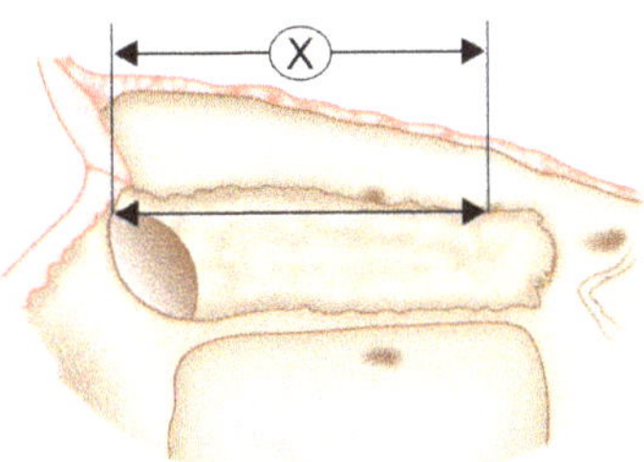

A. 30 mm

B. 35 mm

C. 40 mm

D. 55 mm

Ans: B. 35 mm

Q 73. Which of the following statements related to orbital anatomy is TRUE?

A. The orbital walls are formed by 6 bones

B. The optic foramen is located in the greater wing of the sphenoid bone

C. The anterior ethmoidal foramina is located at 18 mm from the frontoethmoidal suture

D. The posterior ethmoidal foramina is located at 36 mm from the frontoethmoidal suture

Ans: D. The posterior ethmoidal foramina is located at 36 mm from the frontoethmoidal suture

Q 74. The drawing below represents the right bony orbit. Which of the following anatomical structures DOES NOT pass through the opening indicated by the arrow?

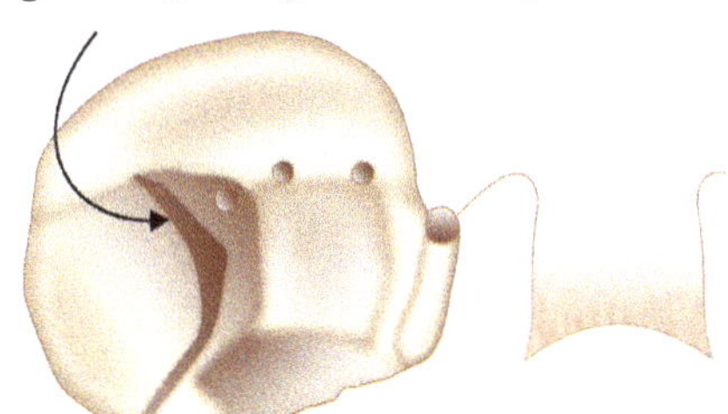

A. Oculomotor nerve

B. Trochlear nerve

C. Abducens nerve

D. Infraorbital nerve

Ans: D. Infraorbital nerve

Q 75. Which of the following indicates the LOCATION in the Orbit of the Optic Foramen?

A. Greater wing of the sphenoid

B. Lesser wing of the sphenoid

C. Orbital roof of the frontal bone

D. Lateral orbital wall of the orbit

Ans: B. Lesser wing of the sphenoid

Q 76. Which of the following statements related to the anatomy of the orbit is FALSE?

A. The optic foramen is located in the lesser wing of the sphenoid bone

B. The lateral orbital wall is formed mainly by the greater wing of the sphenoid bone

C. Lateral to the superior orbital fissure is located the optic foramen

D. Lateral to the superior orbital fissure is located the optic

Ans: C. Lateral to the superior orbital fissure is located the optic foramen

Q 77. Which of the following anatomy terminology is the ONE indicated by the black arrow? Please note that the drawing is related to the internal aspect of the mandible.

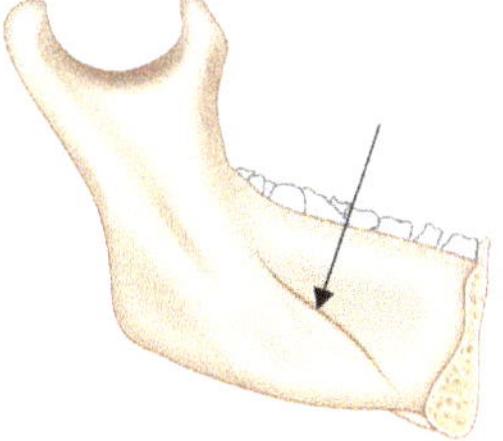

A. Mylohyoid line

B. Mylohyoid groove

C. Oblique line

D. Mental groove

Ans: A. Mylohyoid line

Q 78. Which of the following muscle that exerts a force on the mandible is considered a depressor-retractor?

A. Temporalis

B. Mylohyoid

C. Median pterygoid

D. Lateral pterygoid

Ans: B. Mylohyoid

Q 79. Which of the following muscle is the ONE indicated in the drawing below (medial view of the left hemimandible)?

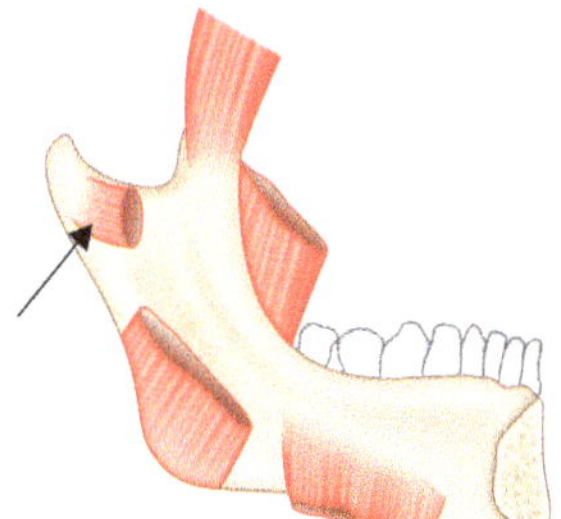

A. Mylohyoid   B. Lateral pterygoid
C. Medial pterygoid   D. Masseter

Ans: B. Lateral pterygoid

Q 80. Which of the following anatomical features related to the frontal sinus is FALSE?

A. The floor of the frontal sinus forms the medial portion of the orbital roof
B. The posterior table forms a portion of the anterior cranial fossa
C. The nasofrontal recess is the outflow tract of the frontal sinus
D. The vascular supply to the frontal sinus is from arteries branches of the external carotid system

Ans: D. The vascular supply to the frontal sinus is from arteries branches of the external carotid system

Q 81. Which of the facial areas represented in the drawing below is the MOST resistant to fracture?

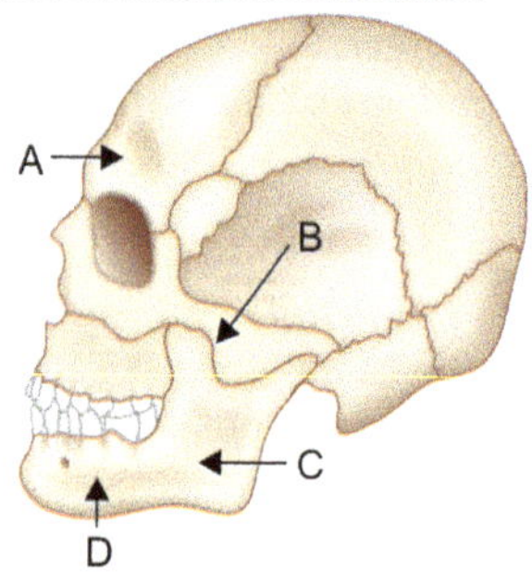

A. A   B. B
C. C   D. D

Ans: A. A

Q 82. Which of the following TREATMENTS IS INCORRECT in the initial management of FACIAL BURNS?

A. The head of the adult represents 9% of the total body surface area to be considered for treatment
B. Tracheotomy rather than in intubation
C. Silver Sulfadiazine topical
D. Skin grafting

Ans: B. Tracheotomy rather than in intubation

Q 83. Which of the following statements is FALSE about MIDFACE DEGLOVING?

A. It will require a sublabial incision through mucosa
B. It will require a full transfixion incision
C. It will require a bilateral intercartilaginous incision
D. It will require a midcolumellar nasal incision

Ans: D. It will require a midcolumellar nasal incision

Chapter 28

Cleft Lip and Palate

Cinzia L Marchica

■ SUMMARY OF EMBRYOLOGY

Facial development arises from the five prominences:
- Paired maxillary prominences
- Paired mandibular prominences
- Single midline frontonasal prominence.

Palate Embryology

Normal

Week 4 of embryonic development:
- Pharyngeal arch formation: First pharyngeal arch gives rise to mandible and maxilla
- The above five prominences emerge from the primitive oral cavity or stomodeum
- *Nasal pits*, or placodes form in the frontonasal prominence
- Inferior frontonasal prominence divides into:
  - 1-Medial nasal prominence ⎫ Form around the
  - 2-Lateral nasal prominence ⎭ nasal pits
- *The nasal ala*:
  - Formed by elevation of the lateral nasal prominence.

Week 6 of embryonic development:
- Fusion of bilateral maxillary prominences with the two medial nasal prominences forms the *upper lip* and *primary palate* at the end of the 6th week.

Weeks 6–7 of embryonic development:
- The *secondary palate*:
  - Originates from the lip and primary palate
  - Produced by growth of bilateral palatal shelves of the maxillary processes
    - » Week 6 → vertical growth phase
    - » Week 7 → transition to horizontal growth phase
  - Fusion of the palatal shelves occurs in the midline, and anteriorly to the primary palate and nasal septum.

Week 8 of embryonic development:
- Ossification of the anterior aspect of the secondary palate occurs
  - Differentiates hard palate from posterior soft palate.

Week 10 of embryonic development:
- Palatal development is complete.

Formation of Cleft (Unilateral and Bilateral)

- Caused by failure of palatal shelf elevation or fusion during embryonic development
- Teratogen exposure and timing of insult are critical factors in palatal clefting
- Embryologic failures may be either unilateral or bilateral
  - Anterior or primary palate clefts:
    - » Occur anterior to incisive foramen
    - » Caused by a failure of the lateral palatine processes to fuse with the primary palate
  - Anterior and posterior palate clefts:
    - » Involve both the primary and secondary palate
    - » Caused by failure of the lateral palatine processes to fuse with each other, the primary palate, and nasal septum
  - Posterior or secondary palate clefts:
    - » Located posterior to the incisive foramen
    - » Caused by a failure of the lateral palatine processes to meet and fuse with each other and the nasal septum.

Lips Embryology

Normal

- *Seventh week of embryonic development*:
  - Fused medial nasal processes expand laterally and inferiorly to form the intermaxillary process
    - » Gives rise to philtrum of upper lip, bridge, and septum of the nose
  - Maxillary swellings grow to meet this process and fuse with it

- Orbicularis oris muscle passes from modiolus to philtrum and then decussates with contralateral fibers.

Formation of Cleft (Unilateral and Bilateral)

- *Unilateral cleft lip:*
  - Failure of maxillary prominence on affected side to join with the merged medial nasal prominences.
- *Bilateral cleft lip*:
  - Failure of the mesenchymal masses of the maxillary prominences to merge with the fused medial nasal prominences.

Nose Embryology

Growth of maxillary prominences and with frontonasal prominence regression pushes the two medial nasal prominences together which fuse and form the midline of the nose and philtrum of the upper lip.

■ MUSCULAR ANATOMY

Normal Soft Palate Muscular Anatomy: Five Paired Muscles

Tensor Veli Palatini

- *Origin/insertion*: From Eustachian tube and greater wing of sphenoid. Tendon courses anteriorly around the hook of hamulus. Inserts medially along the palatine tensor aponeurosis.
- *Function*: Depresses and tenses soft palate, opens Eustachian tube.
- *Innervation*: CN V$_3$.

Levator Veli Palatini

- *Origin/insertion*: From junction of bony and cartilaginous Eustachian tube.
- *Function*: Elevates soft palate, pulls posteriorly to help close nasopharynx.
- *Origin/innervation*: CN X, pharyngeal plexus.

Musculus Uvulae

- *Origin/Insertion*: On tensor aponeurosis in the anterior midline, extends posteriorly to the uvula.
- *Function*: Elevates uvula and pulls it laterally.
- *Innervation*: CN X, pharyngeal plexus.

Palatoglossus

- *Origin/insertion*: Dorsolateral tongue and extends within the anterior tonsillar pillar. Inserts into velum.
- *Function*: Pulls the palate down, narrows pharynx.
- *Innervation*: CN X, pharyngeal plexus.

Palatopharyngeus

- *Origin/insertion*: Posterior border of hard palate, superior pharyngeal constrictor, extends within posterior tonsillar pillar. Inserts in velum.
  - Divides into two heads:
    - » Superior oral head
    - » Inferior nasal head
  - Both heads envelope levator veli palatini (LVP) within the velum.
- *Function*: Pulls the palate down, narrows pharynx and helps close nasopharynx.
- *Innervation*: CN X, pharyngeal plexus.

Deficiencies on Cleft Palate

- Palatal closure begins at incisive foramen at 8 weeks of gestation and completed through the uvula by 12 weeks.
- Clefting of the secondary palate is related to the period of fetal development when the fusion process is interrupted.

Normal Lip Anatomy (Fig. 1)

Components

- *The vermilion*:
  - Dry portion of the lip's red mucous membrane
  - Modified mucosal membrane lacking pilosebaceous units, salivary or eccrine glands, bordered superiorly by the vermilion-cutaneous junction.
- *The philtrum*: Midline area between the base of nose and vermillion border of the upper lip.
- *Lower lip*

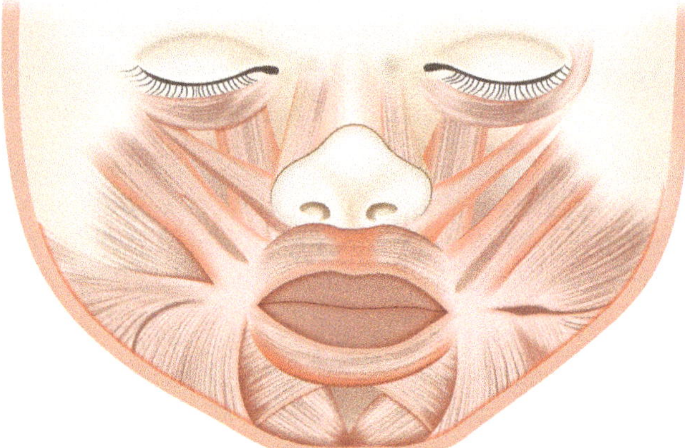

Fig. 1: Normal lip anatomy.

Source: Capone RB, Ames JA, Skyes JM. Evaluation and management of cleft lip and palate disorders. In: Papel ID, Frodel JL, Holt GR, Larrabee Jr WF, Nachlas NE, Park SS, Skyes JM, Toriumi DM (Eds). Facial Plastic and Reconstructive Surgery, 4th edition. New York, Stuttgart: Thieme Publishers, 2016. p. 882.

- Upper lip can be divided into two components:
  - Red: Mucous membrane
  - White: Cutaneous
- *Muscles (Table 1):*
  - Play an important role in the appearance and function of the lips
  - Careful attention required when recreating muscle continuity
  - Orbicularis oris:
    » Encircles the oral opening, creating a sphincter effect
    » The superficial layer arises from the dermis and passes obliquely to insert into inner surface (mucosal membrane) of the lips
    » The deep layer arises from the maxilla and mandible.

Deficiencies in Cleft Lips (Table 2 and Fig. 2)

The deficiencies in cleft lips are described in Table 2.

HISTORY AND PHYSICAL

Pertinent History

- Feeding/eating problems
- Change in nose shape
- Recurrent ear infections
- Misaligned teeth
- Failure to gain weight
- Poor growth
- Speech sound difficulties
- Flow of liquids through nasal passages during feeding/drinking
- Hypernasal voice quality.

Table 1: Characteristics of muscle—orbicularis oris.

Muscle	Orbicularis oris
Origin	*Bone attachments:* Maxilla and mandible along the anterior midline *Muscle attachments:* Muscle fibers blend in with other muscles including levator anguli oris, depressor anguli oris, zygomaticus major and risorius at the angle of the mouth
Insertion	Skin
Innervation	Buccal and marginal mandibular branches: Facial nerve
Function	Acts as a sphincter at oral orifice. Closes mouth. Lip pursing and protrusion
Artery	Superior and inferior labial arteries—branches of facial artery

Table 2: Deficiencies of unilateral cleft lip and bilateral cleft lip.

Cleft lip deficiencies	Unilateral cleft lip	Bilateral cleft lip

Bone		• Premaxilla:
		  – Completely detached from each maxilla
		  – Protrudes more thus the columella of the nose is usually shorter

Muscle—orbicularis oris	• Hypoplastic • Incompletely developed • *Prevented from attaching to normal insertion points* • Abnormally attached to anterior nasal spine at the columellar base on the non-clefted side • Attached to the nasal alar base on the clefted side	• Abnormal insertion of the cleft lip musculature follows the margin of the cleft • Orbicularis oris inserts superiorly • Central prolabium does not contain muscle

Vasculature	Aberrant blood supply which follows the musculature
	• Medial side not developed
	• *Superior labial artery:*
	  – Courses along margin of cleft
	  – Anastomoses with *angular artery* or *lateral nasal arteries*
		Aberrant course of the superior labial artery
		• *Superior labial artery:*
		  – Courses superiorly along the edge of the cleft
		  – Anastomoses with *angular* and *lateral nasal arteries*
		• Prolabial segment receives its blood supply from
		  – Septal, columellar, and premaxillary vessels

Incomplete clefts comments	• Muscles are more hypoplastic on the medial side of the cleft • Upper lip muscles do not cross cleft gap unless skin bridge is at least one-third of the height of the lip • Terminal branch of superior labial artery crosses the skin bridge	• Skeletal continuity • Little protrusion of the premaxilla/prolabium • Some orbicularis oris muscle fibers cross cleft from lateral to medial segment: Amount is variable and related to size of skin bridge

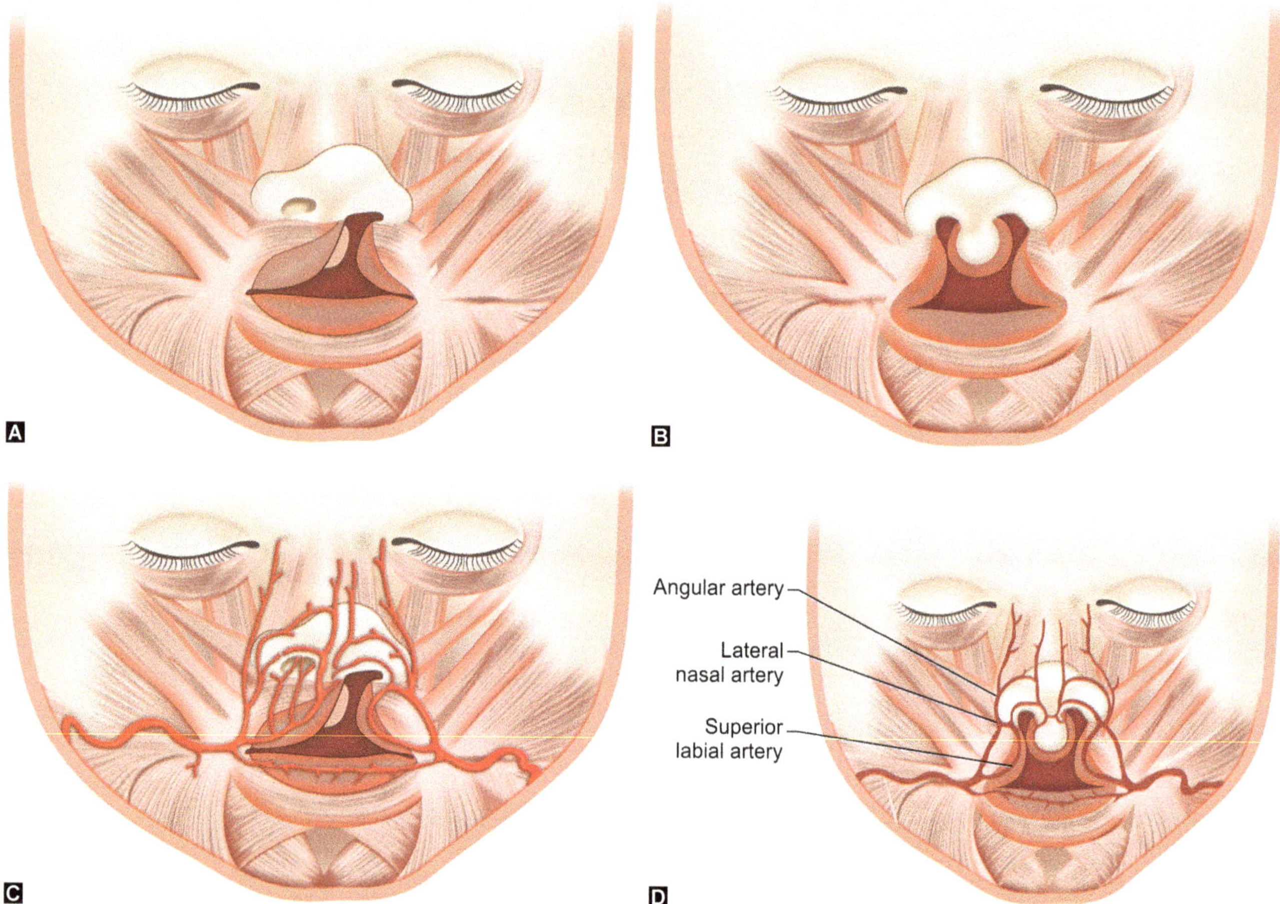

Figs. 2A to D: Lip deformities in cleft lip. (A and B) demonstrate abnormal muscular insertions and aberrant vasculature in unilateral cleft lip, respectively; and (C and D) demonstrate abnormal muscular insertions and aberrant vasculature associated with bilateral cleft lip.

Source: Capone RB, Ames JA, Skyes JM. Evaluation and management of cleft lip and palate disorders. In: Papel ID, Frodel JL, Holt GR, Larrabee Jr WF, Nachlas NE, Park SS, Skyes JM, Toriumi DM (Eds). Facial Plastic and Reconstructive Surgery, 4th edition. New York, Stuttgart: Thieme Publishers, 2016. p. 883-6.

Commonly Associated Syndromes

- Van der Woude syndrome
- Treacher Collins syndrome
- Stickler syndrome
- Apert syndrome
- Crouzon syndrome
- Down syndrome
- 22q11 deletion syndrome
- Goldenhar syndrome
- Pierre Robin sequence (PRS).

Physical Examination

Essential Elements of Physical Examination

- General pediatric assessment including growth
- Assess airway
- *Assess head and facial features*:
  - Presence of facial asymmetry
  - Assess the intercanthal distance and width of the nasal bridge
  - Craniosynostosis
  - Telecanthus
  - Maxillary or mallar hypoplasia
  - Microtia
  - Auricular atresia
  - Ear tags or pits.
- *Assess feeding*:
  - Poor suction
  - Aspiration with feeds
  - Assess for velopharyngeal insufficiency (VPI) and nasal regurgitation.

Evaluating Velopharyngeal Insufficiency

- 20–30% of the cleft palate closures result in VPI
- An otolaryngology and speech pathology evaluation is indicated for all children with a history of cleft palate

- Velopharyngeal insufficiency is due to the lack of complete closure of soft palate to posterior pharyngeal wall during speech
- *History*: Presence of nasal regurgitation, recurrent ear infections, speech sound quality and intelligibility
- *Physical examination*:
  - Ear: Tympanic membrane otoscopy → evaluate for otitis media with effusion or retraction of the drum → indicates Eustachian tube dysfunction (ETD)
  - Oropharyngeal examination → evaluate soft palate, including movement; tonsils, teeth, and occlusion
  - Perceptual evaluation of the patient's speech
  - Instrumental evaluation:
    » Nasometry and aerodynamic instrumentation
    » Videofluoroscopy
    » Nasopharyngoscopy.

Anomalies Found on Nasal Analysis of the Cleft Lip Patient

- *Unilateral cleft*:
  - Alar base → Inferolaterally displaced
  - Lower lateral cartilage
    » Dome blunted: Separated from nonclefted dome
    » Displaced posterolaterally
    » Long lateral crus and shorter medial crus
  - Downward rotation of tip
  - Short columella, deviated to noncleft side
  - Horizontally positioned widened nostril on the cleft side
  - Caudal septum
    » Frequently dislocated from vomer groove and displaced into nonclefted nostril.
- *Bilateral cleft lip*:
  - Alar bases:
    » Flared
    » Displaced posteriorly, laterally, and inferiorly
  - Wide and flat nasal tip
  - Nostrils
    » Wide, horizontally oriented
  - Short columella—deviates toward less involved side.

Classifications: Most Commonly used Classifications for Cleft Lip and Palate

Cleft Lip Classifications (Table 3)

The cleft lip classifications are described in Table 3.

Cleft Palate Classification (Table 4)

The cleft palate classification is described in Table 4.
- *Calnan's triad*: Seen in submucous clefts
  1. Bifid uvula
  2. Notching of posterior hard palate
  3. Zona pellucida.

Table 3: Characteristics of unilateral and bilateral cleft lip.

Extent/Side	Unilateral	Bilateral

Incomplete	• Full-thickness deficit of skin, muscle, and mucosa
	• Does not extend superiorly through entire lip height
	• Ranges:
	  – Thin skin bridge → *Simonart's band*
	  – Substantial musculocutaneous connection
		• Skeletal continuity
		• Little or no protrusion of the premaxilla

Complete	• Full-thickness cleft • Extends through entire height of the lip and floor of nose • Through alveolar ridge	• Premaxilla is detached from each maxilla
Other	Findings	
Microform cleft lip deformity	• Minor malformation with diastasis of central orbicularis oris muscle fibers • No overt clefting of the epidermis of the upper lip	

Table 4: Cleft palate classification.

Bifid uvula	• Mildest form of soft palate cleft • Lack of normal uvular fusion
Submucous cleft palate	• Diastasis of soft palatal musculature • Palatal mucosa is intact • Intrinsic muscle dysfunction caused by the diastasis

- *Veau classification (Figs. 3A to D)*:
  - *Veau I*: Soft palate cleft
  - *Veau II*: Soft and hard palate cleft (posterior to incisive foramen)
  - *Veau III*: Unilateral cleft lip and palate. Involves soft and hard palates and extends through the alveolus
  - *Veau IV*: Bilateral cleft lip extending through hard and soft palates and through the alveolus bilaterally.
- *Kriens' LAHSHAL classification*:
  - *L*: Lip
  - *A*: Alveolus
  - *H*: Hard palate
  - *S*: Soft palate
    » Capital letter: complete cleft
    » Small letter: incomplete
    » No cleft represented with a dot (.)
  - *H*: Hard palate
  - *A*: Alveolus
  - *L*: Lip
- *Kernahan "striped-Y" classification (Fig. 4 and Table 5)*.

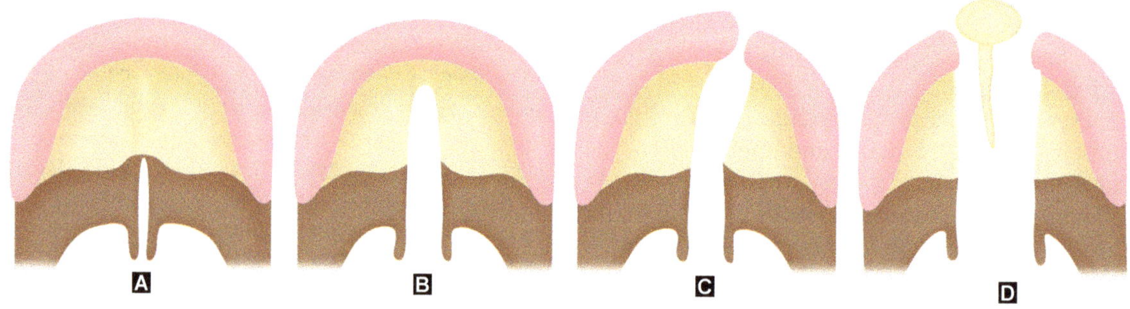

Figs. 3A to D: Veau classification of cleft palate.

Source: Rogers CR, Meara JG. Cleft lip and palate repair. In: Cheney ML, Hadlock TA (Eds). Facial Surgery: Plastic and Reconstructive. CRC Press; 2015.

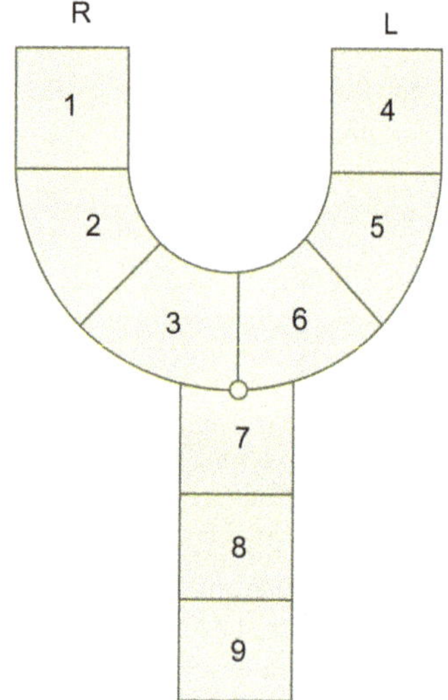

Fig. 4: Kernahan "striped-Y" cleft palate classification. Numbered boxes represent areas of the lip and palate. Shaded boxes would represent cleft areas.

Source: Liu Q, Yang ML, Li ZJ, et al. A Simple and precise classification for cleft lip and palate: A five-digit numerical recording system. Cleft Palate-Craniofacial Journal. 2007;44:465-8.

Kernahan DA. The striped Y—a symbolic classification of cleft lip and palate. Plast Reconstr Surg. 1971;47:469-70.

Table 5: Numbers and anatomical area of Kernahan "striped-Y" cassification

Numbers	Anatomical area
1, 4	Lips
2, 5	Alveolus
3, 6	Premaxilla/hard palate anterior to incisive foramen
7	Hard palate posterior to incisive foramen
8	Soft palate
9	Submucous cleft

■ MANAGEMENT

Timeline of Management for Cleft Lip and Palate

The timeline of management for cleft lip and palate is described in Table 6.

Various Members of the Interdisciplinary Team in Cleft Care

- *Audiologist:* Identification of any hearing abnormalities. Newborn hearing screening test important in cleft patients as pass rates for these patients are only 72%.
- *Cleft surgeon:* Involved in the surgical management of the cleft patient, and the multitude of surgical procedures and techniques performed.
- *Dentist/orthodontist:* Provide good dental hygiene and orthodontic care.

Table 6: Timeline of management for cleft lip and palate.

Age	Procedure
Birth	Consider: Lip adhesion, nasoalveolar molding, Latham appliance Cleft lip repair if wide
3 months	Cleft lip repair Rule of 10's: >10 weeks, >10 lbs, Hbg > 10 g/dL
	Tip rhinoplasty
	Close nasal floor
9–18 months	Palatoplasty
3 years	Speech evaluation
4–6 years	Velopharyngeal insufficiency evaluation ± surgery
9–11 years	Orthodontic surgery: Alveolar bone grafting
12–16 years	Nasal reconstruction, and orthognathic surgery

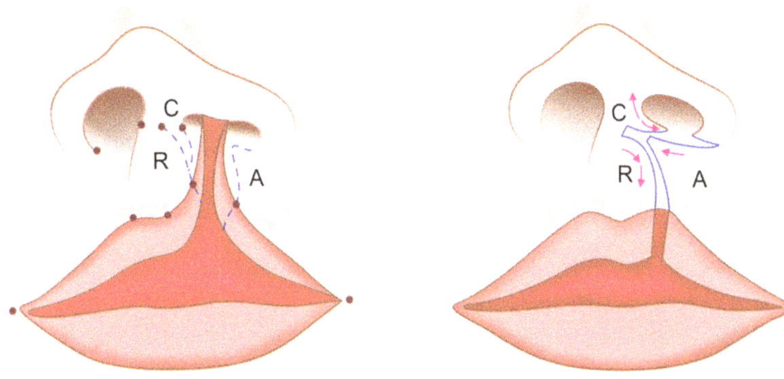

Fig. 5: Millard rotation-advancement flap reference points.

Source: Ness JA, Sykes JM. Basics of Millard rotation-advancement technique for repair of the unilateral cleft lip deformity. Facial Plast Surg. 1993;9:167-76.

- *Geneticist*: Rule out genetic syndromes associated with the cleft.
- *Nutritionist*: Close weight monitoring, help find strategies to maximize growth by increasing formula calories or changing types if warranted.
- *Otolaryngologist*: Provides regular assessments and treatments for otologic issues such as ETD, hearing loss, and cholesteatomas as well as velopharyngeal insufficiency.
- *Pediatrician*: General assessment and care of the patient.
- *Social service*: Provides family with information and support for financial, intellectual, and emotional issues.
- *Speech language pathologist*: Assess oral and pharyngeal function, feeding. Offer support to patients and families with learning appropriate feeding techniques.

Surgical Principles

Most Commonly Used Techniques for Each Type of Cleft and Underlying Principle for Each Deficiency Type

Cleft lip:
- Principles of repair:
  - Reconstitution of the orbicularis oris muscle
  - Alignment of cupids bow and the vermilion border
  - Creation of the nasal sill and floor of the nose
  - Symmetrical placement of the alar bases.
- Repair options and their indications: Unilateral and bilateral cleft lip repair:
  - Nasoalveolar molding
    » Approximates the complete cleft lip (CL) deformity
    » Improves the deformed lower lateral cartilage on cleft lip side.
  - Lip adhesion:
    » Reduces tension for final closure
    » Converts complete to incomplete cleft
  - Millard's rotation-advancement repair (Figs. 5 and 6A to D):
    » Indication: Unilateral or bilateral lip repair (rotation-advancement flap done on each side)
    » Medial segment → downward and lateral rotation
    » Lateral segment advanced medially.
  - Other:
    1. *Mulliken repair and variations:* Single stages bilateral cleft lip repair. Achieve muscular continuity, design a narrow philtral flap and construct median tubercle from the lateral labial elements. Reposition lower lateral cartilage to construct the nasal tip and columella.
    2. *Mohler repair:* For unilateral cleft lip, modification of Miller, extends the incision back into the columella.
    3. *Fisher's anatomical subunit repair*: Lengthens lateral and medial segments of the cleft while observing an anatomic subunit concept.
    4. *Tennison-Randall—triangle cleft lip repair*: For unilateral cleft lip repair. Rotation, advancement and interposition of triangular flaps.

Cleft palate:
- Principles of repair:
  - Separation of the oral cavity from nasal cavity with use of oral and nasal mucosal closures
  - Development of a functional velopharynx
  - Functional and aesthetic restoration development of dentition
  - Preservation of facial growth.

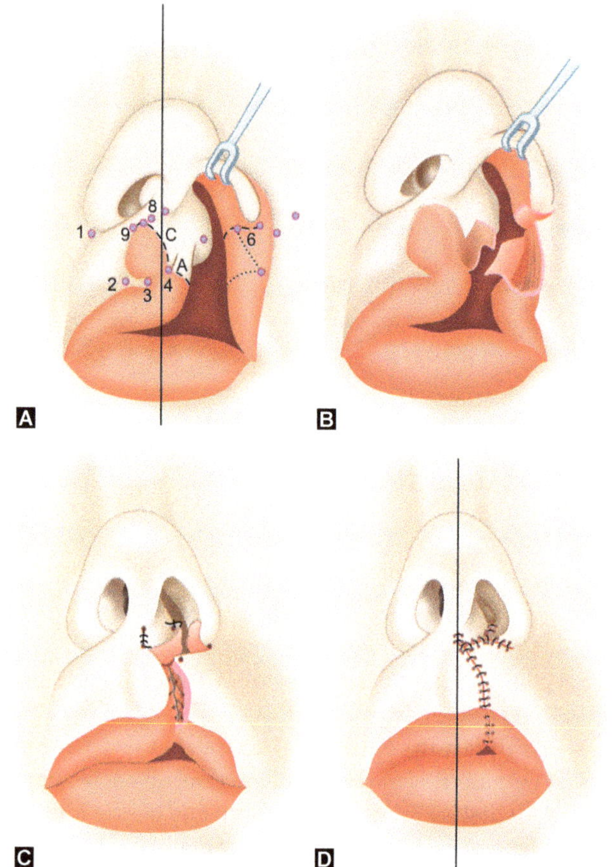

Figs. 6A to D: Millard rotation-advancement repair of a unilateral cleft lip.

Source: Rogers CR, Meara JG. Cleft lip and palate repair. In: Cheney ML, Hadlock TA (Eds). Facial Surgery: Plastic and Reconstructive. CRC Press; 2015.

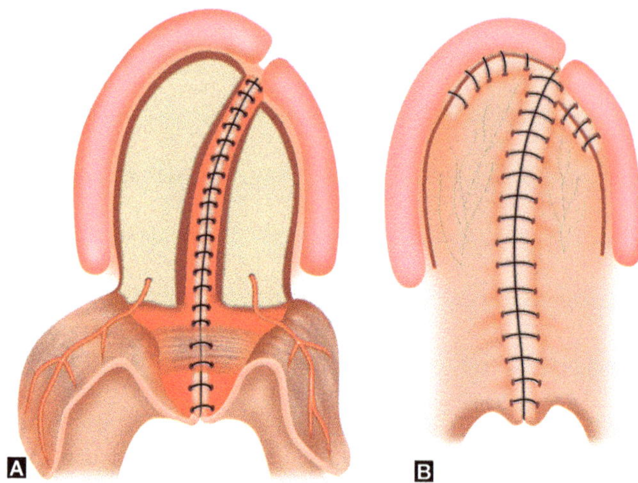

Figs. 7A and B: Two-flap palatoplasty.

Source: Chiang T, Allen GC. Cleft palate repair. In: Goudy S, Tollefson TT (Eds). Complete Cleft Care. New York: Thieme; 2015. p. 103.

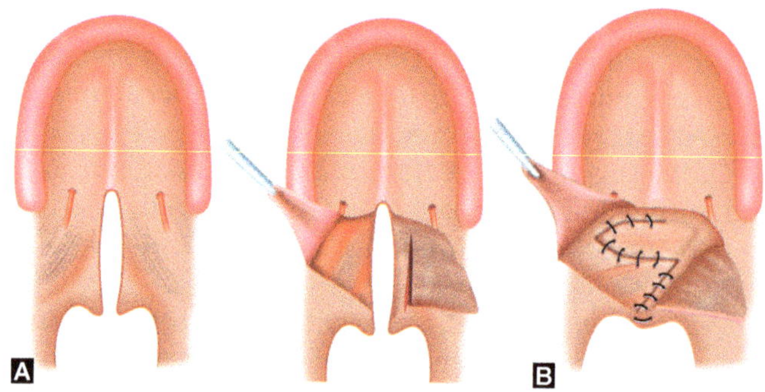

Figs. 8A and B: Furlow Z-palatoplasty.

Source: Chiang T, Allen GC. Cleft palate repair. In: Goudy S, Tollefson TT (Eds). Complete Cleft Care. New York: Thieme; 2015. p. 103.

■ COMMON TECHNIQUES

- *Bardach two-flap palatoplasty technique (Fig. 7):*
  - Indications: Complete unilateral and bilateral clefts (primary and secondary palate)
  - Single pedicle based on greater palatine arteries on each side
  - Utilizes intravelar veloplasty.
- *Furlow palatoplasty (double opposing Z-plasty) (Figs. 8A and B):*
  - Indications: Incomplete secondary, submucous cleft
  - Palatal muscles raised with mucosal flaps, with the oral mucosal flap on one side and nasal mucosal flap on the other
  - Posterior rotation of these flaps to overlap muscles and create a muscular sling
- *Veau-Wardill-Kilner—V to Y advancement (Figs. 9A and B):*
  - Palatal flaps are retropositioned
  - Exposed bone left anteriorly
  - Lengthens the palate.

- *"Von Langenbeck" bipedicled palatoplasty (Figs. 10A and B):*
  - Indication: Isolated complete cleft palate
  - Subperiosteal mobilization of the mucoperiosteal flaps mobilized to midline for palatal closure
  - Levator veli palatine and palatopharyngeus muscles released to close soft palate.
- *Principles of management of alveolar defects:*
  - Bone Grafting goals include:
    » Support for tooth eruption
    » Stabilization of maxilla
  - Can occur as primary or secondary bone grafting
  - Maxillary canine and lateral incisors begin to erupt between 7 and 12 years old
  - Maxillary canine erupts into the alveolar cleft space
  - Lateral incisor erupts either adjacent to cleft or into cleft space
  - Types of grafts used: (Sources = Cortical and cancellous bone)
    » Iliac crest

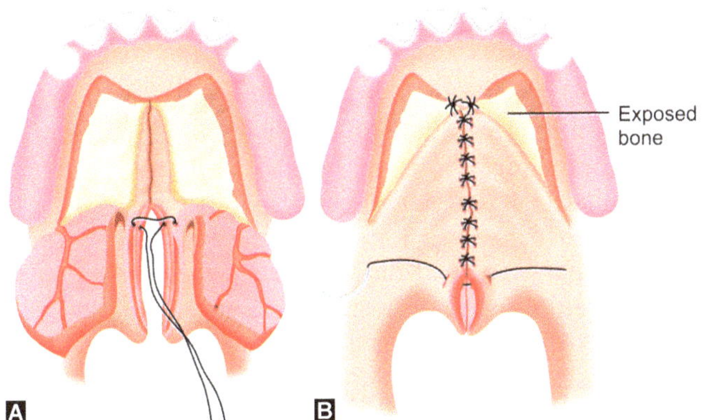

Figs. 9A and B: Veau-Wardill-Kilner—V to Y advancement.

Source: Rogers CR, Meara JG. Cleft lip and palate repair. In: Cheney ML, Hadlock TA (Eds). Facial Surgery: Plastic and Reconstructive. CRC Press; 2015.

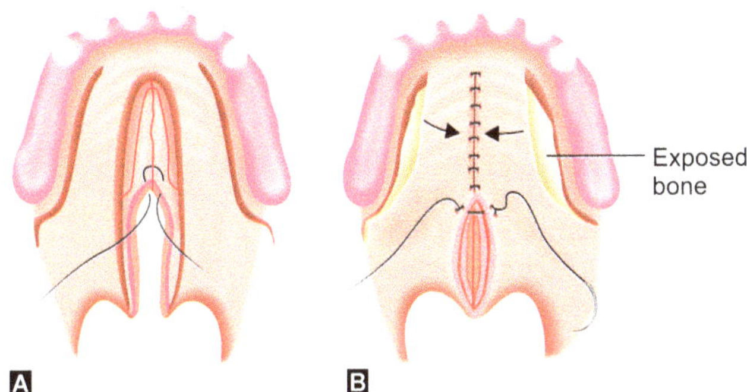

Figs. 10A and B: Bipedicled palatoplasty.

Source: Rogers CR, Meara JG. Cleft lip and palate repair. In: Cheney ML, Hadlock TA (Eds). Facial Surgery: Plastic and Reconstructive. CRC Press; 2015.

- » Cranial bone
- » Mandibular symphysis
- » Tibia
- » Rib (limited).
- *Role and indications for distraction osteogenesis*:
  - Correction of maxilla-mandibular discrepancies with a class III malocclusion that is symptomatic
  - Relieves supraglottic airway obstruction or tongue-based airway obstruction
  - Indication:
    - » Pierre Robin sequence with micrognathia, glossoptosis and cleft palate
    - » Micrognathia with retrodisplacement of the tongue resulting in airway obstruction (Figs. 11A and B).

Cleft Lip Rhinoplasty

- *Basic principles*:
  - Three rhinoplasty, types exist:
    - » Primary rhinoplasty:
      - Timing: At same time as cleft lip repair
      - Goal: Close anterior nasal floor; reposition the displaced alar base; accomplish early symmetry to nasal base and tip
    - » Intermediate:
      - Timing: 1–14 years, between lip repair and definitive rhinoplasty
      - Goals: Stabilize the nasal base, lengthen the columella, septum repositioning if presence of nasal obstruction.
    - » Definitive:
      - Timing: Once nasal and midface growth is complete (woman—14 years and men—16 years)
      - Goals: Reestablish symmetry and give definition to nasal tip and base. Relieve any nasal obstruction.
- *Technique*:
  - Nasal base:
    - » Establish a solid nasal base done by:
      - Rhinoplasty and closure of nasal floor

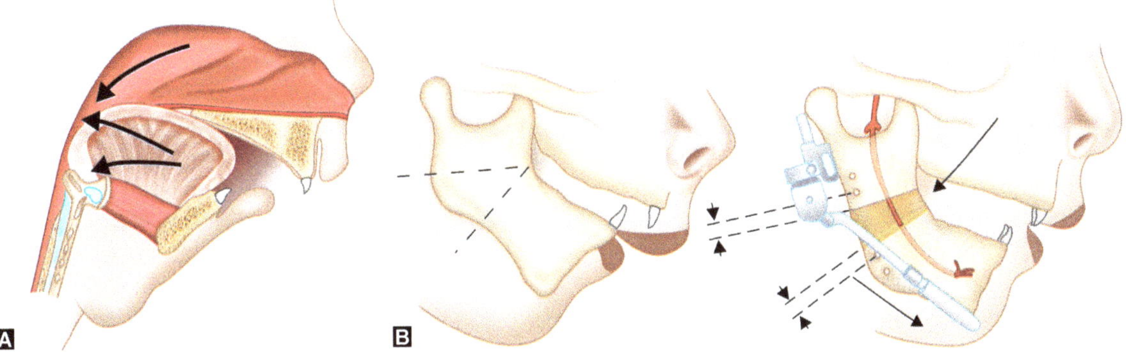

Figs. 11A and B: (A) Demonstrating micrognathia with subsequent retrodisplacement of tongue and upper airway obstruction. (B) Demonstartes the principle of mandibular distraction osteogenesis.

Source: Lander TA, Scott AR. Mandibular distraction. In: Goudy SL, Tollefson TT. Complete Cleft Care: Cleft and Velopharyngeal Insufficiency Treatment in Children. New York: Thieme; 2015.

- Correction of the maxilla and premaxilla bony deficiency
    - Restoring abnormal posterior-anterior position of the alar base
  - Rhinoplasty technique:
    » Alar base:
      - Complete alotomy to release of all the alar attachments to the piriform aperture
      - Placement of the alar base
    » Lower lateral cartilages:
      - Release nasal skin from lower lateral cartilage (LLC) to prevent tethering
      - LLC placement done using interdomal sutures to position dome in more lateral position
      - This increases tip projection and enhances tip symmetry
    » Increasing columellar length:
      - Back cut onto the columella and rotation of a c-flap
      - V-Y closure
    » Septoplasty:
      - Septum can be repositioned onto the nasal spine
    » External nasal valve obstruction improved with:
      - Z-plasty over the alar webbing
      - Increased tip projection
      - Excision of redundant tissue
      - Placement of bolsters
    » Internal valve obstruction improved with spreader graft between septum and upper lateral cartilage
    » Sliding chondrocutaneous flap:
      - Augments vestibular lining
      - Reduces alar-columellar web
      - Contributes to tip refinement and stability
    » Grafts and struts used for refinement and shape:
      - Dorsal and caudal struts
      - Columellar strut grafts
      - Cartilaginous tip graft.

Velopharyngeal Insufficiency

- *Options for management before surgery*:
  » Speech therapy
  » Prosthetic obturation
  » Injection pharyngoplasty
- *Most common surgical techniques*:
  - Furlow palatoplasty, or double-opposing Z-plasty → lengthens the palate
  - Pharyngeal flap: Superiorly-based
  - Dynamic sphincter pharyngoplasty
  - Posterior pharyngeal wall augmentation
- *Principles behind types of surgery*:
  - Surgical considerations:
    » Velopharyngeal gap size
    » Pattern of pharyngeal closure

» Short palatal length
» Central palate defect
» Lateral pharyngeal wall immobility
» Palate scarring and immobility
  - Double opposing Z-plasty: Reorients the levator musculature and increase palatal length
  - Superior-based pharyngeal flap:
    » Performed in patients with adequate lateral pharyngeal wall movement and sagittal or circular velopharyngeal closure patterns
    » Posterior pharyngeal wall musculomucosal flap incised inferiorly and laterally and elevated into soft palate submucosal pocket
  - Sphincter pharyngoplasty:
    » Indications: Patients with coronal velopharyngeal closure patterns and limited/absent lateral pharyngeal wall motion
    » Bilateral superiorly based musculomucosal flaps are rotated medially and set to augment the posterior pharyngeal wall and promote closure
- Postoperative complications.

Most Common Complications of Cleft Lip and Palate Surgery

- *Cleft lip*:
  - Complete dehiscence
  - Mild asymmetry
  - Hypertrophic scarring → addressed with steroid injections
  - Long lip → Excision of excess tissue
  - Short lip "whistle deformity" → dermal graft or a Z-plasty versus complete revision
  - Depression of the philtral column
  - Nostril stenosis.
- *Cleft palate*:
  - Bleeding
  - Airway obstruction
  - Dehiscence → reduced risk if patient put on liquid/soft diet for 2 weeks postoperative, no pacifier use
  - Fistula → prevented by everting nasal and palatal closures with minimal tension. Revision requires two-layered closure. Options: Turn-in flap, advancement or rotational flaps, facial artery musculomucosal (FAMM) flap.
  - Velopharyngeal insufficiency:
    » Treated with speech therapy and surgery
    » Surgical treatment includes: Furlow palatoplasty, superior-based pharyngeal flap, sphincter pharyngoplasty, posterior pharyngeal wall augmentation
    » Complications: Infection, dehiscence, scarring, nasopharyngeal stenosis, obstructive sleep apnea, hyponasality, hemorrhage (rule out medialized carotids), and neck stiffness
  - Disruption of maxillary growth.

■ BIBLIOGRAPHY

1. Capone RB, Sykes JM. Evaluation and management of cleft lip and palate disorder. In: Papel ID (Ed). Facial Plastic and Reconstructive Surgery, 3rd edition. New York: Thieme Medical Publishers; 2009. pp. 1059-78.
2. Coleman JR, Sykes JM. Cleft lip rhinoplasty. In: Papel ID (Ed). Facial Plastic and Reconstructive Surgery, 2nd edition. New York: Thieme Medical Publishers;2002. pp. 830-43.
3. Coots, B.K. Alveolar bone grafting: past, present, and new horizons. Semin Plast Surg. 2012;26:178-83.
4. Davit AJ, Otteson T, Losee JE. Comprehensive cleft care. In: Johnson JT (Ed). Bailey's Head and Neck Surgery: Otolaryngology, 5th edition. Philadelphia: Lippincott Williams and Wilkins; 2014.
5. Emery BE, Sykes JM, Senders CW. Diagnosis and treatment of secondary unilateral cleft lip deformities. Facial Plast Clin North Am. 1996;4:311-21.
6. Furlow LT Jr. Cleft palate repair by double opposing Z-plasty. Plast Reconstr Surg. 1986;78:724-38.
7. Garfinkle JS, Kapadia H. Presurgical tretament. In: Goudy SL, Tollefson TT (Eds). Complete Cleft Care: Cleft and Velopharyngeal Insufficiency Treatment in Children. New York: Thieme; 2015.
8. Glade RS, Deal R. Diagnosis and management of velopharyngeal dysfunction. Oral Maxillofac Surg Clin North Am. 2016;28:181-8.
9. Goudy SL, Buckmiller LM. Genetics, prenatal diagnosis and counseling, and feeding. In: Goudy SL, Tollefson TT (Eds). Complete Cleft Care: Cleft and Velopharyngeal Insufficiency Treatment in Children. New York: Thieme; 2015.
10. Gray SD, Pinborough-Zimmerman J. Diagnosis and treatment of velopharyngeal incompetence. Facial Plast Clin North Am. 1996;4:405-12.
11. Hartzell LD, Kilpatrick LA. Diagnosis and management of patients with clefts: a comprehensive and interdisciplinary approach. Otolaryngol Clin North Am. 2014;47:821-52.
12. Kohli SS, Kohli VS. A comprehensive review of the genetic basis of cleft lip and palate. J Oral Maxillofac Pathol. 2012;16:64-72.
13. Kriens O. LAHSHAL: a concise documentation system for cleft lip, alveolus, and palate diagnoses. In: Kriens O (Ed). What is a Cleft Lip and Palate?: A Multidisciplinary Update. New York, NY: Thieme Medical Publishers; 1989. pp. 30-4.
14. Kummer AW. Speech evaluation for patients with cleft palate. Clin Plast Surg. 2014;41:241-51.
15. Lander TA, Scott AR. Mandibular distraction. In: Goudy SL, Tollefson TT (Eds). Complete Cleft Care: Cleft and Velopharyngeal Insufficiency Treatment in Children. New York: Thieme; 2015.
16. Mulliken JB. Repair of bilateral cleft lip and its variants. Indian J Plast Surg. 2009;42(Suppl):S79-S90.
17. Ness JA, Sykes JM. Basics of Millard rotation-advancement technique for repair of the unilateral cleft lip deformity. Facial Plast Surg. 1993;9:167-76.
18. Pansky B. Congenital malformations of the lip and palate. In: Pansky B (Ed). Review of Medical Embryology. [online] Available from http://discovery.lifemapsc.com/library/review-of-medical-embryology/chapter-56-congenital-malformations-of-the-lip-and-palate [Accessed July, 2017].
19. Rogers CR, Meara JG. Cleft lip and palate repair. In: Cheney ML, Hadlock TA (Eds). Facial Surgery: Plastic and Reconstructive. CRC Press; 2015.
20. Scott AR, Ribesar RJ, Sidman JD. Pierre Robin Sequence: evaluation, management, indications for surgery and pitfalls. Otolaryngol Clin North Am. 2012; 45:695-710.
21. Shah SN, Khalid M, Khan MS. A review of classification systems for cleft lip and palate patients- I. Morphological classifications. JKCD. 2011:1(2).
22. Shaye D, Liu CC, Tollefson TT. Cleft lip and palate: an evidence-based review. Facial Plast Surg Clin North Am. 2015;23:357-72.
23. Siebert RW. Surgical repair of the bilateral cleft lip deformity. Facial Plast Clin North Am. 1996;4:351
24. Sykes JM, Tollefson TT. Management of the cleft lip deformity. Facial Plast Clin North Am. 2005;13:157-67.
25. Sykes JM. Diagnosis and treatment of cleft lip and palate deformities. In: Papel ID (Ed). Facial Plastic and Reconstructive Surgery, 2nd edition. New York: Thieme Medical Publishers; 2002. pp. 813-29.
26. Tollefson TT, Senders CW. Cleft lip repair: bilateral. In: Goudy SL. Tollefson TT (Eds). Complete Cleft Care: Cleft and Velopharyngeal Insufficiency Treatment in Children. New York: Thieme; 2015.
27. Tollefson TT, Sykes JM. Cleft lip repair: unilateral. In: Goudy SL, Tollefson TT (Eds). Complete Cleft Care: Cleft and Velopharyngeal Insufficiency Treatment in Children. New York: Thieme; 2015.

Multiple Choice Questions

Q 1. Which of the following unilateral cleft lip repairs is the ONE represented in the drawing below?

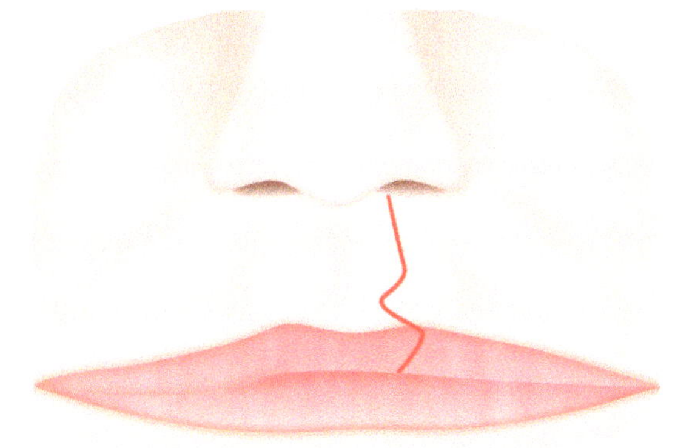

A. LeMesurier
B. Millard
C. Millard with triangular flap inferiorly based
D. Tennison-Randall

Ans: D. Tennison-Randall

Q 2. At which age is a cleft lip repair BEST PERFORMED?

A. 1 month   B. 3 months
C. 6 months   D. 9 months

Ans: B. 3 months

Q 3. Which of the following surgical techniques used for cleft palate repair is REPRESENTED in the drawing below?

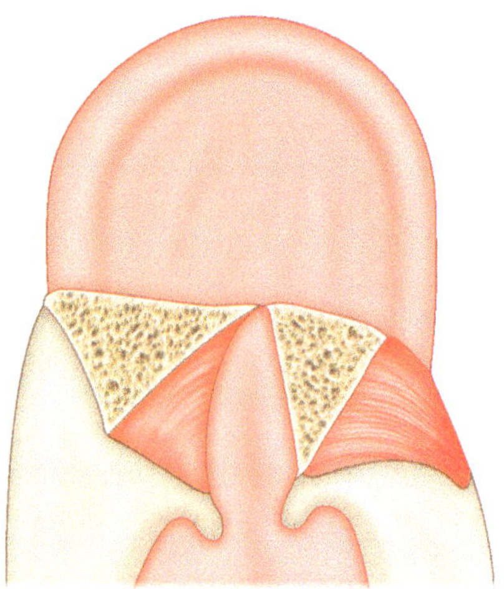

A. Furlow palatoplasty   B. Four-flap palatoplasty
C. Three-flap palatoplasty   D. Two-flap palatoplasty

Ans: A. Furlow palatoplasty

Q 4. Which of the following statements is TRUE about Millard technique for unilateral cleft lip repair?

A. Minimal tissue is discarded
B. The suture line is not well camouflaged
C. The alar base and nasal floor are difficult to reconstruct due to poor access to the nose
D. The procedure will not allow alterations or adjustments during the operation

Ans: A. Minimal tissue is discarded

Q 5. The MOST useful palatoplasty technique for repair of complete unilateral cleft palate deformity is:

A. Furlow technique
B. Von Langenbeck palatoplasty technique
C. Two-flap palatoplasty technique
D. Two-flap palatoplasty technique associated with vomerflap

Ans: C. Two-flap palatoplasty technique

Q 6. The MOST adequate timing for alveolar bone grafting in cleft deformities is:

A. 3 months of age, associated with lip repair
B. 1 year of age, associated with palate repair
C. 3 years of age
D. 10 years of age

Ans: D. 10 years of age

Q 7. Which of the following statements BEST describes the Millard lip repair?

A. The medial segment is rotated superiorly and the lateral segment is advanced medially
B. The medial segment is rotated inferiorly and the lateral segment is advanced medially
C. The medial segment is advanced laterally and the lateral segment is rotated inferiorly
D. The medial and the lateral segments have a rotation and advancement component

Ans: B. The medial segment is rotated inferiorly and the lateral segment is advanced medially

Q 8. Which of the following statements about the triangular flap technique to repair a unilateral cleft lip is TRUE?

A. Minimal tissue is discarded
B. It is a consistent cleft lip repair technique for decreasing vertical lip contraction
C. The suture line is well camouflaged
D. The procedure will allow alterations or adjustments during the operation after the triangular flap has been executed

Ans: B. It is a consistent cleft lip repair technique for decreasing vertical lip contraction

Q 9. Which of the following is the unilateral cleft lip repair REPRESENTED in the drawing below?

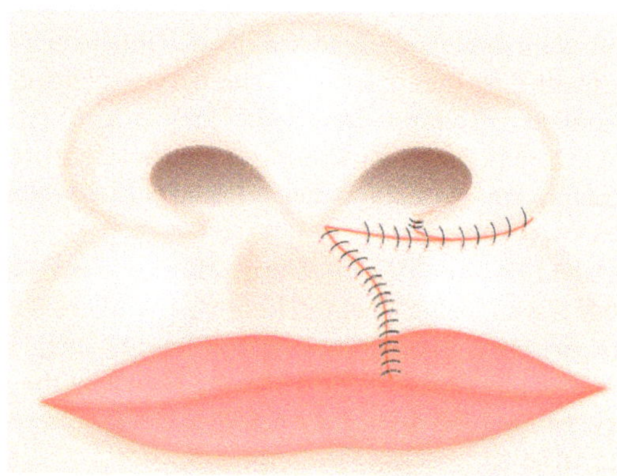

A. Millard   B. LeMesurier
C. Skoog   D. Tennison-Randall

Ans: A. Millard

Q 10. The BEST donor site for a bone graft to close a residual alveolar cleft is the:

A. Allogenic bone   B. Autogenous rib
C. Calvarial bone   D. Iliac crest bone

Ans: D. Iliac crest bone

Q 11. Which of the following statements about Furlow palatoplasty is FALSE?

A. It is indicated for repair of clefts restricted to the soft palate
B. It is indicated for repair of submucous clefts

C. It is indicated for repair of clefts with a width greater than 1 cm

D. It is a double opposing Z-plasty

Ans: C. It is indicated for repair of clefts with a width greater than 1 cm

Q 12. Which of the following areas in a congenital bilateral complete cleft lip represents the PROLABIUM?

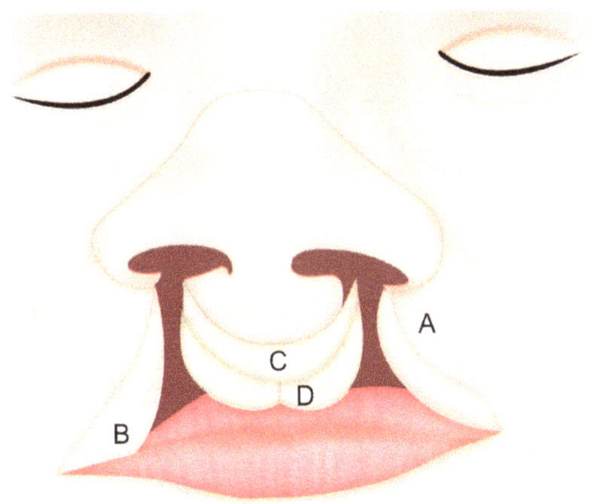

A. A

B. B

C. C

D. D

Ans: C. C

Q 13. Which of the following is the MOST common presentation of cleft lip and palate disorders?

A. Combined cleft lip and palate

B. Isolated cleft palate

C. Isolated cleft lip

D. Isolated unilateral imcomplete cleft lip

Ans: A. Combined cleft lip and palate

Q 14. Which of the following surgical techniques is the MOST useful in the repair of a "whistle" deformity after bilateral cleft lip repair?

A. Unilateral Z-plasty

B. V-Y advancement

C. O-T flap

D. O-Z flap

Ans: B. V-Y advancement

Q 15. Which of the following surgical techniques is the BEST to correct an irregular right Cupid's bow (discrepancy between the level of the vermilion-cutaneous junction of 2 mm on the right side) shown in the drawing?

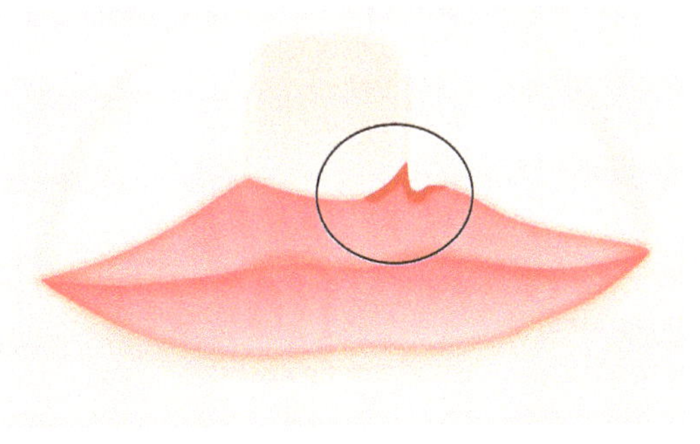

A. Elliptic excision

B. V-Y closure

C. Z-plasty

D. Bilobed flap

Ans: C. Z-plasty

Q 16. Which of the following statements is TRUE about the Millard operative technique in unilateral cleft lip repair?

A. Excessive normal good tissue is discarded

B. It provides a difficult nasal access

C. The resulting lip scar is not well camouflaged

D. Extensive undermining is required to avoid closure with excessive tension

Ans: D. Extensive undermining is required to avoid closure with excessive tension

Q 17. Which of the following statements is RELATED to a unilateral cleft lip nose deformity?

A. Cleft nostril is usually vertically oriented and narrow

B. Caudal septum deflects toward the noncleft side

C. Nasal tip deflects toward the cleft side

D. Internal nasal valve is usually not compromised

Ans: B. Caudal septum deflects toward the noncleft side

Q 18. Which of the following is an ADVANTAGE of the unilateral cleft lip repair technique represented in the drawing below?

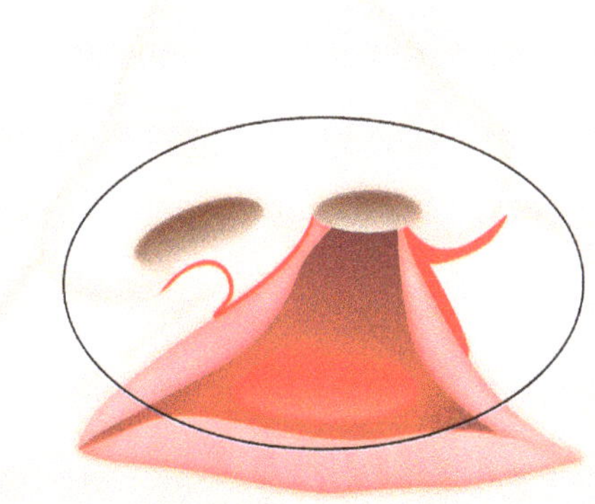

A. Extensive undermining is not required

B. Vertical scar contracture is very uncommon

C. Small nostril does not occur using this technique

D. Good nasal access is provided

Ans: D. Good nasal access is provided

Q 19. Which of the following statements represents the role of the "FORKED FLAP" incisions of the upper lip used in secondary cleft lip-nasal deformities?

A. They provide additional columellar length and increase projection of the bilateral cleft lip-nose deformity

B. They provide additional columellar length and increase projection of the unilateral clef lip-nose deformity

C. They provide reduction in columellar length and decrease projection of the unilateral cleft lip-nose deformity

D. They provide reduction in columellar length and decrease projection of the bilateral cleft lip-nose deformity

Ans: A. They provide additional columellar length and increase projection of the bilateral cleft lip-nose deformity

Q 20. **Which of the following surgical options is the BEST for the management of a "tight upper lip" after repair of a bilateral cleft lip?**

A. Z-plasty

B. V-Y advancement

C. Forked flap procedure

D. Abbé flap

Ans: D. Abbé flap

Q 21. **Which of the following statements regarding repair of cleft lip and palate is FALSE?**

A. 3 months, cleft-lip repair

B. 3 months, myringotomy and tube placement

C. 6 months, palatoplasty

D. 11 years, alveolar cancellous bone grafting

Ans: C. 6 months, palatoplasty

Q 22. **Which of following is CORRECT regarding the preferred palatoplasty techniques?**

A. Complete bilateral palate: Three-flap palatoplasty

B. Submucous cleft: Double reversing Z-plasty

C. Complete secondary palate: Two-flap palatoplasty

D. Complete unilateral: Von Langenbeck palatoplasty

Ans: B. Submucous cleft: Double reversing Z-plasty

Q 23. **Which of the following statements is FALSE regarding the palatoplasty technique represented in the drawing below?**

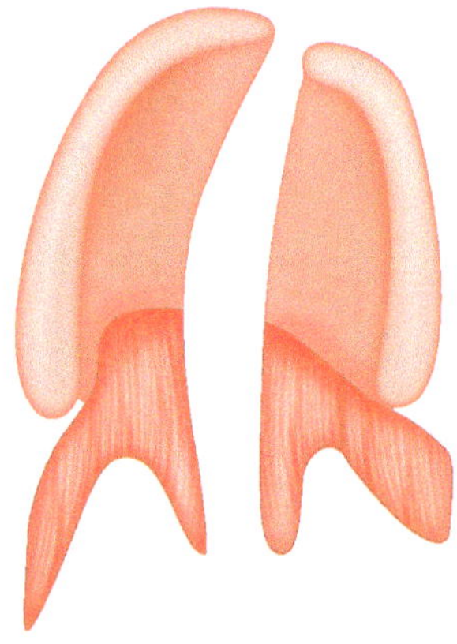

A. The incidence of fistulization at the hard-soft palate junction is high

B. The neurovascular bundle coming from the greater palatine foramen is identified

C. Medial mobility of the soft palate is enhanced by dissecting the posterior extension of the relaxing incision in the plane of the pterygoid and superior constrictor muscles

D. In patients with wider clefts it is necessary to infracture the hamulus process

Ans: A. The incidence of fistulization at the hard-soft palate junction is high

Q 24. **Which of the following statements regarding Two-triangular flap technique for the surgical repair of a complete unilateral cleft lip is FALSE?**

A. The lengthening is calculated by measuring the difference in distance between the base of the columella and the high point Cupid's bow on the noncleft side compared with the cleft side

B. Two triangular flaps are created on the medial aspect of the cleft side of the lip in its lower and upper portion

C. With respect to these two triangular flaps, the lower is greater than the upper

D. The advantage of two triangular flaps technique is that it minimizes the violation of the philtral column and distributes evenly the tension on the lip

Ans: C. With respect to these two triangular flaps, the lower is greater than the upper

Q 25. **Which of the following treatment options is the BEST for an 18 month old child with a submucous cleft palate easily noted on physical examination, but without hipernasality or speech disorder?**

A. No surgical management

B. Two-flap palatoplasty

C. Three-flap palatoplasty

D. Furlow palatoplasty

Ans: A. No surgical management

Q 26. **The area indicated by the arrow in this unilateral cleft lip deformity is:**

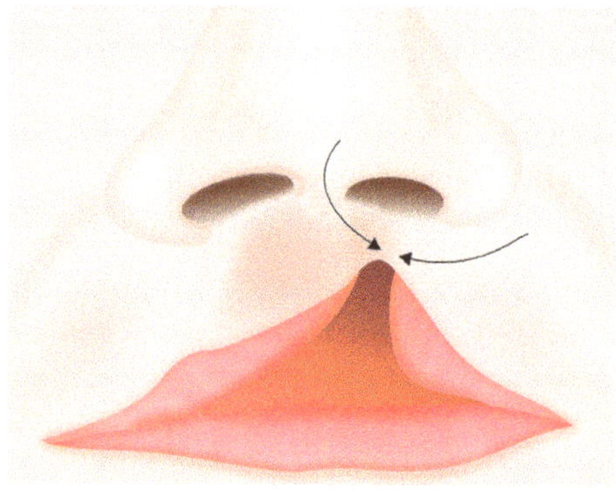

A. The C-flap

B. The M-flap

C. Simonart's band

D. The white roll

Ans: C. Simonart's band

Q 27. **Which of the following is the "OPTIMUM STANDARD" bone graft donor site for repair of an alveolar cleft?**

A. Iliac crest bone (autogenous)

B. Cranial bone (autogenous)

C. Mandibular bone/symphyseal area (autogenous)

D. Rib (autogenous)

Ans: A. Iliac crest bone (autogenous)

Q 28. **Which of the following statements is TRUE regarding cleft lip repair?**

A. Millard's technique will not narrow the nostril

B. Millard's technique will recreate the philtrum
C. Triangular flap technique will narrow the nostril
D. Triangular flap technique will allow modification during surgery

Ans: B. Millard's technique will recreate the philtrum

Q 29. Which of the following is FALSE about the Lip Adhesion?

A. Is performed at 1 month
B. Decreases the tissue to be excised in the definitive lip repair
C. Allows the lip to act as an orthodontic appliance
D. Improves the alignment of the maxillary arches

Ans: B. Decreases the tissue to be excised in the definitive lip repair

Q 30. Which of the following ARE characteristics of unilateral cleft lip and nose?

A. The nasal tip deflects toward the cleft side
B. The columella deviates to the cleft side
C. The cleft side alar base is positioned posteriorly, laterally and inferiorly
D. The caudal septum deflects toward the cleft side

Ans: C. The cleft side alar base is positioned posteriorly, laterally and inferiorly

Q 31. Which of the following is INCORRECT about a Rhinoplasty done for correction of a unilateral cleft lip nasal deformity?

A. Modified columellar incision using bilateral forked flaps is advisable
B. Septoplasty by removing a strip of cartilage inferiorly to allow the "swing" over the nasal spine is advisable
C. Cartilaginous columellar strut graft to enhance projection is advisable
D. Lower lateral cartilages are divided lateral to the dome, reconstructed and sutured to the columellar strut

Ans: A. Modified columellar incision using bilateral forked flaps is advisable

Q 32. Which of the following statements regarding the surgical repair of the bilateral cleft lip is FALSE?

A. Single-stage repair is recommended in symmetrical bilateral cleft lips with moderate protruding prolabium and premaxilla
B. Single-stage repair maximizes symmetry of the lip compared to the two-stage procedure
C. The orbicularis oris muscle from each lateral lip segment is advanced superomedially and sutured to the nasal sills
D. The two lateral prolabial flaps will be sutured to form the nasal sill and the nasal floor on each side of the nose

Ans: C. The orbicularis oris muscle from each lateral lip segment is advanced superomedially and sutured to the nasal sills

Q 33. Which of the following statements is FALSE about Rhinoplasty done for a Bilateral Cleft Lip Nasal Deformity?

A. A columellar approach using an inverted V incision or bilateral forked flaps is advisable
B. Septoplasty to correct any nasal obstruction and to obtain grafting material is advisable
C. A cartilaginous columellar strut graft to enhance projection is advisable
D. The lower lateral cartilages are divided and inverted but not reconstructed or sutured to the columellar strut

Ans: D. The lower lateral cartilages are divided and inverted but not reconstructed or sutured to the columellar strut

Q 34. Which of the following statements regarding care after unilateral cleft lip repair is FALSE?

A. Arm restraints are used for 3 weeks following the surgical procedure
B. Feed during the first 48 hours with an ear bulb syringe then proceed with the usual nursing bottle
C. All sutures are removed on day 7
D. Steri-strips should be applied for 6 weeks after the sutures are removed

Ans: B. Feed during the first 48 hours with an ear bulb syringe then proceed with the usual nursing bottle

Q 35. Which of the following statements regarding management of electrical burns is FALSE?

A. Primary debridement and reconstruction is recommended
B. Delayed eschar demarcation, then reconstruction is advisable
C. Oral splinting as early as possible is recommended in order to prevent contracture
D. Running W-plasty is the most common scar revision used in this particular situation

Ans: D. Running W-plasty is the most common scar revision used in this particular situation

Q 36. Which of the following anatomical structures is the one that comprises the PHARYNGEAL COMPONENT of the velopharyngeal closure?

A. Palatoglossus
B. Inferior constrictor
C. Superior constrictor
D. Tensor veli palatini

Ans: C. Superior constrictor

Q 37. Which of the following methods for Unilateral Primary Cleft Lip Repair will concentrate the closure tension at the UPPER PORTION of the lip?

A. Bardach
B. Millard
C. Skoog
D. Tennison-Randall

Ans: B. Millard

Q 38. Which of the following statements is TRUE about Millard's technique used in the repair of unilateral cleft lip?

A. It involves rotation and transposition flaps

B. It is the best technique for achieving excellent cosmetic results in wider clefts
C. It is used to decrease vertical scar contracture
D. It has a tendency to form small nostril

Ans: D. It has a tendency to form small nostril

Q 39. Which of the following surgical maneuvers is NOT related to the repair of a Unilateral Cleft Lip Nasal Deformity?

A. Forked flap incisions in the upper lip
B. Asymmetric vertical division of the lower lateral cartilages
C. Placement sutures into the cephalic margin of the cleft side alar cartilage to the upper lateral cartilage
D. Nasal tip grafting

Ans: A. Forked flap incisions in the upper lip

Q 40. Which of the following surgical techniques is the IDEAL for repair of a cleft lip greater than 12 mm wide?

A. Millard's repair
B. Triangular repair
C. Rose-Thompson repair
D. Quadrilateral repair

Ans: B. Triangular repair

Q 41. Which of the following techniques to repair Unilateral Cleft Lip involves Upper and Lower Lip Z-plasties?

A. Millard
B. Tennison-Randall
C. Skoog
D. LeMesurier

Ans: C. Skoog

Q 42. Which of the following statement regarding the sphincter pharyngoplasty designed by Orticochea is FALSE?

A. Flaps are raised from the posterior tonsillar pillars
B. Each flap contains a portion of the palatopharyngeus muscle
C. Patients who demonstrate poor velar elevation but good lateral wall motion are good candidates for sphincter pharyngoplasty
D. The flaps are transposed medially and interdigitated on the posterior pharyngeal wall

Ans: C. Patients who demonstrate poor velar elevation but good lateral wall motion are good candidates for sphincter pharyngoplasty

Q 43. Which of the following statements is TRUE regarding the execution of the Rotation-Advancement flap technique for the repair of a Cleft Lip?

A. The A flap is the advancement flap
B. The B flap is the rotation flap
C. The C flap is the columellar flap, noncleft side
D. The D flap is the simonart's band

Ans: C. The C flap is the columellar flap, noncleft side

Q 44. Which of the following measurements related to surgical repair of the cleft lip depicted below is CORRECT? ? In the drawing "X"-*between yellow lines*-is the distance between point 4 and point 5.

A. Millard (3 to 5 + X = 8 to 9)
B. Millard (2 to 6 = 8 to 9)

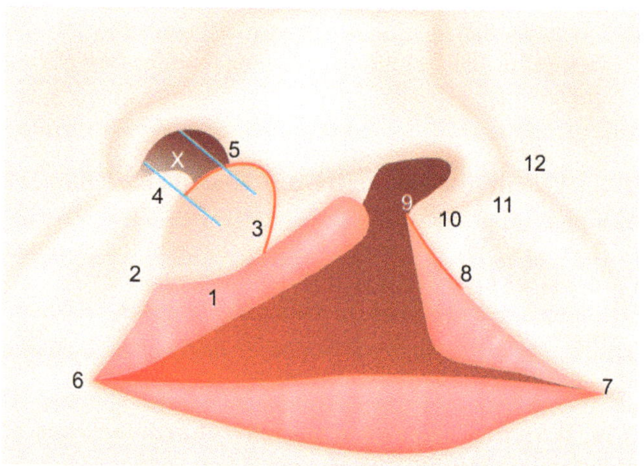

C. Millard (3 to 5 = 8 to 9)
D. Tennison-Randall (3 to 5 + X = 8 to 9)

Ans: A. Millard (3 to 5 + X = 8 to 9)

Q 45. Which of the following statements about Residual Alveolar Ridge Cleft is TRUE?

A. The most common indication for grafting is inadequate oral feeding
B. The most common bone graft used for closure is cranial bone
C. The use of cancellous bone fragments is the ideal choice
D. he best timing for primary repair is at the time of closure of the cleft lip

Ans: A. The most common indication for grafting is inadequate oral feeding

Q 46. Which of the following early postoperative complications is MOST commonly seen with the use of Pharyngeal flap surgery in children?

A. Airway obstruction
B. Aspiration
C. Dehiscence
D. Neck stiffness

Ans: A. Airway obstruction

Q 47. Which of the following statements about Bilateral Cleft Lip repair is FALSE?

A. The prolabium contains muscle
B. The prolabial flap is marked at the midline
C. The prolabial "forked" flaps are marked laterally
D. The "forked" flaps are incised, elevated and sutured laterally into the floor of the nose

Ans: A. The prolabium contains muscle

Q 48. Which of the following statements in the surgical repair of a cleft lip is FALSE?

A. The Millard method is based on the rotation-advancement
B. The Tennison-Randall method is based on the inset of a triangular flap from the cleft side into a releasing incision on the noncleft side

C. The Millard method preserves the Cupid's bow and the philtral dimple

D. The Tennison-Randall method has an excellent access to the nasal deformity

Ans: D. The Tennison-Randall method has an excellent access to the nasal deformity

Q 49. Which of the following palatoplaty technique is the one used in the drawing below?

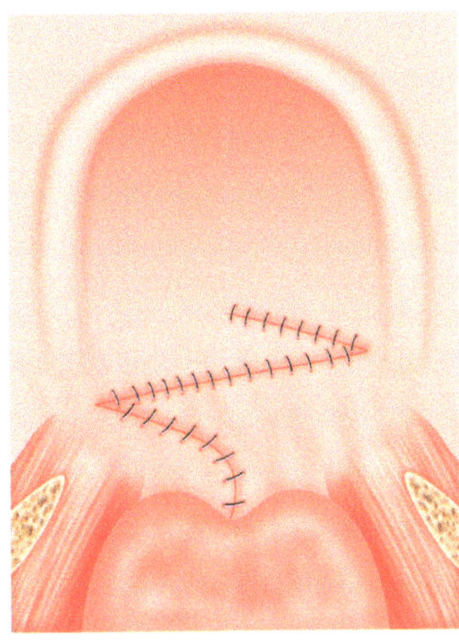

A. Furlow palatoplasty

B. Langenbeck palatoplasty

C. Two-flap palatoplasty

D. Three-flap palatoplaty

Ans: A. Furlow palatoplasty

Q 50. The drawing below represents the Millard technique in ONE-STAGE of a bilateral cleft lip repair. Which of the following flaps is the one indicated by the arrows?

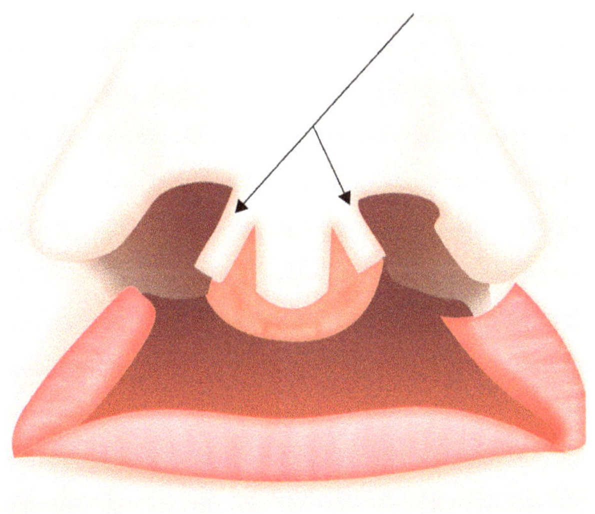

A. Collumellar flap

B. Forked flap

C. Vermillion flap

D. Alar flap

Ans: B. Forked flap

Q 51. Which of the following statements regarding the bilateral cleft lip is FALSE?

A. There is an anterior premaxillary projection

B. There is a deficient, short columella

C. The prolabium contains a well-defined muscle

D. There is a deficient nasal floor present

Ans: C. The prolabium contains a well-defined muscle

Q 52. Which of the following statements regarding Millard unilateral cleft lip repair is FALSE?

A. It is based in a rotation-advancement technique

B. It concentrates the tension at the lower portion of the lip

C. It has its transverse incision at the base of the columella

D. It seeks to restore the Cupid's bow in a normal position

Ans: B. It concentrates the tension at the lower portion of the lip

Q 53. Which of the following techniques in cleft lip repair is MOST effective in the closure of a WIDE unilateral cleft lip that has a difference of 6 mm in height between the two philtral columns?

A. Millard

B. Tennison-Randall

C. Bardach

D. Rose-Thompson

Ans: C. Bardach

Q 54. Which of the following methods of cleft lip repair is based on two triangular flaps?

A. Millard

B. Tennison-Randall

C. Bardach

D. LeMesurier

Ans: C. Bardach

Q 55. Which of the following characteristics of the Unilateral cleft lip nose is FALSE?

A. The nasal tip is deflected toward the noncleft side

B. The length of the lower lateral cartilage on the cleft side is shorter compared to the noncleft side

C. The nasal floor and sill are often absent on the cleft side

D. The caudal septum deflects toward the noncleft side

Ans: B. The length of the lower lateral cartilage on the cleft side is shorter compared to the noncleft side

Q 56. The Furlow double-opposing Z-plasty technique used to repair a cleft of the soft palate will have the following advantage:

A. Less incidence of velopalatal insufficiency

B. Less incidence of palatal fistula

C. Less incidence of airway compromise

D. Less technical difficulties, easy to perform

Ans: A. Less incidence of velopalatal insufficiency

Q 57. **Which of the following surgical techniques is the one represented in the drawing and used in the repair of a bilateral cleft lip? (See drawing below)**

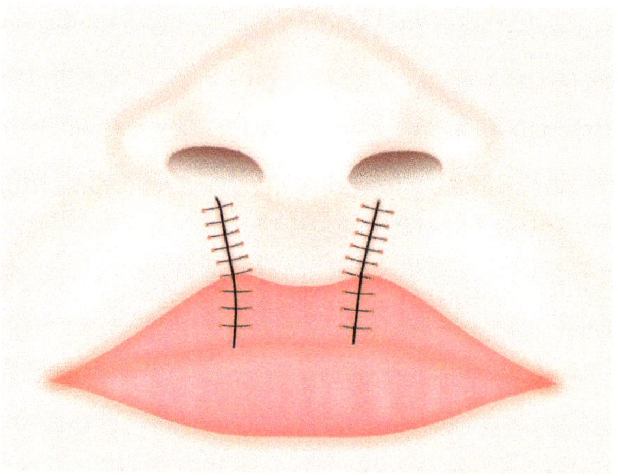

A. Tennison flap technique   B. Millard flap technique
C. Manchester technique   D. Skoog technique

Ans: C. Manchester technique

Q 58. **Which of the following statements is FALSE with respect to the management of bilateral cleft lip repair?**

A. The primary lip repair is performed when the patient is 3 months old
B. In asymmetric clefts, the side to be closed first is the most narrow
C. In symmetrical clefts, it makes no difference which side is closed first
D. In the two-stage lip closure, the second operation is performed 7 weeks after the first

Ans: B. In asymmetric clefts, the side to be closed first is the most narrow

Q 59. **What is the proper classification of the cleft palate presented? (See drawing below)**

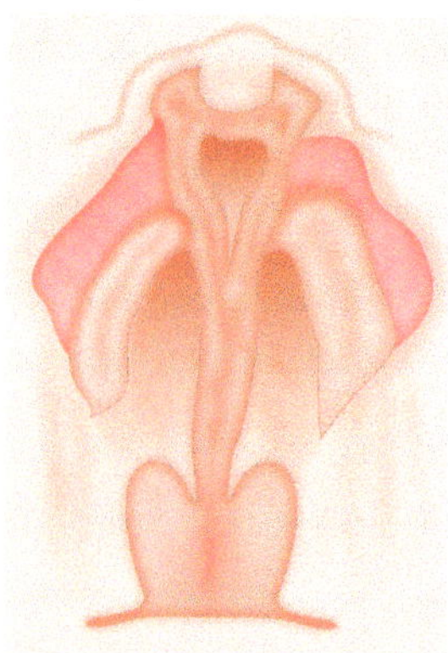

A. Bilateral complete cleft of the secondary palate
B. Bilateral complete cleft of the primary and secondary palate
C. Bilateral incomplete cleft of the primary palate
D. Bilateral incomplete cleft of the secondary palate

Ans: B Bilateral complete cleft of the primary and secondary palate

Q 60. **Which of the following cleft tip deformities is the ONE that can be successfully repair by the Manchester technique?**

A. Complete unilateral cleft lip repair
B. Incomplete unilateral cleft lip repair
C. Bilateral cleft lip repair
D. Bilateral cleft of the soft and the hard palate repair

Ans: C. Bilateral cleft lip repair

Q 61. **Which of the following muscles OPENS the Eustachian tube?**

A. Tensor veli palatini   B. Levator veli palatini
C. Musculus uvulae   D. Glossopalatine

Ans: A. Tensor veli palatini

Chapter 29

Craniofacial Anomalies

Jay J Agarwal

INTRODUCTION

The present chapter represents an overview of the most common craniofacial anomalies with the exception of cleft lip and palate, which are covered in their respective chapter.

EMBRYOLOGY

Facial development occurs between weeks 4 and 8 of gestation.[1] The continuous interaction and signaling from the ectoderm, neural crest cells, mesoderm, and pharyngeal endoderm together allow for the final formation of facial structures. Cranial placodes are ectodermal thickenings that form the sensory organs of the face and develop at the interface of neural and non-neural ectoderm. These can be divided into the anterior (adenohypophyseal, olfactory, and lens placodes), posterior (otic placode), and intermediate (trigeminal placode) groups of cranial placodes.[2] The facial primordia, the most primitive form of the face, are formed by neural crest cells.[3] These small buds of tissue surround the stomodeum, the future mouth, and migrate and divide to form the facial structures listed in Tables 1 and 2 and as seen in Figure 1.[4]

The neurocranium is formed by eight separate bones, the frontal, ethmoid, sphenoid, occipital bones as well as the paired parietal and temporal bones. The frontal, parietal, and occipital bones together form the calvaria by intramembranous ossification. The ethmoid and temporal bone form the cranial skull base by endochondrial ossification of cartilage (Figs. 3 and 4).[5] Fusion of the cranial bones in the calvaria lead to the formation of four sutures lines; the coronal, metopic, sagittal, and lambdoidal sutures.[6] The newborn skull also has an anterior and a posterior fontanel, which is where two cranial bones meet and have widened sutures. The posterior fontanel closes by 2 months of age and the anterior fontanel closes by 18 months (Fig. 2).

ETIOLOGY AND PATHOGENESIS OF CRANIOFACIAL ANOMALIES

Syndromes are defined as a combination of several distinct and recognizable features that have a specific known cause. Causes can be mutations, teratogens, etc. *Sequences*

Table 1: End-results of the development of facial primordial	
Frontonasal prominence	Forehead Dorsum on the nose
Lateral nasal prominence	Ala of the nose
Medial nasal prominence	Nasal septum, philtrum
Maxillary prominence	Maxilla, upper lip, and cheek
Mandibular prominence	Mandible, lower lip, and chin

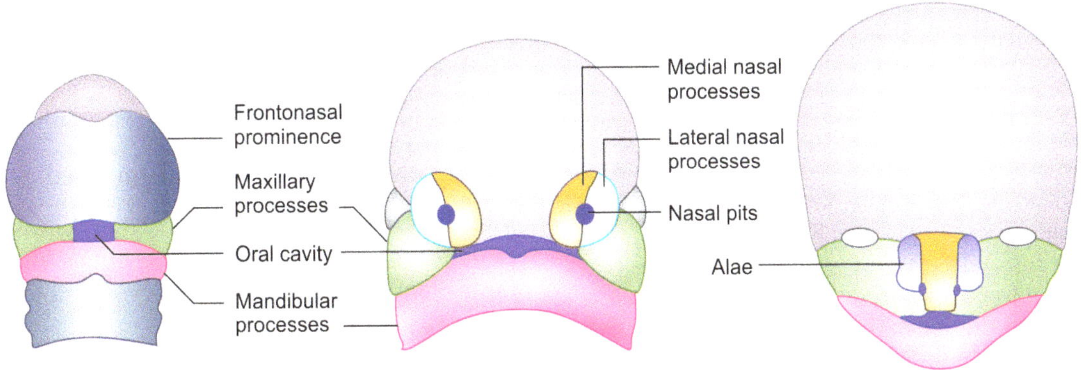

Fig. 1: Illustration of prominences and what they form.

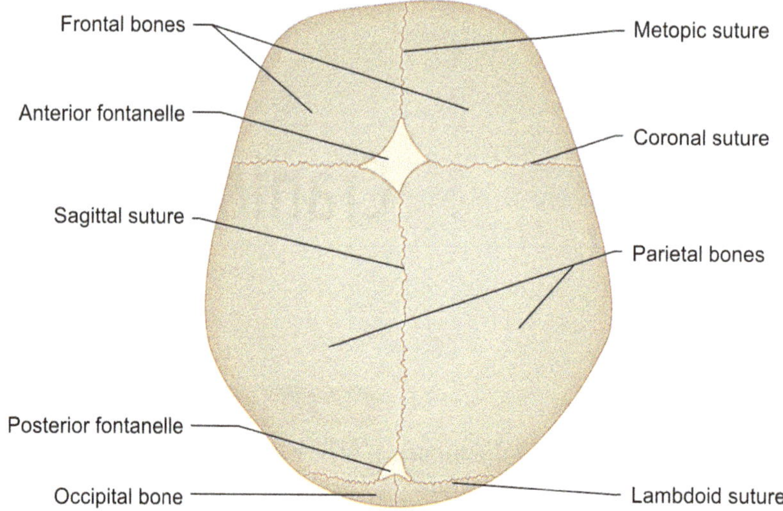

Fig. 2: Normal skull of the newborn and illustration of suture lines.

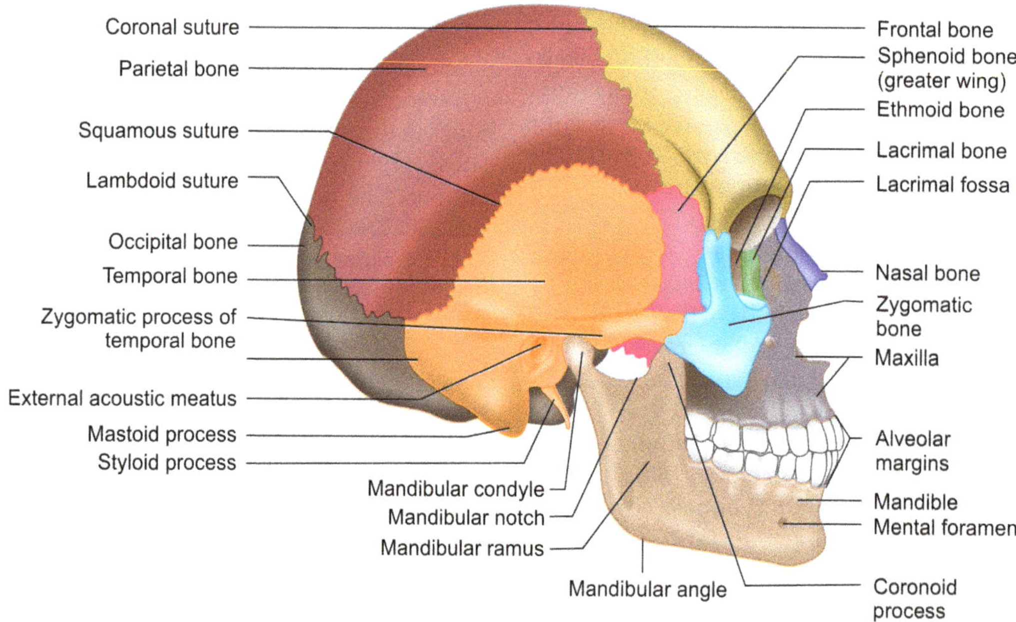

Fig. 3: Basic anatomy of the craniofacial skeleton (cranial vault, orbital framework, maxilla, and mandible).

describe cases when a deformity of some sort leads to the development of other secondary abnormalities as a domino effect. An example would be Pierre Robin sequence in which the initial abnormality is micrognathia, which causes a normal tongue to be displaced disrupting palatal closure which results in the formation of a cleft palate. Lastly, *association* describes multiple anomalies that are frequently seen together, however, there is no single known cause and no sequence of events that lead to the various anomalies.

Most Common Craniofacial Anomalies

Premature closure of suture lines that leads to nonsyndromic craniosynostosis occurs in 1:1000 births.[7] The types of craniosynostoses are classified according to the suture involved.

- Sagittal: Scaphocephaly
- Coronal or lambdoid: Plagiocephaly
- Metopic: Trigonocephaly

- Multiple sutures with trilobe deformity—Kleeblattschadel
- Sagittal, coronal, and lambdoid—acrocephaly.

The most common craniofacial syndromes along with their transmission, genes, and salient features are presented in Table 3.[8-20]

Table 2: End-results of the first and second branchial arches	
Arch	*End-results*
First	• Bones: Maxilla, zygoma, mandible, incus, and malleus • Muscles: Anterior belly of digastric, muscles of mastication, mylohyoid, tensor tympani, and tensor palatine • Nerves: Mandibular branch of trigeminal (V3) • Arteries: Maxillary artery
Second	• Bones: Lesser horn of hyoid and upper body of hyoid, stapes, styloid process, and stylohyoid ligament • Muscles: Stapedius, stylohyoid, posterior belly of digastric, auricular, and muscles of facial expression • Nerves: Facial nerve • Arteries: Hyoid and stapedial arteries

■ TREATMENT

Treatment should always be multidisciplinary.

Indications for Surgical Intervention

There are several indications for surgical intervention that should be considered during the initial assessment of patients with craniofacial anomalies which are listed in Table 4.[21]

Surgical Management

The surgical treatment for craniofacial anomalies depends on the abnormalities present in each patient. Timing for surgical intervention varies based on how extensive the abnormalities are. For single-suture synostosis, treatment should be performed before three months of age. For more involved abnormalities, surgical intervention is usually delayed until 7–9 months of age. However, earlier surgical intervention may be necessary if the patient has elevated intracranial pressure, hypertelorism that can

Table 3: Most common craniofacial syndromes and their features		
Syndrome	*Transmission and gene*	*Main features*
Pierre Robin[8,9]	AD 50% associated with a syndrome (Stickler, velocardiofacial, and Treacher-Collins)	Micrognathia Glossoptosis Airway obstruction (formerly cleft palate)
Stickler[10]	AD COL2A1 gene (chr. 12) for type II collagen	Robin sequence Midfacial hypoplasia Congenital hearing loss (CHL) Eye (myopia, cataracts, and retinal detachment) Joints (hypermobility, spondyloepiphyseal dysplasia, and arthritis)
Treacher-Collins[11]	AD TCOF1 gene-TREACLE protein (chr. 5)	Malformation of first and second branchial arches Malar hypoplasia Downslanting fissures Hair on cheeks Lower lid (coloboma, no lashes) Ear (microtia, aural atresia, and CHL) Nose (flat nasal bridge, narrow nares, and choanal atresia) Robin sequence
Oculo-auriculo-vertebral spectrum (Goldenhar and hemifacial microsomia)[12,13]	Most sporadic, some AD	Classified using *OMENS+* O: Orbital distortion M: Mandibular hypoplasia and Robin spectrum E: Ear anomaly (microtia spectrum, atresia spectrum, and CHL) N: Nerve involvement S: Soft tissue deficiency +: Cleft lip and palate, cardiac, skeletal (cervical fusion), pulmonary, renal, gastrointestinal (GI), and limb
Apert, Crouzon, Pfeiffer, and Saethre-Chotzen[14–20]	AD FGFR-2 gene (chr. 10)	Craniosynostosis Hypertelorism Cervical fusion Low nasal bridge, parrot nose, and choanal atresia Micrognathia and cleft palate *Apert: Syndactyly and CHL* *Pfeiffer: Digital broadening* *Saethre-Chotzen: Partial syndactyly*

Table 4: Indications for surgical intervention	
Psychosocial/cosmetic	Improving a patient's external experience
Ophthalmic	Corneal exposure due to exophthalmos and hypertelorism
Respiratory	Nasal narrowing or complete obstruction of the nasal airway
Neurological	Increased intracranial pressure Cerebral compression
Dental	Malocclusion leading to dental caries Malocclusion severe enough to complicate mastication

lead to corneal ulceration or any other significant surgical indication. Midfacial treatment is usually performed after the age of 4 years old and further smaller anomalies such as malocclusion are treated at older ages (teenage or older) as needed.[6]

Surgical treatment of single suture craniosynostosis is completed with strip craniectomies. These procedures essentially remove the fused sutures with the aim for natural correction of the abnormality. Newer techniques allow for this procedure to be performed endoscopically, resulting in smaller incisions and decreased blood loss. These procedures can be supplemented with molding helmets which aid in normalizing head shape.[22]

Cranial vault reconstruction is performed in patients with more complicated abnormalities and in patients between the ages of 6 months and 12 months. The goals are to remove the abnormally fused sutures and abnormally shaped cranial bone and subsequently reconstruct a normally shaped head. These procedures are more effective at ages greater than 6 months because the infant's bones tend to be firmer and allow for proper fixation.

A fronto-orbital advancement can be performed by bringing the forehead and superior orbits anteriorly with the goal to increase the intracranial volume in the anterior vault. This is performed in patients with metopic or coronal synostosis. Posterior cranial vault reconstruction is performed for sagittal, lambdoid, and complex suture fusion with the goal to advance to posterior segment of the head and possibly increase width.[23]

Distraction osteogenesis is another technique in which typical coronal scalp incisions are made, flaps elevated and craniotomies made and cranial distractors are placed. In the following days to weeks, there is active distraction of the bones with the distractors which results in expansion of the bone and soft tissue. This technique is used for complex craniosynostosis.[23]

Children with Pierre Robin sequence may have frequent desaturations due to obstruction from the tongue. Simple treatments should be tried first as many children outgrow

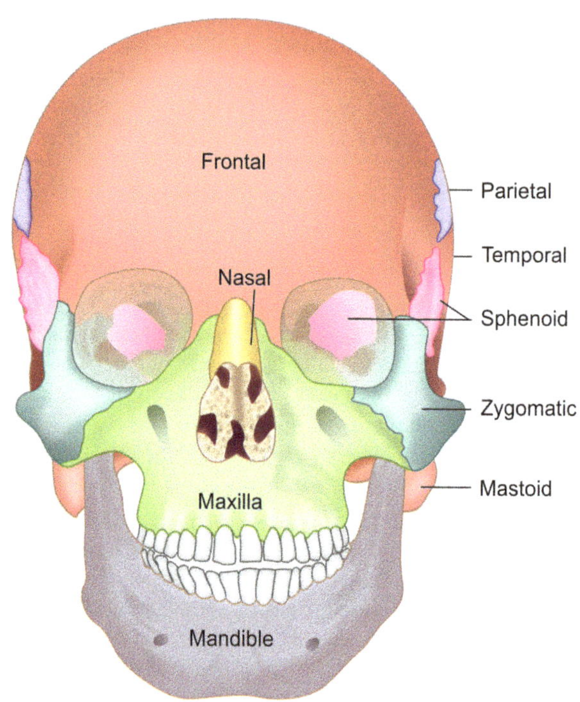

Fig. 4: Frontal view of the facial bones

their airway issues as the mandible develops. The following are the various treatments for airway obstruction in children with Pierre Robin sequence.[11,24,25]

Nonsurgical

- Side or prone positioning (first-line).
- Place nasopharyngeal tube if oxygen saturations or respiratory efforts do not improve.
- Evaluation and treatment for gastric reflux.
- Intubation in the acute setting and if the above maneuvers do not work.

Surgical

- *Glossopexy (tongue-lip adhesion)*: Secures anterior and posterior portions of the tongue to the mandible to prevent airway obstruction.
- *Mandibular distraction*: Bilateral osteotomies with subsequent lengthening of the mandible using distraction hardware.
- *Tracheostomy*: Definitive airway management, but last resort when there are multiple levels of airway obstruction or the above methods fail.

■ COMPLICATIONS

Surgical treatment of craniofacial anomalies is intricate and complicated and has various risks. Electrolyte abnormalities should be prevented and need abrupt treatment and continuous monitoring. Postoperative bleeding can be significant and even require massive transfusions. Common sites of bleeding are from bony donor sites such as the rib or ilium. Facial bleeding and extradural hematomas do not usually lead to extensive bleeding. Pneumothorax is a potential complication when rib resection is required for reconstruction. Diabetes insipidus has been seen in cases where there is traction on brain tissue. Cerebrospinal fluid leak seen in the nose is also a known complication, especially in transcranial approaches.[21]

During these surgeries, the eye and orbital contents may need to be manipulated and retracted which can lead to complications including blindness, decreased visual acuity, and corneal ulcerations.[26]

■ REFERENCES

1. Som PM, Naidich TP. Illustrated review of the embryology and development of the facial region, part 1: Early face and lateral nasal cavities. AJNR Am J Neuroradiol. 2013;34:2233-40.
2. Singh S, Groves AK. The molecular basis of craniofacial placode development. Wiley Interdiscip Rev Dev Biol. 2016;5:363-76.
3. Wedden SE, Ralphs JR, Tickle C. Pattern formation in the facial primordia. Development. 1988;103 Suppl:31-40.
4. Kumar R. Textbook of Human Embryology. Vol 3. I. K. International Pvt Ltd; 2008.
5. Kahn D, Arusoo T, Wright EJ. Neurocranium and facial skeleton. In: Watanabe K, Shoja MM, Loukas M (Eds). Anatomy for Plastic Surgery of the Face, Head and Neck. Thieme,2016.
6. Papel ID, Frodel JL, Holt R, Larrabee Jr WF, Nachlas NE, Park SS, Sykes JM, Toriumi, DM (Eds). Facial Plastic and Reconstructive Surgery, 4th edition. New York: Thieme Medical Publishers; 2016.
7. Garza RM, Khosla RK. Nonsyndromic craniosynostosis. Semin Plast Surg. 2012;26:53-63.
8. Cielo CM, Montalva FM, Taylor JA. Craniofacial disorders associated with airway obstruction in the neonate. Semin Fetal Neonatal Med. 2016;21:254-62.
9. Côté A, Fanous A, Almajed A, et al. Pierre Robin sequence: review of diagnostic and treatment challenges. Int J Pediatr Otorhinolaryngol. 2015;79:451-64.
10. Robin NH, Moran RT, Ala-Kokko L. Stickler Syndrome; 1993.
11. Buchanan EP, Xue AS, Hollier LH. Craniofacial syndromes. Plast Reconstr Surg. 2014;134:128e-153e.
12. Beleza-Meireles A, Clayton-Smith J, Saraiva JM, et al. Oculo-auriculo-vertebral spectrum: a review of the literature and genetic update. J Med Genet. 2014;51:635-45.
13. Passos-Bueno MR, Ornelas CC, Fanganiello RD. Syndromes of the first and second pharyngeal arches: A review. Am J Med Genet A. 2009;149A:1853-9.
14. Preston RA, Post JC, Keats BJ, et al. A gene for Crouzon craniofacial dysostosis maps to the long arm of chromosome 10. Nat Genet. 1994;7:149-53.
15. Kan S, Elanko N, Johnson D, et al. Genomic screening of fibroblast growth-factor receptor 2 reveals a wide spectrum of mutations in patients with syndromic craniosynostosis. Am J Hum Genet. 2002;70:472-86.
16. Forbes BJ. Congenital craniofacial anomalies. Curr Opin Ophthalmol. 2010;21:367-74.
17. McCulloch TM, Makielski KH, McNutt MA, et al. Head and neck liposarcoma. A histopathologic reevaluation of reported cases. Arch Otolaryngol Head Neck Surg. 1992;118:1045-9.
18. Wilkie AO, Slaney SF, Oldridge M, et al. Apert syndrome results from localized mutations of FGFR2 and is allelic with Crouzon syndrome. Nat Genet. 1995;9:165-72.
19. Glaser RL, Jiang W, Boyadjiev SA, et al. Paternal origin of FGFR2 mutations in sporadic cases of Crouzon syndrome and Pfeiffer syndrome. Am J Hum Genet. 2000;66:768-77.
20. Cohen MM. Pfeiffer syndrome update, clinical subtypes, and guidelines for differential diagnosis. Am J Med Genet. 1993;45:300-7.
21. Matthews D. Craniofacial surgery—indications, assessment and complications. Br J Plast Surg. 1979;32:96-105.
22. Kaufman BA, Muszynski CA, Matthews A, et al. The circle of sagittal synostosis surgery. Semin Pediatr Neurol. 2004;11:243-8.
23. Morris L. Management of craniosynostosis. Facial Plast Surg. 2016;32:123-32.
24. Myer CM, Reed JM, Cotton RT, et al. Airway management in Pierre Robin sequence. Otolaryngol Head Neck Surg. 1998;118:630-5.
25. Scott AR. Surgical management of Pierre Robin sequence: Using mandibular distraction osteogenesis to address hypoventilation and failure to thrive in Infancy. Facial Plast Surg. 2016;32:177-87.
26. Whitaker LA, Munro IR, Salyer KE, et al. Combined report of problems and complications in 793 craniofacial operations. Plast Reconstr Surg. 1979;64:198-203.

Multiple Choice Questions

Q 1. The helical rim in microtia repair is created by which number CONTRALATERAL COSTAL RIB?

A. 6   B. 7
C. 8   D. 9

Ans: D. 9

Q 2. Which of the following statements is TRUE about the vertical axis of normal ear architecture?

A. It is inclined anteriorly 5 degrees
B. It is inclined anteriorly 15 degrees.
C. It is inclined posteriorly 5 degrees.
D. It is inclined posteriorly 15 degrees.

Ans: D. It is inclined posteriorly 15 degrees.

Q 3. Where is the IDEAL PLACE from which to harvest the skin graft used in the third stage reconstruction of congenital microtia repair?

A. Buttocks   B. Postauricular
C. Supraclavicular   D. Thigh

Ans: A. Buttocks

Q 4. Which of the following statements regarding proper positioning and orientation of the auricle is TRUE?

A. The ear is tilted at an angle of 30 degrees posteriorly
B. The normal auricle protrudes approximately 30 degrees from the skull
C. The top of the ear is 0.5 cm above the level of the brow
D. The vertical height of a normal adult ear is 8 cm

Ans: B. The normal auricle protrudes approximately 30 degrees from the skull

Q 5. Which of the following statements regarding this stage of the microtia reconstruction (shown in the picture) is TRUE?

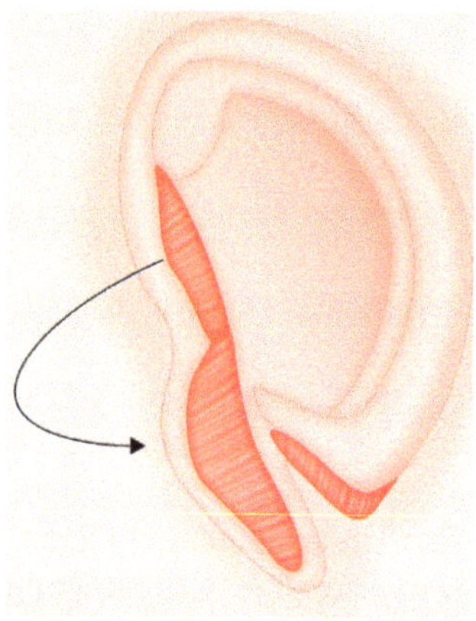

A. The designed flap will require to have an internal cartilage
B. The fibroadipose lobular remnant is transposed posteriorly and inferiorly
C. The flap used can be either superiorly or inferiorly based
D. Usually is done at the time of carving the auricular framework

Ans: B. The fibroadipose lobular remnant is transposed posteriorly and inferiorly

Q 6. Which of the following statements about calvarial bone grafting is TRUE?

A. The calvarial bone graft has a higher incidence of resorption than the iliac crest
B. The place for harvesting the graft is below the temporal line
C. Harvesting the graft above the temporal line will avoid complications because the calvarium is thicker above the temporal line
D. Midline calvarial bone grafts are prone to fewer complications, however, the surgical technique is more

Ans: C. Harvesting the graft above the temporal line will avoid complications because the calvarium is thicker above the temporal line

Q 7. Which following statement is TRUE regarding normal adult anatomy and position of the ear?

A. The ear width is normally about 70% of its height
B. The ear is normally about 75 mm in height
C. The ear sits at a distance of about one ear width from the lateral orbital rim
D. The angle formed by the auricle and the head is 40°

Ans: C. The ear sits at a distance of about one ear width from the lateral orbital rim

Q 8. Which of the following represents the distance indicated by the arrow seen in the drawing below?

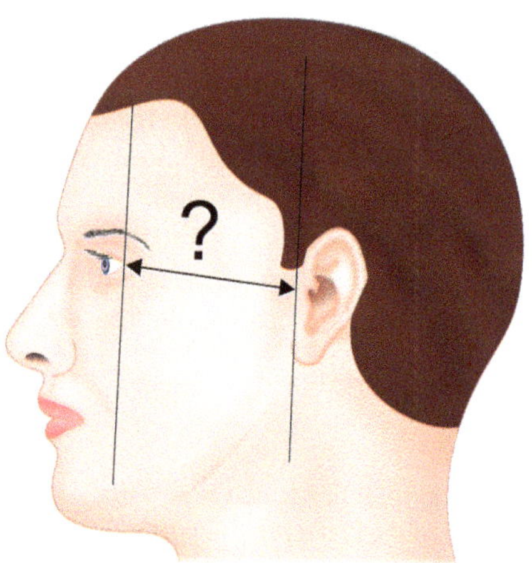

A. 4 cm
B. 6 cm
C. 8 cm
D. 10 cm

Ans: B. 6 cm

Q 9. Which of the following statements about congenital microtia is TRUE?

A. Auricular reconstruction should be performed after atresia
B. The best time to perfom the surgery is after 8 years of age
C. The autogenous costal cartilage is taken from ipsilateral side of the chest
D. The ninth rib is dissected to form the helical rim

Ans: D. The ninth rib is dissected to form the helical rim

Q 10. Which of the following is the MOST COMMON complication related to the use of silastic material for auricular reconstruction?

A. Hematoma
B. Infection
C. Exposure
D. Displacement

Ans: C. Exposure

Q 11. Which of the following represents the SECOND STAGE of BRENT'S technique for microtia reconstruction?

A. Framework placement
B. Lobule transposition
C. Lobule transposition and tragus reconstruction
D. Framework placement, incorporation of tragal component and lobule transposition

Ans: B. Lobule transposition

Q 12. Which of the following craniofacial synostosis syndromes is characterized by the following anatomical features: craniosynostosis, brachycephaly, shallow orbits (exorbitism), maxillary hypoplasia without extremity syndactyly?

A. Apert's syndrome
B. Crouzons syndrome
C. Pfeiffer's syndrome
D. Saethre-Chotzen syndrome

Ans: B. Crouzons syndrome

Q 13. Which of the following statements indicated THE PROPER TIMING of initial surgical midfacial treatment in craniomaxillofacial deformities?

A. 12 months
B. 2 years
C. 4 years
D. 12 years

Ans: C. 4 years

Q 14. Which of the following statements about TESSIER OPERATIVE ADVANCEMENT performed in patients with craniosynostosis is FALSE?

A. Hydrocephalus should be repaired first
B. Procedure should be done at 6 months of age
C. It will allow a maximal advancement of 10 mm
D. It is a fronto-orbital advancement

Ans: C. It will allow a maximal advancement of 10 mm

Q 15. Which of the following types of Calvarial Bone Grafts is MOST USEFUL in the treatment of Cranioplasty/Craniosynostosis?

A. Bone chips
B. Bone strips
C. Partial thickness
D. Full thickness

Ans: D. Full thickness

Q 16. Which of the following auricular congenital malformations is the ONE represented in the drawing below?

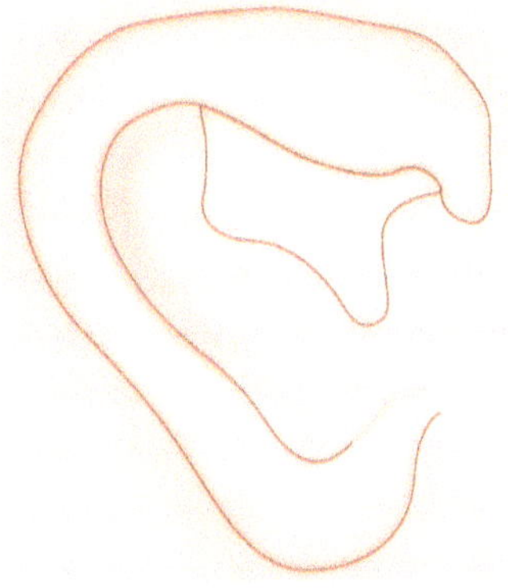

A. Cup ear
B. Microtic ear
C. Macrotic ear
D. Cryptotic ear

Ans: A. Cup ear

Q 17. Which of the following surgical incisions is MOST commonly used in the correction of Craniofacial Deformities?

A. Bilateral rhitidectomy incision
B. Bilateral lateral rhinotomy with infraorbital extension
C. Bicoronal incision
D. Midface degloving incision and bilateral brow incision

Ans: C. Bicoronal incision

Q 18. The ratio of cranial vault to facial skeleton (CRANIOFACIAL RATIO) in an infant is:

A. 8:1
B. 6:1
C. 5:1
D. 4:1

Ans: A. 8:1

Q 19. What is the INCLINATION of the normal ear in relation to the vertical axis of the skull?

A. 5 degrees
B. 10 degrees
C. 20 degrees
D. 30 degrees

Ans: C. 20 degrees

Q 20. Which of the following statements about microtia reconstruction with autologous rib cartilage is FALSE?

A. Age 6 is the ideal age for reconstruction
B. Otologic reconstruction should precede auricular reconstruction
C. Proper positioning is crucial for satisfaction
D. The contralateral costal margin is used for harvesting autologous costal cartilages

Ans: B. Otologic reconstruction should precede auricular reconstruction

Q 21. Which of the following statements about Microtia is FALSE?

A. Girls are more often affected than boys
B. Microtia occurs in approximately 1 in 10,000 live births
C. The right ear is most commonly affected
D. Unilateral occurrence is more common than bilateral

Ans: A. Girls are more often affected than boys

Q 22. Which of the following indicates the "X" measurement in the adult auricle?

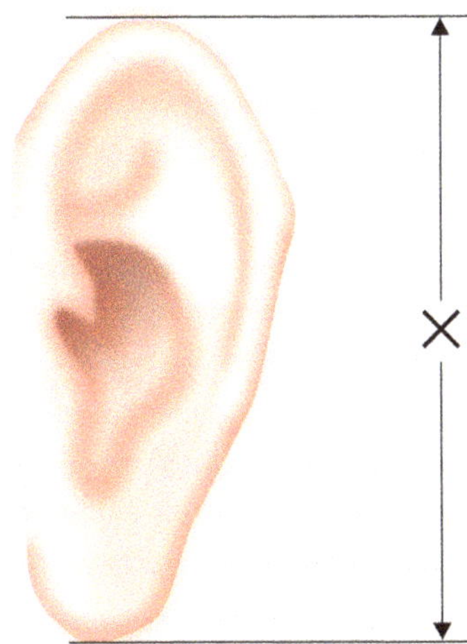

A. 60 mm
B. 70 mm
C. 75 mm
D. 80 mm

Ans: A. 60 mm

Q 23. Which of the following position IS USUALLY found in the vestigial lobule of the ear microtia?

A. Higher and more anterior than normal position
B. Higher and more posterior than normal position
C. Lower and more anterior than normal position
D. Lower and more posterior than normal position

Ans: A. Higher and more anterior than normal position

Q 24. Which of the following implant materials is the one MOST COMMONLY USED in the non-autologous costal cartilage alternative for ear microtia reconstruction?
A. Expanded polytetrafluoroethylene (ePTFE)
B. Hydroxyapatite
C. Polyethylene Terephthalate (Dacron)
D. Porous high-density polyethylene (PHDPE)
Ans: D. Porous high-density polyethylene (PHDPE)

Q 25. Which of the following ear deformities is the MOST common found in protruding ears?
A. Antihelical unfurling
B. Helix unfurling
C. Conchal excess
D. Outstanding lobule
Ans: A. Antihelical unfurling

Q 26. Which of the following condition is MOST likely related to excessive pain in the immediate postoperative period in otoplastic surgery?
A. Hematoma
B. Infection
C. Necrosis of the cartilage
D. Sutures extrusion
Ans: A. Hematoma

Q 27. Which of the following stages is designed for the lobule reconstruction in a microtic ear (Brent technique)?
A. First stage
B. Second stage
C. Third stage
D. Fourth stage
Ans: B. Second stage

Q 28. Which of the following is NOT true regarding ear analysis?
A. The width of the ear is approximately one half its length
B. The ear length should approximate the length of the nose
C. The superior aspect of the ear lies at the level of the eyebrow
D. The ear has a posterior rotation of approximately 30 degrees from the vertical plane
Ans: D. The ear has a posterior rotation of approximately 30 degrees from the vertical plane

Q 29. The RECOMMENDED management of a giant congenital hairy nevus is:
A. Conservative management
B. Laser coagulation
C. Photodynamic therapy
D. Surgical excision
Ans: D. Surgical excision

Q 30. Which of the following represents the FIRST STAGE of Nagata's Method for microtia reconstruction is TRUE?
A. Framework placement
B. Framework placement and lobule transposition
C. Framework placement, incorporation of tragal component and lobule transposition
D. Excision of remnant cartilages and lobule transposition
Ans: C. Framework placement, incorporation of tragal component and lobule transposition

Q 31. With reference to the auricle, which of the following dimensions is INCORRECT?
A. The vertical axis of the auricle is inclined 20 degrees posteriorly
B. The width of the auricle should be 75% of the length
C. The superior aspect of the auricle is at the level of the brow
D. The helical rim has a protrusion of 2 cm from the skull
Ans: B. The width of the auricle should be 75% of the length

Q 32. Which of the following about in head and neck embryology is TRUE?
A. The development of the pharyngeal arches begins at approximately day 20
B. Each pharyngeal arch contains an artery, a nerve, a cartilaginous bar, and a muscle component
C. The stapedius and posterior belly muscles form part of the first pharyngeal arch
D. The stylopharyngeus muscle forms part of the second pharyngeal arch
Ans: B. Each pharyngeal arch contains an artery, a cartilaginous bar, and a muscle component

Q 33. Which of the following anatomical structures is a derivative of the second pharyngeal arch?
A. Zygoma
B. Incus
C. Cricoid
D. Stapes
Ans: D. Stapes

Q 34. Which of the following anatomic structures is NOT innervated by V3?
A. The lateral pterygoid muscle
B. The mylohyoid muscle
C. The posterior belly of the digastric muscle
D. The tensor veli palatini muscle
Ans: C. The Posterior Belly of the Digastric Muscle

Chapter 30

Vascular Anomalies

Neha A Patel

◼ INTRODUCTION AND BRIEF OVERVIEW

Vascular anomalies represent a spectrum of head and neck lesions divided into vascular malformations and vascular tumors. They occur in 4.5% of children.[1] Hemangiomas are the most common vascular anomalies followed by lymphatic and venous malformations. Accurate diagnosis helps guide treatment and depends upon the patient's presentation as well as the tumor's growth rate and pathophysiology. The treatment of patients with vascular anomalies often requires a multidisciplinary collaboration between otolaryngology, interventional radiology, hematology, dermatology, pediatrics, and plastic surgery.

Presentation

History and Physical

Vascular anomalies are organized based on the International Society for the Study of Vascular Anomalies (ISSVA) classification system[2] (Table 1). Briefly children with *vascular malformations* have lesions with *abnormal vascular morphogenesis*. These lesions fail to regress, may grow with the child, and have normal endothelial mitotic activity.[3] Vascular malformations may have any components from capillary, venous, arterial or lymphatic elements.

Table 1: Modified International Society for the Study of Vascular Anomalies (ISSVA) classification system[1,2,7]

Vascular malformations	Vascular tumors
Low-flow	Infantile hemangioma (IH)
Capillary/venular	Congenital hemangioma (CH)
Venous	Rapidly involuting CH (RICH)
Lymphatic malformations (LMs)	Non-involuting CH (NICH)
High-flow	Partially involuting CH (PICH)
Arteriovenous malformations (AVMs)	Kaposiform hemangioendothelioma (KHE)
Arteriovenous fistulae (AVF)	Tufted angioma

Children presenting with benign *vascular tumors* can have lesions that exhibit *cellular proliferation or hyperplasia*. Vascular tumors such as infantile hemangiomas (IHs) rapidly enlarge and then slowly regress.

◼ VASCULAR MALFORMATIONS

Classification

Vascular malformations can be organized into low-flow and high-flow lesions based on the way they behave and their blood vessel type and radiographic appearance. Low-flow lesions are capillary, venular, venous, or lymphatic malformations (LMs) while high-flow lesions are arteriovenous malformations or fistulae.

Capillary Malformations

- *Natural history*:
  - *Epidemiology and associated syndromes*: Capillary malformations occur in about 0.3% of children. While the cause of isolated capillary malformations is unknown, the most common syndrome associated with capillary malformations is Sturge-Weber syndrome (SWS). SWS is associated with capillary malformations in the distribution of the ophthalmic division of the trigeminal nerve, leptomeningeal angiomatosis and choroid angioma.[4]
  - *Presentation*: Capillary malformations red or purple skin lesions made up of dilated channels of abnormal capillary. They are present at birth.
  - *Evaluation*: Patients with signs of SWS need an magnetic resonance imaging (MRI) of the brain and consultation with ophthalmology. These patients may present with seizures, mental retardation and glaucoma.[4]
- *Treatment*: Flashlamp pumped pulsed dye laser (FPDL) and potassium-titanyl-phosphate (KTP) lasers have been used to treat flat capillary malformations. Surgery is reserved for lesions that are more advanced.[4]

Venous Malformations

- *Natural history*:
  - *Epidemiology and associated syndromes*: Abnormal venous morphogenesis creates a low-flow venous malformation system that can lead to thrombosis. While they are more commonly sporadic and unifocal, venous malformations can be associated with autosomal dominant genetic anomalies such as glomuvenous malformations (GVM) and multiple cutaneous and mucosal venous malformations (VMCM).[5] Patients with multiple venous malformations need an extensive preoperative work-up as they can develop severe coagulopathies and have elevated D-dimers.
  - *Presentation*: While venous malformations are present at birth and grow with the child, deep tumors are often only diagnosed after rapid expansion due to various triggers such as infection, trauma, and hormonal changes of puberty and pregnancy. Lesions overlying skin or mucosa appear blue or purple (Figs. 1 and 2).
  - *Evaluation*: Venous malformations are compressible and develop areas with tender phleboliths. These lesions can swell up in the dependent position or with a Valsalva maneuver. Areas of calcification are seen on CT imaging while Doppler ultrasonography is used to evaluate the flow characteristics of the lesion.
  - *Treatment*: Multiple modalities are used to treat venous malformations. Small, asymptomatic venous malformations can be observed while superficial, well circumscribed, symptomatic lesions can be treated surgically or with Nd: YAG laser therapy.[5] More extensive lesions can be reduced with sclerotherapy using agents such as ethanol, bleomycin, doxycycline, and picinabil (OK-432) or a combined approach.

Lymphatic Malformations

- *Natural history*:
  - *Epidemiology and associated syndromes*: Lymphatic malformations (LMs) are an abnormal collection of low-flow lymphatic channels occurring in 1 out of 500–4,000 live births. Microcystic disease and disease with mucosal involvement tends to have worse prognosis. LMs can be associated with syndromes such as Noonan's and Klippel-Trenaunay syndrome.[6,7]
  - *Presentation*: The diagnosis of LM is typically made after swelling secondary to infection or hormonal changes. While some LMs can regress, others can be symptomatic and cause airway obstruction depending on location.
  - *Evaluation*: Magnetic resonance imaging can help evaluate the extent of the lesion while ultrasound imaging can also help guide sclerotherapy treatment.

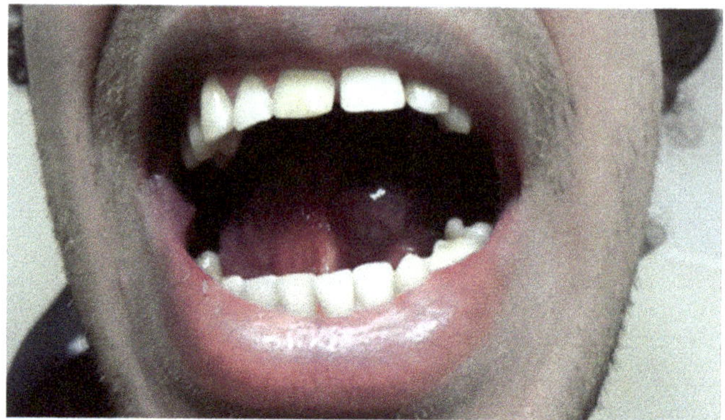

Fig. 1: Patient with a classic venous malformation of the ventral surface of the oral tongue.

Source: Personal collection of author Neha Patel.

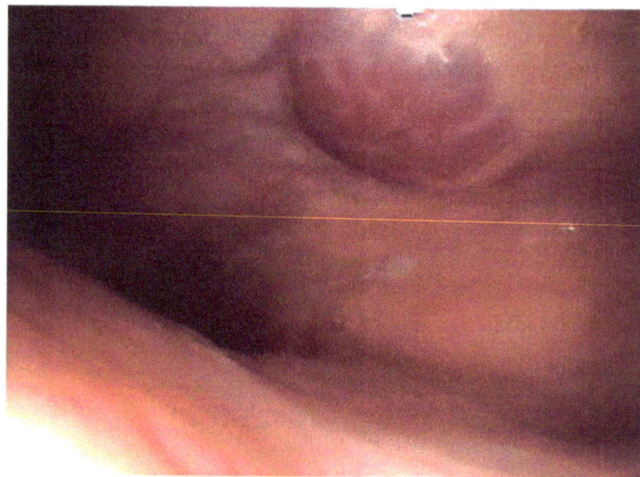

Fig. 2: Flexible nasopharyngoscopy of a patient with a venous malformation of the posterior pharynx at the level of the soft palate

Source: Personal collection of author Neha Patel.

  - *Classification*:
    » Lesions can be classified as microcystic, if they are less than 2 cm in diameter, macrocystic if they are greater than 2 cm in diameter or mixed in components of both exist. All lesions are pathologically the same and are positive for lymphatic endothelial hyaluronan receptor-1 on immunohistochemistry.[7]
    » The de Serres proposal for staging LMs divides LMs into stage 1-tumors that are unilateral infrahyoid (17% complication rate), stage 2-unilateral suprahyoid (41% complication rate), stage 3-unilateral suprahyoid and infrahyoid (67% complication rate), stage 4-bilateral suprahyoid (80% complication rate) stage 5-bilateral suprahyoid, and infrahyoid (100% complication rate).[8]

– *Treatment*: The goal of therapy is to restore or maintain function and aesthetic appearance. Conservative therapy includes treating superimposed infections with antibiotics and steroids and bypassing airway obstruction by means of a surgical tracheostomy or partial tongue resection. Sclerotherapy has been used to treat macrocystic LM but has the potential for cranial nerve injury, skin necrosis, and edema as well as agent specific complications. The use of OK-432 (a mixture of group A *Streptococcus pyogenes* and benzylpenicillin) has the potential for shock-like symptoms in those with penicillin allergies. Bleomycin use can potentially cause interstitial pneumonia and pulmonary fibrosis. Doxycycline use has the potential for electrolyte abnormalities and tooth discoloration (patients younger than 8 years). Absolute ethanol use can cause respiratory depression, arrhythmias, seizures and rhabdomyolysis.[6] Surgical resection and laser ablation of LMs also carry the similar risk of cranial nerve injury.

Arteriovenous Malformations

- *Natural history*:
  - *Epidemiology*: Arteriovenous malformations (AVMs) are high-flow lesions caused by anomalous connections between the venous and arterial system (as opposed to arteriovenous fistulas that cause direct shunting of blood). Early AVMs undergo a quiescent stage but later they can undergo expansion. Ultimately, AVMs with multiple arterial feeders can be diffusely infiltrative, destructive, and have a high recurrence rate.[1]
  - *Presentation*: The skin overlying an AVM can be pulsatile and warm. It can also have a palpable thrill and a slight blush. Skin changes also include erythema, ulceration and bleeding. Like venous malformations, AVMs can also show rapid growth with hormonal changes such as puberty.[1]
  - *Evaluation*: Magnetic resonance imaging shows characteristic arterial flow voids and is helpful to evaluate the extent of the lesion. Angiography can determine the feeding vessels and also help guide treatment.[1]
  - *Treatment*: Arteriovenous malformation treatment consists of embolization and surgical resection alone or in combination. Embolization agents include ethanol, polyvinyl alcohol, coils, and Onyx. Complications of embolization include ulceration, soft tissue necrosis, and nerve injury. Often preoperative embolization is done 24–48 hours prior to surgical resection to help prevent blood loss.[1,4]

VASCULAR TUMORS

Hemangiomas

Natural History

Epidemiology and associated syndromes: Affecting 4–5% of the population, IHs are the most common tumors of infancy. The female to male ratio ranges from 1.4:1 to 3:1.[9] One-third of infants with segmental head and neck IHs have PHACE syndrome (posterior fossa abnormalities, hemangioma, arterial anomalies, cardiac anomalies, eye abnormalities, and sternal cleft/supraumbilical raphe).[10]

Presentation: Infantile hemangiomas are vascular tumors that present in the first months of life and are characterized by a rapid proliferation phase followed by a slower involutional period.[10] Superficial lesions look red while deeper lesions may have a slight bluish tinge. Patients with beard distribution segmental hemangiomas are at increased risk for subglottic hemangiomas. Subglottic hemangiomas present with biphasic stridor which is often worsened with crying or a superimposed upper respiratory tract infection.[11]

Evaluation: Magnetic resonance imaging and MRA imaging is typically reserved for evaluating the extent of deep hemangiomas such as those within the parotid or airway. IHs are positive for GLUT-1 on immunohistochemistry. Patients with signs of PHACE syndrome should have a cardiac and ophthalmology consultation as well as a brain MRI.

Treatment

Medical: Infantile hemangiomas that spontaneously regress and do not cause functional or aesthetic morbidity can be observed. For symptomatic lesions, historically, steroids had been the mainstay of therapy with interferon alpha and vincristine used to treat refractory lesions. A randomized, controlled trial of oral propranolol in IH showed that propranolol, a nonselective beta blocker, was effective at a dose of 3 mg/kg for 6 months. The adverse effects of treatment are infrequent but include hypoglycemia, hypotension, bradycardia, seizures, and bronchospasm.[12] More common adverse effects are sleep disturbances, cold extremities, and diarrhea.[9] Propranolol therapy is useful for lesions that are large, ulcerating, or rapidly growing as well as those near critical structures (nasal and orbital areas as well as the ears and lips).

Laser: Pulsed dye laser treat the superficial component of hemangiomas and has also been used for ulcerated lesions.[13] Laser use can lead to atrophic scarring and hypopigmentation.

Surgery: Surgical treatment is beneficial for exophytic IHs. The modified subunit approach is useful for nasal tip hemangiomas.[14] The bulk of the hemangioma can be excised with conservative resection of affected skin and lesions involute and laser therapy can be used after surgery.

■ REFERENCES

1. Hoff SR, Rastatter JC, Richter GT. Head and neck vascular lesions. Otolaryngol Clin North Am. 2015; 48:29-45.
2. ISSVA (2014). International Society for the Study of Vascular Anomalies: Classification of Vascular Anomalies. [online] Available from http://www.issva.org/classification. [Accessed July, 2017].
3. Mulliken JB, Glowacki J. Hemangiomas and vascular malformations in infants and children: a classification based on endothelial characteristics. Plast Reconstr Surg. 1982;69:412-22.
4. Richter GT, Friedman AB. Hemangiomas and vascular malformations: current theory and management. Int J Pediatr. 2012;2012:645678.
5. Amato MV, Patel NA, Hu S, et al. Sporadic multifocal venous malformations of the head and neck. Case Rep Otolaryngol. 2015;2015:508149.
6. Perkins JA, Manning SC, Tempero RM, et al. Lymphatic malformations: review of current treatment. Otolaryngol Head Neck Surg. 2010;142:795-803, 803 e1.
7. Manning SC, Perkins J. Lymphatic malformations. Curr Opin Otolaryngol Head Neck Surg. 2013;21:571-5.
8. de Serres LM, Sie KC, Richardson MA. Lymphatic malformations of the head and neck. A proposal for staging. Arch Otolaryngol Head Neck Surg. 1995;121:577-82.
9. Darrow DH, Greene AK, Mancini AJ, et al. Diagnosis and management of infantile hemangioma: executive summary. Pediatrics. 2015;136:786-91.
10. Neri I, Balestri R, Patrizi A. Hemangiomas: new insight and medical treatment. Dermatol Ther. 2012;25:322-34.
11. Rahbar R, Nicollas R, Roger G, et al. The biology and management of subglottic hemangioma: past, present, future. Laryngoscope. 2004;114:1880-91.
12. Leaute-Labreze C, Hoeger P, Mazereeuw-Hautier J, et al. A randomized, controlled trial of oral propranolol in infantile hemangioma. N Engl J Med. 2015;372:735-46.
13. Waner M. Recent developments in lasers and the treatment of birthmarks. Arch Dis Child. 2003;88:372-4.
14. Waner M, Kastenbaum J, Scherer K. Hemangiomas of the nose: surgical management using a modified subunit approach. Arch Facial Plast Surg. 2008;10:329-34.

Multiple Choice Questions

Q 1. Which of the following statements regarding steroid therapy for Hemangioma is INCORRECT?

A. Steroid treatment provokes a better response in the involuting hemangioma phase than in the proliferating hemangioma
B. Steroids are given for a rapidly growing hemangioma that seriously distorts facial features
C. Steroids are given for a lesion where there is bleeding, ulceration or infection
D. Steroids are given for a lesion that interferes with essential, normal, and physiological functions

Ans: A. Steroid treatment provokes a better response in the involuting hemangioma phase than in the proliferating hemangioma phase

Q 2. In which of the following areas is the surgical option for hemangioma in favored rather than observation for purpose of Involution?

A. Cheek area
B. Forehead
C. Lower side of the face and neck
D. Nasal tip

Ans: D. Nasal tip

Q 3. Which of the following is NOT a characteristic of Hemangioma?

A. Present at birth
B. Female/male ratio is 3:1
C. Rapid growth proliferation
D. Slow involution

Ans: A. Present at birth

Q 4. The MOST appropriate management of spider telangiectasia is:

A. Electrocautery
B. Incisional biopsy
C. Excision
D. CO_2 laser

Ans: A. Electrocautery

Q 5. Which of the following facial conditions will NOT require treatment?

A. Displastic nevus
B. Actinic keratosis
C. Venous lakes
D. Dermatofibrosarcoma protuberans

Ans: C. Venous lakes

Q 6. Which of the following statements regarding hemangiomas and vascular malformations is FALSE?

A. Hemangiomas are present at birth
B. Hemangiomas are characterized by a rapid postnatal growth for the first 8 to 12 months
C. Hemangiomas have a slow regression over 5–8 years
D. Vascular malformations grow proportional with the child's growth

Ans: A. Hemangiomas are present at birth

Q 7. Which of the following statements regarding PORT WINE STAINS is FALSE?

A. Port wine stains are present at birth
B. Port wine stains grow in proportion to child's growth
C. Port wine stains will not regress spontaneously
D. 60% of patients will require treatment

Ans: D. 60% of patients will require treatment

Q 8. Which is the LASER OF CHOICE in the treatment of port-wine stain (PWS)?

A. Argon laser
B. KTP (Potassium-titanyl-phosphate laser)
C. PDL (Pulsed dye laser)
D. APTDL (Argon-pumped tunable dye laser)

Ans: C. PDL (Pulsed dye laser)

Index

Page numbers followed by *f* refer to figure, *fc* refer to flow chart, and *t* refer to table

EU GSPR Authorised Reprsentative
Logos Europe, 9 rue Nicolas Poussin
1700, La Rochelle, France
Phone: +33 (0) 6 67 93 73 78
E-mail: contact@logoseurope.eu

www.ingramcontent.com/pod-product-compliance
Ingram Content Group UK Ltd.
Pitfield, Milton Keynes, MK11 3LW, UK
UKHW060047170726
7214IPUK00037B/386